Teddy Bear Book

Pediatric Injectable Drugs

Eighth Edition

Stephanie J. Phelps, Pharm.D., BCPS
Emily B. Hak, Pharm.D., BCPS, BCNSP
Catherine M. Crill, Pharm.D., BCPS, BCNSP

American Society of Health-System Pharmacists®
Bethesda, MD

Any correspondence regarding this publication should be sent to the publisher, American Society of Health-System Pharmacists, 7272 Wisconsin Avenue, Bethesda, MD 20814, attention: Special Publishing.

Director, Special Publishing: Jack Bruggeman
Acquisitions Editor: Jack Bruggeman
Senior Editorial Project Manager: Dana Battaglia
Production Editor: Kristin Eckles
Design: David Wade

Library of Congress Cataloging-in-Publication Data

Teddy bear book: pediatric injectable drugs/[edited by] Stephanie J. Phelps, Emily B. Hak, Catherine M. Crill.—8th ed.
p.; cm.
Rev. ed. of: Pediatric injectable drugs. 7th ed. c2004.
Includes bibliographical references and index.
ISBN 978-1-58528-158-9 (alk. paper)
1. Intravenous therapy. 2. Pediatric pharmacology. I. Phelps, Stephanie J. II. Hak, Emily B. III. Crill, Catherine M. IV. American Society of Health-System Pharmacists. V. Pediatric injectable drugs. VI. Title: Pediatric injectable drugs.
[DNLM: 1. Infusions, Intravenous—Guideline. 2. Child. 3. Drug Therapy—Guideline. 4. Infant. 5. Pharmaceutical Preparations—administration & dosage—Guideline. WB 354 T256 2007]

RM170.P47 2007
615.5′8083—dc22

2007002619

ISBN 978-1-58528-158-9

Table of Contents

Dedication

pi•o•neer (noun) a person or group that originates or helps open up a new line of thought or activity or a new method or technical development; one of the first to settle in a territory

leg•a•cy (noun) something transmitted by or received from an ancestor or predecessor or from the past

It became apparent to us as we began our careers in pediatric pharmacy that what we were allowed to do could be largely attributed to those first and second generation pioneers who had been the earliest to define the disciplines of pediatric and neonatal pharmacy practice. This edition is dedicated to those who paved the way and created a legacy that will continue to influence the care of children.*

Stephen J. Allen, B.S.Pharm., M.S.

Jeffery N. Baldwin, Pharm.D.

John A. Bosso, Pharm.D.

Gerald Briggs, B.S.Pharm.

Gilbert J. Burckhart, Pharm.D.

Gary C. Cupit, Pharm.D.

William E. Evans, Pharm.D.

Peter Gal, Pharm.D.

David Grinder, M.S.

Richard A. Helms, Pharm.D.

Leslie Hendeles, Pharm.D.

William H. Kelley, Pharm.D.

Roger Klotz, B.S.Pharm.

Richard D. Leff, Pharm.D.

Robert H. Levin, Pharm.D.

Cliff L. Littlefield, Pharm.D.

Christopher C. Lomax, Pharm.D.

Harvey Miltzner, B.S.Pharm.

Milap C. Nahata, M.S., Pharm.D.

Bruce Parks, Ph.D.

John Piecoro, Pharm.D.

Robert L. Poole, Pharm.D.

Albert Price, D.Ph.

John H. Rodman, Pharm.D.

Rosalie Sagraves, Pharm.D.

Harry C. Shirkey, B.S.Pharm., M.D.

Douglas Smith, Pharm.D.

Hank Wedemeyer, M.S.

Karen E. Zenk, Pharm.D.

*We have done our best to create a list that is all inclusive and apologize if we have omitted any deserving individual.

About the Editors

Stephanie J. Phelps, Pharm.D., is a Professor of Clinical Pharmacy and Pediatrics at The University of Tennessee Health Science Center, Memphis, Tennessee. She is also Vice Chair of Professional Programs for the Department of Clinical Pharmacy. Certified by the Board of Pharmaceutical Specialties in Pharmacotherapy, Dr. Phelps is a fellow of the American College of Clinical Pharmacy (ACCP) and the American Pharmacists Association (APhA). She is an active member of The Pediatric Pharmacy Advocacy Group (PPAG) and is editor of their official publication, *The Journal of Pediatric Pharmacology and Therapeutics.*

Emily B. Hak, Pharm.D., is a Professor of Clinical Pharmacy and an Associate Professor of Pediatrics and Pharmacology at The University of Tennessee Health Science Center, Memphis, Tennessee. Dr. Hak is a fellow of the ACCP and Board of Pharmaceutical Specialties certified in Nutrition Support and Pharmacotherapy. Dr. Hak is a member of the ACCP, the PPAG, the American Society of Health-System Pharmacists (ASHP), the Tennessee Pharmacists Association (TPA), the Society of Critical Care Medicine (SCCM), and the American Society for Parenteral and Enteral Nutrition (ASPEN).

Catherine M. Crill, Pharm.D., is an Associate Professor of Clinical Pharmacy and Assistant Professor of Pediatrics at The University of Tennessee Health Science Center, Memphis, Tennessee. Dr. Crill is certified by the Board of Pharmaceutical Specialties in Pharmacotherapy and Nutrition Support and is an active member of the American Association of Colleges of Pharmacy (AACP), ACCP, ASHP, ASPEN, PPAG, and TPA.

Preface

Those who practice in pediatrics understand that the majority of medications given to children are used off-label because research to validate safety and efficacy has not been conducted in children. The reason for the lack of studies in children is multifactorial and relates to priorities in pharmaceutical industry and federal funding, the need to protect our most vulnerable from medication-associated harm, and ethical considerations such as voluntary participation and informed consent/assent, which in many cases is not possible to obtain due to the patient's young age.

In 1957, the use of thalidomide to prevent nausea and vomiting during early pregnancy resulted in babies who were born with significant birth defects; thalidomide was not tested for teratogenic effects prior to marketing. In December 1983, the intravenous vitamin E supplement, E-Ferol, was marketed. Within three months its use was associated with ascites, liver and renal failure, thrombocytopenia, and death in low birth weight infants. This tragedy was ultimately attributed to the polysorbates added as emulsifiers; a new drug application had not been submitted to the FDA prior to use. Other noteworthy "therapeutic disasters" include sulfanilamide elixir, chloramphenicol Gray syndrome, valproate hepatotoxicity in young children, aspirin and Reye's syndrome, benzyl alcohol and fatal gasping syndrome, and the list goes on.

During the late 1960s, Dr. Harry Shirkey coined the term *therapeutic orphan*. Although pharmacokinetic and pharmacodynamic research has increased our understanding of medication therapy in neonates, infants, and children, unfortunately, the use of the term *therapeutic orphan* continues to be applicable to the pediatric population.

In 1994, the NIH established Pediatric Pharmacology Research Units (PPRUs) whose mission is to support the attainment of pediatric labeling of new and currently marketed drugs. The Food and Drug Administration Modernization Act (FDAMA) of 1998 provided an incentive to study drugs in children by extending the manufacturer's patent right for six months if they conducted pediatric studies. The impact of FDAMA was noted when, from 1998 to 2000, over 90 industry-sponsored primarily pharmacokinetic and pharmacodynamics studies were conducted in children, including neonates. In addition, NIH-supported, investigator-initiated trials have been conducted for older, off-patent drugs routinely used in pediatric patients, thereby validating their use in this population.

The eighth edition of *The Teddy Bear Book* has been revised to include more than 200 parenteral medications. More than 50 of these drugs were not in previous editions, and they include primarily antimicrobial and antineoplastic agents. Information included in this text was compiled in an evidence-based manner from, in most cases, the primary literature including case reports, observational reports, and comparative trials. Limited information is available for some of the frequently used older drugs in which case recommendations may come from textbooks. Importantly, the references are provided in the back of the book according to drug generic name, thereby allowing readers to quickly access and examine the evidence. A new feature of this text is the inclusion of a referenced chart, listing compatibility of medications that may be added to or given concomitantly with parenteral nutrition solutions.

Yes, drugs are used off-label in children all the time. We do hope that this text improves medication use and delivery in children, which will facilitate recovery and improve their quality of life.

Stephanie J. Phelps
Emily B. Hak
Catherine M. Crill
2006

Contributors

Marcia L. Buck, Pharm.D., FCCP
Department of Pharmacy Services
Schools of Medicine and Nursing
University of Virginia Children's Hospital
Charlottesville, VA

Michael Chicella, Pharm.D.
Clinical Coordinator
Children's Hospital of the King's Daughters
Norfolk, VA

Karen D. Dominguez, Pharm.D.
Associate Professor of Pharmacy
Director of Assessment
College of Pharmacy
University of New Mexico Health Sciences Center
Albuquerque, NM

Jaclyn E. Lee, Pharm.D.
Clinical Assistant Professor
Ernest Mario School of Pharmacy at Rutgers University
Piscataway, NJ

Kelley Lee, Pharm.D., BCPS
Clinical Pharmacy Manager
Le Bonheur Children's Medical Center
Professor of Clinical Pharmacy
The University of Tennessee Health Science Center
Memphis, TN

Sherry Luedtke, Pharm.D.
Associate Dean, Professional Affairs
Associate Professor, Pharmacy Practice
Texas Tech University HSC
School of Pharmacy
Amarillo, TX

Holly D. Maples, Pharm.D.
Assistant Professor, Department of Pharmacy Practice and Pediatrics
College of Pharmacy
University of Arkansas for Medical Sciences
Little Rock, AR

Katherine Marks, Pharm.D., BCPS
Assistant Professor, Department of Clinical Pharmacy
University of Tennessee Health Science Center
Memphis, TN

Susannah E. Motl, Pharm.D.
Assistant Professor, Department of Clinical Pharmacy
University of Tennessee Health Science Center
Memphis, TN

Pamela D. Reiter, Pharm.D.
Clinical Pharmacy Specialist, Pediatric Intensive Care and Trauma
The Children's Hospital, Denver Colorado
Clinical Associate Professor
The University of Colorado at Denver Health Sciences Center
School of Pharmacy
Denver, CO

Christine A. Robinson, Pharm.D.
Clinical Assistant Professor
Ernest Mario School of Pharmacy at Rutgers University
Piscataway, NJ

Chasity M. Shelton, Pharm.D., BCPS
Advanced Pediatric Pharmacotherapy Resident
University of Tennessee Health Science Center and
Le Bonheur Children's Medical Center
Memphis, TN

Katherine P. Smith, Pharm.D., BCPS
Acting Director of Continuing Education
Assistant Professor of Pharmacy Practice
University of Southern Nevada College of Pharmacy
Henderson, NV

Introduction

The following guidelines were developed to provide a single authoritative source of information on the parenteral administration of medications to pediatric patients. All recommendations should be individualized in accordance with the clinical situation.

This eighth edition of ASHP'S *Teddy Bear Book: Pediatric Injectable Drugs* provides the following information for updates to 217 drugs and all references that support information contained in the text.

Brand names

Common brand names and, if applicable, other names (synonyms) are listed.

Dosage

Unless otherwise specified, dosages are for all age groups. These age groups are neonates (premature and term) up to 1 month; infants, 1 month to 24 months; children, 2 years to 12 years; and adolescents, 12 years to 18 years. When applicable, adult dosing is also provided. While these age groups provide general guidelines for therapy in pediatric patients, it should be noted that changes in development that affect drug pharmacokinetics and pharmacodynamics and, hence, dosing recommendations, are not confined to the limits of these defined age groups.

Dosage is often expressed as X mg/kg/d divided q Y–Z h, where the total daily dose (X) is given in equally divided doses at evenly spaced intervals, or as X mg/kg q Y–Z h, from which the total daily dose may be extrapolated. Dosage may also be expressed as X mg/m^2, a calculation of body surface area (BSA) as determined from height and mass. See Appendix A for a BSA nomogram.

The presence of obesity may require the practitioner to estimate ideal body mass/weight and calculate an adjusted weight for the dosing of some medications. Appendix B provides a nomogram for estimating total body mass/weight.

Dosage adjustment in organ dysfunction

Drugs requiring dosage adjustment in patients with renal or hepatic dysfunction and serum drug concentration monitoring are indicated. The manufacturer's package insert and specialized references are provided when available.

Maximum dosage

Maximum dosages are referenced to primary literature where available. However, maximum dosages for pediatric patients are often extrapolated from adult data because of a lack of documented experience with pediatric patients. Many manufacturers caution against exceeding the maximum recommended adult dosage (usually expressed as X g/d) in pediatric patients. In this reference, when the maximum dosage is expressed as "mg/kg/d, not to exceed X g/d," "X g/day" is typically the manufacturer's maximum recommended adult dosage and should be used only as an upper limit for pediatric dosing. It should not be inferred that use of these maximum dosages in pediatric patients is recommended and is without risk of toxicity. You should consult the references indicated for information on the use of these maximum dosages in the pediatric population.

IV push

This rate is generally expressed as a period of time over which the dose should be administered (seconds or minutes) or as a quantity of drug per unit of time. In the latter case, the size of the dose determines the administration time. For the purpose of this text, IV push was defined as ≤5 minutes. Drugs for which IV push administration is contraindicated are noted.

Intermittent infusion

The recommended infusion rate is expressed as a period of time over which the dose should be administered (minutes) or as a quantity of drug per unit of time (size of dose determines administration time).

Introduction

Continuous infusion

The recommended infusion rate is usually expressed as a quantity of drug per unit of time; infusion is continued for 24 hours unless otherwise specified (e.g., until the desired therapeutic endpoint is achieved).

Other routes of administration

This section contains information on the appropriateness of other routes of administration, including IM, SC, ET, IT, and IO administration, and the best site for administration. Drugs for which other routes of administration are contraindicated are noted.

Maximum concentration

Generally, any concentration up to the maximum may be administered, taking into consideration the patient's fluid status (and potential for loss of vascular access), administration method (IV push vs. IV infusion), drug administration rate (and drug administration device flow rate range, if applicable), dose (and degree of accuracy required in dose measurement), and drug stability. However, some drugs, as indicated in these guidelines, should not be diluted.

For drugs available as solutions that may be administered undiluted, the maximum concentration is the commercially available concentration. For drugs that must be constituted prior to administration, the maximum concentration should serve as a guide for the minimum dilution required.

Concentrations listed are referenced to literature on drug use in pediatric patients to the extent possible. However, concentrations administered to adults are cited where documentation on use in pediatric patients is insufficient. The references should be consulted. The IV push, Intermittent infusion, Continuous infusion, and Other routes of administration sections all begin with information concerning the concentration or concentration range usual for that method or route of administration.

Drug stability in some of the IV solutions listed is limited. The manufacturer's package insert and specialized references (e.g., Trissel LA. *Handbook on Injectable Drugs,* 13th Edition, Bethesda, MD: American Society of Health-System Pharmacists; 2005) should be consulted for detailed stability information.

Cautions related to IV administration

Warnings are provided where appropriate.

Other additives

Pertinent additives, including sodium and those with a potential for toxicity or adverse effects, are included.

Comments

Miscellaneous information is included where pertinent. Information pertaining to adults is sometimes included because, in the absence of reports on pediatric use, adult data may be relevant and may be cautiously extrapolated to the pediatric population.

Abbreviations

Solutions:

BW	Bacteriostatic water for injection
D-LR	Dextrose—Ringer's injection, lactated, combinations
D-R	Dextrose—Ringer's injection combinations
D-S	Dextrose—saline combinations
D5LR	Dextrose 5% in Ringer's injection, lactated
D2.5½NS	Dextrose 2.5% in sodium chloride 0.45%
D5NS	Dextrose 5% in sodium chloride 0.9%
D5¼NS	Dextrose 5% in sodium chloride 0.225%
D5½NS	Dextrose 5% in sodium chloride 0.45%
D10NS	Dextrose 10% in sodium chloride 0.9%
D5R	Dextrose 5% in Ringer's injection
D5S	Dextrose 5% in sodium chloride 0.9%, 0.45%, or 0.225%
D2.5W	Dextrose 2.5% in water
D5W	Dextrose 5% in water
D10W	Dextrose 10% in water
D15W	Dextrose 15% in water
D20W	Dextrose 20% in water
FE	Fat emulsion
LR	Ringer's injection, lactated
NS	Sodium chloride 0.9% (normal saline)
¼NS	Sodium Chloride 0.225%
½NS	Sodium chloride 0.45% (1/2normal saline)
PN	Parenteral nutrition
R	Ringer's injection
SW	Sterile water for injection
TNA	Total nutrient admixtures

Terms:

AAP	American Academy of Pediatrics
ACT	Activated clotting time
ADH	Antidiuretic hormone
AHA	American Heart Association
AIDS	Acquired Immunodeficiency Syndrome
ALL	Acute Lymphocytic Leukemia
ANC	Absolute neutrophil count
APAP	Acetaminophen
APTT	Activated partial thromboplastin time
ATG	Antithymocyte globulin
AZT	Azidothymidine
BLC	Blood lead concentration
BSA	Body surface area
BUN	Blood urea nitrogen

CDP-1	Crystalline degradation products
CHF	Congestive heart failure
CML	Chronic myelogenous leukemia
CMV	Cytomegalovirus
CNS	Central nervous system
CPK-MB	Serum creatine phosphokinase–MB isoenzyme
CPR	Cardiopulmonary resuscitation
CrCl	Creatinine clearance
CSF	Cerebral spinal fluid
CYP1A2	Cytochrome P450 isoenzyme 1A2
CYP2C19	Cytochrome P450 isoenzyme 2C19
CYP2C9/10	Cytochrome P450 isoenzymes 2C9 and 2C10
CYP3A3/4	Cytochrome P450 isoenzymes 3A3 and 3A4
DEHP	Diethylhexylphthalate
DKA	Diabetic ketoacidosis
DPT	Demerol, phenergan, thorazine
ECMO	Extracorporeal membrane oxygenation
EEG	Electroencephalogram
EKG	Electrocardiogram
EMIT	Enzyme multiplied immunoassay technique
ET	Endotracheal
FAB	Digoxin immune Fab
FDA	Food and Drug Administration
FPIA	Fluorescence polarization immunoassay
FT4	Free thyroxine
GM-CSF	Granulocyte-macrophage colony-stimulating factor
GVHD	Graft versus host disease
H1	Histamine-1 receptor antagonist
H2	Histamine-2 receptor antagonist
Hgb	Hemoglobin
HIV	Human Immunodeficiency Virus
HPLC	High-performance liquid chromatography
IBW	Ideal body weight
ICP	Intracranial pressure
ICU	Intensive care unit
IM	Intramuscular
IO	Intraosseous
IT	Intrathecal
ITP	Idiopathic thrombocytopenic purpura
IQ	Intelligence quotient
IV	Intravenous
IVIG	Intravenous immune globulin
MAC	Mycobacterium avium complex

Abbreviations

MTX	Methotrexate
NAPA	N-Acetylprocainamide
NHL	Non-Hodgkin's lymphoma
NIH	National Institutes of Health
NMTT	N-methyl-thiotetrazole side chain
NSAIDs	Nonsteroidal anti-inflammatory drugs
PALS	Pediatric advanced life support
PCA	Postconceptional age
PDA	Patent ductus arteriosus
PE	Phenytoin equivalents
PID	Pelvic inflammatory disease
PMA	Postmenstrual age
PNA	Postnatal age
PO	Orally
PTT	Partial thromboplastin time
PVC	Polyvinyl chloride
SC	Subcutaneous
SCr	Serum creatinine
SDC	Serum digitalis concentration
TBW	Total body weight
THC	Tetrahydrocannabinol
TPA	Tissue plasminogen activator
TSH	Thyroid stimulating hormone
UGT	Uridine diphosphate-glucuronosyltransferase
USP	United States Pharmacopeia
UTI	Urinary tract infection
Vitamin B12a	Hydroxocobalamin
Vitamin B12	Cyanocobalamin
WBC	White blood cell count

Monographs

Acetazolamide

Brand names	Diamox
Dosage	Because acetazolamide has been administered to only a limited number of pediatric patients, the doses and side effects have not been established. No pediatric-specific problems have been documented to date. **Acute glaucoma:** 20–40 mg/kg/d divided q 6 h.[1] **Edema/diuresis/urinary alkalinization:** 5 mg/kg/dose[1-4] or 150 mg/m^2[4] once daily as required to achieve forced alkaline diuresis.[1] (See Comments section.) **Posthemorrhagic ventricular dilatation:** Studies have shown increased rates of shunt placement and greater neurological morbidity with maximum tolerable doses (100 mg/kg/d); therefore, use of acetazolamide is not recommended.[5,6] **Pseudotumor cerebri:** 40–120 mg/kg/d divided q 6–8 h up to 2 g/d.[7]
Dosage adjustment in organ dysfunction	Adjust dosage in patients with renal dysfunction. If CrCl is 10–50 mL/min, give q 12 h.[8] (See Comments section.) Contraindicated in patients with hepatic cirrhosis due to the risk of encephalopathy.[9]
Maximum dosage	100 mg/kg/d[3] up to 1–2 g/d.[3,9]
IV push	100 mg/mL in SW[10]; also compatible with D2.5W, D5W, D10W, NS, LR, or R.[10]
Intermittent infusion	100 mg/mL in D2.5W, D5W, D10W, NS, LR, or R.[10]
Continuous infusion	No information available to support administration by this method.
Other routes of administration	IM administration not recommended; very painful due to alkaline pH of 9.2.[9] No information available to support administration by other routes.
Maximum concentration	100 mg/mL.[1]
Cautions related to IV administration	None. For PN compatibility, please see Appendix C.
Other additives	2.049 mEq of sodium/500 mg acetazolamide.[9]
Comments	Acetazolamide contains a sulfonamide moiety. Although rare, cross reactivity with other sulfonamides may be associated with severe dermatological reactions (e.g., Stevens-Johnson syndrome), which occurred due to sulfonamide structure.[9] Acetazolamide is a carbonic anhydrase inhibitor that shares the pharmacological actions and toxic potentials of this class of medications.[9] May cause hypokalemia, paresthesia, and kidney stones. Not effective at CrCl <20 mL/min.[2] Overdoses or too frequent dosage may cause a failure to produce diuresis. Acetazolamide should be withheld for 1–2 days to allow for kidney recovery.[9]

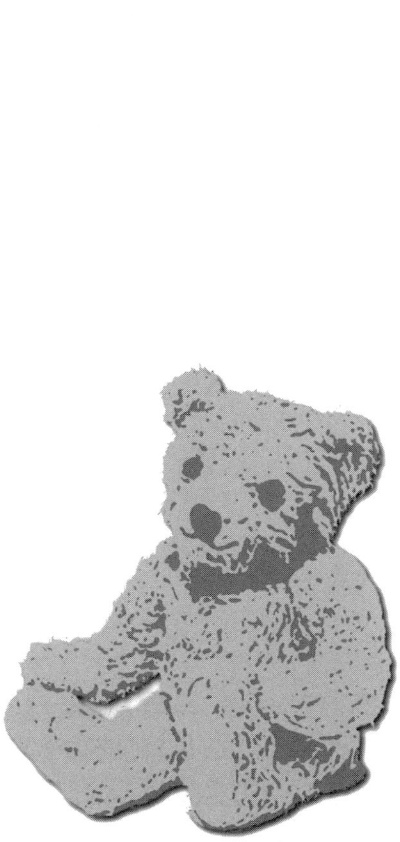

Acetylcysteine (NAC)

Brand names	Acetadote
Dosage	**Acetaminophen overdosage:** Use the Rumack-Matthew nomogram to estimate the potential for hepatotoxicity due to acetaminophen overdose and guide therapy with N-acetylcysteine (NAC).[1] Ideally, administer a dose within 8 h of acetaminophen ingestion; however, it may be effective when given 24 h or longer after ingestion. Infuse loading dose of 150 mg/kg over 15 min (see Intermittent infusion section), followed by 50 mg/kg over 4 h, then 100 mg/kg over 16 h (for a full course consisting of 300 mg/kg administered IV over 20.25 h).[1,2] (See Comments section.) **Prevention of acute renal failure associated with radiographic contrast media:** Most reports of the use of NAC for this purpose involved oral dosing[4,5]; however, it has been given by the intravenous route for this purpose in *adults*.[6] **Prevention of BPD:** When compared to placebo, there was *no* difference in the development of BPD or death in 194 infants (500–999 g) who received a 6-day course of NAC (16–32 mg/kg/d beginning within 36 h of birth) compared to placebo.[4] (See Comments section.)
Dosage adjustment in organ dysfunction	Dosage should not be reduced in hepatic impairment.[1] The manufacturer states that data are not available to determine whether dosage adjustment is needed in patients with moderate or severe renal impairment[1]; however, others suggest that patients with CrCl <10 mL/min should receive 75% of the maintenance dosage.[7]
Maximum dosage	300 mg/kg per treatment.[1]
IV push	No information available to support administration by this method.
Intermittent infusion	Loading dose should be diluted and given over 15 min.[8] Some clinicians recommend infusing the loading dose over 60 min to reduce the potential for a life-threatening anaphylactoid reaction.[2] (See Cautions related to IV administration section.)
Continuous infusion	First (50 mg/kg) and second (100 mg/kg) maintenance doses should be given over 4 h and 16 h, respectively.[2] Infusions of 0.3–4.6 mg/kg/h have been used safely in newborns.[9]
Other routes of administration	No information available to support administration by other routes.
Maximum concentration	Must be diluted in D5W prior to infusion. Loading dose concentrations up to 50 mg/mL and maintenance dose concentrations up to 10 mg/mL.[1] Adjust total volume as needed for patients' weight and those requiring fluid restriction.[2]

Weight	Loading Dose (150 mg/kg)	2nd Dose (50 mg/kg)	3rd Dose (100 mg/kg)
<40 kg	Add dose to a volume of 3–4 mL/kg* of D5W	Add dose to a volume of 7–10 mL/kg* of D5W	Add dose to a volume of 14–20 mL/kg* of D5W
≥40 kg	Add dose to 200 mL of D5W	Add dose to 500 mL of D5W	Add dose to 1000 mL of D5W
*If patient weighs 20 kg, add dose to 60–80 mL.			

Cautions related to IV administration	Serious anaphylactoid reactions and death have been reported causing some to recommend infusing the loading dose over 60 min.[1] Once the anaphylactoid reaction has been treated, NAC can be reinstituted cautiously, but it should be discontinued if anaphylactoid reaction recurs.[1] Caution in patients with asthma or history of bronchospasm. Acute flushing and erythema can occur 30–60 min after initiation of the infusion, with resolution despite continued infusion.[1]
Other additives	None.
Comments	Contact a poison center at 1-800-222-1222 to obtain information about the clinical management of acetaminophen overdoses. No adverse effects were noted following a mean rate of 8.4 mg/kg/h for 24 h in preterm infants (gestational age of 25–31 weeks and weight of 500–1380 g) or following infusion 0.1–1.3 mg/kg/h for 6 days in six neonates (gestational age of 26–30 weeks and weight of 520–1335 g).[3,9,10] NAC crossed the placenta when a mother was treated following an acetaminophen exposure.[11]

Acyclovir Sodium

Brand names	Zovirax

Dosage

Doses generally range from 7.5–60 mg/kg/d or 750–1500 mg/m²/d divided q 8 h depending on the infection.[1-12] Obese patients should be dosed using ideal body weight.[1]

Herpes simplex virus (HSV)

Neonatal HSV: 60 mg/kg/d divided q 8 h for 14–21 days.[11,12]

HSV encephalitis: 60 mg/kg/d divided q 8 h for 14–21 days.[11,12]

Genital HSV (severe cases): 15 mg/kg/d divided q 8 h for 5–7 days.[11]

HSV in immunocompromised host (localized, progressive, or disseminated)

<12 years: 30 mg/kg/d divided q 8 h for 7–14 days.[11]

>12 years: 15 mg/kg/d divided q 8 h for 7–14 days.[11]

HSV-seropositive patients: 15 mg/kg/d divided q 8 h during risk period.[11]

Varicella-Zoster virus (VZV) in immunocompromised hosts

<1 year: 30 mg/kg/d divided q 8 h for 7–10 days.[11]

>1 year: 1500 mg/m²/d (or 30 mg/kg/d) divided q 8 h for 7–10 days.[7-11,13]

Initiate therapy as soon as possible after rash appears. Early initiation therapy (<24–72 h) is associated with more rapid improvement and less dissemination than late initiation therapy (>3–5 days).[8,9,13]

Twenty-six children (1–13 years of age) receiving immunosuppressive therapy who developed VZV were given 1500 mg/m²/d divided q 8 h for 48 h. If able to take oral medications, they were changed to oral therapy after 48 h if there was no ongoing fever, no new skin lesions, and no evidence of systemic desease. Immunosuppressive drugs were discontinued or decreased by 50% during acyclovir treatment.[14]

Sixty-six pediatric renal transplant recipients with VZV were given 1500 mg/m²/d divided q 8 h. Azathioprine was temporarily discontinued until the lesions crusted over and no new lesions appeared; at that time, azathioprine was restarted at the usual dose. Three recipients experienced acute rejection that responded to prednisone. One patient died.[15]

Prevention or suppression of cytomegalovirus infection in allogeneic bone marrow transplant recipients (this use has largely been replaced by ganciclovir): 1500 mg/m²/d divided q 8 h beginning 5 days before transplantation and continuing 30 days after.[4,16]

Aplastic anemia (use not established): 15 mg/kg/d (schedule not provided) for 10 days has been given to two patients (one, a 13-year-old girl) who had severe aplastic anemia refractory to standard treatment.[2]

Dosage adjustment in organ dysfunction

Adjust dosage in patients with renal dysfunction.[1,11,17-19] If CrCl is 25–50 mL/min, give normal dose q 12 h; if CrCl is 10–25 mL/min, give normal dose q 24 h, and if CrCl is <10 mL/min, give 50% of the dose q 24 h.[1,18]

Neonates with hepatic or renal dysfunction and young premature infants may also require dose adjustment.[19]

Maximum dosage

Do not exceed 20 mg/kg q 8 h.[1]

An 11-day-old neonate received a 258 mg/kg of IV acyclovir in a 24-h period that was treated with NS hydration; the patient experienced only a transient increase in serum creatinine.[20]

IV push

Not recommended.[1] Rapid administration (<10 min) can cause crystalluria, elevations in serum urea and creatinine, renal tubular damage, and acute renal failure.[1,21]

Intermittent infusion

≤7 mg/mL in D5NS, D5W, LR, or NS.[1,22] BW for injection containing parabens or benzyl alcohol should not be used to dilute acyclovir sodium powder because precipitation could occur.[22] Although acyclovir has been given over 30 min,[23] the dose should be infused over 1 h to minimize renal dysfunction.[1,21,22] Dilution should be used within 12 h.[1,22] Refrigeration may cause precipitation; however, the precipitate redissolves at room temperature and potency does not appear to be affected.[22]

Continuous infusion

No information available to support administration by this method.

Other routes of administration

Not recommended.[1,22]

Maximum concentration

≤7 mg/mL.[1,22] Infusion of a solution ≥10 mg/mL increases the risk of phlebitis and extravasation.[1,24]

Cautions related to IV administration

To decrease the risk of nephrotoxicity, the patient should be adequately hydrated before and during the infusion.[1,21]

Extravasation may cause inflammation and phlebitis at the injection site.[1,25]

For PN compatibility information, please see Appendix C.

Other additives

Contains 4.2 mEq sodium/g of acyclovir.[22]

Comments

Nonherpetic vesicular eruptions occurred in a child receiving acyclovir for presumed herpes simplex encephalitis.[26]

A 33-week-old infant with HSV encephalitis received IV acyclovir 30 mg/kg/d for 21 days followed by 30 mg/kg/d of oral acyclovir for 25 days. The infant developed neutropenia 5 days after starting a second course of acyclovir. Neutropenia corrected after switching to 30 mg/kg/d of vidarabine (no longer available in the United States) for 7 days and 10 mg/kg/d of oral acyclovir for 7 months.[27]

A 9-year-old child with HSV encephalitis developed nonoliguric acute renal failure after 6 days of 10 mg/kg/dose of IV acyclovir. Renal failure reversed following discontinuation of acyclovir.[28] If CrCl decreases by ≥20%, the authors recommend that acyclovir be discontinued. If the patient has a potentially life-threatening infection, the dosage should be adjusted and the drug continued.

Adenosine

Brand names	Adenocard
Dosage	Contraindicated in heart transplant patients.[1] **Pulmonary hypertension:** 0.05 mg/kg/min improved PaO2 in four of nine infants with persistent pulmonary hypertension without causing hypotension or tachycardia.[2] **Stress test in aortic valve disease:** 0.14 mg/kg/min for 6 min.[3] **Supraventricular tachycardia** **Initial dosing:** 0.04,[4] 0.05,[1,4-9] or 0.1[10-16] mg/kg. Infuse over 1–2 sec, then flush catheter with saline.[1] Initial doses are usually ≤6 mg.[10] The maximum single dose is 0.5 mg/kg in children and 0.3 mg/kg in neonates.[17] One report noted that only 9% of infants responded to a dose of 0.05 mg/kg.[16] **Subsequent dosing:** If no response in 1–2 min, increase dose to 0.1 mg/kg[1,7,10,15] and flush catheter with saline. If no response in 1–2 min, increase in increments of 0.15, 0.2 mg/kg (maximum of 12 mg).[1,10]
Dosage adjustment in organ dysfunction	No dosage adjustment necessary in patients with renal dysfunction.[19]
Maximum dosage	The maximum single dose is 0.5 mg/kg in children and 0.3 mg/kg in neonates[17] up 12 mg.[10] A preterm neonate receiving theophylline required doses of 0.4–0.8 mg/kg to convert to normal sinus rhythm.[20] Over a 14.5-h period, a 3-week-old was given 119 doses of 0.1–0.2 mg/kg.[21] A 14-year-old adolescent who failed to respond to an 18-mg dose was believed to have ventricular tachycardia.[11] (See Comments section.)
IV push	≤3 mg/mL in NS over 1–2 sec, followed by an NS flush.[4,5,11]
Intermittent infusion	IM administration not recommended.[22]
Continuous infusion	Although concentration and solution type was not provided, one child received a continuous infusion.[5] (See Dosage section.)
Other routes of administration	IM administration not recommended.[22] Has been administered intraosseously in emergencies.[10]
Maximum concentration	3 mg/mL (available commercially).[22]
Cautions related to IV administration	Adverse effects are common but transient. They include flushing, dyspnea, headache, complete atrioventricular block, sinus bradycardia, and other rhythm disorders.[4,5,22] Bronchospasm and respiratory failure have occurred in patients with a history of reactive airway disease.[23-25] Aminophylline has been used to relieve bronchospasm associated with adenosine.[25]

Other additives	None.
Comments	Larger doses may be required in patients receiving concomitant methylxanthines (e.g., theophylline, caffeine).[13,22] Lower doses may be required in patients receiving concomitant dipyridamole.[26]

Albumin (Normal Human Serum)

Brand names	**50 mg/mL:** Albumarc, Albuminar-5, Albumin (Human) 5% Solution, Albutein 5%, Buminate 5%, Plasbumin-5 **250 mg/mL:** Albumarc, Albuminar-25, Albumin (Human) 25% Solution, Albutein 25%, Buminate 25%, Plasbumin-25
Dosage	**Hypovolemia:** Rapid infusion of 0.5–1 g/kg.[1] 20 mL/kg of 4.5% (0.9 g/kg)[2] and 5% albumin (1 g/kg)[3] have been given over 20 min in premature neonates. **Hypoalbuminemia**: Albumin deficits have been replaced by intermittent bolus infusions of up to 1 g/kg of albumin 25%.[4] The continuous infusion of albumin results in a more sustained increase in serum albumin concentration.[5] The albumin deficit can be estimated with the following equation: g albumin = weight (kg) x 3 dL/kg x (3.5 - observed serum albumin in g/dL).[6,7] **Nephrotic syndrome (controversial):** 0.25–1 g/kg of albumin 25% infused over $\geq$1 to 12 h keeping in mind that rapid expansion of intravascular volume may increase the risk for congestive heart failure.[8-10] Infusion over a longer time decreases the risk for the development of congestive heart failure.[10] Furosemide (0.5–2-mg/kg)[8-10] infusion may accompany or follow the albumin infusion. **Metabolic acidosis in very low birth weight infants (use not established):** 10 mL/kg of 4.5% albumin (0.45 g/kg).[11] However, sodium bicarbonate was superior to albumin for metabolic acidosis in normotensive neonates.[11]
Dosage adjustment in organ dysfunction	No dosage adjustment required for renal or hepatic impairment.[12]
Maximum dosage	125 g in 24 h or 250 g in 48 h have been given to *adults*.[1,12]
IV push	If clinically indicated, infuse over 30–60 min. In severe hypovolemia, faster rates may be required.[12] (See Cautions related to IV administration section.)
Intermittent infusion	Dilute in suitable volume of D5W, D10W, or NS.[1,13] After rapid infusion to replace plasma volume in *adults* with hypovolemic shock, infuse 1 mL/min of albumin 25% or 2–4 mL/min of albumin 5%.[12] In euvolemic *adults* with hypoproteinemia, infuse 2–3 mL/min of albumin 25% or 5–10 mL/min of albumin 5%.[12] In patients who require sodium restriction, a 5% albumin solution that contains less sodium than manufacturers products can be made by diluting each 1 mL of albumin 25% in 4 mL of D5W or D10W. Infusion of large amounts of albumin diluted with D5W can result in hyponatremia; therefore, when using large volumes of albumin, dilution in NS is preferred.[12]
Continuous infusion	Can be infused continuously.
Other routes of administration	No information available to support administration by other routes.

Maximum concentration	Undiluted.
Cautions related to IV administration	Too rapid infusion may result in acute hypertension[10] or vascular overload, causing pulmonary edema or cardiac failure.[12,13] Premature neonates are at risk for intraventricular hemorrhage from rapid intravascular volume expansion.[14] Allergic reactions may result in chills, fever, nausea, vomiting, or urticaria.[14] Anaphylaxis has been reported in an *adult*.[15]
Other additives	Contains 130–160 mEq sodium/L of albumin.[1,12] Contains no preservatives or antimicrobial.[1,12]
Comments	The infusion should begin within 4 h of opening the bottle.[1] Because of a reduction in tonicity, fatal hemolysis and acute renal failure may occur if sterile water is used as a diluent.[12] Solutions containing >25 g/L of albumin are more likely to occlude 0.22-micron in-line filters; however, PN solutions containing as little as 10.8 g/L caused filter occlusion.[16,17]

Alfentanil

Brand names	Alfenta

Dosage

Not recommended in children <12 years.[1]

An opioid antagonist, resuscitative and intubation equipment, and oxygen should be available.[1]

Alfentanil should only be administered by persons specifically trained in the use of IV anesthetics. Dosages vary depending on the desired degree of analgesia/anesthesia and adjunctive therapies (e.g., halothane, propofol).

When dosing obese (>20% above ideal body weight) patients, use lean body weight.[1] (See Appendix B.)

Anesthesia

Induction

Preterm neonates: 20 mcg/kg over 30 min.[2]

Neonates and infants: 20–25 mcg/kg.[3-5]

Children (<12 years): 20–100 mcg/kg.[5-8] May also give 12.5–25 mcg/kg when combined with halothane.[7]

Children (≥12 years): 130–245 mcg/kg.[1]

Maintenance

Preterm infants: 3–5 mcg/kg/h.[2]

Children (<12 years): 2.5–5 mcg/kg/min.[8]

While on cardiac bypass, infants and children undergoing congenital heart repair surgery have received a loading dose of 20 mcg/kg followed by continuous infusions of 1 mcg/kg/min with supplemental doses of 5 mcg/kg as needed.[9]

Children (≥12 years): 0.5–3 mcg/kg/min.[1]

Intubation (>12 years): 20–50 mcg/kg, repeat 5–15 mcg/kg q 5–15 min.[10]

Dosage adjustment in organ dysfunction

No dosage adjustment required in patients with renal dysfunction.[11] Patients with hepatic dysfunction may require smaller doses to achieve the same therapeutic effect. Average doses may lead to medication accumulation; therefore, caution is warranted on administration of alfentanil to patients with liver dysfunction.

Maximum dosage

Dosages are titrated to the desired level of sedation or analgesia.

IV push

≤80 mcg/mL diluted in D5W, NS, or LR over 3–5 min.[1,12] Doses ≤100 mcg/kg have been given over 30 sec.[7,8] (See Cautions related to IV administration section.)

Intermittent infusion

≤80 mcg/mL diluted in D5W, NS, or LR over 10–30 min.[3,4,6,12]

Continuous infusion

≤80 mcg/mL diluted in D5W, NS, or LR at a rate ≤5 mcg/kg/min. (See Dosage section.)[2,7,8,12] After the first hour, rates may need to be decreased by 30% to 50% in some patients.[1]

Other routes of administration

No information available to support administration by other routes.

Maximum concentration	≤80 mcg/mL.[12]
Cautions related to IV administration	Significant bradycardia, muscle or chest wall rigidity, and apnea may occur early in administration of alfentanil or following rapid administration.[3] Pretreatment with atropine and a nondepolarizing neuromuscular blocking agent may aid in minimizing these adverse effects. Ventilatory support is indicated.
Other additives	None.
Comments	Epileptiform activity has occurred in patients receiving alfentanil during epilepsy surgery.[13,14]

Allopurinol Sodium

Brand names	Aloprim

Dosage

Prevention/treatment of hyperuricemia secondary to neoplastic disorders: Treatment is started 24–48 h prior to chemotherapy.[1,2] It is important to maintain adequate hydration to avoid potential formation of xanthine calculi and prevent renal precipitation of urates.[2]

<10 years of age: 200 mg/m^2 either as a single dose, in divided doses, or as a continuous infusion.[1,2]

10 years of age and older: 200–400 mg/m^2 (5–10 mg/kg/d) divided q 4–12 h[1-4] or as a continuous infusion.[1]

In outpatients, the daily dose has been diluted in 25–50 mL of dextrose and infused over 15–30 min.[1]

Inhibition of free radical production

Postasphyxial brain injury in newborns: 20 mg/kg given within 4 h of life and again 12 h later.[5]

Severely hypoxic neonates on ECMO: 10 mg/kg prior to cannulation followed by 5 mg/kg q 8 h for 72 h after initiation of bypass.[6]

Cardiopulmonary bypass (CPB) or deep hypothermic circulatory arrest: The percent reduction in uric acid concentrations was not different in neonates who received 5 (n = 6) or 10 mg (n = 6).[7] A placebo controlled trial in 350 infants reported that 5 mg/kg given at least 16 h preoperatively, 5 mg/kg given 8 h preoperatively, 10 mg/kg given at 0700 the morning of surgery, 20 mg/kg intraoperatively via CPB circuit, and nine postoperative doses of 5 mg/kg q 8 h decreased morbidity in neonates with hypoplastic left-heart syndrome.[8]

Dosage adjustment in organ dysfunction

Adjust dosage in patients with renal dysfunction.[9] If CrCl is 10–50 mL/min, give 50% of a normal dose; if CrCl is <10 mL/min, give 25% of a normal dose.[9]

Maximum dosage

Not established.[2] However, doses >600 mg in *adults* have not been associated with increased benefit.[2] In one study, the median prophylactic daily dose was 180 mg/dose (range: 15–700 mg), the median therapeutic daily dose was 175 mg/d (range: 3–514 mg), and the average daily doses ranged from 5.2–10.7 mg/kg.[10] Neonates have been given single doses as large as 20 mg/kg.[5] In children with acute lymphocytic leukemia (ALL), a 3-year old received 410 mg/m^2 daily for 11 days, and a 4-year-old received a cumulative dose of 8.8 g/m^2 over a 6-month period as an outpatient.[4]

IV push

No information available to support administration by this method.

Intermittent infusion

5 mg/mL over 15–20 min.[4,6,7]

Continuous infusion

The daily dose can be given as a continuous infusion.[1]

Other routes of administration	Not indicated.
Maximum concentration	Usually 6 mg/mL in D5W or NS.[1-3,12] The pH of the reconstituted vial (500 mg in 25 mL of sterile water for injection) ranges from 11.1 to 11.8 and further dilution is recommended.[2] Although the final concentration was not specified, a single daily dose was added to 25–50 mL of dextrose.[3] A single 20-mg/mL solution was infused over 2 min[12] and 10 mg/mL in D5W solution was given over 15 min to healthy *adult* volunteers.[13]
Cautions related to IV administration	None known.
Other additives	Contains ~85 mg sodium/500-mg vial. Contains no preservatives.

Comments

Ensuring adequate urine flow by providing sufficient fluid intake is recommended.[1,2]

Should a rash occur the drug should be discontinued.[1,2] The use of allopurinol with ampicillin or amoxicillin increases the incidence of rash.[1]

A 15-year-old boy with Williams syndrome receiving oral allopurinol for 6 weeks developed acute pure red-cell aplasia that resolved when the drug was discontinued.[14]

Drug interactions: Because allopurinol inhibits the metabolism of azathioprine and mercaptopurine, doses of these drugs should be reduced by 25% to 33% and subsequent dosage based on patient response and occurrence of toxicity.[1] The dose may need to be increased with concomitant use of drugs that increase urate concentration.[1]

Other drug interactions have been proposed and appropriate resources for dosing recommendations should be consulted.

Alprostadil

Brand names	Prostin VR Pediatric

Dosage

Hepatic veno occlusive disease: 0.075 mcg/kg/h increasing q 12 h until the maximum tolerated dose of 0.3–0.5 mcg/kg/h has been reached.[1] Used in conjunction with 100 units/kg/d of heparin.

Patent ductus arteriosus (PDA): Short-term maintenance of PDA in neonates with ductal-dependent cyanotic and acyanotic congenital heart disease until surgery can be performed. 0.01–0.1 mcg/kg/min.[2-8] Dosages exceeding 0.1 mcg/kg/min generally do not provide additional benefit.[9]

Peripheral gangrene secondary to ischemia: 0.05 mcg/kg/min reversed acrocyanosis of the hands and feet within 4 days.[10,11]

Pulmonary hypertension

Heart transplant: 0.05 mcg/kg/min during ECMO. After releasing aortic cross clamps, increase to 0.1–0.15 mcg/kg/min.[12,13]

Liver transplant: Prior to unclamping infuse 0.0125 mcg/kg/min. If hypotension occurs, double infusion to 0.025 mcg/kg/min.[14-18]

Dosage adjustment in organ dysfunction

No dosage adjustment required in renal dysfunction.

Maximum dosage

0.4–0.75 mcg/kg/min has been used without adverse effects, but doses of >0.1 mcg/kg/min have not improved efficacy in PDA.[2,8]

IV push

Not recommended because of short half-life.[19]

Intermittent infusion

Not recommended because of short half-life.[19]

Continuous infusion

2–20 mcg/mL in D5W, D10W, or NS[19] infused using a controlled-infusion device (i.e., IV infusion pump) to ensure precise control of the flow rate. If using a volumetric infusion chamber (e.g., buretrol) for dilution, the dose of alprostadil should be added to the appropriate amount of solution and infused through a large vein or an umbilical artery catheter.[19] (See Comments section.) Final concentration is based on the infusion device's flow-rate range and the patient's ability to tolerate fluid. The manufacturer suggests the following dilutions and infusion rates to provide 0.1 mcg/kg/min.[19]

Add 1 Ampul (500 mcg) to	Approximate Concentration of Resulting Solution	Infusion Rate (mL/kg/min)	Infusion Rate (mL/kg/h)
250	2 mcg/mL	0.05	3.0
100	5 mcg/mL	0.02	1.2
50	10 mcg/mL	0.01	0.6
25	20 mcg/mL	0.005	0.3

Start with 0.1 mcg/kg/min.[2,19] Once a therapeutic response is attained, gradually decrease the infusion rate to the lowest effective dose.[2,19,20]

Other routes of administration

No information available to support IM administration; however, extravasation of alprostadil may cause tissue sloughing and necrosis.[19,21]

Maximum concentration

Alprostadil for injection concentrate containing 500 mcg/mL must be diluted prior to infusion.[22] The highest concentration recommended is 20 mcg/mL.[23]

Cautions related to IV administration

Theoretically, intra-aortic or intra-arterial infusion should be the preferred route since it allows for the greatest concentration to the ductus; however, clinical studies have shown these routes to be no more effective than IV infusion.[19]

Apnea occurs in 10% to 12% of neonates weighing <2 kg, usually within the first hour of therapy.[19] Infusion rate should be slowed if fever or hypotension develops until resolution.[19] If apnea or bradycardia occur during the infusion, it is recommended to discontinue therapy and provide supportive therapy.[19]

Reposition intra-arterial catheter if cutaneous flushing develops since this side effect usually results from improper catheter placement. Rapid reversal of cutaneous vasodilation generally occurs with repositioning.[19]

Because of alprostadil's high osmolality, extravasation may cause tissue sloughing and necrosis.[21] Osmolality (by freezing-point depression) of undiluted solution (500 mcg/mL) is 23,250 mOsm/kg.[23]

Other additives

None.

Comments

Reports of an urticarial rash[24] and "harlequin color change"[25] have been documented during prostaglandin infusions in neonates with cardiac heart defects. The rashes may be described as erythematous, migratory, primarily limited to the upper torso, self-limiting, and resolve upon drug discontinuation.[24,25]

Direct contact of the concentrated alprostadil with the wall of the plastic volumetric infusion chamber should be avoided because the drug may interact with the plastic chamber to produce a hazy solution. If this occurs, the chamber and solution should be discarded.[19,23]

A "pseudo-Barter syndrome" has been reported during infusions characterized by severe hyponatremia and polyuria, which resolves upon drug discontinuation.[1,19,26] In addition to the other well-established adverse infusion reactions such as apnea and hyperthermia,[1,19] leukocytosis has been reported.[27] Likewise, the leukocytosis resolves with discontinuation of therapy.

Several adverse effects have been associated with the long-term use of alprostadil. Cortical proliferation may develop as easily as 9 days into therapy (usually 4–6 weeks) and present as soft tissue swelling, peripheral hard edema, and cortical hyperostosis.[19,28-30] The changes are reversible upon discontinuation of the infusion but have been reported to take up to 38 weeks to resolve completely.[28] It is believed that the effects are dose and duration dependent.[28-30]

Several case reports described gastric outlet obstruction in neonates receiving alprostadil. The effect appears to be related to the duration of therapy (i.e., >120 h) and cumulative dose.[31,32] Ectopic calcifications in the deep tissues of the axillae, thoracic inlet, and neck were noted on the chest x-ray of an infant who had received a cumulative alprostadil dose of 5654 mcg/kg for documented transposition. Brown fat necrosis was confirmed on autopsy.[33]

Amikacin Sulfate

Brand names Amikin

Dosage

Except in neonates, dosage should be based on the following equation in any obese patient.[1,2] Dosing weight = IBW + 0.4 (TBW – IBW). (See Appendix B.)

Loading dose: Although limited data are available, some advocated an initial 10-mg/kg dose in neonates.[3-6] If once-a-day dosing is used, some have suggested a dose of 25 mg/kg in infants <1 year and a dose of 20 mg/kg in infants ≥1 year.[7]

Maintenance dose: The maintenance dose is estimated using age and weight,[5] gestational age,[13] or postmenstrual and postnatal age[14]:

Based on age and weight

PNA	<1200 g	1200–2000 g	≥2000 g
<7 d	7.5 mg/kg q 18–24 h[5]	7.5 mg/kg q 12 h[5-11]	7.5–10 mg/kg q 12 h[5-11]
≥7 d	7.5 mg/kg q 18–24 h[5]*	7.5–10 mg/kg q 8–12 h[5-7]	7.5–10 mg/kg q 8 h[5]

*Until 4 weeks of age.

Based on gestational age[13]

Gestational Age	Dose
≤26 weeks	7.5 mg/kg q 24 h
27–34 weeks	7.5 mg/kg q 18 h
35–42 weeks	10 mg/kg q 12 h
≥43 weeks	10 mg/kg q 8 h

Based on postmenstrual and postnatal age[14]

Postmenstrual Age	Postnatal Age	Dose
≤29 weeks	≤7 d	18 mg/kg q 48 h
	8–28 d	15 mg/kg q 36 h
	≥29 d	15 mg/kg q 24 h
30–34 weeks	≤7 d	18 mg/kg q 36 h
	≥8 d	15 mg/kg q 24 h
≥35 weeks	ALL	15 mg/kg q 24 h

Infants and children: 7.5 mg/kg q 8 h[4-5,7] or 420 mg/m^2 q 8 h.[15]

Several investigators have reported that once-daily dosing has comparable efficacy and perhaps less toxicity than classical 8–12 h dosing.[6,16] A single dose of 15–20 mg/kg has been given once daily (over 20–30 min) in critically ill infants and children with severe gram-negative infections,[9,17,18] bone marrow transplantation,[19] or in febrile neutropenic patients with cancer.[21-23] Once-daily therapy has also been used to treat UTI on an outpatient basis.[24] At this time, the use of once-daily dosing in infants and children is controversial.[25] Once-daily dosing should only be done in combination with an appropriate beta-lactam antibiotic in neutropenic patients and in those with *Pseudomonas aeruginosa* or *Serratia marcescens*.[6]

Dosage adjustment in organ dysfunction

Adjust dosage in patients with renal dysfunction.[26] If CrCl is >50 mL/min, give a normal dose q 12–24 h.[26] If CrCl is 10–50 mL/min, give a normal dose q 24–48 h.[26] If CrCl is <10 mL/min, give normal dose q 48–72 h.[26] Dosage adjustment should be based on serum concentrations, pharmacokinetic parameters, and clinical response.

Maximum dosage

<30 mg/kg/d,[4] 20 mg/kg/dose in CF,[6] up 1.5 g/d in *adults*.[3] Larger doses or shorter dosing intervals of aminoglycosides are sometimes required in patients with cystic fibrosis, major thermal burns or dermal loss, ascites, or in patients with febrile granulocytopenia.[26-30] Based on similarities between aminoglycosides, prolonged dosing interval may be required in those receiving ECMO.[31] Individualize dosage based on serum concentrations.

IV push	Although aminoglycosides have been safely administered over 15 sec,[32] 1 min,[33] and 3–5 min,[34] rapid infusion is not recommended.
Intermittent infusion	Dilute in sufficient volume (e.g., 10 mg/mL) of D5¼NS, D5½NS, D5W, LR, or NS and infuse over 30 min.[3]
Continuous infusion	Although aminoglycosides have been given by continuous infusion,[35-37] this method of administration is not recommended.[6] Administration of a normal daily dose over 24 h results in low serum concentrations[36] and nephrotoxicity may occur more frequently.[37]
Other routes of administration	May be administered undiluted by the IM route.[6,8] No information available to support administration by other routes.
Maximum concentration	10 mg/mL for intermittent infusion[38]; however, the diluted volume must allow for accurate measurement and administration over 30–60 min.
Cautions related to IV administration	None. For PN compatibility information, please see Appendix C.
Other additives	**Sulfites:** The 50-mg/mL and 250-mg/mL products contain 0.064 mEq/L and 0.319 mEq/mL of sodium bisulfite, respectively.[39] Sulfites may cause hypersensitivity reactions, which are more common in *adults* with asthma. Most reactions are mild but can include anaphylactic symptoms and life-threatening or less severe asthma episodes.[40,41] Epinephrine may be required in severe cases; and if the sulfite-free product is not available, the sulfite-preserved epinephrine should be used.[40]

Comments

Because large variability exists in patient response to therapy, individualize dosage based on serum concentrations, clinical response, and renal function. Recommended peak and trough serum amikacin concentrations are 20–30 mg/L and <10 mg/L, respectively.[6]

Serum concentrations may be falsely elevated when samples are collected through central venous Silastic catheters.[42]

Although serum concentration monitoring has become routine practice in many institutions, not all patients require monitoring.[43,44] Monitoring is indicated if the patient is not clinically responding, is ≤3 months of age, has disease that requires large doses or high concentrations (CNS infections, endocarditis, pneumonia, ascites, burns), has decreased or unstable renal function, or will be treated more than 10 days.

The beta-lactam ring of penicillins can link with an amino sugar of the aminoglycoside and inactivate the aminoglycoside.[39] This is dose-dependent and particularly problematic in patients with renal failure. To avoid this potential interaction, administer penicillins 1 h before or after an aminoglycoside, adequately flush the infusion line between each infusion, or infuse them through separate lines.

Cochlear and/or vestibular ototoxicity has been associated with all aminoglycoside antibiotics.[6] Total AUC is a better indicator of ototoxic risk than either peak or trough serum concentration.[45,46] Use with caution if other drugs (e.g., macrolide antibiotics, loop diuretics, and platinum-based chemotherapeutic agents) are known to cause ototoxicity.

Aminoglycosides accumulate in renal cortical tissue and may damage proximal tubule cells leading to oliguric renal failure. This has been associated with elevated trough serum concentrations. Risk of nephrotoxicity may increase if aminoglycosides are combined with other potentially nephrotoxic drugs.[6]

May cause neuromuscular blockade that is pronounced in patients with renal insufficiency, neuromuscular disease, and hypocalcemia.[47,48] The effects of nondepolarizing neuromuscular blockers may be prolonged during aminoglycoside use.[47]

Aminocaproic Acid

Brand names	Amicar
Dosage	**Loading dose:** 100–200 mg/kg or 3 g/m^2 over 1 hour.[1-11] **Maintenance dosing:** 100–200 mg/kg q 4–6 h[7,10] or by continuous infusion at a rate of 10–33.3 mg/kg/h or 1 g/m^2/h.[1-11] In children undergoing surgery for scoliosis, the infusion was discontinued when the wound was closed.[2,8] In high-risk patients (those expected to undergo surgery while on ECMO, with severe acidosis or hypoxia, <35 weeks gestation, prior intracranial hemorrhage, or profound coagulopathy), the infusion was continued until decannulation or up to 72 h during ECMO.[3]
Dosage adjustment in organ dysfunction	Use with caution in patients with cardiac, renal, or hepatic disease.[11] Some recommend administering 25% of the normal dose to patients with oliguria or end-stage renal dysfunction.[10]
Maximum dosage	The loading dose is not to exceed 5 g.[2,12] Usually, 18 g/m^2/d in children or 30 g/d in *adults*.[1,10,11] However, 36 g/d were given to a 12-year-old with acute lymphocytic leukemia.[13] (See Comments section.)
IV push	Not recommended.[11,12,14] (See Cautions related to IV administration section.)
Intermittent infusion	Over 1 h.[1,10,14] However, loading doses of 100 mg/kg have been infused over 15–20 min in children 11–18 years of age.[2]
Continuous infusion	Can be given by continuous infusion.
Other routes of administration	No information available to support administration by other routes.
Maximum concentration	20 mg/mL.[4,12]
Cautions related to IV administration	Hypotension, bradycardia, and cardiac arrhythmias may occur with rapid or undiluted administration.[1,7,12] Thrombophlebitis may occur.[1,12]
Other additives	Contains benzyl alcohol 0.9% as a preservative.[1,11,12,14] Benzyl alcohol in small doses as a preservative in drugs is considered safe in newborns.[15] However, a 3-week-old, very low birth weight (710 g) infant who received clindamycin experienced a profound desaturation that required resuscitation after the third and fourth doses, which was subsequently related to the benzyl alcohol preservative.[16] Administration of saline flushes containing benzyl alcohol (bacteriostatic water for injection) was associated with a fatal gasping syndrome, intraventricular hemorrhage, metabolic acidosis, and increased mortality in preterm infants.[17] This should not be used in neonates.

Other additives (cont.)

Hypersensitivity reactions to benzyl alcohol in parenteral products have been reported in *adults*.[18,19]

Comments

Prophylactic aminocaproic acid in children undergoing cardiac surgery reduced intraoperative blood loss, but did not significantly decrease blood product transfusions.[6] Perioperative blood loss was reduced in patients during posterior spinal fusion and segmental spinal instrumentation.[2,8]

Reports on the ability of aminocaproic acid to decrease the incidence of intracranial hemorrhage and other hemorrhagic complications in neonates on ECMO are conflicting.[3-5]

A 12-year-old child with refractory thrombocytopenia after bone marrow transplantation developed myopathy after 98 days of treatment with doses ranging from 4 to 36 g/d.[13]

Serum creatine phosphokinase concentrations, particularly in patients with myalgia, may be a useful indicator of muscle injury. Myopathy is usually reversible on discontinuation of therapy.[1,13]

A pharmacokinetics study found that children require larger loading and maintenance doses than *adults*.[20]

Aminophylline

Brand names Various manufacturers

Dosage

Aminophylline product contains varying amounts of theophylline (check manufacturers information). The following doses are reported as THEOPHYLLINE.

Apnea and bradycardia of prematurity (usual therapeutic range 6–12 mcg/mL)

Loading dose (LD): 5–6 mg/kg over 20–30 min.[1-4] If the patient is already receiving theophylline, a serum concentration must be obtained and the LD based on that concentration[5] using the equation:

LD (mg/kg) = (desired concentration - measured concentration) / 2

(See Comments section for more information about the equation.)

Initial maintenance doses

Postconceptional age <55 weeks: 1–3 mg/kg q 8–12 h.[4]

Postconceptional age >55 weeks: 4–6 mg/kg q 6–12 h.[4]

Neonates and infants up to 3 months of age eliminate 50% of theophylline unchanged in the urine. The dosage should be adjusted in newborns with renal dysfunction.[5]

Because of large variability in patient response to initial doses,[6-12] individualize dosage based on serum concentrations and clinical response.

Severe acute asthma (usual therapeutic range 5–15 mcg/mL): The role of IV aminophylline in acute asthma is controversial.[13-15] Many *adult*[16-20] and pediatric[21-24] studies have shown that patients responsive to beta-agonist and systemic glucocorticoid experience no additional benefit from IV aminophylline. However, recent evaluations in critically ill children with severe acute asthma and impending respiratory failure who are unresponsive to aggressive beta-agonist and systemic glucocorticoids suggest that the addition of aminophylline may be beneficial.[25,26]

Loading dose (no theophylline use in the past 24 h): 5–6 mg/kg over 20–30 min.[5,27-29]

Loading dose (theophylline use in the past 24 h): A theophylline serum concentration must be obtained prior to theophylline administration. The loading dose (LD) is then estimated based on the following equation:

LD (mg/kg) = (desired concentration - measured concentration) / 2

(See Comments section.)

Maintenance dose (initial dose to achieve a target serum concentration of 10 mcg/mL): Dose should be based on ideal body weight in children who are overweight or obese.[5,29] (See Appendix B.)

Infants 6–52 weeks: [0.008 (age in weeks) + 0.21] = mg/kg/h.[27,30]

Children 1–<9 years: 0.8 mg/kg/h.[31]

Children 9–12 years: 0.7 mg/kg/h.[31]

Children 12–16 years (smoker): 0.7 mg/kg/h.[31]

Children 12–16 years (nonsmoker): 0.5 mg/kg/h.[31]

Not to exceed 900 mg/d unless a subtherapeutic serum concentration combined with an inadequate response indicate the need for larger doses.[31]

Large variability exists in patient response to initial doses[27,29,32,33]; therefore, individualize dosage based on serum concentrations and clinical response.

Dosage adjustment in organ dysfunction	Neonates and infants up to 3 months of age eliminate 50% of theophylline unchanged in the urine. The dosage should be adjusted in newborns with renal dysfunction.[5] Adjust dose in patients with cardiac failure, hepatic dysfunction, acute hepatitis, or sustained high fever; in neonates with renal dysfunction; and in asphyxiated neonates.[5,12,15,31,34,35]
Maximum dosage	Individualize dosage based on serum concentrations and clinical response.[5]
IV push	Contraindicated. (See Cautions related to IV administration section.)
Intermittent infusion	≤25 mg/mL over 15–30 min[5] not to exceed 0.36 mg/kg/min or 25 mg/min.[2] Doses are given q 12 h in neonates[4,31] and q 4–6 h in infants and children.[4,31,36-39]
Continuous infusion	1–25 mg/mL in D–LR, D–R, D–S, D5LR, D5NS, D5¹/₄NS, D5W, D10W, D20W, LR, NS, ¹/₂NS, or R.[40] (See Dosage section.)
Other routes of administration	No information available to support administration by other routes.
Maximum concentration	25 mg/mL (commercially available).[40]
Cautions related to IV administration	Rapid administration may result in toxic serum concentrations[43] and circulatory failure.[29] For PN compatibility information, please see Appendix C.
Other additives	None.
Comments	Because large variability exists in patient response to initial and maintenance doses, individualize dosage based on attainment of a therapeutic serum concentration and clinical response. The equation to calculate loading dose (LD) is based on the following: LD = desired concentration x volume of distribution (assuming a normal volume of distribution of 0.5 L/kg). As a general rule, 1 mg/kg of theophylline will increase the serum theophylline concentration by 2 mg/L.[43] Because theophylline is primarily metabolized by the CYP1A2 isoenzyme, and to a lesser extent by CYP3A4, it may be associated with many potentially fatal drug interactions.[44-47] Consult appropriate resources for dosing recommendations before combining any drug with theophylline.

Amphotericin B

Brand names	Fungizone, Amphocin

Dosage

Initial and maintenance: 0.25–0.5 mg/kg q 24 h infused over 2–6 h. Increase daily dose as tolerated by 0.25–0.5 mg/kg up to 0.5–1.5 mg/kg q 24 h.[1-18]

Early studies, many administering amphotericin B in combination with flucytosine, used smaller initial doses and slower dose titration.[19-26] Recent data supports the use of larger doses initially (0.25–0.5 mg/kg q 24 h) followed by a more rapid dose titration to achieve the desired therapeutic dose.[1,3,6,8]

Test dose (to minimize anaphylactic response in susceptible individuals): Although one study in *adults*, who were frequently premedicated, failed to show that a test dose predicted anaphylactic reactions,[27] a single dose of 0.1 mg/kg, up to 1 mg, infused over 20–30 min is often used.[19,22,25,28-30] Vital signs should be monitored q 30 min for 2 h. If a test dose is done, therapy should commence the same day with the remainder of a recommended therapeutic dose.[31]

Pharmacokinetic data suggest great variability in clearance, volume of distribution, and half-life in neonates, particularly premature neonates.[8,30,32] Some papers have advocated smaller and/or less frequent doses in neonates.[30,33-34] Doses of 0.5 mg/kg and dosing intervals >24 h may be appropriate for these patients.[23,26,30] One study used an every-other-day dosing regimen with 0.5 mg/kg in neonates <1 kg or 1 mg/kg in neonates ≥1 kg.[35]

Dosage adjustment in organ dysfunction

Dose adjustment is not necessary in patients with renal insufficiency[1]; however, if renal insufficiency occurs during therapy, the dosing interval should be increased.[36] Alternately, therapy may be changed to an amphotericin B lipid product.[36]

Maximum dosage

Total daily dose should not exceed 1.5 mg/kg.[1,29] Doses of 1.5 mg/kg/d for an unspecified time[30] and 1.3 mg/kg/d for 31 d[17] have been used in children. Reported cumulative doses in pediatric patients have ranged from 2.5 to 52 mg/kg.[4,8-10,12-13,20,22-24,37]

Larger doses (>1 mg/kg) may be associated with increased risk of nephrotoxicity, which can present as oliguria, azotemia, increased serum creatinine, potassium wasting, and renal tubular acidosis. Glomerular filtration rate was reduced permanently in *adults* who received >4 g over the course of therapy.[31,38-39] Pediatric patients have received total cumulative doses of 30–52 mg/kg without evidence of "permanent" nephrotoxicity.[10,12-13] Evidence does not support serum drug concentration or cumulative dose monitoring as a marker of toxicity.[40] (See Comments section regarding nephrotoxicity.)

Three children who inadvertently received doses of 3.8, 4.6, or 5 mg/kg and two premature neonates who received 25 and 40.8 mg/kg experienced cardiac arrest during or shortly after the infusion. Only one child survived.[41]

IV push

No information available to support administration by this method.

Intermittent infusion

0.1 mg/mL in D5W, D10W, D15W, or D20W[42] over 2–6 h.[28,31,43] Although amphotericin B is incompatible with fat emulsions,[43] it has been reconstituted in a small volume of D5W and then diluted in IV fat emulsion 20% in order to improve tolerance and decrease infusion-related side effects in *adults*.[44,45] (See Comments section regarding premedication.)

Continuous infusion

No information available to support administration by this method.

Other routes of administration

No information available to support administration by other routes.

Maximum concentration

0.1 mg/mL.[29,43] The osmolality of this solution (0.1 mg/mL in D5W) is 256 mOsm/kg.[43] While one reference states that a concentration of 0.5 mg/mL may be given in fluid-restricted patients via a central catheter,[46] more concentrated solutions increase the risk of phlebitis.[47] Concentrations as high as 0.5–1 mg/mL have been found to be chemically stable for up to 120 h when stored at 4°C.[48]

Cautions related to IV administration

Hypersensitivity reactions, including anaphylaxis, have been reported.[27,49,50]

Arrhythmias have been reported during infusion in a neonate.[55]

Although cardiovascular collapse has occurred in animals after rapid injection,[31,51] it has been infused over 45–60 min without problems in *adults*.[52-54]

For PN compatibility information, please see Appendix C.

Other additives

Each 50-mg vial also contains 41 mg sodium desoxycholate and 20.2 mg sodium phosphates (including mono- and d-basic sodium phosphate, phosphoric acid, and sodium hydroxide).[29]

Comments

Nephrotoxicity: Concomitant nephrotoxic drugs may increase the potential for nephrotoxicity.[34,56] Hydration and sodium repletion, either through sodium loading with 0.9% saline over 30 min prior to administration or with sodium intakes of >4 mEq/kg/d, may reduce the risk of nephrotoxicity.[1,56,57] Because rifampin acts synergistically with amphotericin B, they have been given concomitantly to reduce the amphotericin B dose and, hence, the risk of nephrotoxicity.[58]

Premedication: Patients have been premedicated with acetaminophen, codeine, diazepam, diphenhydramine, hydroxyzine, meperidine, or prochlorperazine.[39,59,60] Corticosteroids have been added to amphotericin B solutions to decrease the incidence and severity of febrile response during infusion.[16,39] However, congestive heart failure was reported in *adults* who received 25–40 mg/d of hydrocortisone with amphotericin B.[39]

Phlebitis: Adding 1 unit of heparin to each mL of solution may reduce pain at the injection site and phlebitis.[61]

Filtration: If in-line filtration is indicated, use filters with a pore size ≥1 micron.[43]

Amphotericin B Cholesteryl Sulfate Complex

Brand names	Amphotec
Dosage	Amphotericin B cholesteryl sulfate complex has also been referred to as amphotericin B colloidal dispersion (ABCD) in clinical studies and case reports. **Systemic fungal infections (*Aspergillus* sp., *Candida* sp., and *Cryptococcus* sp.) in patients refractory or intolerant to conventional amphotericin B because of adverse effects, including nephrotoxicity** **Children and adolescents:** 3–6 mg/kg/d.[1-6] One study in premature neonates gave 3 mg/kg/d on day 1 followed by 5 mg/kg/d thereafter.[7] The manufacturer recommends administration of a test dose (10 mL of the final preparation containing between 1.8 and 8.3 mg) to be given over 15–30 min while observing the patient for tolerance.[8]
Dosage adjustment in organ dysfunction	No dosage adjustment recommended for hepatic or renal impairment (CrCl ≥35 mL/min). No information on dosage adjustment in more severe hepatic or renal disease.[8]
Maximum dosage	6 mg/kg/d.[1] However, doses as high as 7.5 mg/kg/d have been used.[8]
IV push	Not recommended.[8]
Intermittent infusion	Reconstitute with SW to a concentration of 5 mg/mL, then further dilute with D5W to a final concentration of 0.6 mg/mL (range 0.16–0.83 mg/mL).[8,9] Infuse at a rate of 1 mg/kg/h.[1,8,9] May infuse over a minimum of 2 h in patients exhibiting no adverse effects.[8,9]
Continuous infusion	No information available to support administration by this method.
Other routes of administration	No information available to support administration by other routes.
Maximum concentration	0.83 mg/mL.[8,9]
Cautions related to IV administration	Acute reactions (hypotension, fever, chills) may occur within 1–3 h after administration. Infusion related reactions may be managed by decreasing the rate of infusion or by premedicating with antihistamines or corticosteroids.[8] Anaphylaxis has been reported.[8]

Other additives	None.
Comments	Hepatotoxicity has been reported.[1] Do not mix lipid-based amphotericin B products with other IV medications or saline or coadminister with other parenteral solutions containing saline or electrolytes.[8] Do not filter or use an in-line filter during administration.[8,9] There is some evidence that the colloidal dispersion formulation may be the least tolerable of the available amphotericin B lipid formulations.[10]

Amphotericin B Lipid Complex

Brand names	Abelcet
Dosage	**Empiric treatment of febrile neutropenic patients:** 5 mg/kg/d has been studied in children 2–16 years of age.[1] **Systemic fungal infections (*Aspergillus* sp., *Candida* sp., and *Cryptococcus* sp.) in patients refractory or intolerant to conventional amphotericin B because of adverse effects, including nephrotoxicity** **Neonates, infants, and children 2–17 years:** 2.5–5 mg/kg/d.[2-7] One study in neonates gave up to 6.5 mg/kg/d.[8]
Dosage adjustment in organ dysfunction	The need for dosage adjustment with amphotericin B lipid complex in hepatic or renal impairment is not known.
Maximum dosage	5 mg/kg/d.[2,3] However, doses as high as 6.5–13 mg/kg have been given to children and *adults*.[3,6,8-10]
IV push	Not recommended.[3]
Intermittent infusion	Add desired dose of amphotericin B lipid complex, using the 5-micron filter needle supplied with each vial, to D5W to make a final concentration of 1–2 mg/mL. Infuse at a rate of 2.5 mg/kg/h. If >2 h is required to administer a given dose, shake the bag to mix contents q 2 h.[3]
Continuous infusion	No information available to support administration by this method.
Other routes of administration	No information available to support administration by other routes.
Maximum concentration	2 mg/mL.[3]
Cautions related to IV administration	Acute reactions (hypotension, fever, chills) may occur within 1–2 h after administration.[3] Infusion related reactions may be managed by decreasing the rate of infusion or by premedicating with antihistamines or corticosteroids. Chest discomfort has been reported.[1] Anaphylaxis has been reported.[3] Hypertension has been reported in an *adult*.[11]
Other additives	Each mL contains 9 mg NaCl.[3]
Comments	Hepatotoxicity has been reported.[2] Do not mix lipid-based amphotericin B products with other IV medications, saline, or coadminister with other parenteral solutions containing saline or electrolytes.[3] Do not use an in-line filter during administration.[3] Shake bag thoroughly before infusion.[3]

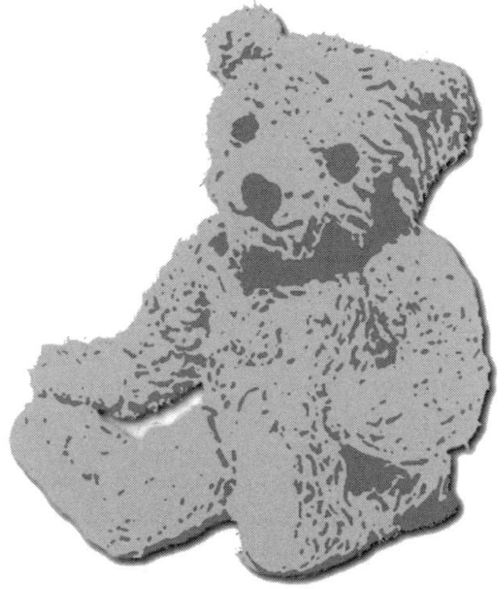

Amphotericin B Liposomal

Brand names	AmBisome

Dosage

Empiric treatment of febrile neutropenic patients

Children and adolescents: 3 mg/kg/d.[1,2]

Solid bone marrow transplant prophylaxis/treatment

Children and adolescents: 2–6 mg/kg/d over a mean of 25 days (range 5–90 days).[3-6]

10 mg/kg once weekly may provide useful prophylaxis against fungal infections as described in 14 children (4.5 months to 9 years of age) undergoing hematopoietic stem cell transplant.[7]

Systemic fungal infections (*Aspergillus* sp., *Candida* sp., and *Cryptococcus* sp.) in patients refractory or intolerant to conventional amphotericin B because of adverse effects, including nephrotoxicity

Neonates, infants, children, and adolescents: 3–5 mg/kg/d.[8-16]

Doses in neonates have been reported as high as 7 mg/kg/d.[14-16] Up to 10 mg/kg/d in pediatric patients and 15 mg/kg/d in *adults* has been found to be well-tolerated and effective for treatment of aspergillosis and other filamentous fungal infections.[17,18]

Visceral leishmaniasis

Immunocompetent children and adolescents[18-21]: 3 mg/kg/d on days 1–5 and on days 14 and 21 of therapy. Alternatively, 4 mg/kg has been given on days 1–5 and on day 10 of therapy. Mediterranean visceral leishmaniasis has been successfully treated with 20 mg/kg given either as 4 mg/kg for 5 days or 10 mg/kg for 2 days.[21]

Immunocompromised children and adolescents[18]: 4 mg/kg/d on days 1–5 and on days 10, 17, 24, 31, and 38 of therapy.

Dosage adjustment in organ dysfunction	The need for dosage adjustment in hepatic or renal impairment is not known. It has been given successfully to patients with pre-existing renal impairment.[18]
Maximum dosage	10 mg/kg/d in children; 15 mg/kg/d in *adults*.[17,18]
IV push	Not recommended.[18]
Intermittent infusion	After reconstituting with SW and shaking vigorously, add desired dose of liposomal amphotericin B, using the 5-micron filter needle provided with each vial, to D5W to make a final concentration of 1–2 mg/mL (more dilute concentrations of 0.2–0.5 mg/mL may also be used). Infuse over 2 h. May infuse over 1 h in patients exhibiting no adverse effects.[18]
Continuous infusion	No information available to support administration by this method.
Other routes of administration	No information available to support administration by other routes.

Amphotericin B Liposomal

Maximum concentration	2 mg/mL.[18]
Cautions related to IV administration	Acute infusion related reactions (chest pain; dyspnea; hypoxia; severe abdomen, flank, or leg pain; and flushing and urticaria) may occur within the first 5 min of infusion and are not related to infusion rate. Use diphenhydramine and infusion interruption to manage these acute reactions. Acute reactions (hypotension, fever and chills) that occur with conventional amphotericin B may still occur within 1–2 h after the administration of liposomal amphotericin B, but with decreased frequency.[18,22,23] Anaphylaxis has been reported.[18]
Other additives	Each vial contains 0.64 mg alpha tocopherol.[18]
Comments	Hepatotoxicity has been reported.[8] Do not mix lipid-based amphotericin B products with other IV medications or saline or coadminister with other parenteral solutions containing saline or electrolytes.[18] An in-line filter that is ≥1 micron may be used.[18]

Ampicillin Sodium

Brand names	Omnipen-N, Polycillin-N, Totacillin-N

Dosage

Serious anaphylactoid reactions may require immediate emergency treatment with epinephrine, oxygen, IV steroids, and airway management.

Neonates

PNA	≤1200 g	≤ 1200–2000 g	≥2000 g
<7 d	50–100 mg/kg/d divided q 12 h[1,2]*	50–100 mg/kg/d divided q 12 h[2,3]	75–150 mg/kg/d divided q 8–12 h[2,3]
≥7 d		75–150 mg/kg/d divided q 8–12 h[2,3]	100–200 mg/kg/d divided q 6 h[2,3]

*Until 4 weeks of age.

Infants and children

Mild-to-moderate infections: 100–150 mg/kg/d divided q 6 h up to 4 g/d.[2]

Severe infections: 200–400 mg/kg/d divided q 6 h up to 12 g/d.[2]

Bacterial endocarditis (prophylaxis)

Dental, oral, respiratory tract, or esophageal procedures: 50 mg/kg up to 2 g within 30 min of starting a procedure.[2]

Genitourinary and gastrointestinal procedures: 50 mg/kg up to 2 g within 30 min of starting procedure. High-risk patients should also be given 1.5 mg/kg of gentamicin plus another 25-mg/kg dose of ampicillin in 6 h.[2]

Bacterial endocarditis (treatment)

Enterococcal endocarditis (sensitive to penicillin, gentamicin and vancomycin): 300 mg/kg/d divided q 4–6 h plus gentamicin 3 mg/kg/d divided q 8 h.[4] If resistant to gentamicin, give penicillin G potassium (300,000 units/kg/d divided q 4–6 h) plus streptomycin (20–30 mg/kg/d divided q 12 h).[4] If symptom ≤3 months treat for 4 weeks and if >3 months treat for 6 weeks.[4]

Enterococcus faecalis (resistant to penicillin, gentamicin and vancomycin): Imipenem/cilastatin 60–100 mg/kg/d divided q 6 h or ceftriaxone 100 mg/k q 24 h plus ampicillin 300 mg/kg/d divided q 4–6 h for 4–6 weeks.[4]

Meningitis

≤1200 g: 100 mg/kg/d divided q 12 h.[1]

≤7 days and >1200 g: 100–300 mg/kg/d divided q 8–12 h.[2,4]

>7–28 days and ≥1200 g: 150–300 mg/kg/d divided q 6–8 h.[2,4]

Infants and children: 200–400 mg/kg/d divided q 6 h up to 6–12 g/d.[2,5-10]

Dosage adjustment in organ dysfunction

Adjust dosage in patients with renal dysfunction.[11] If CrCl is <10 mL/min administer normal dose q 12–24 h.[12]

Maximum dosage

400 mg/kg/d,[2,13-15] not to exceed 14 g.[2,13-15]

IV push

100 mg/mL.[16] Doses <500 mg generally given over 3–5 min.[11,16] Not to exceed 10 mg/kg/min in infants and children[3] or 100 mg/min in *adults*.[16] More rapid administration may result in seizures. (See Cautions related to IV administration section.)[11]

Intermittent infusion	≤30 mg/mL in LR, NS, or SW over 10–15 min for doses >500 mg.[16]
Continuous infusion	Although 5 mg/mL has been added to PN solution,[17] not recommended to be given by this method.
Other routes of administration	≤250 mg/mL in SW or BW has been given IM.[11,16] No information available to support administration by other routes.
Maximum concentration	100 mg/mL[11,16,18] in NS or 200 mg/mL in SW for central-line delivery; 50 mg/mL for peripheral infusion[19]; 200 mg/mL in SW[19] for IV push; 30 mg/mL for intermittent infusion[16,19,20]; and up to 112 mg/mL in SW for peripheral infusion in fluid restricted patients.[11,16]
Cautions related to IV administration	None. For PN compatibility information, please see Appendix C.
Other additives	Contains 2.9 mEq sodium/g of ampicillin.[16]

Comments

Patients with a history of type I reaction to penicillin should not receive beta-lactam antibiotics. From 5% to 15% of patients allergic to penicillin will also be allergic to cephalosporins. Certain infections (e.g., syphilis) require penicillin for cure. It is recommended that a desensitization protocol for penicillin-allergic individuals should be performed in a hospital setting. This can usually be completed in about 4 h, at which time the first dose of penicillin can be given.[2]

The beta-lactam ring of penicillins can link with an amino sugar of the aminoglycoside and inactivate the aminoglycoside.[21-23] To avoid this potential interaction, administer penicillins 1 h before or after an aminoglycoside, adequately flush the infusion line between each infusion, or infuse them through separate lines. *In vivo* inactivation that is dose dependent can also occur particularly in patients with renal failure.[23-25] In patients with end-stage renal failure, gentamicin half-life was decreased by 22–31 h after carbenicillin or ticarcillin was added to the drug regimen.[24]

In a study of 14 very low birth weight neonates (<750 g and <28 weeks gestational age), the authors concluded that doses of 50 mg/kg q 18–24 h sufficiently killed bacteria while reducing the risk of ampicillin-associated seizures.[26]

A false-positive urinary glucose results when cupric sulfate solution-based tests (Clinitest, Benedict's solution, Fehling's solution) are used. Glucose oxidase methods (Clinistix) are not associated with false-positive test results.[15]

Ampicillin Sodium–Sulbactam Sodium

Brand names	Unasyn

Dosage

Serious anaphylactoid reactions may require immediate emergency treatment with epinephrine, oxygen, IV steroids, and airway management.

Dosage based on ampicillin component.[1] 1.5 g contains 1 g of ampicillin and 0.5 g of sulbactam. Sulbactam is a beta-lactamase inhibitor that extends the spectrum of ampicillin but has little antibacterial activity.

The manufacturer does not recommend use in those <1 year of age[1]; however, the American Academy of Pediatrics suggests doses for those older than 1 month of age.[2] Pediatric patients who weigh ≥40 kg may receive the usual *adult* dose of ampicillin–sulbactam.[1]

Mild-to-moderate infections: 100–150 mg/kg/d of ampicillin divided q 6 h.[2-5]

Severe infections: 200–400 mg/kg/d of ampicillin divided q 6 h.[2,6-13]

Bacterial endocarditis (treatment)

Culture negative and native valve: 200 mg/kg/d of ampicillin divided q 4–6 h plus gentamicin (3 mg/kg/d divided q 8 h) for 4–6 weeks.[14]

Enterococcal endocarditis (resistant to penicillin and susceptible to aminoglycoside and vancomycin): 200 mg/kg/d of ampicillin divided q 6 h plus gentamicin (3 mg/kg/d divided q 8 h) for 6 weeks.[14] If resistant to gentamicin >6 weeks of ampicillin–sulbactam will be needed.

HACEK* microorganisms: 200 mg/kg/d of ampicillin divided q 4–6 h.[14] Treat for 4 weeks unless prosthetic material is present then treat for 6 weeks.[14]

Gynecologic infections (e.g., acute gonococcal and nongonococcal PID): Adolescents should receive 2 g of ampicillin q 6 h plus doxycycline.[15]

Meningitis: 400 mg/kg/d of ampicillin divided q 4–6 h.[2,15,16]

Perioperative prophylaxis: Although ampicillin–sulbactam has been used to reduce the incidence of infections in patients undergoing contaminated or potentially contaminated surgery,[17] other antibiotics are generally preferred.

Dosage adjustment in organ dysfunction

Adjust dosage in patients with renal dysfunction. If CrCl is 15–29 mL/min, administer normal dose q 12 h and if CrCl is 5–14 mL/min, give normal doses q 24 h.[1] The elimination of ampicillin–sulbactam is affected to the same degree by renal impairment; hence, the recommended 2:1 ratio of the drugs remains.[15]

Maximum dosage

400 mg/kg/d of ampicillin[2] up to 8 g/d of ampicillin.[1]

IV push

Although ampicillin–sulbactam has been given over 2–3 min,[18] this method of delivery is not recommended because rapid administration may cause seizures.[1]

Intermittent infusion

2–30 mg/mL of ampicillin in D5½NS, D5W, LR, NS, or SW over 10–15 min.[1,19] If diluted in 50–100 mL of solution, give over 15–30 min.[1,10]

Continuous infusion

No information available to support administration by this method.

Other routes of administration

250 mg/mL of ampicillin in SW or lidocaine 0.5% to 2% may be given IM.[1] Because IM administration is painful, administer deep into a large muscle within 1 h of reconstitution.[1]

*Haemophilus influenzae, H aphrophilus, Actinobacillus actinomycetemcomitants, Cardiobacterium hominis, Eikenelia corrodens, and Kingella kingae.

Ampicillin Sodium–Sulbactam Sodium

Maximum concentration	20 mg/mL of ampicillin in D5W is stable at room temperature for 2 h and 30 mg/mL in NS, SW, and LR is stable at room temperature for 8 h.[1] 2 mg/mL of ampicillin in D5½NS is stable at room temperature for 4 h.[1] 250 mg/mL of ampicillin in SW or lidocaine 0.5% to 2% for IM administration should be used within 1 h.[1]
Cautions related to IV administration	If a decision is made to give this medication to a patient with known penicillin hypersensitivity, the patient should be closely observed for allergic reactions. (See Comments section.) For PN compatibility information, please see Appendix C.
Other additives	Contains 115 mg (5 mEq) of sodium/g of ampicillin.[19]
Comments	Patients with a history of type I reaction to penicillin should not receive beta-lactam antibiotics. From 5% to 15% of patients allergic to penicillin will also be allergic to cephalosporins. Certain infections (e.g., syphilis) require penicillin for cure. It is recommended that a desensitization protocol for penicillin-allergic individuals should be performed in a hospital setting. This can usually be completed in about 4 h, at which time the first dose of penicillin can be given.[2] The beta-lactam ring of penicillins can link with an amino sugar of the aminoglycoside and inactivate the aminoglycoside.[20-22] To avoid this potential interaction, administer penicillins 1 h before or after an aminoglycoside, adequately flush the infusion line between each infusion, or infuse them through separate lines. *In vivo* inactivation that is dose dependent can also occur particularly in patients with renal failure.[22-24] In patients with end-stage renal failure, gentamicin half-life was decreased by 22–31 h after carbenicillin or ticarcillin was added to the drug regimen.[24] Thrombophlebitis may occur.[1] A false-positive urinary glucose results when cupric sulfate solution-based tests (Clinitest, Benedict's solution, Fehling's solution) are used.[1] Glucose oxidase methods (Clinistix) are not associated with false-positive test results. Ampicillin-sulbactam may cause falsely increased serum uric acid concentration when copper-chelate method is used; phosphotungstate and uricase methods appear to be unaffected by ampicillin.[10] Ampicillin-sulbactam may cause false-positive Coombs' test results.[25]

Anidulafungin

Brand names	Eraxis
Dosage	Experience with anidulafungin in children, particularly neonates, is limited[1]; currently there is no established dose range for pediatric patients.[2] **Children 2–17 years (treatment/prophylaxis)** **Loading dose[3]:** 1.5 mg/kg (not to exceed 100 mg) or 3 mg/kg (not to exceed 200 mg). **Maintenance dose[1,3]:** 0.75 mg/kg (not to exceed 50 mg) or 1.5 mg/kg (not to exceed 100 mg) given once daily. The above dosage regimens were found to produce similar concentrations as that seen in *adults* receiving maintenance therapy with 50 or 100 mg/d.[3]
Dosage adjustment in organ dysfunction	No dosage adjustment in renal or hepatic dysfunction.[4,5]
Maximum dosage	**Loading dose[3,4]:** 200 mg/d in children and *adults*. **Maintenance dose[3,4]:** 100 mg/d in children and *adults.*
IV push	Not recommended.
Intermittent infusion	Reconstitute with companion diluent (15 mL 20% w/w Dehydrated Alcohol in Water for Injection), then further dilute with D5W or NS to a concentration of 0.36–0.43 mg/mL.[4] Infuse over 45 min to 3 h at a rate not to exceed 1.1 mg/min.[3,4]
Continuous infusion	No information available to support administration via this method.
Other routes of administration	No information available to support administration by other routes.
Maximum concentration	0.43 mg/mL.[4]
Cautions related to IV administration	Histamine-mediated symptoms (rash, urticaria, flushing, pruritus, dyspnea, and hypotension) have been reported. These symptoms occur infrequently if infusion rate is ≤1.1 mg/min.[4]

Other additives	None.

Comments

Anidulafungin has been given empirically to neutropenic children (2–17 years) for 1–23 days (mean 8.7 days); none of the children developed a fungal infection.[3] The most common adverse drug effects included fever, feeling abnormal, rash/erythema, increased BUN, and hypotension. Most adverse effects in children receiving larger doses occurred in children <11 years of age.[3]

A 16-year-old developed moderate facial erythema and rash at the start of anidulafungin infusion that resolved within 1.5 h of stopping the infusion. These symptoms did not reoccur with repeat infusion and continuation of therapy.[3]

The labeling reports that clinically significant hepatic abnormalities (hepatic dysfunction, hepatitis and hepatic failure) may occur.[4]

Aprotinin

Brand names	Trasylol

Dosage

Aprotinin doses are expressed in terms of Kallikrein Inhibitor (KI) Units. 10,000 KI units/mL = 1.4 mg/mL.[1,2]

Aprotinin is a proteinase inhibitor from bovine lung and hypersensitivity reactions can occur.[1] A test dose of 10,000 KI units should be given ≥10 min prior to the loading dose due to the risk of hypersensitivity reactions.[1,2] The full test dose has been used in infants and children.[3-6] A prick test or skin test is only about 20% predictive of a hypersensitivity reaction.[5]

Loading dose: 10,000–50,000 KI units/kg[3,6-13] over 15 min.[3] Alternatively, 140,000 KI units/m^2 in those <1.16 m^2 and 250,000 KI units/m^2 in those >1.16 m^2[14] up to 1,700,000 KI units/m^2.[4,5]

Pump priming dose: Usually 10,000–50,000 KI units/kg.[7-13] A total dose of 500,000 KI units (not weight based) has been used in children <10 kg.[6] Alternatively, 240,000 KI units/m^2 in those <1.16 m^2 and 280,000 KI units/m^2 in those >1.16 m^2[14] up to 1,700,000 KI units/m^2.[5]

Continuous infusion: 10,000–30,000 KI units/kg/h during cardiopulmonary bypass[9-12] or for 3 h after weaning from cardiopulmonary bypass.[7] Alternatively, 56,000 KI units/m^2 in those <1.16 m^2 and 70,000 KI units/m^2 in those >1.16 m^2[14] up to 400,000 KI units/m^2.[4,5]

Dosage adjustment in organ dysfunction

Studies have not been conducted in patients with renal or hepatic disease.[1,2] Serum creatinine concentrations did not change after treatment in patients with mildly elevated values prior to aprotinin administration.[1,2] However, the risk of renal failure in *adults* was significantly increased in patients undergoing coronary-artery bypass surgery who received aprotinin compared to other treatments.[15] (See Comments section.)

Maximum dosage

Not established. In *adults,* up to 17.5 million KI units have been administered within 24 h.[1,2]

IV push

Not recommended.[1,2]

Intermittent infusion

The loading dose should be infused over 20–30 min.[1,2]

Continuous infusion

10,000–30,000 KI units/kg/h[9-12] for up to 136 ± 44 min.[9] Some do not use a continuous infusion.[3,6,8]

Other routes of administration

Not indicated.

Maximum concentration

Undiluted. 10,000 KI units/mL (1.4 mg/mL) solution for central line infusion.[1,2]

Cautions related to IV administration

Aprotinin should only be administered through a central venous line.[1,2]

Aprotinin is incompatible with other medications. Heparin and aprotinin should be administered separately in the priming solution to allow recirculation and dilution prior to the other drug being administered.[1,2]

Other additives Contains 9 mg sodium chloride mL.[1,2]

Comments

A test dose should always be given due to the risk of hypersensitivity reactions.[1,2] Patients re-exposed to aprotinin have a higher incidence of hypersensitivity reactions and anaphylaxis.[1,2] Hypersensitivity reactions to the test dose[16] or subsequent doses may occur in children.[3] Children are re-exposed to aprotinin sooner than *adults* and in one study two of 46 children compared to one of 77 *adults* studied experienced a hypersensitivity reaction.[3]

Pharmacokinetics in children is highly variable. Despite weight–based dosing, aprotinin concentrations are lower after the loading dose and 5 min after the start of cardiopulmonary bypass in children <10 kg.[11] Neonates and infants are more likely to have subtherapeutic aprotinin concentrations, and this may be related to the discrepancy in volume between the priming volume and the patient's blood volume.[11]

Aprotinin may prolong activated clotting time (ACT) tests assessed using the celite ACT test. The kaolin-based ACT test may be affected to a much lesser degree. Thus, additional heparin may be needed even when ACTs appear adequate.[1,2]

The risk of renal failure, myocardial infarction, stroke, and encephalopathy was significantly increased in *adults* undergoing revascularization who received aprotinin compared to those receiving aminocaproic acid or tranexamic acid.[15]

Aprotinin is primarily used to reduce perioperative bleeding and the requirement for blood transfusion during cardiopulmonary pulmonary bypass.[1,2] Its use did reduce transfusion requirements in children <12 years of age undergoing complicated craniofacial surgery,[4] but did not decrease the requirement for blood transfusions in patients 15–64 years old who underwent orthotopic liver transplantation.[17]

Argatroban

Brand names Generic

Dosage

Argatroban is for use during heparin induced thrombocytopenia (HIT) and in patients with a history of HIT.

Children[1-3]

Prophylaxis or treatment of thrombosis: Infusion rates range from 0.1–12 mcg/kg/min (usually <6) with doses titrated to activated partial thromboplastin time (aPTT) above 50 sec (2 × baseline) (n = 14, six of them <6 months of age).

Hemodialysis or ECMO: Infusion rates ranged from 0.1–24 mcg/kg/min (usually <6) titrated to activated clotting time (ACT) of at least 160 up to 200 sec for anticoagulation during hemodialysis or ECMO (n = 17).

Cardiac catheterization: 150 or 250 mcg/kg bolus followed by infusion rates of 7.5–15 mcg/kg/min titrated to an ACT of 300 (n = 5).

Data on file with the manufacturer includes results from an ongoing phase IV study of the pharmacokinetics and pharmacodynamics of argatroban in pediatric patients from birth to 16 years.[4] The initial infusion rate was 1 mcg/kg/min and for those undergoing cardiac catheterization or surgery, a bolus dose of 250 mcg/kg followed by infusion rates of 15–20 mcg/kg/min was used. Based on pharmacokinetic data from 10 patients, infusion rates of 0.25–1 mcg/kg/min for patients <6 months and infusion rates of 0.5–2 mcg/kg/min for patients 6–16 years should achieve an aPTT 1.7–2.7 × baseline. There were no patients between 6 months and 6-years-old enrolled.

Adults[5]

Prophylaxis or treatment of thrombosis: 2 mcg/kg/min by continuous infusion, dose adjusted up to 10 mcg/kg/min to steady-state aPTT of 1.5–3 × baseline value (not to exceed 100 sec).

Percutaneous coronary interventions (requires larger doses): Bolus of 350 mcg/kg via large bore IV line over 3–5 min followed by an infusion of 25 mcg/kg/min. ACT should be measured 5–10 min after the bolus dose with a goal ACT of 300–450 sec. If the ACT <300 sec, an additional bolus dose of 150 mcg/kg should be given and the infusion rate increased to 30 mcg/kg/min. If the ACT is >450 sec, the infusion rate should be decreased to 15 mcg/kg/min. Another ACT should be checked 5–10 min after changes in infusion rate.

Dosage adjustment in organ dysfunction

No dosage adjustment is needed for impaired renal function.[5] A decrease in the initial dosage is needed for patients with hepatic impairment. Start with a lower dose and titrate to desired level of anticoagulation. For patients with moderate hepatic impairment, an initial dose of 0.5 mcg/kg/min is recommended.[5]

Maximum dosage

In *adults*, 10 mcg/kg/min for HIT or 40 mcg/kg/min for percutaneous coronary interventions.[5,6] A 5-month-old required 15 mcg/kg/min to reach a target ACT of 300 sec during cardiac catheterization.[1] A 15-month-old on ECMO required 24 mcg/kg/min to attain an aPTT 2 × baseline; the rate subsequently stabilized at 13–15 mcg/kg/min.[7] (See Comments section.)

IV push

Over 3–5 min (loading dose).[4]

Intermittent infusion

Infused for the length of percutaneous coronary intervention or cardiac catheterization.[4]

Continuous infusion

1 mg/mL in D5W, NS, or LR.[4,6,8]

Other routes of administration	No information available to support administration by other routes.
Maximum concentration	1 mg/mL.[4,6]
Cautions related to IV administration	All parenteral anticoagulants should be discontinued before use of argatroban.[4]
Other additives	Each 250 mg/2.5 mL vial contains D-sorbitol 750 mg and dehydrated alcohol 1000 mg.[4,6,8]
Comments	The seventh American College of Chest Physicians' conference on antithrombotic and thrombolytic therapy guidelines notes that danaparoid sodium, hirudin, and argatroban are alternatives to heparin in the treatment of children with HIT.[9]

Arginine HCl

Brand names	R-Gene 10

Dosage

Growth hormone reserve test (pituitary function test): 500 mg/kg (adult dose= 300 mL or 30 g) over 30 min.[1-4]

Inborn errors of urea synthesis[5,6]

Management of argininosuccinic acid lysase or argininosuccinic acid synthetase disorders: Loading dose of 600 mg/kg (12 g/m^2) infused over 90 min followed by 600 mg/kg/d (12 g/m^2/d) as a continuous infusion.

Management of carbamyl phosphate synthetase or ornithine transcarbamylase disorders: Loading dose of 200 mg/kg (4 g/m^2) followed by 200 mg/kg/d (4 g/m^2/d) as a continuous infusion.

Severe metabolic alkalosis: Recommended only after sodium and potassium chloride supplementation have failed (serum pH >7.55).[1,10] Estimate deficit/dosage by[1]

Arginine dose (g) = [Desired decrease in plasma bicarbonate concentration (mEq/L) × weight (kg)] ÷ 9.6

or

Arginine dose (mEq Cl) = 0.2 × weight (kg) × [103 – actual chloride concentration (mEq/L)][3]

One-half to two-thirds of the calculated deficit is given initially and the patient is re-evaluated prior to infusion of the remainder.[3]

Pulmonary hypertension (use not established): 500 mg/kg over 30 min.[7-9]

Dosage adjustment in organ dysfunction	No information available to support the need for dosage adjustment; however, arginine is metabolized to produce nitrogen products for urinary elimination. This should be considered in patients with renal insufficiency.[4] (See Comments section.)
Maximum dosage	60 g/h.[1]
IV push	Not recommended.[1] (See Cautions related to IV administration section.)
Intermittent infusion	300 mL over ≥30 min in *adults*[1] not to exceed 1 g/kg/h.[3]
Continuous infusion	No information available to support administration by this method.[1]
Other routes of administration	No information available to support administration by other routes.
Maximum concentration	100 mg/mL (commercially available).[1] This solution is hypertonic (950 mOsm/L).[1]

Cautions related to IV administration	Hyperchloremic metabolic acidosis, cerebral edema, or death may occur with overdose.[4] A child who inadvertently received 2000 mg/kg of arginine butyrate over 6 h suffered a grand mal seizure. It was not known whether the arginine or butyrate component was responsible.[11] A 21-month-old girl inadvertently received 3.9 g/kg (300 mL of 10% arginine) over 30 min. She experienced gasping respirations and immediate cardiopulmonary arrest with acute metabolic acidosis and transient hyponatremia. Thirty-six hours later, she experienced fatal central pontine and extrapontine myelinolysis.[12] Three anaphylactic reactions have been reported, two in children.[13,14] Hypotension, within 10 min of drug administration, was reported in 11 children (9.4 ± 4.1 years) receiving 500 mg/kg of arginine for pituitary function testing. Blood pressure returned to normal within 30 min.[15] Flushing, nausea, vomiting, numbness, headache, and local venous irritation have been associated with rapid infusion.[1] Extravasation, causing tissue necrosis, has been reported in three children (ages: 3.5–7 years) who received a 10% solution.[16-18]
Other additives	Contains 0.475 mEq/mL of chloride.[1,4]
Comments	May produce significant and symptomatic hyperkalemia in renal failure[19] with severe hepatic disease or with moderate renal impairment.[20]

Asparaginase

Brand names	Elspar

Dosage

Consult institutional protocol for complete dosing information.

Asparaginase is used as a component of combination therapy to treat childhood acute lymphocytic leukemia (ALL).[1] To reduce the incidence of adverse effects, asparaginase should be administered after other chemotherapeutic agents, specifically vincristine and prednisone.

Test dose: Hypersensitivity reactions commonly occur and intradermal testing is recommended in all patients prior to asparaginase therapy.[1] Inject 0.1 mL of a 20-units/mL solution (2 units) intradermally and observe injection site for 1 h.[1] A wheal or erythema represents a positive reaction; false negative reactions may occur.[1]

Patients with a positive skin test may undergo desensitization therapy if the benefits of therapy outweigh the risks. The labeling contains a desensitization protocol in which patients receive 1 unit of asparaginase IV that is doubled q 10 min until the total amount of the daily total dosage has been met (provided no adverse events occur).[1]

Induction therapy (combination therapy)

IV: 1000 units/kg/d for 10 days.[1-3]

IM: 6000 units/m^2/d every third day for 3 weeks.[1,4,5] A high dose of 25,000 units/m^2 has also been administered once weekly for 9 weeks.[6]

Induction therapy (monotherapy—not recommended if patient can tolerate combination therapy): 200 units/kg/d for 28 days.[1,7]

Maintenance therapy: Not recommended.[1]

Dosage adjustment in organ dysfunction

Asparaginase has been associated with hepatic dysfunction. However, no dosage adjustments have been recommended with any pre-existing organ dysfunction, including hepatic.[1]

Maximum dosage

Not established.

IV push

Not recommended.[1,8]

Intermittent infusion

Further dilute the appropriate dose from the reconstituted 2000-units/mL solution by administering via an infusion of D5W or NS. Give over at least 30 min.[1,8]

Continuous infusion

Intermittent infusion or IM administration are preferred routes of administration. Continuous infusions of asparaginase have been reported.[9]

Other routes of administration

May be given via IM administration (reconstitute to a 5000-units/mL solution). Do not exceed 2 mL at each injection site.[1] Two injection sites should be used if the volume of required dose is >2 mL. IM administration is associated with a lower incidence of anaphylaxis compared to IV administration.[1,10]

IT and intraventricular administration of asparaginase has been reported in patients with CNS lymphoblastic leukemia.[11,12] However, these routes have not demonstrated superiority over conventional treatments.

Asparaginase

Maximum concentration	2000 units/mL (IV) and 5000 units/mL (IM).[1,8]
Cautions related to IV administration	Asparaginase carries a boxed warning about the severity and incidence of anaphylaxis.[1] The following administration parameters are associated with an increased risk of hypersensitivity reactions: IV route of administration, IV dosages >6000–12,000 units/m^2, previous regimens containing asparaginase, and intermittent therapy.[13] When administering asparaginase, emergency treatment, including IV diphenhydramine, epinephrine, and hydrocortisone with a freely running IV in place, should be available.[14] Patients should be monitored for 30–60 min following administration and the drug should not be administered at night. Gelatinous fiber-like particles may develop after reconstitution; administration with a 5-micron filter will remove any particles without loss of potency.[1]
Other additives	Mannitol (80 mg/vial).[1,8]
Comments	Pancreatitis and hepatic dysfunction have been reported.[1] When handling asparaginase, avoid inhaling aerosols or dust or contact with the mucous membranes or skin.[1]

Asparaginase–pegylated (Pegaspargase)

Brand names	Oncaspar
Dosage	Consult institutional protocol for complete dosing information. IM injection is the preferred form of administration due to a lower incidence of hepatotoxicity, coagulopathy, renal and gastrointestinal disorders compared to IV administration.[1] **BSA ≥0.6 m²:** 2500 international units/m² q 14 d.[1,2] **BSA <0.6 m²:** 82.5 international units/kg q 14 d.[1] Induction therapy with weekly doses of pegaspargase 2500 international units/m² IM q 7 d, with or without intensification therapy (an additional 2500 international units/m² IM dose), has also been studied, although the use of these regimens is not established.[2-4] Dosing based on BSA limits was not discussed.
Dosage adjustment in organ dysfunction	Not established.
Maximum dosage	Not established. Three *adult* patients received IV infusions of 10,000 international units/m² with no major adverse events.[1]
IV push	Not recommended.
Intermittent infusion	Administer over 1–2 h in 100 mL of NS or D5W.[1]
Continuous infusion	Not recommended.
Other routes of administration	IM administration is the preferred route of administration.[1,5] Do not exceed 2 mL at each injection site.[1] Two injection sites should be used if the volume of required dose is >2 mL.
Maximum concentration	Not established.
Cautions related to IV administration	Due to risk of hypersensitivity reaction, IV diphenhydramine, epinephrine, hydrocortisone, and a freely running IV should be in place when administering pegaspargase.[6] Patients should be monitored for 60 min following administration and the drug should not be administered at night.

Asparaginase–pegylated (Pegaspargase)

Other additives	Each mL contains approximately 8.5 mg NaCl.[1]

Comments

Pegaspargase is used as a component of combination therapy to treat acute lymphocytic leukemia (ALL) in patients who are hypersensitive to the native forms of L-asparaginase (Elspar).[1] It may also be used in blast crisis of chronic lymphocytic leukemia (CLL) and salvage therapy of non-Hodgkin's lymphoma, although use has not been established.[6]

Pegaspargase may be a contact irritant. Professionals should wear gloves while handling and administering and should avoid inhalation of pegaspargase. If contact occurs with eyes, skin, or mucous membranes, wash with water for at least 15 min.[1]

Freezing destroys the activity of pegaspargase; do not use if the product has been frozen.[1]

Unlike asparaginase therapy, no test dose is required with pegaspargase as there is less risk for hypersensitivity reactions. The manufacturer reports an incidence of hypersensitivity reactions between 3% to 73%; however, this includes patients that had previous reactions to L-asparaginase.[1]

Pegaspargase is contraindicated in patients with a history of pancreatitis.[1]

Atenolol

Brand names	Tenormin I.V.
Dosage	Little information is available on intravenous atenolol in pediatric patients. Labetalol is the most useful beta-blocker for treatment of severe hypertension.[1,2] (See Labetalol monograph.) 0.1 mg/kg/dose[3] up to 5 mg/dose in older adolescents and *adults*. If necessary, the dose may be repeated in 10 min.[4]
Dosage adjustment in organ dysfunction	No significant accumulation occurs until CrCl is ≤35 mL/min/1.73 m^2.[4] If CrCl is 10–50 mL/min, give a normal dose q 48 h; if CrCl is <10 mL/min, give a normal dose q 96 h.[5]
Maximum dosage	Up to 15 mg/dose have been used in *adults*.[6,7]
IV push	0.5 mg/mL[4] or dilute in D5W or NS[4,8] and infuse over 5 min,[3,4] not to exceed 1 mg/min.[4]
Intermittent infusion	No information available to support administration by this method.
Continuous infusion	No information available to support administration by this method.
Other routes of administration	No information available to support administration by other routes.
Maximum concentration	0.5 mg/mL.[4]
Cautions related to IV administration	Monitor heart rate, blood pressure, and EKG during infusion.[4]
Other additives	None.
Comments	Studies in breast-fed patients of mothers receiving atenolol noted that premature infants or infants with impaired renal function may be more likely to develop adverse effects.[4]

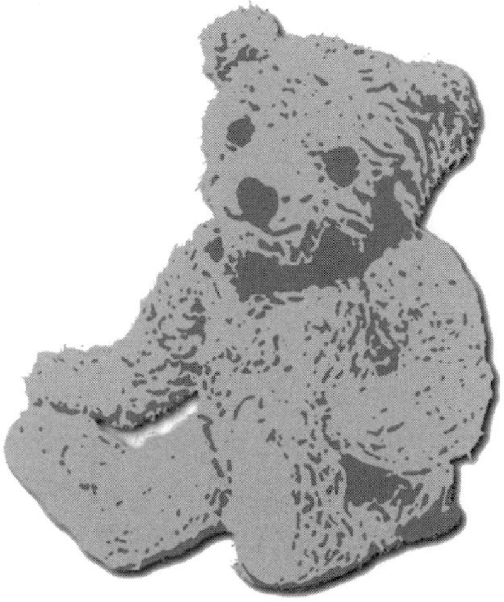

Atracurium Besylate

Brand names	Tracrium

Dosage

Respiratory function must be supported and concurrent administration of a sedative is also necessary. Monitoring of neuromuscular transmission with a peripheral nerve stimulator is recommended during continuous infusion or with repeated dosing.[1]

Endotracheal intubation and maintenance of neuromuscular blockade

Loading dose: Not recommend in infants 1 month–2 years of age who are receiving halothane.[2]

Neonates (≤1 month): 0.2–0.5 mg/kg.[2-4] (See Comments section.)

Infants and children (1 month–2 years): 0.3–0.4 mg/kg given as a single dose.[1,5-12] If the patient has a history of histamine sensitivity (anaphylactoid reactions or asthma), the dose should be given over 1 min.[2] (See Cautions related to IV administration section.)

Children (≥2 years): 0.3–0.5 mg/kg given as a single dose.[2,5-12] If the patient has a history of histamine sensitivity (anaphylactic reactions or asthma), the dose should be divided over 1 min.[2] (See Cautions related to IV administration section.)

Maintenance dose

Intermittent: 0.08–0.1 mg/kg as needed to maintain desired effects.[2] Children may require more frequent administration than *adults*.[2]

Continuous infusion: Not recommended in infants <2 years of age.[2] A continuous infusion (following loading dose) of 0.08–0.12 mg/kg/h (1.3–2 mcg/kg/min) has been safely used in neonates.[3] A continuous infusion of 0.15–1.2 mg/kg/h (2.5–20 mcg/kg/min) has been used in infants, children, and *adults*.[2,13-17] In a study with 20 children (1 month–13 years old), the dose of atracurium ranged from 0.44–2.4 mg/kg/h (7.3–40 mcg/kg/min).[16] (See Maximum dosage section.)

Larger doses have been required to facilitate mechanical ventilation in critically ill children.[17] Mean doses were 1.6–1.72 mg/kg/h (starting rate of 0.5 mg/kg/h) and increase until desired effect is achieved.[17] Infusion requirement may increase with prolonged administration.[18] (See Maximum dosage section.)

Dosage adjustment in organ dysfunction

No dosage adjustment required in renal[2,19] or hepatic dysfunction.[2]

Maximum dosage

0.6 mg/kg has been used safely in infants with severe hepatic dysfunction under halothane/nitrous oxide/oxygen anesthesia.[20] 0.53 ± 0.01 mg/kg/h (8.8 mcg/kg/min) has been used in those >1 month of age and 0.4 ± 0.01 mg/kg/h (6.7 mcg/kg/min) has been given to neonates.[21]

Occasionally, continuous infusion doses as large as 4.5 mg/kg/h (75 mcg/kg/min) may be required.[2,16,22] In one study, seven pediatric patients required a mean infusion of 1.72 mg/kg/h (28.7 mcg/kg/min) for up to 72 h.[17] In other studies, a pediatric patient required 2.4 mg/kg/h,[16] and a 19-year-old received 4.5 mg/kg/h (75 mcg/kg/min).[22] (See Comments section.)

IV push

10 mg/mL given over 1 min.[2]

Intermittent infusion

No information available to support administration by this method. Too slow of an injection may cause bradycardia.[2,5]

Continuous infusion	0.2–0.5 mg/mL in D5NS, D5W, or NS.[2]
Other routes of administration	Should not be given IM due to tissue irritation.[2] No information available to support administration by other routes
Maximum concentration	10 mg/mL for IV push or 0.5 mg/mL for continuous infusion.[2]
Cautions related to IV administration	Histamine release resulting in flushing, erythema, pruritus, urticaria, bronchospasm, hypotension, and changes in heart rate may occur.[2,5,23-25] Caution should be taken when administering this agent to patients who may be histamine sensitive (e.g., cardiovascular disease, previous anaphylactoid reactions, asthma). Asystole has occurred in *adults*.[26] For PN compatibility information, please see Appendix C.
Other additives	Multidose vials contain benzyl alcohol 0.9% as a preservative.[2] Administration of flushes containing benzyl alcohol (bacteriostatic water for injection) was associated with a fatal gasping syndrome, intraventricular hemorrhage, metabolic acidosis, and increased mortality in preterm infants.[27] While benzyl alcohol in small doses as a preservative in drugs is considered safe in newborns,[28] a 3-week-old, very low birth weight (710 g) infant experienced a profound desaturation that required resuscitation after receiving clindamycin (third and fourth doses), which was subsequently related to the benzyl alcohol preservative.[29] Hypersensitivity reactions to benzyl alcohol in parenteral products have been reported in *adults*.[30,31]
Comments	Neonates and infants generally require smaller doses than children; however, they recover more rapidly.[3] One report noted a 25% smaller dose.[21] Prolonged paralysis lasting 81 days was reported following atracurium infusion (20–75 mcg/kg/min) for 2 weeks in a 19-year-old patient.[22] The patient was also receiving corticosteroids, which may be a risk factor for this adverse effect. Prolonged paralysis has also been reported after long-term use of other neuromuscular blocking agents.[6,32] Concomitant administration of atracurium with certain antibiotics (e.g., aminoglycosides, clindamycin, vancomycin) may prolong neuromuscular blockade.[2,8] Consult appropriate resources for additional information on drug interactions. Enflurane and isoflurane anesthesia potentiate effects of atracurium; therefore, reduce atracurium dose by approximately 33% in these patients.[2,33] Also reduce atracurium dose in patients receiving succinylcholine or halothane.[2] Prolonged administration of atracurium may also lead to the accumulation of its laudanosine metabolite. This metabolite has been associated with CNS irritation and seizures in animal models. Accumulation of laudanosine has been reported in patients with renal failure as well as those with hepatic failure, before and after liver transplantation, but generally at concentrations significantly lower than those associated with CNS excitation.[2,34,35]

Atropine Sulfate

Brand names	Various manufacturers

Dosage

Cardiopulmonary resuscitation/bradycardia

Neonates: Vagal stimulation is not the cause of bradycardia in neonates; therefore, atropine should not be used during the acute phase of resuscitation.[1-3] Atropine is not included in current neonatal resuscitation guidelines.[4]

Infants, children, and adolescents[5]**:** 0.02 mg/kg (minimum 0.1 mg) IV or intraosseous; repeat if needed.

Chemical warfare/nerve agent poisoning in children[13]**:** 0.05–0.1 mg/kg up to 4 mg unless symptoms of apnea, convulsions, cardiopulmonary arrest, or rapid progression of symptoms. Repeat dose q 5–10 min until respiratory status (e.g., bronchospasm) improves or secretions resolve.

Auto-injector Dosing

10–20 kg: 0.5 mg.

20–40 kg: 1 mg.

40 kg or greater: 2 mg.

Organophosphate insecticide exposure in children[12]**:** 0.05 mg/kg (2–5 mg in *adults*) slowly (IV); may be doubled and repeated q 10–20 min until desired response achieved (e.g., drying of excessive secretions). Larger doses may be needed for large exposures. Atropine will not reverse nicotinic effects from organophosphate poisonings (e.g., muscular weakness, diaphragmatic weakness).

Physostigmine toxicity: 0.5 mg for each 1 mg of the last dose of physostigmine administered.[6]

Preanesthesia (to decrease secretions and block cardiac vagal reflexes during surgery)

Infants: 0.02–0.04 mg/kg 30–60 min preoperatively and then q 4–6 h as needed.[6-8]

Children: 0.01–0.02 mg/kg (0.1–0.4 mg) 30–60 min preoperatively and then q 4–6 h as needed.[7,9,10]

Other dosing recommendations include the following[11]

<20 kg: 0.1 mg for 3 kg, 0.2 mg for 7–9 kg, 0.3 mg for 12–16 kg given 30–60 min before anesthesia.

>20 kg: 0.4 mg given 30–60 min before anesthesia.

Dosage adjustment in organ dysfunction	No information available for dosage adjustment in hepatic or renal insufficiency.[11]

Maximum dosage

Cardiopulmonary resuscitation/bradycardia: 0.4–0.5 mg (child), 1 mg (adolescent).[5,6]

Nerve agent exposure: 4 mg maximum dose unless symptoms include apnea, convulsions, cardiopulmonary arrest, or rapid progression of symptoms.[13]

Organophosphate poisonings: May require larger doses.[12] In a pediatric study, one patient received 86 doses and another patient received 61 doses (0.005–0.1 mg/kg/dose) in 24 h. Another patient received 26 doses totaling 25 mg/kg over several days.[14] *Adults* with severe organophosphate poisoning may require up to 100 mg over several hours or several grams over several days.[12]

IV push	Infuse rapidly.[11,15] If administered into a peripheral vein for resuscitation, follow dose with a flush to increase drug circulation time.[11]
Intermittent infusion	Not recommended.
Continuous infusion	Used for some cases of severe organophosphate poisonings when atropine is required for several days.[11,12,16] Suggested dosing is 0.02–0.08 mg/kg/h of undiluted atropine begun after the initial bolus dose.
Other routes of administration	0.05, 0.1, 0.4, 0.5, or 1 mg/mL (available commercially) may be given IM.[11] If injected in an extremity, it should be elevated for 10–20 sec.[11] In preanesthesia induction, a faster onset of heart rate acceleration was reported following submental glossal injection than with deltoid or vastus lateralis injection.[17] May be given SC when used preoperatively.[11]
Maximum concentration	1 mg/mL.[11]
Cautions related to IV administration	Slow administration may cause paradoxical bradycardia.[11]
Other additives	9 mg sodium chloride/mL.[11,15] Multiple-dose vials may contain methylparaben or benzyl alcohol.[11,15] Paraben preservatives may cause hypersensitivity reactions that are more common with cutaneous exposure.[18] However, one case of pruritus and bronchospasm that occurred following infusion of hydrocortisone, which contained a paraben, has been reported.[19] Benzyl alcohol in small doses as a preservative in drugs is considered safe in newborns.[20] However, a 3-week-old, very low birth weight (710 g) infant who received clindamycin experienced a profound desaturation that required resuscitation after the third and fourth doses, which was subsequently related to the benzyl alcohol preservative.[21] Hypersensitivity reactions to benzyl alcohol in parenteral products have been reported in *adults*.[22,23]
Comments	A 2-month-old given a 0.1-mg dose for bradycardia during ophthalmologic surgery subsequently had spontaneous extrusion of the lens and vitreous.[24] Children with accidental wartime exposures to atropine doses ranging from 0.01–0.17 mg/kg had few adverse events.[13] Adverse events were primarily dilated pupils, tachycardia, dry mucous membranes, flushed skin, temperature above 37.8°C, and neurologic abnormalities. There were no fatalities or life-threatening dysrhythmias.

Azithromycin

Brand names	Zithromax
Dosage	The manufacturer does not recommend the use of IV azithromycin in patients <16 years of age.[1] **Community-acquired pneumonia (moderate to severe):** 500 mg IV q 24 h for a minimum of 2 days followed by 500 mg/d orally for a total of 7–10 days.[1-4] These reports in *adults* (>16 years of age) supported the use of azithromycin as monotherapy for community-acquired pneumonia.[2,3] **Pelvic inflammatory disease (PID):** 500 mg IV as a single dose for the first 2 days, followed by 250 mg/d orally to complete 7 days of therapy.[1] If anaerobic organisms are suspected, an antimicrobial agent with anaerobic activity should be given concurrently.[1]
Dosage adjustment in organ dysfunction	While azithromycin is hepatically eliminated, no dosage adjustment is required in patients with hepatic or renal dysfunction.[1,5,6]
Maximum dosage	Little information is available, but generally 10 mg/kg/dose up to 500 mg.[1,7] A large IV dose (4 g) of azithromycin was well-tolerated in healthy *adult* males with serum concentrations persisting for >10 days.[8]
IV push	Not recommended.[1]
Intermittent infusion	1 mg/mL should be given over 3 h.[1] A 2-mg/mL concentration should be given over 1 h.[1] Any dose larger than 500 mg should be given over at least 1 h.[1] Dose should be diluted in NS, ½NS, LR, D5W, D5LR, D5W⅓NS, D5W½NS, or D5W½NS + 20 mEq KCl.[1,9]
Continuous infusion	No information available to support administration by this method.
Other routes of administration	Not recommended.[1,9]
Maximum concentration	2 mg/mL.[1,9] Patients receiving azithromycin in concentrations >2 mg/mL have experienced pain and local inflammation at the site during administration.[1,8]
Cautions related to IV administration	None.
Other additives	None.
Comments	One case of ototoxicity occurred in an *adult* receiving IV azithromycin for 8 days.[10]

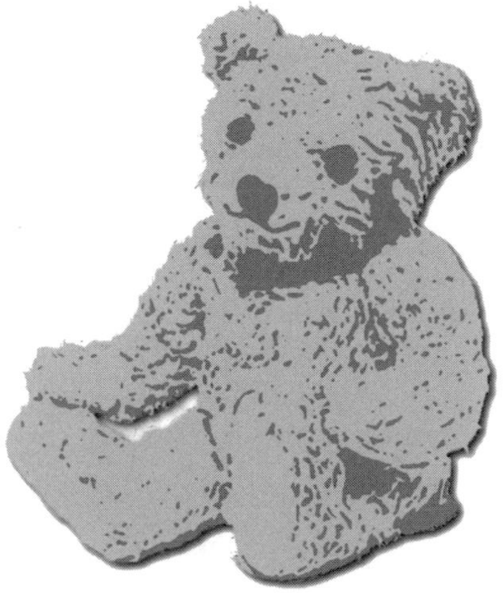

Aztreonam

Brand names Azactam

Dosage

Neonates

PNA	<1200 g	≤2000 g	>2000 g
≤7	60 mg/kg/d divided q 12 h*[1]	60 mg/kg/d divided q 12[1-4]	90 mg/kg/d divided q 8 h[1-4]
>7		90 mg/kg/d divided q 8 h[1,2,5]	120 mg/kg/d divided q 6 h[1,3]

*Until 4 weeks of age.

Infants and children

Mild-to-moderate infections: 90 mg/kg/d divided q 8 h[1-6] up to 3 g/d.[1]

Severe infections: 120 mg/kg/d divided q 6 h[1-6] up to 8 g/d.[1]

Cystic fibrosis *(Pseudomonas aeruginosa)*: 200 mg/kg/d divided q 6 h.[3,4,7,8]

Dosage adjustment in organ dysfunction Adjust dosage in patients with renal dysfunction. If CrCl is 10–50 mL/min, give 50% to 75% of normal dose; if CrCl is <10 mL/min, give 25% of normal dose.[9] Some clinicians recommend that aztreonam doses be reduced by 20% to 25% in patients with cirrhosis; however, others do not recommend any dosage adjustment in hepatic impairment.[10]

Maximum dosage 200 mg/kg/d divided q 6 h in cystic fibrosis patients,[7,8] not to exceed 8 g/d.[1]

IV push Reconstitute 500 mg, 1 g, or 2 g vials with 6–10 mL SW and administer over 3–5 min.[11,12]

Intermittent infusion ≤20 mg/mL in D5LR, D5¼NS, D5½NS, D5W, D10W, and NS administered over 20–60 min.[11,12]

Continuous infusion Not recommended.[12]

Other routes of administration May be given IM in a concentration of <333 mg/mL in SW or BW, NS, or bacteriostatic NS.[11] Should be given by deep injection into a large muscle.[11,12] The dose should be given IV in patients with septicemia, localized parenchymal abscess, peritonitis, or when doses >1 g are administered.[12]

Maximum concentration ≤20 mg/mL for IV infusion, and 333 mg/mL for IM administration.[11,12]

Cautions related to IV administration The manufacturer recommends that caution be taken when giving aztreonam to patients who have had immediate hypersensitivity reactions to penicillins or cephalosporins.[12] (See Comments section.)

Local reactions such as phlebitis, thrombophlebitis, discomfort, and swelling at the injection site have been reported.[12]

For PN compatibility information, please see Appendix C.

Other additives None.

Comments

The cross-reactivity between cephalosporins and penicillins does not appear to extend to the monobactams; patients with penicillin hypersensitivity have been given aztreonam without incident.[15] Similarly, those who experience hypersensitivity to aztreonam may not be hypersensitive to other beta-lactam antibiotics.[13]

Aztreonam may cause false-positive urinary glucose results when cupric sulfate solution–based tests (Clinitest, Benedict's solution, or Fehling's solution) are used.[10] Glucose oxidase methods (Clinistix) are not associated with false-positive test results.[10]

Baclofen

Brand names	Lioresal Intrathecal
Dosage	**Intrathecal administration** **Spasticity** **Test dose for response to intrathecal baclofen:** Usual test dose 50 mcg into intrathecal space via barbotage (≥1 min).[1-8] Test doses have ranged from 25–100 mcg.[9] Some would begin with 10 mcg[10] or 25 mcg[1,8] in very small children. If the response is not sufficient within 4–8 h, then a second test dose (75 mcg) should be given[4,6,8]; however, this dose should not be administered until 24 h after initial test dose.[1,2] If response to the second test dose is inadequate, a third test dose (100 mcg)[3,8,10] may be given; however, this dose should not be administered until 24 h after the second test dose.[1,2] If the response continues to be inadequate, the patient is not a candidate for chronic intrathecal baclofen therapy.[1] **Maintenance therapy:** An initial daily dose is based on the effective test dose and duration of its effects.[11] If the response to the test dose lasted ≤8 h, then the initial daily dose should be twice the test dose.[8] If the response lasted >8 h, the initial daily dose should be the same as the test dose.[1] The dose should be increased daily by 5% to 15% until desired results are achieved.[1] The infusion rate is the total daily dose divided by 24 h. Children ≤12 years generally require about 270 mcg/d.[1] Doses used in one study ranged from 65–320 mcg/d.[4] A retrospective review reported an average dose of 110–1050 mcg/d[3] with a range of 25–1500 mcg/d.[6] Adolescents (>12 years) whose spasticity has a spinal cord origin should be given 300–800 mcg/d.[1,7] If spasticity is of cerebral origin doses ranging from 90–1000 mcg/d have been used.[1,9,11] Doses up to 1400 mcg/d have been given to children.[4]
Dosage adjustment in organ dysfunction	No specific information is available regarding dosage adjustment, but the manufacturer suggests that a patient with renal impairment may require a smaller dose.[1]
Maximum dosage	Although doses up to 1500 mcg/d have been given, there is limited experience with dosages >1000 mcg/d.[1]
IV push	Not intended for IV administration.[1]
Intermittent infusion	Not applicable.
Continuous infusion	Administered *intrathecally* via implantable pump device. Total daily dose in mcg divided by 24 h = infusion rate.[1]
Other routes of administration	Not intended for IM, IV, SQ, or epidural administration.[1]

Baclofen

Maximum concentration	50 mcg/mL for test dose; 2 mg/mL for maintenance use.[12] Both are commercially available.[1,12] Intrathecal refill kit concentration 0.5 mg/mL in 20-mL ampuls or 2 mg/mL in 5-mL ampuls.[1] Screening kit concentration (50 mcg/mL) can dilute with sterile, preservative-free NaCl 0.9% injection.[1,12]
Cautions related to IV administration	Not intended for IV use.
Other additives	0.15 mEq sodium/L of baclofen.[12]

Comments

Baclofen withdrawal syndrome can develop quickly into an emergent, life-threatening situation if not recognized and treated.[13] It can be difficult to diagnose because symptoms can be similar to sepsis,[14] meningitis, autonomic dysreflexia,[13,15] and neuroleptic malignant syndrome.[16] Patients can present with fever, tachycardia, seizures, and spasticity.[13,14,17,18] Even with early diagnosis and treatment of baclofen, withdrawal patients can become refractory to therapy, and withdrawal can lead to morbidity and mortality[17,18] including rhabdomyolysis, elevated plasma creatine kinase, elevated LFTs, organ failure, DIC, and death.[13,16,18,19] This syndrome has been reported in *adults* and pediatric patients.[16]

Standard treatment for intrathecal baclofen withdrawal is to reinitiate therapy as soon as possible.[13,18] Other treatment options for intrathecal baclofen withdrawal include oral baclofen replacement, benzodiazepines,[13,18] dantrolene sodium, and cyproheptadine.[20] Dantrolene infusion has been shown to improve muscle rigidity but has little to no effect on other symptoms of withdrawal.[13] However, withdrawal symptoms in an *adult* responded to dantrolene.[21] Four *adult* cases reported resolution of symptoms following cyproheptadine.[24] There are also reports of baclofen withdrawal symptoms despite use of oral baclofen replacement therapy.[21,22] It is important to recognize the signs and symptoms early and try to pre-empt withdrawal by using an alternative therapy (i.e., oral baclofen) if withdrawal is suspected to occur.

One should carefully consider pump/catheter failure in patients who appear to be developing drug tolerance. There have been several case reports of intrathecal baclofen withdrawal due to catheter leakage,[15,18,23] dislodgment,[18] or pump failure.[18,24,25]

One study recommends that CSF pressure should be measured prior to implantation to decrease risk of postoperative CSF leaks in patients with elevated CSF pressures.[26]

A study with *adult* patients demonstrated that intrathecal baclofen increased risk of seizures in patients with multiple sclerosis.[27,28] However, a pediatric study reported no change in the incidence/frequency of seizures in patients with spasticity of cerebral origin receiving intrathecal baclofen.[4]

The use of intrathecal baclofen pumps has also been associated with rapid progression of scoliosis in pediatric and *adult* patients.[29,30]

Intrathecal baclofen has also been used successfully in treating muscle rigidity associated with tetanus in *adults*.[31,32]

Bretylium Tosylate

Brand names	Bretylol
Dosage	Bretylium is not contained in the current pediatric advanced life support guidelines[1] due to limited drug availability, high prevalence hypotension and other adverse reactions, and the availability of safer and more effective therapies.[2] "The safety and effectiveness in children has not been established. Its limited use in pediatric patients has been inadequate to fully define proper dosage and limitations for use."[3] Previous PALS Guidelines recommended 5 mg/kg followed by defibrillation, then 10 mg/kg and defibrillation continuing to alternate until a total dose of 30 mg/kg is reached.[4] **Initial dose:** 2.5–5 mg/kg.[5-12] If necessary, 10 mg/kg may then be given q 15–30 min.[5,11] However, the total initial dose per episode should not exceed 30–35 mg/kg.[5,11] **Maintenance dose:** 5–10 mg/kg q 6–8 h to a maximum dose of 40 mg/kg/d.[5] In *adults*, 1–2 mg/min have been used.[12,13]
Dosage adjustment in organ dysfunction	Adjust dosage in patients with renal dysfunction.[14,15] If CrCl is 10–50 mL/min, administer 25% to 50% of normal dose; if CrCl is <10 mL/min, give 25% of normal dose or consider an alternative antiarrhythmic.[15] Bretylium is not metabolized; therefore, do not reduce dose in hepatic dysfunction.[5]
Maximum dosage	10 mg/kg/dose.[5] The total initial dose per episode should not exceed 30–35 mg/kg[5,11] to a maximum of 40 mg/kg/d.[5]
IV push	In life-threatening situations, undiluted bretylium (50 mg/mL) should be administered over 30–60 sec.[5] Infusion of the dose in <8 min is associated with nausea, vomiting, and hypotension.[5,9]
Intermittent infusion	10 mg/mL in LR, D5LR, D5W, D5$^1/_4$NS, D5NS, or NS over ≥8 min.[5,9]
Continuous infusion	1–2 mg/min for 6 h have been used in *adults*.[13]
Other routes of administration	2.5–5 mg/kg not to exceed 5 mL (*adult*) as a single IM dose.[5] Undiluted solution should be used. Because pharmacodynamic effect may not occur for up to 2 h, IM administration is not recommended for ventricular fibrillation. Muscle atrophy and necrosis may occur with repeated IM injections; hence, injection site should be rotated.[5,16] No information available to support administration by other routes.
Maximum concentration	50 mg/mL (available commercially).[5,16]
Cautions related to IV administration	Although hypotension occurs in about 50% to 75% of patients following prolonged use,[1,4,12] tachycardia, hypertension, flushing, and syncope may occur because bretylium interferes with norepinephrine reuptake.[13]

Other additives	None.
Comments	Contraindicated in arrhythmias induced by digoxin.[5] Hyperthermia has been associated with bretylium infusion.[17] Inadvertent administration of 12 mg/kg/h resulted in what resembled clinical brain death in a 3-day-old neonate.[18] The effects were reversible after the bretylium infusion was discontinued.

Bumetanide

Brand names	Bumex
Dosage	0.01–0.1 mg/kg/dose (up to 2 mg) twice a day, daily, or every other day.[1-11] Acutely ill infants had maximum diuresis after receiving 0.035–0.4 mg/kg.[2] (See Comments section.) In *adults* with chronic renal insufficiency, a 1-mg loading dose followed by 0.912 mg/h for 12 h was more effective than two 6-mg bolus doses given 6 h apart.[12] Another study in *adults* reported administering between 1 and 4 mg/h.[13] (See Comments related to IV administration section.)
Dosage adjustment in organ dysfunction	No dosage decrease required in patients with renal dysfunction.[14] Larger doses (e.g., >2 mg in *adults*) may be needed in patients with CrCl <5 mL/min to produce the desired diuresis.[15] May need to reduce dosage in patients with hepatic impairment.[16] During ECMO, term neonates given 0.1 mg/kg had a half-life of 3.2 ± 3.8 h[6] compared to about 6 h in preterm and term neonates not on ECMO who were given 0.05[4,8] or 0.1[8] mg/kg.
Maximum dosage	Although infants may not benefit from doses >0.05 mg/kg,[2] 0.1 mg/kg up to 10 mg/d have been used in *adults* with normal renal function.[15] 20 mg/d have been given to *adults* with renal dysfunction.[15]
IV push	0.25 mg/mL over 1–2 min.[7-11,15,16]
Intermittent infusion	Dilute in D5W, LR, or NS[15,16] and infuse over 5 min.[12]
Continuous infusion	0.024 mg/mL in D5W.[12]
Other routes of administration	May be given IM using same dose as IV.[15,16]
Maximum concentration	0.25 mg/mL (available commercially).[15,16]
Cautions related to IV administration	Ototoxicity may occur with large doses or prolonged IV therapy and may be additive when bumetanide is combined with aminoglycosides.[15] Musculoskeletal symptoms (e.g., muscle tenderness, cramping, tightness, pain, weakness, and loss of mobility) have been documented during continuous infusion in *adults*. This is especially prominent with doses >2 mg/h.[13] For PN compatibility information, please see Appendix C.

Other additives

Each mL contains 8.5 mg NaCl and 4 mg ammonium acetate as buffers and 0.1 mg disodium edetate and 10 mg benzyl alcohol as preservatives.[16]

Benzyl alcohol in small doses as a preservative in drugs is considered safe in newborns.[17] However, a 3-week-old, very low birth weight (710 g) infant who received clindamycin experienced a profound desaturation that required resuscitation after the third and fourth doses, which was subsequently related to the benzyl alcohol preservative.[18]

Administration of saline flushes containing benzyl alcohol (BW) was associated with a fatal gasping syndrome, intraventricular hemorrhage, metabolic acidosis, and increased mortality in preterm infants.[19] This should not be used in neonates.

Hypersensitivity reactions to benzyl alcohol in parenteral products have been reported in *adults*.[20,21]

Comments

Electrolyte abnormalities, including hypokalemia, can occur; therefore, monitoring serum potassium concentration is important.[15]

Cross-allergenicity may occur in those allergic to sulfonamides but not in those allergic to furosemide.[15]

Use cautiously in jaundiced neonates at risk for kernicterus. *In vitro* studies have shown bilirubin displacement in pooled cord blood samples from critically ill neonates.[16,22]

Discolors when exposed to light.[15,16]

Bupivacaine

Brand names	Marcaine, Sensorcaine, Sensorcaine-MPF

Dosage

Not for IV infusion. Administered by local infiltration, peripheral or sympathetic nerve block, lumbar epidural, or caudal block. [1]

Dose varies with the anesthetic procedure, the area to be anesthetized, the vascularity of the tissues, the number of neuronal segments to be blocked, the depth and duration of anesthesia required, as well as individual response.[1,2] Once the catheter is placed, negative aspiration of blood or cerebrospinal fluid[3-6] with the absence of cardiovascular changes following a test dose indicates correct position of the catheter.[7,9,10]

Caudal block (preservative-free solution only): Children 1–3.7 mg/kg[2] or 0.5–1 mL/kg of the 0.25% solution (1.25 or 2.5 mg/kg).[3-8]

Epidural block (preservative-free solution only): Children 1.25 mg/kg/dose.[1,2]

Peripheral nerve block: 5 mL of 0.25% or 0.5% (12.5–25 mg).[2]

Sympathetic nerve block: 20–50 mL of 0.25% solution (without epinephrine).[1,2]

Continuous epidural (caudal or lumbar) infusion (preservative-free solution only)

Loading dose: 1.25–2.5 mg/kg (0.8–1 mL/kg) of the 0.25% bupivacaine.[1,2,9]

Infusion[2]

<4 months of age: 0.2–0.25 mg/kg/h (equivalent to 0.08–1 mL/kg/h of the 0.25% solution).[3-6] Use with caution in infants due to reduced levels of alpha$_1$-acid-glycoprotein leading to higher concentrations of unbound drug.[9,10]

>4 months and children: 0.375–0.5 mg/kg/h (equivalent to 0.16–0.2 mL/kg/h of the 0.25% solution).

Dosage adjustment in organ dysfunction	Reduce dosage and use with caution in patients with hepatic disease.[1,2] There is a potential for increased toxicity in patients with renal impairment, but no specific dosage adjustment is recommended.[2] Reduce dosage in patients with cardiac disease or in those who are acutely ill.[1,2]
Maximum dosage	In *adults*, do not exceed a maximum of 400 mg within a 24-h period.[1,2]
IV push	Do not administer IV. Accidental IV injection may result in seizures, coma, or cardiac or respiratory arrest.[1,2]
Intermittent infusion	Do not administer IV.[1,2]
Continuous infusion	Do not administer IV.[1,2]
Other routes of administration	Do not administer IM.[1,2]
Maximum concentration	0.75% (7.5 mg/mL) is available. However, the maximum recommended concentration varies by indication.[1,2,10] (See Dosage section.)

Cautions related to IV administration

Do not administer IV. Accidental IV injection may result in seizures, coma, or cardiac and respiratory arrest.[1,2]

Other additives

Available with epinephrine 1:200,000. Products containing epinephrine should not be used for sympathetic nerve blocks.[2]

Multidose vials contain paraben preservatives and should not be used for epidural or caudal blocks.[1,2] Paraben preservatives may cause hypersensitivity reactions that are more common with cutaneous exposure.[12] However, one case of pruritus and bronchospasm that occurred following infusion of hydrocortisone, which contained a paraben, has been reported.[13]

Epinephrine containing solutions contain metabisulfite.[1] Sulfites may cause hypersensitivity reactions and these are more common in *adults* with asthma. Most reactions are mild but can include anaphylactic symptoms and life-threatening or less severe asthma episodes.[14-16] Epinephrine may be required in severe cases; and if the sulfite-free product is not available, the sulfite-preserved epinephrine should be used.[14]

Comments

The manufacturer does not recommend the use of bupivacaine with or without epinephrine in children <12 years or the use of bupivacaine in dextrose in children <18 years.[1] However, epinephrine containing solutions of bupivacaine have been used in neonates, infants, and children.[6,9,10]

Peripheral facial nerve paralysis lasting 8 h has been reported after peritonsilar infiltration of bupivacaine in a 4-year-old.[17]

Systemic absorption of local anesthetics may result in toxic plasma concentrations, resulting in cardiovascular adverse effects, including decreased cardiac output, heart block, hypotension, bradycardia, ventricular arrhythmias, and cardiac arrest. Patients should be carefully monitored during injection. Use with caution in patients with underlying cardiovascular disease.[2]

Products containing epinephrine may produce an exaggerated vasoconstrictor response resulting in ischemic injury or necrosis. Use with caution in areas with restricted or limited blood flow, such as the fingers.[2]

Caffeine Citrate

Brand names Cafcit

Dosage

The dose of caffeine base is one-half the dose of caffeine citrate.

Apnea and bradycardia of prematurity[1-10]

Loading dose: 10–40 mg/kg (as caffeine citrate) or 10–20 mg/kg (as caffeine base).

Maintenance dose: 5–8 mg/kg (as caffeine citrate) q 24 h or 2.5–5 mg/kg (as caffeine base) q 24 h. Begin maintenance dose 24 h after loading dose.

Facilitate extubation in neonatal apnea (use not established)[1,4,5,11]

Loading dose: 20–80 mg/kg (as caffeine citrate) or 10–40 mg/kg (as caffeine base) 24 h prior to planned extubation.

Maintenance dose: 10–30 mg/kg (as caffeine citrate) or 5–15 mg/kg (as caffeine base). Begin maintenance dose 24 h after loading dose.

Dosage adjustment in organ dysfunction

In neonates, approximately 86% of drug is excreted unchanged in the urine, with the remainder metabolized by the CYP1A2 hepatic enzyme system.[7,10] Dose adjustment may be required in neonates with renal/hepatic dysfunction or those suffering from birth asphyxia.[10]

Maximum dosage

Individualize dosage based on serum concentration and clinical effect. A study evaluating caffeine citrate used to facilitate extubation reported that a loading dose of 80 mg/kg followed by a maintenance dose of 20 mg/kg resulted in a lower rate of extubation failure than the usual loading dose of 20 mg/kg followed by a maintenance dose of 5 mg/kg/d.[11] (See Cautions related to IV administration section.)

IV push

Not recommended.

Intermittent infusion

The loading dose is usually infused over 30 min[2,4,6-9,12]; however, infusions of 15 and 20 min have been used.[5,10] The maintenance dose is usually infused over 10–15 min[2,8,9,12]; however, the maintenance dose has been infused over 3 min.[4]

Continuous infusion

D5W¼NS, D5W¼NS and 20 mEq KCl/L.[12]

Other routes of administration

No information to support administration by other routes.

Maximum concentration

20 mg/mL (as citrate) or 10 mg/mL (as base, commercially available).

Cautions related to IV administration

None.

For PN compatibility information, please see Appendix C.

Other additives	Each mL of caffeine citrate provides citric acid monohydrate (5 mg) and sodium citrate dehydrate (8.3 mg).[10]

Comments

Caffeine exhibits single-compartment, linear pharmacokinetics where both weight and age influence caffeine clearance.[4,5] Using standard dosage guidelines, a predicted concentration-time curve can be easily generated and routine monitoring of serum concentrations during treatment is probably not necessary unless a clinical problem arises.[4]

If serum concentrations are monitored, the desired serum trough concentration ranges from 5–25 mcg/mL. Concentrations >50 mcg/mL are considered toxic.[7,10]

Caffeine is known to increase metabolic rate and oxygen consumption and may place treated neonates at risk for growth failure.[3]

During a double-blind, placebo-controlled clinical trial, cases of necrotizing enterocolitis were higher in the caffeine citrate group.[2]

Calcitriol

Brand names Calcijex

Dosage

Hyperparathyroidism in hemodialysis patients: Initial dose based on PTH concentration.[1,2] Dose given immediately after dialysis session.

PTH Concentration	Dose
<500 pg/mL	0.5 mcg
500–1000 pg/mL	1.0 mcg
>1000 pg/mL	1.5 mcg

Dose can be increased by 0.25 mcg q 2 weeks until ≤30% decrease in PTH or Ca >11 mg/dL or Ca×P product >75.

Mean maintenance doses[2]

2–12 years: 0.04 mcg/kg (range = 0.5–2 mcg).

13–18 years: 0.02 mcg/kg (range = 0.25–2.25 mcg).

Hyperparathyroidism in peritoneal dialysis patients: In a 12-month study, 16 patients (12.5 ± 1.1 years) had an initial dose of 1 mcg added to 50–100 mL residual dialysate volume that was instilled into the peritoneal cavity after overnight exchanges 3 × week.[3] Dose was increased by 0.5 mcg if Ca <10.0 mg/dL and P <6 mg/dL. If Ca >11 mg/dL, the dose was held until Ca was <11 mg/dL at which time calcitriol was restarted at 50% of the previous dose. Average maintenance dose was 1.3 ± 0.08 mcg.

Seizures associated with hypocalcemia: An 8-month-old African-American girl was given 0.25 mcg two times a day for ≤2 days when she was changed to oral vitamin D.[4]

Of note: Nineteen hypocalcemic neonates (≤32 weeks GA) failed to respond to large doses.[5]

Dosage adjustment in organ dysfunction No dosage adjustment necessary in renal dysfunction.

Maximum dosage Usually ≤0.05 mcg/kg.[6] 0.06 mcg/kg was given as single dose to adolescents.[7]

IV push 1 or 2 mcg/mL over 15 sec[7] or at end of hemodialysis through venous catheter.[1,6]

Intermittent infusion 0.5 mcg/mL diluted in D5W, NS, or SW[8] or 1–2 mcg/mL undiluted infused over 15 min.[9]

Continuous infusion No information available to support administration by this method.

Other routes of administration 1 or 2 mcg/mL has been added to a small volume of peritoneal dialysate and instilled intraperitoneally after nightly peritoneal dialysis.[3]

Maximum concentration 2 mcg/mL.[1]

Cautions related to IV administration	Hypercalcemia can cause cardiac arrhythmias in patients receiving digoxin; therefore, calcitriol should be used cautiously in these patients.[1]
Other additives	Each mL (1 or 2 mcg/mL) of aqueous solution contains 4 mg polysorbate 20 and 2.5 mg sodium ascorbate.[1]
Comments	Hypercalcemia, hyperphosphatemia, and hypercalcuria can occur.[1,6] Monitor serum calcium and phosphorous concentrations once or twice a week during the first 12 weeks of treatment and during dose titration. If hypercalcemia occurs, discontinue therapy (including oral calcium phosphate binders) until serum calcium concentration normalizes.[1] Antacids containing magnesium should not be used during calcitriol treatment because of the potential for hypermagnesemia.[1] Is stable undiluted or diluted in polypropylene (tuberculin) syringes under room light at ambient temperature for ≤8 h; use of PVC bags and sets is not recommended.[10]

Calcium Chloride

Brand names	Various manufacturers
Dosage	Information is expressed as milligrams of a 10% (100 mg/mL) calcium chloride (CaCl) solution, which provides approximately 1.36 mEq/mL or 27.3 mg/mL of elemental calcium.[1,2] 1 mEq is equivalent to 20 mg (elemental calcium). **Hypocalcemia in critically ill infants and children:** 10–20 mg/kg q 4–6 h.[3] Base subsequent doses on calcium deficit.[2] **Hypocalcemia secondary to infusion of blood products:** 33 mg/100 mL of citrated blood.[2] $CaCl_2$ infusion during FFP administration decreased hypocalcemia in children with thermal injury.[4] **Neonatal tetany:** 2.4 mEq/kg/d in divided doses.[2] **Cardiopulmonary resuscitation (see Comments section)** **Neonates, infants, and children:** 18–26 mg/kg[2,5] over 5–10 min.[2] In cardiac arrest, a second dose can be given after 10 min; base subsequent doses on calcium deficit.[2] Using a 10% $CaCl_2$ solution, 20 mg/kg = 0.2 mL/kg. **Adolescents and adults:** 2–4 mg/kg repeated in 10 min if needed.[2]
Dosage adjustment in organ dysfunction	Calcium is renally eliminated; however, dosing is based on serum calcium concentrations so no dosage adjustment is necessary in renal dysfunction.
Maximum dosage	35–75 mg/kg/dose as an intermittent infusion.[6] 1000 mg/dose in *adults*.[1]
IV push	Not indicated.[1]
Intermittent infusion	35–75 mg/kg over 10–30 min; monitor for bradycardia.[6] 10% $CaCl_2$ (undiluted) at 1 mL (100 mg)/min in *adults*.[1] (See Cautions related to IV administration section.)
Continuous infusion	Can be diluted in most standard dextrose and/or saline-containing IV fluids that do not contain bicarbonate or phosphate and infused continuously.[7] Because of the potential for serious sequelae following infiltration of calcium-containing fluids, infusion through a large vein (central line) is preferred.[1]
Other routes of administration	Contraindicated.[1,2]
Maximum concentration	Undiluted, 100 mg/mL.[1,2]

Calcium Chloride

Cautions related to IV administration

IV calcium should be used cautiously in patients receiving cardiac glycosides because of the potential for development of arrhythmias.[1]

Bradycardia, hypotension, and cardiac arrhythmias may occur.[2] If symptomatic bradycardia occurs, the injection should be stopped.

Because extravasation may cause tissue sloughing and necrosis, the infusion should be stopped if the patient complains of discomfort.[8-10] A 15-unit dose of a 1:10 dilution of a 150-unit vial of hyaluronidase in NS should be injected with a fine hypodermic needle (e.g., 25 gauge) into the extravasation area within 12 h of extravasation.[1,9,11]

Because of extravasation and infiltration risk, infusion into scalp veins should be avoided if at all possible.[2]

Other additives

Contains aluminum as a contaminant.[1]

Comments

$CaCl_2$ dissociates rapidly in solution and increases the risk of calcium phosphate precipitation in parenteral nutrition solutions.

Routine administration during cardiopulmonary resuscitation/arrest is not indicated.[5]

Calcium EDTA (Edetate Calcium Disodium)

Brand names	Calcium Disodium Versenate

Dosage

Treatment of lead poisoning: Dosing is based on blood lead concentration (BLC) and clinical presentation.

Acute lead encephalopathy: 1500 mg/m²/d for 5 days.[1,2] Patients with lead encephalopathy and cerebral edema may experience a lethal increase in intracranial pressure following IV infusion. IM administration is the preferred route in these patients.[1,3]

Combine with dimercaprol (British anti-lewisite or BAL); second course may be required after 2–4 day interval; give third course if BLC ≥50 mcg/dL within 48 h (wait 5–7 days before third course).[1,2,4]

Symptomatic and/or BLC ≥70 mcg/dL (symptomatic or asymptomatic): 1500 mg/m²/d[2] or 50 mg/kg/d[4] for 5 days via an 8–24 h infusion.[1-4] One reference recommends 1000 mg/m²/d if BLC ≥70 mcg/dL and patient is asymptomatic.[1]

Combination therapy with BAL until BLC is ≤50 mcg/dL.[1] Second and third courses may be given depending on BLC and severity of symptoms.[1-4]

BLC of 45–69 mcg/dL (asymptomatic): 1000 mg/m²/d[2] or 25 mg/kg/d[4] for 5 days via an 8–24 h infusion[1-4] or in divided doses q 4–12 h (IV/IM)[2,5]; a second course may be required if BLC rebounds.[2]

BLC 25–44 mcg/dL: Chelation therapy not routinely given.[2,4]

Provocative chelation test: No longer recommended by the AAP.[4] After patient empties bladder, infuse 500 mg/m² in D5W over 1 h[1-2,6] and collect urine for the following 8 h. Dose may also be given IM. Urinary excretion ≥200 mcg of lead or a ratio of urinary lead (mcg) to calcium EDTA dose (mg) of ≥0.6 (children <36 months) or ≥0.7 (children >36 months) identifies patients who will respond to chelation therapy.[1,7] A 5-h lead mobilization test has also been validated.[8] With IM therapy, infusing IV fluids after administration ensures a greater diuresis.[9]

Continuation of therapy should be based on BLC. Patients who require >5 days of therapy should have a 2–4 day drug-free period between courses.[1,2,4]

Measure BLC 7–21 days after therapy to determine if retreatment is necessary.[2]

Dosage adjustment in organ dysfunction	Reduce dose with pre-existing renal disease.[3] Stop therapy if anuria or severe oliguria develop.[3] Avoid in patients with inadequate urine flow.[1,2]
Maximum dosage	75 mg/kg/d (reserved for severely symptomatic patients) not to exceed 1 g/24 h.[10] Five times the recommended dose infused over 24 h in a 16-month-old without adverse effects.[3]
IV push	Not recommended.[3-5]
Intermittent infusion	Dilute to a concentration of <0.5%[2] or 2–4 mg/mL in NS, D5W.[5] Although 15–60 min infusions have been used,[1,2,5] 4 h or greater is recommended[4] and usually given over 8–12 h; however, continuous infusion is preferred.[1,4]
Continuous infusion	Preferred method of administration in hospitalized patients.[1,2] Dilute to a concentration of <0.5%[2] or 2–4 mg/mL in D5W or NS.[5]

Calcium EDTA (Edetate Calcium Disodium)

Other routes of administration	IM administration is extremely painful. Must be given with procaine or lidocaine (final anesthetic concentration = 0.5%) at 8–12 h intervals.[1-3,5]
Maximum concentration	0.5% or 5 mg/mL.[1,2,4,5]
Cautions related to IV administration	Supplied from the manufacturer as a 200-mg/mL solution that has an osmolality of 1514 mOsm/kg.[5] Rapid infusion may result in thrombophlebitis or precipitation of encephalopathy.[3,4] Diluted solutions (≤5 mg/mL) infused over at least 4 h may decrease the risk of thrombophlebitis.[4]
Other additives	Contains 5.3 mEq sodium/g of calcium EDTA.[5]

Comments

Never use disodium EDTA (edetate disodium) to treat lead poisoning, because it chelates calcium and induces tetany and potential fatal hypocalcemia.[2,11]

Renal toxicity is dose-related and reversible, and it rarely occurs at daily doses <1500 mg/m^2 if the patient is adequately hydrated.[1-3] Calcium EDTA is renally excreted; adequate hydration and urine output must be maintained to reduce nephrotoxicity.[1-4] Beginning 1–2 days after 5 days of calcium EDTA and BAL therapy, about 16% of children developed increased serum creatinine lasting for ≤22 days and oliguria lasting for 2–4 days.[12]

Animal studies found a redistribution of lead from bone to target organs (e.g., brain and kidneys) following calcium EDTA administration.[13]

Neonatal lead poisoning has been treated with calcium EDTA in combination with BAL, with and without exchange transfusion within the first week of life.[14,15]

Hypercalcemia has been reported in children treated with calcium EDTA.[16]

A falsely elevated lead concentration may occur if blood is drawn during a continuous infusion of calcium EDTA; therefore, the infusion should be stopped at least 1 h before a test is performed.[17]

Calcium Gluconate

Brand names	Various manufacturers

Dosage

Doses are expressed as milligrams of a 10% (100 mg/mL) calcium gluconate solution, which provides approximately 0.465 mEq/mL or 9.3 mg/mL of elemental calcium.[1,2] 1 mEq is equivalent to 20 mg (elemental calcium).

Hypocalcemia

Neonates: 200 mg/kg[3,4] to 400 mg/kg as continuous infusion or divided q 6–8 h.[5-8] Doses as large as 800 mg/kg.[7]

Infants and children: 200–500 mg/kg either by continuous infusion or intermittent infusions q 6 h.[9]

Adolescents and adults: 10–15 g as a continuous infusion or divided q 6 h.[9]

Dosing should be guided by monitoring serum calcium concentrations.

Hypocalcemia secondary to infusion of blood products

Neonates: 98 mg/100 mL of citrated blood.[2]

Adults: 500 mg/100 mL of citrated blood.[9]

Tetany

Neonates: 500 mg/kg divided q 6 h.[2]

Children: 100–140 mg/kg given three to four times a day until tetany resolves.[2]

Dosage adjustment in organ dysfunction

Calcium is renally eliminated; however, dosing is based on serum calcium concentrations so no dosage adjustment is necessary in renal dysfunction.

Maximum dosage

For term neonates, 800 mg/kg either continuously or in four divided doses.[9] For older infants and children, 500 mg/kg either continuously or in four divided doses.[9]

IV push

Not indicated.[2]

Intermittent infusion

200 mg/kg over 10–30 min in symptomatic neonates.[10]

Continuous infusion

Dilute in D5LR, D5NS, D5W, D10W, D20W, LR, NS, or PN.[9] Because of the potential for serious sequelae following infiltration of calcium-containing fluids, infusion through a central line is preferred.[1] For peripheral infusion, the final concentration should be limited.

Other routes of administration

IM not recommended.

Maximum concentration

Undiluted, 100 mg/mL.[1,2]

Calcium Gluconate

Cautions related to IV administration

IV calcium should be used cautiously in patients receiving cardiac glycosides because of the potential for development of arrhythmias.[1]

Bradycardia, hypotension, and cardiac arrhythmias may occur.[1,2] If symptomatic bradycardia occurs, the injection should be stopped.[10]

Extravasation may cause tissue sloughing and necrosis.[11-14] Because of extravasation and infiltration risk, infusion into scalp veins should be avoided if at all possible.[2]

A 15-unit dose of a 1:10 dilution of a 150-unit vial of hyaluronidase in NS should be injected with a fine hypodermic needle (e.g., 25 gauge) into the extravasation area within 12 h of extravasation.[15]

Calcinosis cutis occurred in an 11-year-old boy within 3 weeks of calcium gluconate infusion.[16]

Should not be administered through an arterial catheter because of the potential for vasospasm.[8,17]

Other additives

Aluminum is present as a contaminant. (See Comments section.)

Comments

Calcium gluconate bioavailability is considered to be less than that of calcium chloride. In 49 critically ill children an average age of 3.7 ± 5 years, ionized calcium concentrations were increased 30 min after calcium gluconate and calcium chloride infusions.[18] Serum calcium concentrations were greater in the calcium chloride group compared to the calcium gluconate group.[18] In stable burn patients an average age of 5.5 ± 4.4 years, ionized calcium concentrations were not different 10 min after infusion of either calcium chloride or calcium gluconate.[19]

Calcium gluconate is the preferred calcium source in parenteral nutrition solutions, but it can have a significant amount of aluminum present as an inherent contaminant.[20] Calcium gluconate in polyethylene vials contains significantly less contaminant aluminum than calcium gluconate in glass vials.[21]

Caspofungin

Brand names	Cancidas
Dosage	**Neonates and infants:** 1 mg/kg/d for 2 days followed by 2 mg/kg/d.[1-3] One report has given 5 mg/kg/d (50 mg/m^2) for 3 days followed by 2.5 mg/kg/d (25 mg/m^2).[4] **Children 2–17 years of age:** 50 mg/m^2/d (maximum 70 mg/d).[3,5-9] 70 mg/m^2/d for the first day of therapy followed by 50 mg/m^2/d has also been recommended.[5,8] BSA-based dosing regimens are recommended in children 2–17 years of age since 1 mg/kg/d resulted in suboptimal concentrations.[6] 2 mg/kg/d for 1 day followed by 1.5 mg/kg/d has been used successfully in combination with liposomal amphotericin B in a 24-month-old.[10] **Adults:** 70 mg/d for 1 day followed by 50 mg/d.[3,5,11]
Dosage adjustment in organ dysfunction	No dosage adjustment is recommended with renal impairment or mild hepatic impairment. With moderate to severe hepatic impairment (Child Pugh score of >7–9), dose adjustment is recommended.[12,13]
Maximum dosage	70 mg/d.[6] 100 mg/d has been given to *adults* and a 13-year-old.[12,14]
IV push	No information available to support administration by this method.
Intermittent infusion	Prepare solution by adding 10.5 mL NS, SW, or BW (see Other additives section) to the vial of caspofungin. Further dilute solution with NS, ½NS, ¼NS, or LR to a final concentration of 0.14–0.47 mg/mL. Infuse slowly over 1 h.[12] Do not use dextrose-containing solutions as diluents.[12]
Continuous infusion	No information available to support administration by this method.
Other routes of administration	No information available to support administration by other routes.
Maximum concentration	0.47 mg/mL.[12]
Cautions related to IV administration	Possible histamine-mediated symptoms (flushing, urticaria, pruritus and bronchospasm), including anaphylaxis, have been reported.[12] Do not admix or infuse concomitantly with other drugs.[12]

Other additives

May contain parabens (methylparaben and propylparaben) or 0.9% benzyl alcohol if BW is used as diluent for solution preparation.

Paraben preservatives may cause hypersensitivity reactions that are more common with cutaneous exposure.[15] However, one case of pruritus and bronchospasm that occurred following infusion of hydrocortisone, which contained parabens, has been reported.[16]

Benzyl alcohol in small doses as a preservative in drugs is considered safe in newborns.[17] However, a 3-week-old, very low birth weight (710 g) infant who received clindamycin experienced a profound desaturation that required resuscitation after the third and fourth doses, which was subsequently related to the benzyl alcohol preservative.[18]

Administration of saline flushes containing benzyl alcohol (bacteriostatic water for injection) was associated with a fatal gasping syndrome, intraventricular hemorrhage, metabolic acidosis, and increased mortality in preterm infants.[19] This should not be used in neonates.

Hypersensitivity reactions to benzyl alcohol in parenteral products have been reported in *adults*.[20,21]

Comments

Hepatic effects, including transient elevations in ALT, hepatic dysfunction, hepatitis, and hepatic failure, have been reported.[12] ALT elevations are more likely when used concomitantly with cyclosporine.[12,22]

Drug interactions are possible when used with tacrolimus and cyclosporine.[12] Concomitant use of inducers of drug clearance (rifampin, efavirenz, nevirapine, phenytoin, dexamethasone and carbamazepine) may decrease caspofungin concentrations. A dose of 70 mg/d in *adults* has been recommended when used with rifampin.[12] Consult appropriate resources for dosing recommendations before combining any drug with caspofungin.

Cefazolin Sodium

Brand names	Ancef, Kefzol, Zolicef

Dosage

Neonates: Safety in patients <1 month has not been established.[1] However, the following doses have been used:

PNA	≤2000 g	>2000 g
≤7 d	40 mg/kg/d divided q 12 h[2,3]	40 mg/kg/d divided q 12 h[2,3]
>7 d*		60 mg/kg/d divided q 8 h[2,3]

*Until 4 weeks of age.

Infants and children

Mild-to-moderate infections: 25–50 mg/kg/d divided q 6–8 h.[1,6-8]

Severe infections: 50–100 mg/kg/d divided q 6–8 h.[1,3,8,9]

Bacterial endocarditis

Prophylaxis (for dental, oral, respiratory tract, or esophageal procedure): A single 25-mg/kg dose not to exceed 1 g given 30 min prior to a procedure.[4]

Treatment (oxacillin-susceptible staphylococci in nonanaphylactoid penicillin-allergic patient)

Absence of prosthetic material: 100 mg/kg/d divided q 8 h with or without gentamicin for 3–5 days.[5]

Prosthetic valve endocarditis: 100 mg/kg/d divided q 8 h plus rifampin for ≥6 weeks; plus gentamicin for 2 weeks.[5]

Perioperative prophylaxis: 20–30 mg/kg administered 30 min to 1 h prior to the start of surgery. For lengthy operative procedures (≥2 h), may need to redose during surgery.[1]

Dosage adjustment in organ dysfunction

Adjust dosage in patients with renal dysfunction.[1,10] In pediatric patients with mild-to-moderate renal impairment (CrCl 70–40 mL/min), give 60% of the normal daily dose divided doses q 12 h. In patients with moderate impairment (CrCl 40–20 mL/min), give 25% of the normal daily dose divided doses q 12 h. Pediatric patients with severe renal impairment (CrCl 20–5 mL/min) give 10% of the normal daily dose q 24 h. All dosage recommendations apply after an initial loading dose.[1]

Maximum dosage

100 mg/kg/d,[1,3,5] not to exceed 6 g/d in children and 12 g/d in *adults*.[1]

IV push

Dilute the reconstituted product with 5 mL of SW (50–100 mg/mL) and give over 3–5 min.[1,11]

Intermittent infusion

5–20 mg/mL in D5LR, D5NS, D5½NS, D5¼NS, D5W, D10W, LR, NS, or R.[1,11] Give over 10–60 min.[11,12]

Continuous infusion

Although no specific information is available, other beta-lactam antibiotics have been given by this method.[13] Manufacturer states that cefazolin may be administered by continuous infusion.

Other routes of administration	Reconstitute in SW and give by deep IM administration using same doses as those given IV.[1]
Maximum concentration	77 mg/mL (in D5W), 69 mg/mL (in NS), and 138 mg/mL in SW.[14]
Cautions related to IV administration	If a decision is made to give this medication to a patient with known penicillin hypersensitivity, the patient should be closely observed for allergenicity. (See Comments section.) For PN compatibility information, please see Appendix C.
Other additives	Contains 2 mEq sodium/g of cefazolin.[1]
Comments	Patients with a history of type I reaction to penicillin should not receive beta-lactam antibiotics. From 5% to 15% of patients allergic to penicillin will also be allergic to cephalosporins. Certain infections (e.g., syphilis) require penicillin for cure. It is recommended that a desensitization protocol for penicillin-allergic individuals should be performed in a hospital setting. This can usually be completed in about 4 h, at which time the first dose of penicillin can be given.[8] Thrombophlebitis after 36–48 h of intermittent infusion has been reported.[7] A false-positive urinary glucose results when cupric sulfate solution-based tests (Clinitest, Benedict's solution, Fehling's solution) are used. Glucose oxidase methods (Clinistix) are not associated with false-positive test results.[1]

Cefepime

Brand names	Maxipime
Dosage	**Neonates** **≤14 days (term and preterm):** 60 mg/kg/d divided q 12 h.[1] **>14 days:** 100 mg/kg/d divided q 12 h.[1] **Infants and children (2 month–16 years)** **Mild-to-moderate infection:** 100–150 mg/kg/d divided q 8 h.[2] **Severe infections:** 150 mg/kg/d divided q 8 h.[2] **Adolescents or patients >40 kg:** 1–4 g/d divided q 12 h.[3] **Bacterial endocarditis (treatment of culture negative within 1 year of prosthetic valve infection):** 150 mg/kg/d divided q 8 h for 6 weeks (plus gentamicin, vancomycin and rifampin).[4] **Cystic fibrosis (acute pulmonary exacerbation):** 150 mg/kg/d (up to 2 g/dose) divided q 8 h.[5,6] **Febrile neutropenia** **Infants and children (2 month–16 years):** 150 mg/kg/d divided q 8 h.[3,7,8] **Adolescents or those >40 kg:** 6 g/d divided q 8 h.[3,9] **Meningitis:** Although cefepime has been given to treat meningitis (150 mg/kg/d divided q 8 h),[10,11] the manufacturer recommends that patients with suspected or documented meningitis should receive an alternate antibiotic with demonstrated clinical efficacy.[3] **Skin and soft tissue infections, urinary tract infections (including pyelonephritis), pneumonia, and lower respiratory tract infections:** Infants and children should receive 150 mg/kg/d divided q 8–12 h.[3,12-16]
Dosage adjustment in organ dysfunction	Adjust dosage in patients with renal dysfunction. Patients with renal impairment who received large doses have developed encephalopathy and/or seizures.[3] CrCl is >50 mL/min, give normal dose q 12 h; if CrCl is 10–50 mL/min, give normal dose q 16–24 h; if CrCl is <10 mL/min, give dose q 24–48 h.[17] Unlike other cephalosporins, no dosage adjustment is needed for burn patients.[18]
Maximum dosage	2 g/dose.[3]
IV push	Although not generally administered by this method, doses of 2 g have been given over 3–5 min in *adults*.[19]
Intermittent infusion	10–40 mg/mL diluted in D5W, D10W, D5NS, LR or NS, or Normosol-M or -R and administered over 30 min.[3,20]
Continuous infusion	Total daily dose of 3–4 g was delivered over 24 h (125–167 mg/h) at a concentration of 3–4 mg/mL in *adults*.[21]

Other routes of administration	Has been given by IM administration.[3] Dilute dose in D5W, 0.5 or 1% lidocaine, BW, SW, or NS.[3,13] Maximum concentration for IM administration is 280 mg/mL. No information available to support administration by other routes.
Maximum concentration	280 mg/mL for IM[3,20] and 160 mg/mL for IV administration.[3,20]
Cautions related to IV administration	Although rare, anaphylactoid reactions may require immediate emergency treatment with epinephrine, oxygen, steroids, antihistamines, pressor amines, and airway management.[3] Pain or phlebitis may occur at the injection site.[3] For PN compatibility information, please see Appendix C.
Other additives	None.
Comments	Caution is warranted in administering cefepime to patients with a history of hypersensitivity reactions to cephalosporin or beta-lactam antibiotics.[3] Patients with a history of type I reactions to penicillin should not receive beta-lactam antibiotics. From 5% to 15% of patients allergic to penicillin will also be allergic to cephalosporins. Certain infections (e.g., syphilis) require penicillin for eradication. It is recommended that a desensitization protocol for penicillin-allergic individuals should be performed in a hospital setting. This can usually be completed in about 4 h, at which time the first dose of penicillin can be given.[2] The beta-lactam ring of penicillins can link with an amino sugar of the aminoglycoside and inactivate the aminoglycoside.[22-24] To avoid this potential interaction, administer penicillins 1 h before or after an aminoglycoside, adequately flush the infusion line between each infusion, or infuse them through separate lines. *In vivo* inactivation that is dose dependent can also occur particularly in patients with renal failure.[24-26] In patients with end-stage renal failure, gentamicin half-life was decreased by 22–31 h after carbenicillin or ticarcillin was added to the drug regimen.[25] A false-positive urinary glucose results when cupric sulfate solution-based tests (Clinitest, Benedict's solution, Fehling's solution) are used. Glucose oxidase methods (Clinistix) are not associated with false-positive test results.[3,27] Positive direct Coombs' tests have been reported during treatment with cefepime.[3]

Cefoperazone Sodium

Brand names	Cefobid
Dosage	**Neonates:** Although a dose of 100 mg/kg/d divided q 12 h has been suggested,[1] other cephalosporins are more appropriate in this population. **Infants and children** **Mild-to-moderate infections:** 100–150 mg/kg/d (up to 4 g) divided q 8–12.[2-5] **Serious infections:** No information available. **Adolescents and adults:** 2–4 g/d divided q 12 h.[7] (See Maximum dosage section.)
Dosage adjustment in organ dysfunction	No need to adjust dose in renal failure.[6] Decrease dose by 50% in patients with hepatic disease or biliary obstruction.[7] In general, in *adults* the dose should not exceed 4 g/d.[7] The dose should not exceed 1–2 g/d in patients with combined renal and hepatic dysfunction.[7]
Maximum dosage	400 mg/kg/d[4,5] up to 4 g/d in children[3] and 12 g/d in *adults*.[7] However, 16 g/d has been given by continuous infusion to immunocompromised *adults*.[7]
IV push	Not recommended.[1,8] However, 2 g/20 mL has been given over 3–5 min to *adults*.[4,8]
Intermittent infusion	2–50 mg/mL in D5LR, D5NS, D5¼NS, D5W, D10W, LR, or NS[1,8] over 15–60 min.[1,9,10]
Continuous infusion	Diluted to 2–25 mg/mL in D5LR, D5NS, D5¼NS, D5W, D10W, LR, or NS.[8-10] Other beta-lactam antibiotics have been given by this method.[11]
Other routes of administration	Give by deep IM injection.[7] <250 mg/mL reconstituted with SW, BW, D5LR, D5NS, D5½NS, D5W, D10W, LR, or NS.[7,8] For concentrations >250 mg/mL, add SW and gently agitate vial until dissolved. Then add required amount of 2% lidocaine HCl to achieve a final lidocaine concentration in the solution of 0.5%.[7]
Maximum concentration	50 mg/mL for intermittent infusion.[7] In *adults*, 100 mg/mL in NS resulted in a recommended osmolality for peripheral infusion in fluid-restricted patients.[12] 113 mg/mL in D5W and 202 mg/mL in SW resulted in recommended osmolality for peripheral infusion in fluid-restricted patients.[8,12]
Cautions related to IV administration	If a decision is made to give this medication to a patient with known penicillin hypersensitivity, the patient should be closely observed for allergenicity.[13-17] Phlebitis may occur at the injection site.[7] For PN compatibility information, please see Appendix C.
Other additives	Contains 1.5 mEq sodium/g of cefoperazone.[7]

Comments

Patients with a history of type I reactions to penicillin should not receive beta-lactam antibiotics. From 5% to 15% of patients allergic to penicillin will also be allergic to cephalosporins. Certain infections (e.g., syphilis) require penicillin for eradication. It is recommended that a desensitization protocol for penicillin-allergic individuals should be performed in a hospital setting. This can usually be completed in about 4 h, at which time the first dose of penicillin can be given.(3)

Cefoperazone contains an N-methyl-thiotetrazole (NMTT) side chain that causes a disulfiram-like reaction (e.g., flushing, sweating, headache, and tachycardia) when combined with alcohol.(7) The side chain may also be responsible for an increased risk of bleeding.(7,18)

A false-positive urinary glucose results when cupric sulfate solution-based tests (Clinitest, Benedict's solution, Fehling's solution) are used. Glucose oxidase methods (Clinistix) are not associated with false-positive test results.(1)

Cefotaxime Sodium

Brand names Claforan

Dosage

Neonates

PNA	<1200 g	1200–2000 g	≥2000 g
<7 d	100 mg/kg/d divided q 12 h[1,2]*	100 mg/kg/d divided q 12 h[2,3]	100–150 mg/kg/d divided q 8–12 h[2-4]
≥7 d		150 mg/kg/d divided q 8 h[2,3]	150–200 mg/kg/d divided q 6–8 h[2-4]

*Until 4 weeks of age.

Doses as small as 50 mg/kg given as a single dose or divided q 12 h may provide effective serum concentrations for non-CNS infections in very low birth weight infants.[5,6]

Infants and children

Mild-to-moderate infections: 75–100 mg/kg/d (up to 4–6 g) divided q 6–8 h.[2,7-9]

Severe infections: 150–300 mg/kg/d (up to 8–10 g) divided q 6–8 h.[2]

Adolescents and adults: Usual dose 2 g given as a single dose or divided q 12 h.[7] Severe infections may be treated with 3–4 g q 6–12 h up to 12 g/d.[7]

Gonococcal infection

Complicated: 25–50 mg/kg q 24 h (up to 1 g) for 7 days.[2,10] If meningitis or endocarditis, give 50 mg/kg/d divided q 12 h (up to 2 g/d) for 10–14 days and 28 days, respectively.[2,10]

Ophthalmia: Neonates born to mothers with known gonorrhea should receive a single 125-mg IV/IM dose.[2] Premature and VLBW infants should be given 25–50 mg/kg as a one-time dose up to 125 mg.[2]

Prophylaxis: Neonates born to mothers with gonococcal infections should be given 25–50 mg/kg (up to 125 mg) as a one-time dose.[2,10] Regardless of weight, children should receive 125-mg IM.[2] If providing prophylaxis after sexual victimization, add appropriate therapies for chlamydia trachomatis, hepatitis B, and trichomoniasis.[2,10]

Uncomplicated: 125 mg as a single dose.[2,10]

Meningitis: For neonates see maximum doses in above table. 225–300 mg/kg/d divided q 6–8 h[2,3,11-14] up to 8–12 g/d divided 4–6 h.[11]

Dosage adjustment in organ dysfunction

Adjust dosage in patients with renal dysfunction.[7,15] If CrCl is 10–50 mL/min, give q 6–12 h; if CrCl is <10 mL/min, give q 24 h.[16] The manufacturer recommends halving the dose when CrCl is <20 mL/min.[7]

Maximum dosage

300 mg/kg/d in neonates, infants, and children with meningitis.[2,9,11] Total daily dose should not exceed 12 g.[7]

IV push

200 mg/mL via central catheter and 60 mg/mL via peripheral vein over 3–5 min.[3,7] A 25-mg/kg dose has been infused over 1 min in neonates.[8] Rapid IV push (<1 min) of a cephalosporin has been associated with potentially life-threatening arrhythmias.[17]

Intermittent infusion

10–60 mg/mL[7] in D5NS, D5¼NS, D5½NS, D5W, D10W, LR, or NS[7,19] over 10–30 min.[19]

Continuous infusion	May be infused by continuous infusion in compatible solutions.[7]
Other routes of administration	230–330 mg/mL[7,18] in BW may be given IM at same doses as IV.[7]
Maximum concentration	200 mg/mL in SW for IV push.[7] 86 mg/mL in D5W, 73 mg/mL in NS, and 147 mg/mL in SW results in a recommended osmolality for peripheral infusion in fluid-restricted patients.[18,19]
Cautions related to IV administration	If a decision is made to give this medication to a patient with known penicillin hypersensitivity, the patient should be closely observed for allergenicity. For PN compatibility information, please see Appendix C.
Other additives	Contains 2.2 mEq sodium/g of cefotaxime.[7]
Comments	Patients with a history of type I reactions to penicillin should not receive beta-lactam antibiotics. From 5% to 15% of patients allergic to penicillin will also be allergic to cephalosporins. Certain infections (e.g., syphilis) require penicillin for eradication. It is recommended that a desensitization protocol for penicillin-allergic individuals should be performed in a hospital setting. This can usually be completed in about 4 h, at which time the first dose of penicillin can be given.[2] May cause false-positive urinary glucose results when cupric sulfate solution-based tests (Clinitest, Benedict's solution, or Fehling's solution) are used.[17] Glucose oxidase methods (Clinistix) are not associated with false-positive test results.[17]

Cefotetan Disodium

Brand names	Cefotan
Dosage	Because cefotetan has been administered to only a limited number of pediatric patients, the doses and side effects have not been established in neonates, infants, and children. **Neonates:** No information available. **Infants and children:** For severe infections, 40–80 mg/kg/d divided q 12 h.[1,2] Inappropriate for mild-to-moderate infections.[1] **Adolescents and adults:** 2–6 g divided q 12 h.[3] **Pelvic inflammatory disease:** 2 g q 12 h (plus doxycycline 100 mg orally or IV q 12 h) for at least 48 h after the patient clinically improves.[4,5] **Surgical prophylaxis:** 20–40 mg/kg (up to 1–2 g) 30–60 min prior to surgery.[1,3]
Dosage adjustment in organ dysfunction	Adjust dosage in renal failure.[3] The manufacturer recommends if CrCl is 10–30 mL/min, give the normal dose q 24 h; if CrCl is <10 mL/min, administer a normal dose q 48 h.[3]
Maximum dosage	6 g/d in *adults*.[3]
IV push	≤182 mg/mL in SW, D5W, or NS over 3–5 min.[3,6]
Intermittent infusion	≤40 mg/mL in D5W or NS over 20–60 min.[3]
Continuous infusion	Although no specific information is available to support administration of cefotetan by this method, other beta-lactam antibiotics have been given by continuous infusion.[7]
Other routes of administration	500 mg/mL in SW, BW, NS, 0.5, or 1% lidocaine by deep IM injection.[3,6] Although 100% absorbed,[8] cefotetan should not be given by this route to patients with septicemia, bacteremia, or life-threatening infections.[3] Cefotetan in Galaxy plastic containers should not be used for IM administration.[3]
Maximum concentration	182 mg/mL for IV infusion and 500 mg/mL for IM administration.[3] A solution with a concentration of 200 mg/mL has an osmolarity of 800 mOsm/L.[6] Concentrations used for IM injection are very hypertonic and have osmolarities >1500 mOsm/L.[6]
Cautions related to IV administration	Although rare, anaphylactoid reactions may require immediate emergency treatment with epinephrine, oxygen, IV steroids, antihistamines, pressor amines, and airway management.[3] For PN compatibility information, please see Appendix C.
Other additives	Contains approximately 3.5 mEq (80 mg) of sodium/g of cefotetan.[6]

Comments

Patients with a history of type I reactions to penicillin should not receive beta-lactam antibiotics. From 5% to 15% of patients allergic to penicillin will also be allergic to cephalosporins. Certain infections (e.g., syphilis) require penicillin for eradication. It is recommended that a desensitization protocol for penicillin-allergic individuals should be performed in a hospital setting. This can usually be completed in about 4 h, at which time the first dose of penicillin can be given.[1]

Cefotetan, along with other cephalosporins, has been associated with hemolytic anemia.[3] If anemia occurs within 2–3 weeks of beginning cefotetan, a diagnosis of cephalosporin-associated anemia should be considered and the drug should be stopped.[3]

Cefotetan contains an N-methyl-thiotetrazole (NMTT) side chain that causes a disulfiram-like reaction (e.g., flushing, sweating, headache, and tachycardia) when combined with alcohol.[3] The side chain may also be responsible for an increased risk of bleeding. Prolongation of the prothrombin time, with or without bleeding, has been reported to occur more frequently with cefotetan (3.8%) than with equivalent antibiotics (0.8%).[9]

Cefotetan may cause false-positive urinary glucose results when cupric sulfate solution-based tests (Clinitest, Benedict's solution, or Fehling's solution) are used. Glucose oxidase methods (Clinistix) are not associated with false-positive test results.[3]

When the Jaffe reaction is used to determine creatinine, high concentrations of cefotetan may cause falsely elevated serum or urinary creatinine values.[3]

Cefoxitin Sodium

Brand names	Mefoxin
Dosage	Safety and efficacy in infants <3 months old have not been established.[1] **Neonates:** 75–90 mg/kg/d divided q 8 h.[2-4] **Infants and children** **Mild-to-moderate infections:** 80–100 mg/kg/d up to 3–4 g/d.[1,5,6] May be divided q 4–6 h[1,5,6-8] or given q 8 h.[5] **Severe infections:** 80–160 mg/kg/d (up to 6–12 g/d) divided q 4–6 h.[1,5,7-9] **Adolescents and adults:** 3–12 g/d divided q 6–8 h.[1] Dosage should be guided by susceptibility of organisms, severity of the infection, and clinical status of the patient. The larger dosages should be reserved for more severe or serious infections. **Pelvic inflammatory disease (PID):** 2 g q 6 h (plus doxycycline 100 mg orally or IV q 12 g) for at least 48 h after the patient clinically improves.[5,10] **Surgical prophylaxis:** 30–40 mg/kg (up to 1–2 g) given 30–60 min prior to surgery and continued q 6 h for no longer than 24 h.[1,2,11] One study gave 150 mg/kg/d divided q 8 h (first dose at anesthesia induction) for 5 days for acute appendicitis.[12]
Dosage adjustment in organ dysfunction	Adjust dosage in patients with renal dysfunction.[1] If CrCl is 30–50 mL/min give normal dose q 8–12 h; if CrCl is 10–29 mL/min, give normal dose q 12–24 h; if CrCl is 5–9 mL/min, decrease dose by 50% and give q 12–24h, if CrCl <5 decrease by 50% and give q 24–48h.[1]
Maximum dosage	160 mg/kg/d, not to exceed 12 g/d.[1] Large doses have been associated with an increased incidence of eosinophilia and elevated liver function test.[1]
IV push	180 mg/mL in SW over 3–5 min via central catheter and 50 mg/mL via peripheral vein.[1,6,13]
Intermittent infusion	10–40 mg/mL in D5LR, D5NS, D5¼NS, D5½NS, D5W, D10W, LR, NS, or R over 15–40 min.[1,14,15]
Continuous infusion	10–40 mg/mL in D5W, NS, or D5NS.[1] Other beta-lactam antibiotics have been given by this method.[16]
Other routes of administration	400 mg/mL by IM administration.[1] Add 2 mL of SW for injection or 0.5% to 1% lidocaine HCl injection (without epinephrine) to each gram of cefoxitin.[1] No information available to support administration by other routes.
Maximum concentration	200 mg/mL for IV push, 40 mg/mL for IV infusion, and 400 mg/mL for IM administration.[1] 112 mg/mL in SW results in a maximum recommended osmolality for peripheral infusion in fluid-restricted patients.[13]
Cautions related to IV administration	If a decision is made to give this medication to a patient with known penicillin hypersensitivity, the patient should be closely observed for allergenicity. For PN compatibility information, please see Appendix C.

Other additives Contains 2.3 mEq sodium/g of cefoxitin.[15]

Comments Patients with a history of type I reactions to penicillin should not receive beta-lactam antibiotics. From 5% to 15% of patients allergic to penicillin will also be allergic to cephalosporins. Certain infections (e.g., syphilis) require penicillin for eradication. It is recommended that a desensitization protocol for penicillin-allergic individuals should be performed in a hospital setting. This can usually be completed in about 4 h, at which time the first dose of penicillin can be given.[5]

The beta-lactam ring of penicillins can link with an amino sugar of the aminoglycoside and inactivate the aminoglycoside.[17-19] To avoid this potential interaction, administer penicillins 1 h before or after an aminoglycoside, adequately flush the infusion line between each infusion, or infuse them through separate lines. *In vivo* inactivation that is dose dependent can also occur particularly in patients with renal failure.[19-21] In patients with end-stage renal failure, gentamicin half-life was decreased by 22–31 h after carbenicillin or ticarcillin was added to the drug regimen.[20]

A false-positive urinary glucose results when cupric sulfate solution-based tests (Clinitest, Benedict's solution, Fehling's solution) are used. Glucose oxidase methods (Clinistix) are not associated with false-positive test results.[1]

When the Jaffe reaction is used to determine creatinine, high concentrations of cefotetan may cause falsely elevated serum or urinary creatinine values.[1]

Ceftazidime

Brand names Ceptaz, Fortaz, Tazicef, Tazidime

Dosage

Neonates

PNA	<1200 g	≤2000 g	>2000 g
≤7	100 mg/kg/d divided q 12 h[1]*	50–100 mg/kg/d divided q 12–18 h[1-6]	100–150 mg/kg/d divided q 8–12 h[1,2,4,6-9]
>7		150 mg/kg/d divided q 8 h[1,2,8,9]	150 mg/kg/d divided q 8 h[1,2,8,9]

*Until 4 weeks of age.

One report suggested 25 mg/kg q 24 h in those with a gestational age <32 weeks.[10,11]

Infants and children

Mild-to-moderate infections: 75–100 mg/kg/d divided q 8 h up to 3 g/d.[1]

Severe infections (including meningitis): 125–150 mg/kg/d divided q 8 h up to 6 g/d.[1,12-18]

Adolescents and adults: 250 mg to 1 g q 8–12 h up to 6 g/d.[1,18] Dose is dependent on type and severity of infection.[19]

Cystic fibrosis: 150–320 mg/kg/d divided q 6–8 h[19-24] or a loading dose of 100 mg/kg up to 2000 g followed by 3.4–12.5 mg/kg/h.[25]

Neutropenia and fever (empiric therapy): 100–150 mg/kg/d divided q 8–12 h as monotherapy.[15-17,26]

Dosage adjustment in organ dysfunction Adjust dosage in patients with renal dysfunction.[19,27-29] If CrCl is 31–50 mL/min, give q 12 h; if CrCl is 16–30 mL/min, give q 24 h; if CrCl is 6–15 mL/min, give 50% of the normal dose q 24 h; if CrCl is <5 mL/min, give 50% of the normal dose q 48 h.[19] No dosage adjustment necessary in patients with hepatic dysfunction.[19]

Maximum dosage 240 mg/kg/d in normal children[14,30] or 320 mg/kg/d in patients with cystic fibrosis,[22] not to exceed 6 g/d.[1,2,13,19,24,31]

IV push 100–200 mg/mL in SW over 3–5 min.[19,32] A 25-mg/kg dose has been infused over 1–2 min in a neonate.[9] Generally, give at a rate ≤10 mg/kg/min.[2]

Intermittent infusion 1–40 mg/mL in D5NS, D5¼NS, D5½NS, D5W, D10W, LR, NS, or R[19] infused over 10–30 min.[31] Reconstituted solutions are stable for 24 h at room temperature and for 7 days when refrigerated.[19]

Continuous infusion Although concentration and solution type are usually not specified, ceftazidime has been given by this method.[25,33-35] 200 mg/kg/d in 100 mL D5W has been given to febrile neutropenic children.[35]

Other routes of administration 280 mg/mL in SW, BW, or 0.5% to 1% lidocaine has been given IM.[9,19,31,32]

Maximum concentration	200 mg/mL for administration via a central catheter.[2,19] Although one reference noted a maximum concentration of 40 mg/mL for administration via peripheral vein,[2] 126 mg/mL in SW results in a maximum recommended osmolality for peripheral infusion in fluid-restricted patients.[36]
Cautions related to IV administration	If a decision is made to give this medication to a patient with known penicillin hypersensitivity, the patient should be closely observed for allergenicity. (See Comments section.) For PN compatibility information, please see Appendix C.
Other additives	Contains 2.3 mEq sodium/g of ceftazidime.[19]
Comments	Patients with a history of type I reactions to penicillin should not receive beta-lactam antibiotics. From 5% to 15% of patients allergic to penicillin will also be allergic to cephalosporins. Certain infections (e.g., syphilis) require penicillin for eradication. It is recommended that a desensitization protocol for penicillin-allergic individuals should be performed in a hospital setting. This can usually be completed in about 4 h, at which time the first dose of penicillin can be given.[1] A false-positive urinary glucose results when cupric sulfate solution-based tests (Clinitest, Benedict's solution, Fehling's solution) are used. Glucose oxidase methods (Clinistix) are not associated with false-positive test results.[19] May need to adjust dosage in premature neonates receiving indomethacin.[37] When ceftazidime is reconstituted, carbon dioxide is produced, resulting in bubbles and positive pressure in the vial. The pressure is reduced by removing air from the vial with a syringe. Bubbles remaining in the solution must be expelled prior to infusion.[19]

Ceftriaxone Sodium

Brand names	Rocephin

Dosage

Neonates: Ceftriaxone may displace bilirubin from binding sites on albumin and increase the risk for kernicterus in neonates with physiologic jaundice.[1] Cefotaxime is not recommended for neonates with hyperbilirubinemia.[2]

PNA	<1200 g	≤2000 g	>2000 g
≤7	50 mg/kg/d q 24–36 h[2-5]*	50 mg/kg divided q 24–36 h[2,4,5]	50 mg/kg divided q 24 h[2,4,5]
>7		50 mg/kg divided q 24 h[2,4,5]	50–100 mg/kg/d q 24 h[2,3,5]

*Until 4 weeks of age.

Infants and children

Mild-to-moderate infections: 50–75 mg/kg (up to 2 g/d) given q 12 h.[2,5,6]

Severe infections (including meningitis): 80–100 mg/kg (up to 4 g/d) given q 12 h.[4,6,8-22]

Gonococcal infection

Complicated: 25–50 mg/kg (up to 1 g/d) q 24 h for 7 days.[2,23] If meningitis or endocarditis, give 50 mg/kg/d (up to 2 g/d) divided q 12 h for 10–14 days and 28 days, respectively.[2,23]

Opthalmia: Neonates born to mothers with known gonorrhea should receive a single 125-mg IV/IM dose.[2] Premature and VLBW infants should be given 25–50 mg/kg as a one-time dose up to 125 mg.[2]

Prophylaxis: Neonates born to mothers with gonococcal infections should be given 25–50 mg/kg up to 125 mg as a one-time dose.[2,23] Regardless of weight, children should receive 125 mg IM.[2] If providing prophylaxis after sexual victimization, add appropriate therapies for chlamydia trachomatis, hepatitis B, and trichomoniasis.[2,23]

Uncomplicated: 125 mg as a single dose up to 1 g/d.[2,23]

Otitis media: 50 mg/kg up to 1 g as a single dose. Generally administered IM.[24-26]

Dosage adjustment in organ dysfunction

Most patients with renal dysfunction who receive ≤2 g/d do not require dosage adjustment.[6,27,28] However, some patients with end-stage renal disease receiving hemodialysis may accumulate ceftriaxone.[6,28]

Maximum dosage

100 mg/kg/d,[6,8,10,17-20] not to exceed 4 g/d.[6,8,12,27,28]

IV push

10–40 mg/mL in D5NS, D5½NS, D5W, D10W, NS, or SW.[6,29] Doses have been given over 2–4 min in ambulatory patients >11 years of age[30] or over 5 min in children with meningitis.[15] However, 10 min after ceftriaxone was infused over 5 min, an *adult* being treated for presumed meningitis became diaphoretic, hypertensive, and tachycardic and developed palpitations.[31] Subsequent infusions over 30 min were uneventful.[31]

Intermittent infusion

10–40 mg/mL in D5NS, D5½NS, D5W, D10W, NS, or SW[6,29] infused over 10–30 min.[6,29]

American Society of
Health-System Pharmacists
7272 Wisconsin Avenue
Bethesda, Maryland 20814
301-657-3000
Fax: 301-652-8278

*** P861-NOTICE ***

Important Correction Notice

Pediatric Injectable Drugs Eighth Edition (The Teddy Bear Book)

The publishers wish to inform you of a correction in the monograph for Ceftriaxone Sodium

Page 92 – Ceftriaxone Sodium

"Dosage" section – Infants and Children

Mild to moderate infections: 50 – 75 mg/kg (up to 2 g/d) given once daily or divided q12h.

Severe infections (including meningitis): 80 – 100 mg/kg (up to 4 g/d) given once daily or divided q12h.

Continuous infusion	Although no specific information is available to support administration by this route, other beta-lactam antibiotics have been given by this method.[22]
Other routes of administration	100–350 mg/mL in SW, NS, D5W, BW, or 1% lidocaine (without epinephrine) by deep IM injection.[6,29]
Maximum concentration	40 mg/mL for IV administration and 350 mg/mL for IM use.[6]
Cautions related to IV administration	If a decision is made to give this medication to a patient with known penicillin hypersensitivity, the patient should be closely observed for allergenicity. For PN compatibility information, please see Appendix C.
Other additives	Contains 3.6 mEq sodium/g of ceftriaxone.[30]
Comments	Patients with a history of type I reactions to penicillin should not receive beta-lactam antibiotics. From 5% to 15% of patients allergic to penicillin will also be allergic to cephalosporins. Certain infections (e.g., syphilis) require penicillin for eradication. It is recommended that a desensitization protocol for penicillin-allergic individuals should be performed in a hospital setting. This can usually be completed in about 4 h, at which time the first dose of penicillin can be given.[2] Ceftriaxone may cause false-positive urinary glucose results when cupric sulfate solution-based tests (Clinitest, Benedict's solution, or Fehling's solution) are used. Glucose oxidase methods (Clinistix) are not associated with false-positive test results.[6] Ceftriaxone has been reported to cause primary cholelithiasis,[6,32] nephrolithiasis,[33] and hemolytic anemia.[34] Gallstones spontaneously resolved after discontinuation of the drug.[32]

Cefuroxime Sodium

Brand names Kefurox, Zinacef

Dosage

Safety and efficacy in infants <3 months old have not been established.[1]

Neonates

PNA	<2000 g	>2000 g
<7 d	100 mg/kg/d divided q 12 h[2-4]	150 mg/kg/d divided q 8 h[2]
≥7 d	150 mg/kg/d divided q 8 h[2]*	150 mg/kg/d divided q 8 h[2]

*Until 4 weeks of age.

Infants ≥3 months and children

Mild-to-moderate infections: 50–100 mg/kg/d divided q 6–8 h.[1,5-10]

Severe infections: 100–150 mg/kg/d divided q 8 h.[5] Cefuroxime should not be used to treat bacterial meningitis. (See Comments section.)

Dosage adjustment in organ dysfunction

Adjust dosage in patients with renal dysfunction.[1] If CrCl is 10–20 mL/min, give a normal dose q 12 h and if CrCl is <10 mL/min, q 24 h.[1]

Maximum dosage

300 mg/kg/d,[11,12] not to exceed 4–6 g/d in children[2,5] and 3 g/dose or 9 g/d in *adults*.[1]

IV push

50–100 mg/mL in SW over 3–5 min.[1]

Intermittent infusion

≤30 mg/mL in D5NS, D5¼NS, D5½NS, D5W, D10W, LR, NS, or R over 15–60 min.[1,13]

Continuous infusion

7.5–15 mg/mL in D5NS, D5½NS, D5W, D10W, and NS.[1]

Other routes of administration

220 mg/mL reconstituted with SW and administered into large muscle mass (gluteus or lateral thigh).[1,10,13]

Maximum concentration

100 mg/mL for IV push and 220 mg/mL for IM administration.[1] 137 mg/mL in SW (489 mOsm/kg) resulted in a maximum recommended osmolality for peripheral infusion in fluid-restricted patients.[14]

Cautions related to IV administration

If a decision is made to give this medication to a patient with known penicillin hypersensitivity, the patient should be closely observed for allergenicity. (See Comments section.)

Phlebitis may occur.[1]

For PN compatibility information, please see Appendix C.

Other additives	Contains 2.4 mEq sodium/g of cefuroxime.[1]

Comments

Patients with a history of type I reactions to penicillin should not receive beta-lactam antibiotics. From 5% to 15% of patients allergic to penicillin will also be allergic to cephalosporins. Certain infections (e.g., syphilis) require penicillin for eradication. It is recommended that a desensitization protocol for penicillin-allergic individuals should be performed in a hospital setting. This can usually be completed in about 4 h, at which time the first dose of penicillin can be given.[5]

Infants and children with meningitis who were treated with cefuroxime had an increased incidence of hearing loss[12,15] and an increased time to sterilization of their cerebrospinal fluid.[15] The AAP does not recommend cefuroxime for meningitis.[5]

Cefuroxime may cause false-positive urinary glucose results when cupric sulfate solution-based tests (Clinitest, Benedict's solutions, or Fehling's solution) are used.[1] Glucose oxidase methods (Clinistix) are not associated with false-positive test results.[1] May also cause false-positive direct Coombs' test results.[1]

Concomitant use of probenecid may increase the AUC of cefuroxime.[1]

Chloramphenicol Sodium Succinate

Brand names	Chloromycetin Sodium Succinate

Dosage

Inappropriate for mild-to-moderate infections. When used, dosing should be optimized by measuring serum concentrations.[1-3]

Neonates (see Comments section)

Loading dose: One paper suggests a 20-mg/kg loading dose followed in 12 h by maintenance doses.[4]

Maintenance dose, neonates

Premature, ≤1200 g: 22 mg/kg given q 24 h.[5]

Premature, ≤2000 g and ≤1 week: 25 mg/kg given q 24 h.[5]

Term, <2 weeks: 25 mg/kg/d divided q 12 h.[2,3,6-10]

Term, 2–4 weeks: 25–50 mg/kg/d divided q 12 h.[2,3,6-10]

Maintenance dose, infants and children: 50–100 mg/kg/d divided q 6–8 h.[1-3,7-20] Because of the emergence of vancomycin-resistant *Enterococcus*, some investigators have recommended 75–100 mg/kg/d divided q 6 h for the treatment of meningitis.[18-20] Other investigators noted that 100 mg/kg/d may be unnecessary and only increases the incidence of toxicity.[3,13,14]

Dosage adjustment in organ dysfunction

Adjust dosage in patients with hepatic[7-10] or renal[21-23] dysfunction.

Dose adjustments should be based on plasma concentrations (5–20 mcg/mL).[23,24]

Maximum dosage

100 mg/kg/d.[7-14] In neonates <2 weeks of age, 25 mg/kg/d[24] and 50 mg/kg/d in neonates <4 weeks of age.[25] Maximum *adult* dose should not exceed 2–4 g/d.[1] When large doses are used, serum concentration monitoring is imperative.

IV push

100 mg/mL in D5W, NS, or SW over ≥1 min.[26]

Intermittent infusion

20–25 mg/mL in D–LR, D–R, D–S, D5LR, D5NS, D5W, D10W, LR, R, NS, or ½NS infused over 15–60 min.[5,16,26]

Continuous infusion

Although concentration and solution type were not provided, chloramphenicol has been given by this method.[27]

Other routes of administration

Although chloramphenicol can be administered IM,[24,28] the drug may be less effective when given by this route.[24]

Chloramphenicol has been administered intraventricularly in an *adult.*[29]

Maximum concentration

100 mg/mL.[26]

Cautions related to IV administration

None known.

For PN compatibility information, please see Appendix C.

Other additives	Contains 2.25 mEq sodium/g of chloramphenicol sodium succinate.[26]
Comments	Gray syndrome (e.g., circulatory collapse, acidosis, myocardial depression, and abdominal distension) may result from drug accumulation in patients with immature or impaired hepatic or renal function.[30-36] Because it is generally associated with serum concentrations >50 mcg/mL, individualize dosage based on serum concentrations.[25,28-35] Bone marrow depression, including aplastic anemia, thrombocytopenia, and granulocytopenia, has occurred with short and long term therapy.[24] Chloramphenicol inhibits the metabolism of several drugs (e.g., phenytoin, phenobarbital, tolbutamide, dicumarol, cyclosporine, and tacrolimus).[36-38] Likewise, many drugs (e.g., rifampin, phenobarbital, and phenytoin) decrease chloramphenicol concentrations. Consult appropriate resources for dosing recommendations before combining any drug with chloramphenicol.

Chlorpromazine HCl

Brand names	Thorazine

Dosage

Because of hypothermia and eosinophilia, do not use in children <6 months of age, except where potential exists to save the child's life.[1]

Amphetamine-induced hyperactivity

Children: 1 mg/kg q 6 h as needed. If a barbiturate has been ingested, <4 mg/kg/d should be used.[2]

Adolescents: 25 mg q 6 h as needed.[2]

Hypoxia, neonatal: A loading dose of 0.13–0.88 mg/kg infused over 1 h, followed by 0.03–0.21 mg/kg/h for up to 47 h, has been used in severe hypoxia.[3]

Nausea and vomiting: 0.55 mg/kg IM q 6–8 h prn.[1]

During surgery

IM: 0.275 mg/kg; if nausea and vomiting persist after 30 min and hypotension has not occurred, the regimen may be repeated.[1]

IV: 1 mg at 2-min intervals; do not exceed IM dosage.[1]

Chemotherapy-induced: 1–3.3 mg/kg/d divided q 3–6 h[4-6] or 30 mg/m^2[7] infused over 15 min and given 30 min before chemotherapy.[6,7]

Neonatal abstinence syndrome/withdrawal: While phenobarbital is preferred, IM chlorpromazine has been used for this indication. If used, initial IM doses range from 0.5 to 0.7 mg/kg q 6 h.[8] Chlorpromazine 0.5 mg/kg q 6 h has been used to treat neonatal withdrawal after in utero SSRI exposure.[9]

Presurgical apprehension: 0.55 mg/kg IM 1–2 h before surgery.[1]

Sedation/hypnosis: For infants and children, 0.2–0.5 mg/kg q 4–6 h.[10,11]

Severe behavioral problems: 0.55 mg/kg IM q 6–8 h prn; for severe disorders, larger doses may be necessary; start low and increase gradually up to maximum doses (see Maximum dosage section); older patients may require 200 mg or more daily (further behavior improvement not seen with doses >500 mg/d).[1]

Tetanus: 0.55 mg/kg IM/IV q 6–8 h.[1]

Dosage adjustment in organ dysfunction

Although one reference suggests that no dosage adjustment is necessary in renal dysfunction,[12] the manufacturer recommends chlorpromazine be administered cautiously in patients with renal disease.[1] It should also be used cautiously in patients with cardiovascular, liver, or chronic respiratory disease.[1]

Maximum dosage

6 months–5 years or <23 kg: 40 mg/d.[1]

5–12 years or 23–45 kg: 75 mg/d.[1]

IV push

Dilute to ≤1 mg/mL in NS[1,13] not to exceed 0.5 mg/min in children and 1 mg/min in *adults.*[1,13]

Intermittent infusion

Dilute to ≤1 mg/mL in NS[1,13] not to exceed 0.5 mg/min in children and 1 mg/min in *adults.*[1,13]

Continuous infusion

No information available to support administration by this method.

Other routes of administration	May be given via IM injection. Inject slowly, deep into large muscle.[1,13] If irritation is a problem, dilute with NS or 2% procaine.[1,13]
Maximum concentration	1 mg/mL.[13]
Cautions related to IV administration	Systemic hypotension has occurred in neonates.[14] Because of the risk of hypotension, patients should continue to lie down for 30 min after the injection.[1] Thrombophlebitis may occur.[9] For PN compatibility information, please see Appendix C.
Other additives	**1- and 2-mL ampuls (25 mg/mL chlorpromazine) contain per mL:** 2 mg ascorbic acid, 1 mg sodium bisulfite, 6 mg sodium chloride, and 1 mg sodium sulfite.[1] **10-mL multidose vials (25 mg/mL chlorpromazine) contain per mL:** 2 mg ascorbic acid, 1 mg sodium bisulfite, 1 mg sodium chloride and 1 mg sodium sulfite.[1] Sulfites may cause hypersensitivity reactions, and these are more common in *adults* with asthma. Most reactions are mild but can include anaphylactic symptoms and life-threatening or less severe asthma episodes.[15-17] Epinephrine may be required in severe cases; and if the sulfite-free product is not available, the sulfite-preserved epinephrine should be used.[15] Multidose vials (not ampuls) also contain benzyl alcohol 2% as a preservative.[1] Benzyl alcohol in small doses as a preservative in drugs is considered safe in newborns.[15] However, a 3-week-old, very low birth weight (710 g) infant who received clindamycin experienced a profound desaturation that required resuscitation after the third and fourth doses, which was subsequently related to the benzyl alcohol preservative.[18] Administration of saline flushes containing benzyl alcohol (bacteriostatic water for injection) was associated with a fatal gasping syndrome, intraventricular hemorrhage, metabolic acidosis, and increased mortality in preterm infants.[19] This should not be used in neonates. Hypersensitivity reactions to benzyl alcohol in parenteral products have been reported in *adults*.[20,21]
Comments	Meperidine, promethazine, and chlorpromazine have been used in combination (Demerol, Phenergan, Thorazine [DPT] cocktail) to sedate pediatric patients.[11,22-26] However, with the availability of safer and more effective agents,[24,27-28] this combination is no longer recommended.[26] In one study in *adults*, incremental IV administration of 12.5 mg to a maximum of 37.5 mg was as effective as sumatriptan for the pain of acute migraine.[29] Larger doses (4.6 ± 1.8 mg/kg) have been used for systemic vasodilation during cardio-pulmonary bypass in neonates.[30] An association has been found between chlorpromazine use and acute and clinically relevant liver injury.[31] Chlorpromazine poisoning (17 mg/kg up to 100 mg/kg) has occurred in children; ingestions in children of ≤15 mg/kg producing clinical effects or >15 mg/kg should be referred to the hospital for therapy.[32] Because chlorpromazine is associated with several drug interactions, consult appropriate resources for dosing recommendations before combining any drug with chlorpromazine.[1]

Cimetidine

Brand names	Tagamet
Dosage	**Premature neonates:** 8–10 mg/kg/d divided q 6–12 h.[1-3] **Term neonates:** 8–24 mg/kg/d divided q 6–12 h.[1,2,4-7] **Infants and children:** 20–40 mg/kg/d up to 1.2 g divided q 4–6 h.[8-14] In *adults*, a loading dose of 150–300 mg infused over ≥5 min has been followed by a continuous infusion of 37.5–100 mg/h diluted in a compatible fluid.[15-17] (See Maximum dosage section.)
Dosage adjustment in organ dysfunction	Adjust dosage in patients with severe renal dysfunction.[18,19] If CrCl is 10–50 mL/min, give 50% of normal dose; if CrCl is <10 mL/min, give 25% of normal dose.[18] Dosage adjustment may also be necessary in hepatic impairment.[20] Clearance is increased in children with burns,[12,21] cystic fibrosis,[22] or critical illness.[9,11]
Maximum dosage	40 mg/kg/d,[8-11] not to exceed 2.4 g/d in *adults*.[20,23]
IV push	15 mg/mL[20] has been infused over 5 min.[10,24-26] (See Cautions related to IV administration section.)
Intermittent infusion	6 mg/mL in D5LR, D5NS, D5¼NS, D5½NS, D10NS, D5W, D10W, LR, NS, R, or sodium bicarbonate 5%[20,27] infused over 15–30 min.[9,11,24]
Continuous infusion	6 mg/mL cimetidine in 100–1000 mL of D5LR, D5NS, D5¼NS, D5½NS, D10NS, D5W, D10W, LR, NS, R, or sodium bicarbonate 5%.[20,27] Visually compatible with PN and stable in PN and TNA solutions for 24 h at room temperature.[28,29]
Other routes of administration	150 mg/mL (undiluted) may be given IM.[27]
Maximum concentration	15 mg/mL for slow IV push,[20] 6 mg/mL for IV infusion.[20,27] 150 mg/mL for IM injection.[27]
Cautions related to IV administration	In *adults*, rapid administration over 1–5 min has resulted in cardiac dysrhythmias,[30] hypotension,[25,31] and cardiac arrest,[26] particularly in individuals with myocardial disease. For PN compatibility information, please see Appendix C.
Other additives	None.

Comments

Reversible confusional states have been observed in *adults*.[20] Reversible cerebral toxicity (inattention, lack of spontaneous movements, no crying, and decreased ability to track objects or respond to verbal stimuli) has been reported in a 2-month-old infant receiving 40 mg/kg/d.[32] These effects did not reappear at doses of 25 mg/kg/d. A 4-year-old child on 15 mg/kg/d of cimetidine in combination with two other CNS-active drugs was reported to have dysarthria, hallucinations, and was picking at bedclothes.[33]

Cimetidine has been associated with hypoxemia in a neonate receiving concomitant tolazoline therapy.[34]

The use of H2-blocker therapy has been associated with the incidence of necrotizing enterocolitis in very low birth weight infants.[35]

Because cimetidine inhibits a variety of isoenzymes and is associated with numerous drug interactions,[20] consult appropriate resources for dosing recommendations before combining any drug with cimetidine.

Ciprofloxacin Lactate

Brand names Cipro I.V.

Dosage

Because ciprofloxacin causes arthropathy in immature animals, the manufacturer states that it should not be used in children <18 years.[1] Several investigators were unable to prove ciprofloxacin-induced arthropathy in pediatric patients following IV or oral dosing.[2-5] Two retrospective safety studies of 1795[6] and >1700[7] children report arthralgia rates of 1.5% and 0%, respectively. An extensive review of the issue has been published.[8] (See Comments section.) The American Academy of Pediatrics recommends that the use of ciprofloxacin is not appropriate in mild-to-moderate infections, but should be restricted to severe infections.[9]

Neonates: Thirteen neonates with *Klebsiella pneumoniae* septicemia were treated with 10–40 mg/kg/d divided q 12 h for 10–20 days.[10] A neonate with multiple brain abscesses was given 10 mg/kg/d for 33 days.[11] Twenty-eight preterm or low birth weight neonates received 4–40 mg/kg/d for infections with multiresistant organisms (*Enterobacter cloacae, Pseudomonas aeruginosa, Klebsiella pneumoniae).*[12] Twelve cases of neonatal and infant nosocomial meningitis were treated with doses of 10–60 mg/kg/d for up to 28 days.[13] One hundred and sixteen septic neonates treated with 10 mg/kg/d of ciprofloxacin showed no evidence of immediate hematologic, renal, or hepatic adverse events, and no evidence of arthropathy or growth impairment at 1 year of life.[14]

Infants and children

Mild-to-moderate infections: Inappropriate.[9]

Severe infections: 18–30 mg/kg/d divided q 8–12 h up to 400–800 mg q 12 h.[9] Some patients with sepsis may require 30 mg/kg/d divided q 8 h.[15]

An infant with ventriculitis was given 35 mg/kg/d divided q 12 h for four doses.[16] These doses resulted in an unacceptable increase in serum concentrations and the dosage was decreased (25 mg/kg/d divided q 12 h) and continued for 21 days.

Biologic warfare or bioterrorism: The CDC and other experts recommend that treatment of inhalational anthrax spores due to biologic warfare or bioterrorism should be started on a multiple-drug parenteral regimen that includes ciprofloxacin or doxycycline and one or two additional anti-infective agents (e.g., chloramphenicol, clindamycin, rifampin, vancomycin, clarithromycin, imipenem, penicillin, or ampicillin).[17,18] Strains of *Bacillus anthracis* associated with cases that occurred in the U.S. during September and October 2001 following bioterrorism-related anthrax exposures were susceptible to clindamycin *in vitro*.[18]

Burns: Children with burn or burn-type wound infections have been given 20–30 mg/kg/d (interval not provided) for 7–10 days and had no radiographic evidence of arthropathy.[19]

Cystic fibrosis: 20–30 mg/kg/d divided q 8–12 h up to 1.2 g/d.[20] Two pharmacokinetic studies in children with cystic fibrosis recommend dosages of 20–30 mg/kg/d divided q 8–12 h.[21,22]

Typhoid fever: Eighteen children with severe typhoid fever were given 10 mg/kg/d divided q 12 h initially and then changed to oral therapy as tolerated. The total duration of therapy was 7–14 days.[23] In a separate study, 16 children received doses ranging from 7–24 mg/kg/d; all but one were eventually changed to oral therapy.[24]

Dosage adjustment in organ dysfunction

Adjust dosage in patients with renal or severe hepatic dysfunction.[1,25-28] If CrCl is 10–50 mL/min, give 50% to 75% of a normal dose; if CrCl is <10 mL/min, give 50% of a normal dose.[25]

Maximum dosage

800 mg/d divided q 12 h in *adults*.[1] A 9-year-old child with cystic fibrosis received 76.9 mg/kg/d for 5 days; the only adverse effect noted was mild gastrointestinal distress.[29] A 5-year-old child with multidrug-resistant extrapulmonary tuberculosis received 16 mg/kg/d for 9 months without side effects, but the route of administration was not reported.[30]

Ciprofloxacin Lactate

IV push	Not recommended.[1]
Intermittent infusion	0.5–2 mg/mL in D5W or NS infused over 60 min.[1,31] (See Cautions related to IV administration section.)
Continuous infusion	No information available to support administration by this method.
Other routes of administration	No information available to support administration by other routes.
Maximum concentration	2 mg/mL.[1]
Cautions related to IV administration	Anaphylaxis has occurred even after the first dose.[32,33] (See Comments section.) Thrombophlebitis, burning, pain, erythema, and swelling occur more frequently when infusion time is <30 min.[1,34] For PN compatibility information, please see Appendix C.
Other additives	None.
Comments	The Committee on Infectious Diseases of the American Academy of Pediatrics states that ciprofloxacin seems to be well-tolerated and does not appear to cause arthropathy.[9] Use of ciprofloxacin in pediatric patients is justifiable in some circumstances: no other agent is available,[1] and infection is caused by multidrug-resistant, gram-negative, enteric, or one of several other pathogens.[2] Possible uses include treatment of UTI caused by *P. aeruginosa* or other multidrug-resistant, gram-negative bacteria; chronic suppurative otitis media; or malignant otitis externa, chronic osteomyelitis, exacerbation of cystic fibrosis, mycobacterial infections, or other gram-negative bacterial infections in immunocompromised hosts in which prolonged oral therapy is desired.[9] There may be an increased risk of hypersensitivity reactions in HIV-seropositive patients.[33] A hypertensive reaction has been reported in an infant following IV ciprofloxacin 10 mg/kg/d.[35] Two desensitization regimens have been described: one in a 29-month-old infant[36] and one in a 15-year-old patient with cystic fibrosis.[37] Ciprofloxacin decreases the clearance of several drugs.[1]

Cisatracurium Besylate

Brand names	Nimbex
Dosage	Respiratory function must be supported during use of this agent. Concurrent administration of a sedative is also necessary. Monitoring of neuromuscular transmission with a peripheral nerve stimulator is recommended during continuous infusion or with repeated dosing.[1,2] **Continuous infusion:** 1–4 mcg/kg/min.[1,3-6] Clearance is higher in healthy pediatric patients compared to healthy *adult* patients.[1] **Intermittent dosing:** 0.1–0.15 mg/kg administered over 5 sec followed by 0.03 mg/kg given as needed to maintain pharmacological paralysis.[1,3-6] Onset of action is faster and there is a longer duration of action in infants 1–23 months compared to children 2–12 years of age.[1]
Dosage adjustment in organ dysfunction	No dosage adjustment is required in patients with hepatic or renal dysfunction.[1]
Maximum dosage	The maximum dosage has not been established. In a study of 19 infants and children receiving cisatracurium, the maximum infusion rate was 10 mcg/kg/min.[6] Response may vary over time, resulting in the need for dosage adjustment.[1] Patients with burns may develop resistance to nondepolarizing neuromuscular blocking agents.[1] The extent of resistance is affected by the size of the burn and time since the burn injury.
IV push	2 mg/mL administered over 5–10 sec.[1]
Intermittent infusion	Not administered by this method.
Continuous infusion	0.1–0.4 mg/mL in D5W, NS, or D5NS.[1,7]
Other routes of administration	IM administration is not recommended due to the potential for tissue irritation.[1] No information available to support administration by other routes.
Maximum concentration	2 mg/mL for IV push; 0.4 mg/mL for infusion.[1]
Cautions related to IV administration	Hypersensitivity reactions, bronchospasm, and laryngospasm have been reported[8] but are rare.[1]
Other additives	The 2-mL concentration (10-mL vial) contains benzyl alcohol as a preservative.[1,7] Benzyl alcohol in small doses as a preservative in drugs is considered safe in newborns.[9] However, a 3-week-old, very low birth weight (710 g) infant who received clindamycin experienced a profound desaturation that required resuscitation after the third and fourth doses, which was subsequently related to the benzyl alcohol preservative.[10] Administration of saline flushes containing benzyl alcohol (BW) was associated with a fatal gasping syndrome, intraventricular hemorrhage, metabolic acidosis, and increased mortality in preterm infants.[11] This should not be used in neonates. Hypersensitivity reactions to benzyl alcohol in parenteral products have been reported in *adults.*[12,13]

Comments

Prolonged paralysis has been reported after long-term infusion of neuromuscular blocking agents, including cisatracurium.[3,14,15] Concomitant administration of corticosteroids with neuromuscular blockers is a risk factor for this adverse effect.[16] Likewise, concomitant administration of certain antibiotics (e.g., aminoglycosides, clindamycin, vancomycin) may prolong neuromuscular blockage.[1,3] Consult appropriate resources for additional information on drug interactions. Other factors that potentiate the duration of neuromuscular blockade include acidosis, hyponatremia, hypocalcemia, hypokalemia, and hypermagnesemia.[1,3]

Patients with neurological diseases such as myasthenia gravis may exhibit increased sensitivity. Decreased sensitivity to cisatracurium may occur in patients with severe burns, muscle trauma, demyelinating lesions, peripheral neuropathies, or infection.[1]

Cisplatin

Brand names	Platinol

Dosage

Consult protocol for complete dosing information. Cisplatin should be administered with a regimen of hydration (with or without mannitol and/or furosemide). (See Comments section.) Should not be given to patients with pre-existing renal or hearing impairment or myelosuppression.

The following dosing regimens have been used in pediatric patients

Intermittent dosing: 37–75 mg/m^2 q 2–3 weeks or 50–100 mg/m^2 q 3–4 weeks.[1,2]

Bone marrow transplantation: 55 $mg/m^2/d$ for 72 h by continuous infusion (165 mg/m^2).[1,2]

Brain tumor (recurrent): 60 $mg/m^2/d$ for 2 days q 3–4 weeks.[1-3]

Neuroblastoma: 60–100 mg/m^2 once q 3–4 weeks[1,4-6] or 30 mg/m^2 q week.[1,2]

Osteogenic sarcoma: 60–100 mg/m^2 once q 3–4 weeks[1,2,7-9] or 30 mg/m^2 q week.[1,2]

A repeat course should not be given until the patient's renal, hematologic, and otic functions are within acceptable limits.[1]

Daily dosing: 15–20 $mg/m^2/d$ for 5 days q 3–4 weeks.[1,2,10,11]

Dosage adjustment in organ dysfunction

If CrCl is 10–50 mL/min, administer 75% of the normal dose; if CrCl is <10 mL/min, administer 50% of the normal dose.[12]

The manufacturer states that cisplatin is contraindicated in patients with pre-existing renal dysfunction.[2]

Manufacturer recommends that repeat dosages be held until SCr <1.5 mg/dL, WBC ≥4000/mm^3, platelets ≥100,000/mm^3, BUN <25.[2]

Decrease dosage in infants <6 months of age due to decreased renal tubular secretion and decreased renal function.[13]

Maximum dosage

Occasionally, fatal dosing errors have occurred when cisplatin has been inadvertently substituted for carboplatin. Verify any cisplatin dose exceeding 100 mg/m^2/course.[2] Single doses of 100 mg/m^2 per course q 3 weeks are rarely used.[2]

IV push

Although rapid administration over 1–5 min has been used, it is associated with an increased risk of ototoxicity and nephrotoxicity.[1]

Intermittent infusion

Concentration not specified. Diluted in compatible fluid, it has been given over 15–20 min without adverse effects.[1,3-11]

Continuous infusion

The manufacturer recommends diluting the dose in 2 L of D5W and sodium containing fluid with 18.75 g mannitol/L and infusing over 6–8 h.[1,14] Other studies have reported stability at concentrations of 20, 50, 200, and 500 mg/L.[14] Although cisplatin has been infused over 6–8 h, 8–12 h, or as a 24-h infusion in order to decrease nephrotoxicity,[1] these various rates of administration have generally not been associated with a reduction in renal toxicity.[1]

Other routes of administration

Not administered IM. Has been given intra-arterial and intraperitoneal.[1]

Maximum concentration

Not established. The 1-mg/mL solution has an osmolality of 285 mOsm/kg.[14]

Cautions related to IV administration

Anaphylactic-like reactions, including facial edema, bronchoconstriction, tachycardia, and hypotension, may occur within minutes of administration. Epinephrine, corticosteroids, and antihistamines have been used.[1]

Because extravasation may cause tissue sloughing and necrosis, the infusion should be stopped if the patient complains of discomfort.[1,15] If extravasation occurs, attempt to remove any residual drug from tissues. Because of extravasation and infiltration risk, small veins in the dorsum of the hand or foot and scalp veins should be avoided if at all possible. Severity of tissue damage appears to occur more often when concentration of solution is >0.5 mg/mL.[1]

Skin reactions may occur following exposure; therefore, wear gloves when preparing and administering.[1] If exposure occurs, wash area with soap and water.

For PN compatibility information, please see Appendix C.

Other additives

None.

Comments

Aggressive hydration should be given to ensure good urinary output and reduce the likelihood of nephrotoxicity associated with cisplatin.[16] Several protocols have been advocated. One regimen consists of administration of 1–2 L of an NS-containing fluid over 8–12 h before cisplatin.[14] The manufacturer recommends diluting the dose in 2 L of compatible fluid containing 37.5 mg of mannitol and infusing over 6–8 h.[2] Others have given infusion over 15–120 min and by continuous infusion over 1–5 days.[14]

Renal function tests (e.g., SCr, BUN, CrCl) and electrolytes (e.g., magnesium, calcium, and potassium) should be monitored. Electrolyte supplementation may be necessary.[2]

Nephrotoxicity, neurotoxicity, and ototoxicity increase with cumulative doses.[16-24] Renal toxicity has been noted in 28% to 36% of patients treated with a single 50 mg/m^2/dose.[2]

Cisplatin is associated with a high (>90%) risk of emesis.[25] Patients should receive antiemetic therapy to prevent acute and delayed nausea and vomiting. The recommended therapy is a 5HT3 receptor antagonist in combination with dexamethasone on every day chemotherapy is administered.[25,26] These agents may be continued for up to 4 days after chemotherapy administration for the prevention of delayed nausea and vomiting. Breakthrough medications should also be offered, such as a phenothiazine (e.g., prochlorperazine), a butyrophenone (e.g., droperidol), a substituted benzamide (e.g., metoclopramide), or a benzodiazepine (e.g., lorazepam).

Ototoxicity (high-frequency hearing loss) is especially pronounced in children and is related to a cumulative cisplatin dose >200 mg/m^2.[1] An audiometric test should be performed before therapy is initiated and prior to each subsequent dose of medication.[2]

Needles, syringes, catheters, or IV administration sets that contain aluminum parts that may come in contact with cisplatin should not be used for preparation or administration of the drug, because this may result in precipitate formation.[14]

Clindamycin Phosphate

Brand names Cleocin Phosphate

Dosage

Neonates: Dose is based on postnatal age and weight[1-5] or postmenstrual and postnatal age.[6]

Postnatal Age and Weight[1-5]

PNA	<1200 g	1200–2000 g	>2000 g
<7 d	10 mg/kg/d divided q 12 h[1,2]*	10 mg/kg/d divided q 12 h[1,2]	15 mg/kg/d divided q 8 h[1,2]
≥7 d		15 mg/kg/d divided q 8 h[1,2]*	20–30 mg/kg/d divided q 6–8 h[1-5]

*Until 4 weeks of age.

or

5–7.5 mg/kg/dose using interval below.[6]

Postmenstrual Age and Postnatal Age[6]

Postmenstrual Age (weeks)	Postnatal Age (d)	Interval (h)
≤29	0 to 28	12
	>28	8
30 to 36	0 to 14	12
	>14	8
37 to 44	0 to 7	12
	>7	8
≥45	ALL	6

Infants and children

Mild-to-moderate infection: 15–30 mg/kg/d divided q 6–8 h.[1,7]

Severe infection: 25–40 mg/kg/d divided q 6–8 h.[1,2,8]

Bacterial endocarditis (dental, oral, respiratory tract, or esophageal procedures in penicillin-allergic patients): A single 20-mg/kg dose not to exceed 600 mg given 30–60 min prior to a procedure.[1]

Biochemical warfare or bioterrorism: The CDC and other experts recommend that treatment of inhalational anthrax spores due to biologic warfare or bioterrorism should be started on a multiple-drug parenteral regimen that includes ciprofloxacin or doxycycline and one or two additional anti-infective agents (i.e., chloramphenicol, clindamycin, rifampin, vancomycin, clarithromycin, imipenem, penicillin, or ampicillin).[9,10] Strains of *Bacillus anthracis* associated with cases that occurred in the U.S. during September and October 2001, following bioterrorism-related anthrax exposures, were susceptible to clindamycin *in vitro*.[10]

Surgical (colorectal, appendectomy, incision through the oral mucosa, ruptured viscus): 10 mg/kg/dose preoperative.[11-13]

Dosage adjustment in organ dysfunction

No dosage adjustment required in renal dysfunction.[14,15] Although dosage adjustment is recommended in severe hepatic dysfunction, no specific recommendations are available.

Maximum dosage

20 mg/kg up to 600 mg, not to exceed 4.8 g/d in *adults*.[1,16] Do not give more than 1.2 g in 1 h.[15]

IV push

Not recommended.[15] Hypotension and cardiopulmonary arrest may occur following rapid IV administration.[15]

Clindamycin Phosphate

Intermittent infusion	6–12 mg/mL in D5W, LR, or NS[13,15] or 18 mg/mL in D5W[17] given over 10–60 min.[17] Infusion rate should not exceed 30 mg/min,[13,15] or 1.2 g in an hour.[17]
Continuous infusion	Although solution concentration and type were not specified, 0.75–1.2 mg/min has been given by this method.[15]
Other routes of administration	Has been given IM, but induration, pain, and sterile abscesses are possible.[15] No information available to support administration by other routes.
Maximum concentration	18 mg/mL.[15]
Cautions related to IV administration	Thrombophlebitis and local erythema, pain, and swelling may occur.[15] Induration, pain, and sterile abscesses are possible with IM injection.[15] For PN compatibility information, please see Appendix C.
Other additives	**Benzyl alcohol:** Each mL contains 9.45 mg/mL of benzyl alcohol as a preservative.[15] Benzyl alcohol in small doses as a preservative in drugs is considered safe in newborns.[18] However, a 3-week-old, very low birth weight (710 g) infant who received clindamycin experienced a profound desaturation that required resuscitation after the third and fourth doses, which was subsequently related to the benzyl alcohol preservative.[19] Administration of saline flushes containing benzyl alcohol (bacteriostatic water for injection) was associated with a fatal gasping syndrome, intraventricular hemorrhage, metabolic acidosis, and increased mortality in preterm infants.[20] This should not be used in neonates. Hypersensitivity reactions to benzyl alcohol in parenteral products have been reported in *adults*.[21,22]
Comments	Intravenous clindamycin or vancomycin are recommended for antistaphylococcal coverage. In addition to MIC testing, a D-test should be performed by the clinical laboratory. A negative D-test suggests that the methicillin/oxacillin–resistant organism will not induce resistance to clindamycin during therapy; hence, the patient can be managed with clindamycin.[23] Severe and fatal *Clostridium difficile*–associated diarrhea and colitis (i.e., antibiotic-associated pseudomembranous colitis) has occurred in patients receiving clindamycin.[13] If bowel frequency changes and diarrhea persist, discontinue clindamycin, screen for *C. difficile* toxin, and treat accordingly. Although clindamycin may antagonize the bactericidal activity of several antibiotics (aminoglycosides, erythromycin) *in vitro*, antagonism has not been demonstrated *in vivo*.[16]

Co-Trimoxazole (Trimethoprim-Sulfamethoxazole)

Brand names	Bactrim IV, Septra IV
Dosage	Dosage is based on trimethoprim component. Each mL contains 16 mg trimethoprim and 80 mg sulfamethoxazole.[1] **Neonates:** Not recommended for those <2 months of age.[1] Sulfonamides may cause kernicterus in neonates by displacing bilirubin from plasma protein binding sites. **Infants and children** **Mild-to-moderate infections:** 8–12 mg/kg/d divided q 6–12 h.[1,2] Give up to 14 days for severe UTI and 5 days for shigellosis.[1] **Severe infections (for use in *Pneumocystis carinii* only):** See dosing below.[2] **Meningitis (not first-line; alternative therapy for *Listeria monocytogenes*):** 15–20 mg/kg/d divided q 6 h.[3-7] ***Pneumocystis carinii* pneumonia:** 15–20 mg/kg/d divided q 6 h for 14–21 days.[1,2,7-15]
Dosage adjustment in organ dysfunction	Adjust dosage in patients with renal dysfunction.[1,16-18] If CrCl is 15–30 mL/min, give 50% the normal dose; not recommended if CrCl <15 mL/min.[1]
Maximum dosage	20 mg/kg/d for *P. carinii* pneumonia[1,8-10] up to 4 g/d.[1]
IV push	Not recommended.[1]
Intermittent infusion	Dilute each 5 mL of drug in 125 mL D5W and infuse over 60–90 min.[1] May be added to 75 mL in fluid-restricted individuals[19]; however, it should be prepared and infused within 2 h.[1,20]
Continuous infusion	No information available to support administration by this method.
Other routes of administration	Not recommended.[1]
Maximum concentration	Diluted 5 mL of the concentrate (80 mg of trimethoprim) with 125 mL of D5W. May be added to 75 mL of D5W in fluid-restricted patients.[21]
Cautions related to IV administration	Skin necrosis may occur following extravasation.[1] Pain, local irritation, inflammation, and rarely thrombophlebitis may occur.[21] For PN compatibility information, please see Appendix C.

Co-Trimoxazole (Trimethoprim-Sulfamethoxazole)

Other additives

Sulfites: Contains sodium metabisulfite.[1] Sulfites may cause hypersensitivity reactions, which are more common in *adults* with asthma. Most reactions are mild but can include anaphylactic symptoms and life-threatening or less severe asthma episodes.[22-24] Epinephrine may be required in severe cases; and if the sulfite-free epinephrine product is not available, the sulfite-preserved epinephrine should be used.[22]

Propylene glycol: Contains propylene glycol,[1] which is added to parenteral drugs as a solubilizer. Rapid infusion of medications that contain propylene glycol has resulted in respiratory depression and cardiac dysrhythmias.[25] Its half-life is three times longer in neonates than in *adults*[22] and has caused hyperosmolality[26] and refractory seizures[27] in preterm neonates receiving 3 g/d.

Benzyl alcohol: Contains 1% benzyl alcohol as a preservative.[1] Benzyl alcohol in small doses is considered safe in newborns.[22] However, a 3-week-old, very low birth weight (710 g) infant who received clindamycin experienced a profound desaturation that required resuscitation after the third and fourth doses, which was subsequently related to the benzyl alcohol preservative.[28] Administration of saline flushes containing benzyl alcohol (BW) was associated with a fatal gasping syndrome, intraventricular hemorrhage, metabolic acidosis, and increased mortality in preterm infants.[29] This should not be used in neonates. Hypersensitivity reactions to benzyl alcohol in parenteral products have been reported in *adults*.[30,31]

Comments

Although rare, fatalities associated with sulfonamides have occurred due to severe hypersensitivity reactions, including Stevens-Johnson syndrome, toxic epidermal necrolysis, hepatic necrosis, agranulocytosis, and aplastic anemia.[1,21] Discontinue at first sign of rash.[1,21]

Can cause hemolysis in individuals with G6PD deficiency.[1]

Because folate depletion may worsen the psychomotor regression associated with the fragile X chromosome disorder, co-trimoxazole should be used with caution in these children.[21] Administration of folic acid will not affect the antibacterial effects of co-trimoxazole.[21]

Because co-trimoxazole is associated with numerous drug interactions, consult appropriate resources for dosing recommendations before combining any drug with co-trimoxazole.

Coagulation Factor VIIa (Recombinant) (rFVIIa)

Brand names NovoSeven

Dosage

Hemophilia A or B with inhibitors to Factor VIII or IX[1,2]

Prophylaxis for surgery/invasive procedures: 90 mcg/kg immediately prior to surgery; repeat at 2 h intervals during the procedure and continue for 48 h postsurgery. The interval should be extended to 2–6 h until healing. For major surgery, continue q 2 h dosing for 5 days followed by q 4 h intervals until healing.

Treatment: 90 mcg/kg q 2 h until hemostasis occurs or treatment is felt to be ineffective. Doses of 35–120 mcg/kg have been effective; therefore, the dose and interval may be adjusted based on bleeding severity. After severe bleeds, dosing at q 3–6 h intervals may continue after hemostasis is achieved.

Congenital factor VII deficiency

Treatment and prophylaxis for surgery/invasive procedures: 15–30 mcg/kg q 4–6 h until hemostasis.[1,2] A 3-year-old with cleft palate received 15 mcg/kg beginning 20 min prior to surgery for repair and q 12 h for 3 days and did not have any bleeding events.[3]

Use of rFVIIa in patients without hemophilia may be associated with an increased risk for development of thrombosis.[4] However, several reports of its use in children without hemophilia have been described. In most cases, the use of rFVIIa was only after aggressive use of standard therapies had failed.

Cardiac surgery with cardiopulmonary bypass

Surgery related bleeding: Eight children from 5 days to 8 years of age received 30 or 60 mcg/kg repeated in 15 min and again in 2 h if bleeding continued.[5] A single 70-mcg/kg dose was effective in a 4-month-old with bleeding after atrial septal defect (ASD) repair.[6] A series of five patients that included a 2½-year-old child reported that 30 mcg/kg was effective in decreasing blood loss during and postcardiac surgery.[7] A 9-month-old received two doses of 90 mcg/kg for intraoperative bleeding during cardiopulmonary bypass. In this child, additional fresh frozen plasma was given, and hemostasis was achieved 2 h after the rFVIIa was given.[8]

Bleeding during ECMO: An 11-year-old and a 13-year-old were given 90 mcg/kg q 4 h for three doses or q 2 h for 10 doses to control bleeding.[9] Four children from age 6 days to 33 months were given two doses of 90–120 mcg/kg 4 h apart.[10] All except the 13-year-old were on ECMO after open heart surgery. (See Comments section.)

Miscellaneous bleeding: Four days after cardiac surgery, a 10-month-old male with Noonan syndrome developed gastrointestinal bleeding that was unresponsive to standard treatment.[11] He initially responded to a 90-mcg/kg dose but began bleeding again after about 8 h. Two more doses were given and the bleeding stopped. Another 16-month-old being treated for acute megakaryoblastic leukemia developed severe gastrointestinal tract bleeding that responded to 100 mcg/kg given at 0, 2, and 12 h.[12]

Liver failure coagulopathy

Bleeding management: Twenty-two children with liver disease received doses ranging from 36–118 mcg/kg to treat a variety of bleeding episodes.[13,14] One child was thought to have portal vein thrombosis; however, this could not be confirmed.[14] A 3-month-old, a 9-year-old, and an 11-year-old received 67 mcg/kg × 3, 130 mcg/kg × 2, and 200 mcg/kg to control bleeding from various sources.[15] Following a right hepatectomy, a 5-month-old boy with internal bleeding was given a single 90-mcg/kg dose followed by an infusion of fibrinogen concentrate, and bleeding stopped shortly thereafter.[16]

Prior to invasive procedure: Six children (2 months to 15 years) received doses of 34–163 mcg/kg prior to liver biopsy and other invasive procedures.[14]

Coagulation Factor VIIa (Recombinant) (rFVIIa)

Dosage (cont.)

During transplant: 100- and 300-mcg/kg doses were given prior to transplant in a 7-month-old, a 2½-year-old, and a 7-year-old.[15,17] A second dose was given after 2 h and during transplant in one of these.[17] Seven children with bleeding after liver graft reperfusion received 37–168 mcg/kg that resulted in improved hemostasis.[18] While no postoperative thrombotic events were noted in these children, one group described four *adults* undergoing liver transplantation who received 90 mcg/kg preoperatively and intraoperatively. One developed portal vein thrombosis and another myocardial ischemia leading the authors to express concern over the potential for thrombotic complications.[19]

Congenital platelet disorders: A 15-year-old girl with Bernard Soulier syndrome received 98 mcg/kg × 2 that controlled severe menorrhagia. On a separate occasion she received two doses of 98 and 122.5 mcg/kg that controlled severe epistaxis and mild menorrhagia.[20] In a report describing four children with Glanzmann's thrombasthenia, 89–116 mcg/kg q 2 h was given until bleeding stopped.[21] In a study evaluating use as a primary therapy in seven children with Bernard Soulier syndrome or Glanzmann's thrombasthenia, 100 mcg/kg q 90 min × 3 was more effective in preventing bleeding from a planned intervention than treating an established bleed.[22]

Use in preterm neonates

Intraventricular hemorrhage (IVH): Ten neonates received 100 mcg/kg q 4 h for 3 days to prevent IVH.[26] Two infants developed IVH; one progressed from Grade II to III, and one with Grade III died. The two with umbilical artery catheters developed thrombi at the catheter tip. The incidence of IVH was not different from that seen in neonates who did not receive rFVIIa leading the authors to conclude this should not be used prophylactically but rather should be studied in placebo-controlled trials. One other group described a neonate with an apparent IVH who was given 80 mcg/kg.[24] The bleeding stopped; however, the IVH was Grade IV and the infant did not survive.

Necrotizing enterocolitis (NEC): During surgical management of NEC, four very low birth weight infants with intraoperative bleeding received either 90 mcg/kg as a single dose, 100 mcg/kg × 2, 300 mcg/kg × 2, or 400 mcg/kg × 2.[27] Bleeding was controlled in three of the four infants. One infant developed a brachial artery thrombus necessitating thrombectomy and arterial reconstruction. Another of these infants had transient ischemia of the distal phalanges. (See Comments section.)

Pulmonary hemorrhage: One very low birth weight infant received two daily doses of 50 mcg/kg given 3 h apart for 3 days and another received 50 mcg/kg q 3 h for 48 h.[23] In both neonates coagulation parameters were stabilized, and both survived to be discharged home. Two other preterm neonates with pulmonary hemorrhage received 80 mcg/kg or 120 mcg/kg × 3 given 2 h apart, had resolution of bleeding, and did not experience any complication.[24,25] Of note, one of these preterm infants developed pulmonary hemorrhage 8 h after the dose.[24]

Dosage adjustment in organ dysfunction

No dose modification for renal dysfunction is recommended.

Maximum dosage

Not established. Overdoses of 246–986 mcg/kg have been reported without thrombotic complications.[1] Antibodies against rFVIIa were detected in a newborn with congenital factor VII deficiency who received 800 mcg/kg rFVIIa.[1]

IV push

Over 3–5 min.[1]

Intermittent infusion

No information available to support administration by this method.

Coagulation Factor VIIa (Recombinant) (rFVIIa)

Continuous infusion	Not recommended. However, a bolus dose followed by a short-term (24 h–5 days) continuous infusion has been reported in patients with hemophilia, factor VII deficiency, and platelet disorders who experience severe bleeding or require surgery.[28-30] Factor VII concentration monitoring is recommended to determine maintenance infusion rate (target concentration 10 international units/mL).[29] (See Cautions related to IV administration section.)
Other routes of administration	No information available to support administration by other routes.
Maximum concentration	600 mcg/mL.[1]
Cautions related to IV administration	Reconstituted solution must be administered within 3 h.[1] Anaphylactic reactions may occur in patients with known hypersensitivity reactions to mouse, hamster, or bovine proteins.[1] Thrombophlebitis occurs when undiluted rFVIIa is infused via continuous infusion.[29] It has been suggested that a parallel infusion of saline (20 mL/h) into same vein as undiluted rFVIIa will minimize the thrombophlebitis.[29] Selection of infusion pump devices appears to be crucial to success of continuous infusions with greatest experience reported with the CADD®-Plus minipump (Pharmacia Deltec, St Paul, MN).[28]
Other additives	Each mg contains 0.44 mEq sodium and 0.06 mEq calcium.[1] Reconstituted vials contain 0.1 mg polysorbate 80/mL and 30 mg mannitol/mL.[1]
Comments	Pharmacokinetics studies indicate a shorter half-life, more rapid clearance, and larger volume of distribution at steady state in children than in *adults*.[31] A review of the thromboembolic adverse events reported to the Food and Drug Association suggested that rFVIIa might be more thrombogenic in those without hemophilia.[4] Those at increased risk of thrombotic events may include patients with disseminated intravascular coagulation (DIC), atherosclerosis, crush injury, sepsis, or who are undergoing concomitant treatment with activated or nonactivated prothrombin complex concentrates.[1] An infant on ECMO developed thrombotic occlusions of both subclavian arteries and truncus brachiocephalicus after receiving rFVIIa for uncontrollable bleeding.[32] The infant had received numerous other coagulation products prior to receipt of rFVIIa. Avoid mixing with other infusion solutions.[1] Incompatibility with heparin was reported when used in continuous infusions.[28]

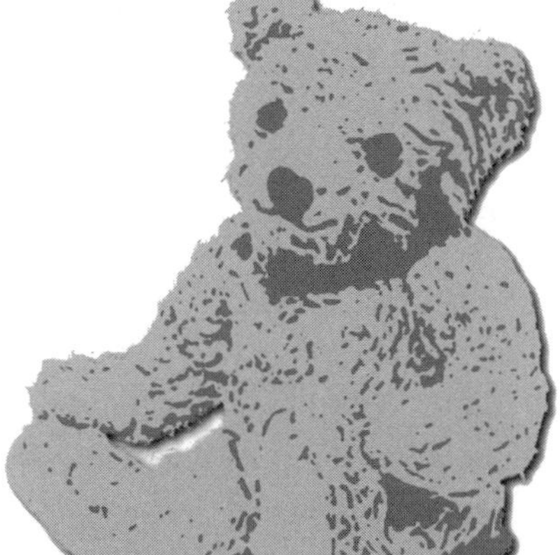

Cyclophosphamide

Brand names	Cytoxan, Neosar
Dosage	Consult institutional protocol for complete dosing information. Cyclophosphamide is used as a component of combination therapy to treat both oncologic and nononcologic diseases. Specifically, it is approved by the Food and Drug Administration (FDA) for the oncologic treatment of lymphomas, Hodgkin's disease, multiple myeloma, leukemias, mycosis fungoides, neuroblastoma, ovarian adenocarcinoma, retinoblastoma, and breast cancer.[1] Nononcologic FDA indications include pediatric minimal change nephritic syndrome.[1] It may also be used in systemic lupus erythematosus, juvenile rheumatoid arthritis and vasculitis, and in consolidation therapy prior to an autologous bone marrow transplantation, although its use here is not established.[2] Selected dosage regimens include the following: **Pediatric solid tumors:** 40–50 mg/kg IV (1.5–1.8 g/m^2) in divided doses over 2–5 days.[1,3,4] Other regimens include 10–15 mg/kg (350–550 mg/m^2) given q 7–10 d or 3–5 mg/kg (110–185 mg/m^2) twice weekly.[1,3-5] **SLE:** 500–750 mg/m^2 every month, maximum dose: 1 g/m^2.[4,6] Continuous daily doses: 60–120 mg/m^2 (1–2.5 mg/kg) every day.[2,7] **BMT conditioning regimen**: 50 mg/kg IV once daily for 3–4 days.[4,8]
Dosage adjustment in organ dysfunction	If CrCl is <10 mL/min, administer 75% of the usual dosage.[1]
Maximum dosage	Not established.
IV push	Dilute with NS for direct injection/IV push.[1] The vial should be shaken to dissolve all cyclophosphamide powder.
Intermittent infusion	Dilute cyclophosphamide with SW and shake vial to dissolve all powder. Further dilute solution with NS, ½NS, D5W, D5NS, D5R, LR, or sodium lactate injection ⅙ M.[1,3,9] Most infusions occur over 30–60 min.[4] If the dosage is >1800 mg/m^2, the infusion should last 4–6 h.
Continuous infusion	Although cyclophosphamide may be administered continuously,[2,7,9] its use is not established.
Other routes of administration	Cyclophosphamide has been administered IM,[9] but use is not established. IM administration may be less effective as this route bypasses the liver.[3] May also be given intraperitoneally or intrapleurally.[9] Reconstitute with NS if administering via IM, intraperitoneal, or intrapleural route.[1]

Maximum concentration	20–25 mg/mL.[1,9]
Cautions related to IV administration	Hypotonic solution should not be directly injected.[1] For PN compatibility information, please see Appendix C.
Other additives	Mannitol 75 mg/100 mg cyclophosphamide.[9]
Comments	Cyclophosphamide is associated with hemorrhagic cystitis.[1] Patients should be encouraged to drink excess fluids and void frequently starting 24 h before therapy and continuing 24 h after therapy.[1,3] Mesna therapy has also been used with high dosages of cyclophosphamide (i.e., dosages >1 g/m^2/d).[3] The urine should be examined for the presence of red blood cells, an indicator of hemorrhagic cystitis. Although rare, cardiac toxicity has been reported at dosages ranging from 2.4–26 g/m^2.[1] Cyclophosphamide is associated with long-term gonadal function damage and infertility in pediatric patients.[1,3] Cyclophosphamide is associated with a high (>90%) risk of emesis in IV dosages >1500 mg/m^2 and a moderate (30% to 90%) risk of emesis with IV dosages ≤1500 mg/m^2.[10] Patients should receive antiemetic therapy to prevent acute and delayed nausea and vomiting. The recommended therapy is a 5HT3 receptor antagonist in combination with dexamethasone every day chemotherapy is administered.[10,11] These agents may be continued for up to 4 days after chemotherapy administration for the prevention of delayed nausea and vomiting. Breakthrough medications should also be offered, such as a phenothiazine (e.g., prochlorperazine), a butyrophenone (e.g., droperidol), a substituted benzamide (e.g., metoclopramide), or a benzodiazepine (e.g., lorazepam).

Cyclosporine

Brand names	Sandimmune
Dosage	Change to oral therapy as soon as possible. **Transplant immunosuppression (bone marrow transplant (BMT), cardiac, liver, and renal):** 2 mg/kg q 8 h beginning prior to transplant[1] or 1–10 mg/kg/d divided q 8–24 h[1-8] or via continuous infusion.[9-14] In renal transplant, a 24-h intraoperative continuous infusion of 165 mg/m^2/d was given to those <6 years of age and 4.5 mg/kg/d to those ≥6 years of age.[14] **Recurrent nephrotic syndrome post transplant:** Continuous infusion of 3 mg/kg/d titrated to maintain desired serum concentrations.[15] **Prevention of graft vs. host disease:** 1–5 mg/kg/d either continuously or in two divided doses beginning up to 7 days before transplant with or without titration to desired trough concentrations.[16-21] **Acute myeloid leukemia:** 10 mg/kg followed by a continuous infusion of 30 mg/kg/d for a period of 98 h as part of a mitoxantrone, etoposide, and cyclosporine (MEC) induction regimen.[22] **Inflammatory bowel disease refractory to steroids:** 1.3–4 mg/kg/d by continuous infusion or 5 mg/kg/d by intermittent infusion.[23-28] (See Comments section.) **Atypical sprue:** Diarrhea resolved and histology improved in a 23-month-old started on 2 mg/kg q 12 h that was increased to 4 mg/kg q 12 h.[29]
Dosage adjustment in organ dysfunction	No dosage adjustment required in renal dysfunction.[30] However, nephrotoxicity occurs in 25% to 38% of patients.[31] This appears to be dose related and may be associated with high trough concentrations.[31] (See Comments section.)
Maximum dosage	Not established.
IV push	Contraindicated.[31,32]
Intermittent infusion	0.5–2.5 mg/mL in D5W or NS[31,32] over 2–8 h.[2,3,7,23-28,31,32] Cyclosporine reconstituted with D5W is stable for 24 h in glass or PVC. Cyclosporine reconstituted with NS is stable for 12 h in glass and 6 h in PVC.[33] Storage of reconstituted drug in glass bottles has been recommended.[33,34] (See Comments section.)
Continuous infusion	1.2–4.5 mg/kg have been given over 24 h.[9-14]
Other routes of administration	No information available to support administration by other routes.
Maximum concentration	2.5 mg/mL.[32]

Cautions related to IV administration

Anaphylaxis has occurred.[35-38]

For PN compatibility information, please see Appendix C.

Other additives

Contains polyoxyethylated castor oil 650 mg (Cremophor EL) and 32.9% alcohol by volume.[32] Anaphylaxis may be a result of the Cremophor EL vehicle.[35-37] In phase I/II trials of high-dose cyclosporine (13–30 mg/kg) for multidrug-resistant tumors in 21 children, anaphylactoid reactions occurred in five patients due to improper mixing of the Cremophor EL vehicle.[38] With high-dose cyclosporine, it was recommended that a homogenous mixture be achieved and premedication with antihistamine and corticosteroid be administered.[38,39] Anaphylaxis requires immediate emergency treatment with epinephrine, oxygen, IV steroids, and airway management.

Comments

Serum concentration monitoring is essential to determining the appropriate dosage. Trough concentrations should be maintained within therapeutic range for the specific assay and transplant type[40-42]; however, trough concentration monitoring is being replaced by C2 (a 2-h concentration), as it better approximates AUC_{0-4}, which has been correlated with the risk of rejection.[43,44] Use the same analytical methodology and sample matrix (i.e., whole blood vs. plasma) consistently. HPLC assays are specific for cyclosporine. Cyclosporine metabolites cross-react with polyclonal radioimmunoassay[45] and fluorescence polarization immunoassay (FPIA), which may result in an overestimation of serum concentrations compared to other methods.[40,41,45,46] The FPIA assay may not be reliable in liver dysfunction.[40,42]

In renal transplant patients, it is often difficult to determine if a decrease in renal function is due to nephrotoxicity or allograft rejection.[31]

Cyclosporine is adsorbed to silicone; blood samples drawn through central venous lines made from silicone may be falsely elevated if cyclosporine has been infused through them.[47]

Concentrations drawn through a second lumen may be erroneously increased when the patient is receiving cyclosporine as a continuous infusion through the other lumen.[49]

Cyclosporine is principally metabolized by the CYP3A4 isoenzyme and is associated with numerous drug interactions.[31] Consult appropriate resources for dosing recommendations before combining any drug with cyclosporine.

Cyclosporine is adsorbed to PVC; up to 10% of a dose may be bound to PVC tubing during infusion. If PVC bags are also used, up to 30% of a dose may be lost to adsorption. In addition, the Cremophor EL vehicle can leach diethylhexylphthalate (DEHP), a known hepatotoxin, from PVC. If PVC bags are used, solutions should be administered immediately to minimize patient exposure to DEHP.[50] One study found that DEHP was not detectable until >4.5 h of contact with PVC using 0.5–2.5 mg/mL of cyclosporine.[51]

The IV dose is approximately one-third of the oral dose.[31,32]

Cytomegalovirus Immunoglobulin

Brand names	CytoGam

Dosage

HIV-infected patients: 200 mg/kg alternating biweekly with IV immune globulin.[1]

Transfusions (multiple) in neonates: 150 mg/kg.[2]

Transplantation

Bone marrow: 200 mg/kg given 6 and 8 days prior to transplant and on days 1, 7, 14, 21, 28, 42, 56, and 70 after transplant.[3]

Heart, liver, lung, and pancreas: 150 mg/kg within 72 h prior to transplant, 150 mg/kg at 2, 4, 6, and 8 weeks after transplant, and 100 mg/kg at 12 and 16 weeks after transplant.[4-6]

Liver and intestine: 100 mg/kg (on alternating day from ganciclovir) followed by 150 mg/kg at weeks 6 and 8 followed by 100 mg/kg at 12 and 18 weeks after transplant.[6]

Renal: 150 mg/kg within 72 h prior to transplant, 100 mg/kg at 2, 4, 6, and 8 weeks after transplant, and 50 mg/kg at 12 and 16 weeks after transplant.[4,7,8]

Infantile cytomegalovirus-associated autoimmune hemolytic anemia: one dose of 500 mg/kg.[9]

Dosage adjustment in organ dysfunction

Use with caution in patients with renal insufficiency or in those at risk for developing renal insufficiency.[4] In order to decrease the risk of renal dysfunction, patients should be well-hydrated prior to administration.[4]

Maximum dosage

For transplant patients, the manufacturer recommends a 150 mg/kg maximum dose. 200 mg/kg has been given in HIV infection and multiple transfusions in neonates.[1,3] 500 mg/kg has been administered to two infants for autoimmune hemolytic anemia.[9]

IV push

Not recommended.[4]

Intermittent infusion

May piggyback into existing infusions of NS or D2.5W, D5W, D10W, D20W (all with or without NaCl) and deliver via an infusion device at no more than 1:2 dilution.[4]

Initial dose[4]: 15 mg/kg/h for 30 min. If no adverse effects are noted, increase to 30 mg/kg/h for 30 min and then to maximum rate of 60 mg/kg/h. (See Comments section.)

Subsequent infusions[4]: 15 mg/kg/h for 15 min. If no adverse effects are noted, increase to 30 mg/kg/h for 15 min and then to a maximum rate of 60 mg/kg/h. (See Comments section.)

Volume should not exceed 75 mL/h.[4]

Continuous infusion

No information available.

Other routes of administration

Not recommended.[4]

Cytomegalovirus Immunoglobulin

Maximum concentration	50 mg/mL.[4]
Cautions related to IV administration	Monitor vital signs during infusion. Flushing, chills, muscle cramps, back pain, fever, vomiting, arthralgias, and wheezing are usually related to infusion rate and may be managed by interrupting the infusion temporarily and restarting at a lower rate. Epinephrine should be available in case of anaphylaxis.[4]
Other additives	Each mL contains 50 mg sucrose and 10 mg human serum albumin. Sodium content is 20–30 mEq/L.[4]
Comments	Cytomegalovirus immune globulin does not contain any preservatives; thus, the infusion should be initiated within 6 h of entering the vial.[4] The product should be infused through an in-line filter with a pore size of 15 microns. A 0.2-micron filter is also acceptable.[4] An initial dose of 150 mg/kg requires infusion over approximately 3 h and 10 min; subsequent doses of 150 mg/kg can be infused in about 20 min less time.[4] Vaccinations with live virus vaccines (measles, mumps, rubella, varicella) should be deferred for 6 months after CytoGam infusion.[10]

Dactinomycin

Brand names	Cosmegen
Dosage	Consult institutional protocol for complete dosing information. Dactinomycin is used as a component of combination therapy for several malignant pediatric solid tumors. Dactinomycin has also been used in patients with nephroblastoma, malignant melanoma, and osteosarcoma. Dosage should be based on body surface area (BSA) for obese or edematous patients.(1) Suggested regimens for different disease states include the following: **Wilms' tumor, rhabdomyosarcoma, Ewing's sarcoma:** 15 mcg/kg/d IV for 5 days in combination with chemotherapeutic agents.(1-5) **Metastatic nonseminatous testicular cancer:** 1000 mcg/m^2/d IV on day 1 with cyclophosphamide, bleomycin, vinblastine, and cisplatin.(1,6) **Gestational trophoblastic neoplasia**: 12 mcg/kg/d IV for 5 days as monotherapy or 500 mcg IV on days 1 and 2 as part of a combination regimen with etoposide, methotrexate, folinic acid, vincristine, cyclophosphamide, and cisplatin.(1,7,8) **Regional perfusion in locally recurrent and locoregional solid malignancies:** 50 mcg/kg for lower extremity or pelvis; 35 mcg/kg for upper extremity.(1)
Dosage adjustment in organ dysfunction	Not established.
Maximum dosage	The manufacturer recommends that dosages should not exceed 15 mcg/kg/d or 400–600 mg/m^2/d for 5 days per 2-week cycle.(1)
IV push	Reconstitute with 1.1 mL of SW to a concentration of 500 mcg/mL. Use of SW containing preservatives is not recommended as it results in precipitation formation.(1,9) The desired dose may be injected into the tubing of a running infusion of NS or D5W.(1,9) Filters should not be used.(9)
Intermittent infusion	Reconstitute with 1.1 mL of SW to a concentration of 500 mcg/mL. Use of SW containing preservatives is not recommended as it results in precipitation formation.(1,9) Further dilute reconstituted solution with NS or D5W or the desired dose may be injected into the tubing of a running infusion of NS or D5W.(1,9) Filters should not be used.(9)
Continuous infusion	No information available to support administration by this method.
Other routes of administration	Do not administer as IM or SC injection.(9) Dactinomycin is highly corrosive and will damage soft tissue.
Maximum concentration	500 mcg/mL.(1)
Cautions related to IV administration	A black box warning exists summarizing the highly toxic nature of dactinomycin.(1) Both the powder and solution can cause severe damage when in direct contact with the skin or through inhalation. Extravasation will result in severe soft tissue damage. If extravasation occurs, ice should be applied to the affected area immediately for 30–60 min.(1) It has been suggested to ice 15 min four times daily for 3 days.

Other additives	Contains 20 mg mannitol/vial.[1]

Comments

Dactinomycin has been associated with the development of hepatic veno-occlusive disease in children <48 months.[1,10]

Dactinomycin has been associated with an increased risk of dermatological adverse effects when used concomitantly with or after radiation.[1] Risks may be increased when radiation involves mucous membranes or when dactinomycin is administered within 2 months of radiation for right-sided Wilms' tumors.

Dactinomycin should not be used in infants <6 months based on a higher incidence of side effects.[1]

Dactinomycin is associated with a moderate (30% to 90%) risk of emesis.[11] Patients should receive antiemetic therapy to prevent acute and delayed nausea and vomiting. The recommended therapy is a 5HT3 receptor antagonist in combination with dexamethasone every day chemotherapy is administered.[11,12] These agents may be continued for up to 4 days after chemotherapy administration for the prevention of delayed nausea and vomiting. Breakthrough medications should also be offered, such as a phenothiazine (e.g., prochlorperazine), a butyrophenone (e.g., droperidol), a substituted benzamide (e.g., metoclopramide), or a benzodiazepine (e.g., lorazepam).

Darbepoietin

Brand names	Aranesp

Dosage

To ensure the erythropoietic response, iron status should be evaluated and supplemental iron prescribed if stores are low. Transferrin saturation should be ≥20% and ferritin should be ≥100 ng/mL.[1]

Anemia in (nonmyeloid or solid tumor) cancer [7-12]: Safety and efficacy of darbepoietin in anemia of childhood cancer has not been established. The following dosages have been used in *adults:*

1–4.5 mcg/kg SC once weekly[9,10]

3–9 mcg/kg SC q 2 weeks[11]

4.5–15 mcg/kg q 3 weeks[12]

A dose-response relationship has been established in *adults* with respect to hemoglobin (Hb) response. Adjust dosage (weekly) to achieve target Hb concentration.

If Hb has increased by <1 g/dL during initial 6 weeks of therapy (with adequate iron stores), then increase dose by 25% every week (up to 4.5 mcg/kg/dose) until at target Hb concentration. If Hb has increased >1 g/dL over a 2-week period or the Hb concentration exceeds 12 g/dL, then decrease dose by 25%. If Hb exceeds 13 g/dL, then temporally hold therapy.

Anemia of chronic renal insufficiency[1-8]

1–16 years: 0.25–0.75 mcg/kg IV or SC once weekly.[2-4] (See Comments section.)

Adjust dosage (monthly) to achieve and maintain a Hb concentration of 12 g/dL or less.

If Hb has increased <1 g/dL during initial 4 weeks of therapy (with adequate iron stores), then increase dose by 25% q 4 weeks until at target Hb. If the Hb increases by more than 1 g/dL in 2 weeks or the Hb is increasing and approaching 12 g/dL, then decrease dose by 25%.[1]

<8 kg (use not established): 0.5 mcg/kg once weekly was given to six infants with renal dysplasia, three on peritoneal dialysis.[5] Doses were increased or decreased by 25% to maintain Hb concentrations 10–11 g/dL. After 20 weeks, in three stable patients (one on peritoneal dialysis) Hb ranged from 11.7–13.5 g/dL, and doses were 0.17 or 0.25 mcg/kg q 4 weeks or 0.34 mcg/kg q 3 weeks. In three medically unstable patients, Hb ranged from 8.5–9.7 g/dL, and doses were 1.06–1.24 mcg/kg weekly. Investigators concluded that individualized dosing was warranted.

Anemia of prematurity (use not established): Erythropoid progenitor cells in cord blood, fetal marrow, and fetal liver were equally stimulated by erythropoietin and darbepoietin.[13] In a pharmacokinetics study, a single dose of 1 or 4 mcg/kg SC increased erythropoiesis in preterm infants <1500 g.[14] Another pharmacokinetic study evaluated a 4-mcg/kg IV dose in 10 neonates 704–3025 g and found a shorter half-life and more rapid clearance than has been noted in children.[15] In addition, both the immature reticulocyte count and the absolute reticulocyte count increased.[15]

Dosage adjustment in organ dysfunction	Patients with chronic renal insufficiency who are not on dialysis may require lower maintenance doses.[1]
Maximum dosage	Not established. Doses up to 8 mcg/kg once weekly and 15 mcg/kg q 3 weeks have been used in *adults* with cancer.[11,12]
IV push	Rapid, within 15 sec.[2]

Intermittent infusion	No information to support this method of administration.
Continuous infusion	No information to support this method of administration.
Other routes of administration	SC route is preferred except in patients on hemodialysis when IV administration is preferred.(1) IM is not indicated.
Maximum concentration	500 mcg/mL.(1,7,8)
Cautions related to IV administration	Rare serious allergic reactions have been reported.(1,8) While not fully evaluated, darbepoietin may act as a growth factor for myeloid malignancies.(1,8) Do not administer with any other IV drug.
Other additives	Each mL contains 2.5 mg of human albumin, 2.23 mg sodium phosphate monobasic monohydrate, 0.53 mg sodium phosphate dibasic anhydrous, and 8.18 mg sodium chloride in water for injection (albumin solution) *or* 0.05 mg polysorbate 80, 2.12 mg sodium phosphate monobasic monohydrate, 0.66 mg sodium phosphate dibasic anhydrous, and 8.18 mg sodium chloride in water for injection (polysorbate solution).(1,8)
Comments	One study in children with chronic renal insufficiency based the initial dose on current recombinant human erythropoietin dosing (rHuEPO dose/200 = darbepoietin weekly dose).(4) Investigators noted an excessive increase in Hb in six of seven children evaluated. The two youngest received 3.6 and 2.79 mcg/kg weekly and developed hypertension (Hb was >13 g/dL). The dose was held for 2 weeks and restarted at half the previous dose. At the end of 6 months, doses in all seven patients ranged from 0.37–0.69 mcg/kg weekly. This is consistent with the manufacturers' current recommendations.(1) Vigorous shaking and/or exposure to light may physically denature the glycoprotein and inactive the molecule.(1) Monitor Hb weekly until target is achieved, then monthly.(1)

Deferoxamine Mesylate

Brand names	Desferal Mesylate

Dosage

Iron exposure

Acute iron ingestion: While the manufacturer states that IM administration is the preferred route and should be used for all patients not in shock,[1] toxicology literature supports the IV administration of deferoxamine for acute iron poisoning.[2]

15 mg/kg/h by continuous infusion[1-5] until urine is a normal color for 24 h[4,5] or until clinical status and laboratory values normalize. Alternatively, an initial dose of 20 mg/kg or 600 mg/m^2 (IM or slow IV infusion) followed by 10 mg/kg or 300 mg/m^2 q 4 h for two doses.[6] Subsequent doses of 10 mg/kg or 300 mg/m^2 q 4–12 h are given as clinically needed.[6]

Chronic iron overload due to transfusion-dependent anemias: 14–98 mg/kg/d over 8–12 h.[7-9] Individualize dose based on the degree of iron overload. Doses that exceed a "therapeutic index" (ratio of mean daily dose in mg/kg divided by serum ferritin) >0.025 increase the risk for sensorineural hearing loss.[9]

Aluminum-related disorders in kidney disease (use not established): To avoid deferoxamine induced adverse effects (neurotoxicity), it should not be given to patients with an initial serum aluminum >200 mcg/L. Treat these patients with intensive high flux dialysis until serum aluminum <200 mcg/L.[10]

Deferoxamine test: 5 mg/kg given during last hour of dialysis session. Measure serum aluminum before infusion and 2 days later (before next dialysis session). Doses as low as 0.5 mg/kg have also been used.[10]

Aluminum rise <300 mcg/L and no side effects after test: 5 mg/kg IV over last hour of hemodialysis, once per week for 2 months; high flux hemodialysis 44 h after dose.

Aluminum rise >300 mcg/L or side effects after test: 5 mg/kg IV over 1 h; give 5 h before hemodialysis, once per week for 4 months; high flux hemodialysis after deferoxamine.

Dosage adjustment in organ dysfunction

While one reference reports no adjustment in dosage in patients with renal dysfunction,[11] the manufacturer states that deferoxamine is contraindicated in patients with severe renal dysfunction or anuria because the drug and the iron chelate are renally eliminated.[1] Another reference states that therapy should continue in renal failure; however, the infusion rate should be adjusted. No guidelines for adjusting rate are given.[2]

Maximum dosage

Although the manufacturer recommends that total amounts should not exceed 6 g/24 h,[1] these doses may be exceeded in clinical practice.[2]

16 g was infused to an *adult* with transfusion-related iron overload over 24 h without apparent adverse effects.[12] While doses >50 mg/kg/d (up to 235 mg/kg/d) have been used,[7-9,13-15] doses <50–60 mg/kg/d are recommended to avoid neurotoxicity. (See Comments section.)[16]

IV push

Not recommended.[1] (See Cautions related to IV administration section.)

Intermittent infusion

250 mg/mL in D5W, LR, or NS.[1] Not to exceed 15 mg/kg/h.[1]

Continuous infusion	250 mg/mL in D5W, LR, or NS.[1] Not to exceed 15 mg/kg/h.[1]
Other routes of administration	IM is preferred route of administration in acute iron ingestion in patients not in shock.[1] 50 mg/kg IM q 6 h as clinically indicated.[1] Not to exceed 6 g/d.[1]
Maximum concentration	250 mg/mL.[1]
Cautions related to IV administration	Flushing, urticaria, hypotension, and shock may occur,[18] particularly with rapid IV administration.[1,17-19] Anaphylaxis may occur.[1]
Other additives	None.

Comments

Protect from light.

Patients with chronic iron overload usually become vitamin-C deficient. *Adults* with chronic iron overload have developed cardiac impairment following concomitant treatment with deferoxamine and high doses of vitamin C. The abnormalities reversed when vitamin C was discontinued.[1] Recommended daily vitamin C doses should not be exceeded.

Urine may not always be vin rosé color with administration of deferoxamine, even when iron overload is present.[20]

Vision and hearing impairment has been attributed to chronic chelation treatment with deferoxamine.[3,9,14-16,18,21-22] Cessation of chelation therapy and/or dosage reduction frequently leads to improvement.[15,18,19,21]

A pulmonary syndrome has been associated with prolonged continuous infusion[14,18,23-26] and total daily doses >6 g.[27] Another study suggests that the pulmonary abnormalities are related to inadequate chelation.[28] Intermittent infusions for <24 h have been recommended[24,29] but are investigational.

Nephrotoxicity has also been reported.[22] Adequate hydration decreases the incidence of this adverse effect.[22]

Neurotoxicity has been reported.[3,7-9,15,16,18,21] Large doses may exacerbate neurologic dysfunction (i.e., seizures) in patients with aluminum-related encephalopathy.[1]

Growth retardation has occurred in patients with low ferritin concentrations who receive large doses of deferoxamine. Following reduction in the deferoxamine dose, growth velocity may partially return to pretreatment rate. Pediatric patients should be monitored for body weight and growth q 3 mo.[1]

Although rare, deferoxamine has been associated with an increased risk of infection. This is particularly true for *Yersinia enterocolitica* and *Yersinia pseudotuberculosis*. Mucormycosis has also been reported, particularly in dialysis patients.[1,10] The drug should be discontinued until any suspected or documented infection resolves.[1]

Dexamethasone Sodium Phosphate

Brand names	Decaject, Solurex, Decadron, generic

Dosage

Prevention of chronic lung disease in very low birth weight infants (VLBW): 0.25–0.5 mg/kg/d tapered over 14–42 days.[1,2] Alternatively, 0.5 mg/kg/d for 3 days followed by 0.25 mg/kg/d for 3 days and then 0.1 mg/kg/d on day 7.[3] Of note, a multicenter study was stopped early because of concerns over side effects in the steroid group.[4] The AAP recommends limited use of dexamethasone in this group because of the association with serious complications.[5] (See Comments section.)

Extubation

Preterm infants: 0.25 mg/kg q 8 h for three doses[6] or 0.15 mg/kg/d for 3 days followed by 0.1 mg/kg/d for 3 days and then 0.05 mg/kg/d for 2 days.[7] (See Comments section.)

Infants and children: 0.5 mg/kg (≤10 mg) q 6 h for six doses beginning 6–12 h before anticipated extubation.[8] (See Comments section.)

Emesis prevention

Highly emetogenic chemotherapy (in addition to ondansetron): 10 mg/m^2 q 12 h on chemotherapy days[9] or 8 mg/m^2 prior to chemotherapy and 8 mg/m^2 4 and 8 h after.[10]

Postoperative nausea and vomiting

Strabismus surgery: After induction, 0.25 mg/kg was as effective as 0.5 and 1 mg/kg in preventing postoperative nausea and vomiting.[11] In one study in 135 children, 0.5 mg dexamethasone (maximum of 25 mg) was as effective as ondansetron.[12]

Tonsillectomy: A single preoperative dose of 0.5 mg/kg (≤8 mg)[13] and 1 mg/kg (≤50 mg) has been reported.[14]

Acute laryngotracheitis (croup): For those who are unable to take PO dexamethasone, 0.6 mg/kg IM or IV as a single dose can be used.[15,16]

Meningitis, bacterial: 0.15 mg/kg q 6 h for 2–4 days of antibiotic therapy was effective in reducing hearing loss in those with *Haemophilus influenza* type b (Hib) disease. However, the outcome in patients with pneumococcal meningitis treated with dexamethasone has either been worse or found to be no different than controls.[17,18] With the use of the Hib and pneumococcal conjugate vaccines, both Hib and pneumococcal meningitis has decreased. Where dexamethasone fits in the treatment of meningitis is unclear.[19]

Asthma: Methylprednisolone sodium succinate is the recommended parenteral glucocorticoid for asthma.[20]

Cerebral edema/elevated ICP: Not recommended for traumatic brain injury in pediatric patients.[21]

Dosage adjustment in organ dysfunction	Those with cirrhosis of the liver or who are hypothyroid may have an exaggerated response.[22]
Maximum dosage	Not established.[22]
IV push	Over 1 to several min.[23]
Intermittent infusion	The dose can be diluted in dextrose or sodium chloride fluids.[22,23] BW should not be used.[22]

Dexamethasone Sodium Phosphate

Continuous infusion	No information available to support administration by this method.
Other routes of administration	4 or 10 mg/mL may be used IM or IV.[23-25] 4 mg/mL can be given intra-articular, intra-synovial, intralesional, or as a soft tissue injection.[22,23] 24 mg/mL for IV infusion.
Maximum concentration	Undiluted (24 mg/mL).[22]
Cautions related to IV administration	Premature ventricular contractions have occurred in *adults*.[22] For PN compatibility information, please see Appendix C.
Other additives	Contains sodium bisulfite, methyl paraben, and propylparaben. Some products contain benzyl alcohol. **Benzyl alcohol:** Benzyl alcohol in small doses as a preservative in drugs is considered safe in newborns.[26] However, a 3-week-old, very low birth weight (710 g) infant who received clindamycin experienced a profound desaturation that required resuscitation after the third and fourth doses, which was subsequently related to the benzyl alcohol preservative.[31] Administration of saline flushes containing benzyl alcohol (BW) was associated with a fatal gasping syndrome, intraventricular hemorrhage, metabolic acidosis, and increased mortality in preterm infants.[32] This should not be used in neonates. Hypersensitivity reactions to benzyl alcohol in parenteral products have been reported in *adults*.[33,34] **Paraben:** Paraben preservatives may cause hypersensitivity reactions that are more common with cutaneous exposure.[29] However, one case of pruritus and bronchospasm that occurred following infusion of hydrocortisone, which contained a paraben, has been reported.[30] **Sulfites:** Sulfites may cause hypersensitivity reactions and these are more common in *adults* with asthma. Most reactions are mild but can include anaphylactic symptoms and life-threatening or less severe asthma episodes.[26-28] Epinephrine may be required in severe cases; and if the sulfite-free product is not available, the sulfite-preserved epinephrine should be used.[26]
Comments	While early dexamethasone facilitates extubation of the VLBW infant, The Vermont Oxford Network Steroid Study Group concluded that neither chronic lung disease nor mortality was favorably affected with its use.[4] Additionally, postnatal exposure is associated with a worse neurological outcome[2] and poor weight gain.[4] On the other hand, 15 years after treatment, a group of ventilator-dependent VLBW infants given a 42-day course beginning at 2 weeks of age (n = 9) had improved neurological outcome compared to infants who received an 18-day treatment (n = 9) or a control group (n = 5).[1] This investigator speculated that steroids might be of benefit in some situations. Extremely low birth weight infants who received dexamethasone were more likely to have decreased growth and intestinal perforation and no decrease in mortality or chronic lung disease than controls.[35] Avoiding dexamethasone in the first 10 days of life has been suggested.[36] If it must be used, recommendations were 0.2–0.3 mg/kg/d divided q 12 h for 48 h; if treatment is extended beyond 48 h, the dose should be halved q 48 h with a maximum treatment length of 10 days.[36]

Dexamethasone Sodium Phosphate

Comments *(cont.)*

Dexamethasone given prior to extubation was not beneficial during uncomplicated airway management.[37]

Patients on chronic steroid therapy may require increased doses during stress.[22]

Supraphysiologic doses of corticosteroids may result in suppressed pituitary-adrenal function, so therapy of more than a few days should be decreased gradually.[22,38]

Important adverse effects include immunosuppression and increased risk for infection.[22]

Other adverse effects include musculoskeletal effects, fluid and electrolyte abnormalities, cataracts, and hyperglycemia.[22]

Drugs that enhance hepatic clearance (e.g., phenytoin, phenobarbital, ephedrine, rifampin) may decrease blood levels and lessen physiologic activity. Drugs that inhibit hepatic clearance may increase dexamethasone concentrations.[22]

Delay live virus (MMR, varicella, rotavirus) vaccinations for 1 month after ending a ≥2-week course of high-dose systemic corticosteroids (2 mg/kg/d of prednisone or its equivalent; or 20 mg/d if >10 kg).[39]

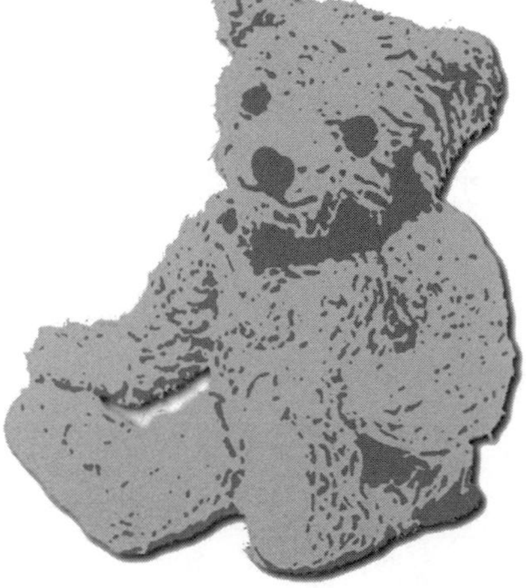

Dexmedetomidine HCl

Brand names	Precedex
Dosage	Little information is available on the use of dexmedetomidine in children. **Procedural sedation:** Forty-eight children from 5 months–16 years received a 0.92 ± 0.36 mcg/kg (range, 0.3–1.9 mcg/kg) loading dose over 10.3 ± 4.7 min followed by maintenance infusion rates of 0.69 ± 0.32 mcg/kg/h (range, 0.25–1.14 mcg/kg/h) for noninvasive procedures lasting 47 ± 16 min.[1] Thirty-two of 40 children given a loading dose of 1 mcg/kg over 10 min followed by 0.5–0.7 mcg/kg/h for 45 ± 11.7 min achieved adequate sedation for MRI compared to eight of 40 children given midazolam.[2] **Critically ill children requiring mechanical ventilation:** 0.25 mcg/kg (n = 10) over 5 min followed by 0.25 mcg/kg/h for 21 ± 10 h or 0.5 mcg/kg over 5 min followed by 0.5 mcg/kg/h for 22 ± 9 h was compared to standard therapy with midazolam (n = 10). If three to four doses of rescue analgesia were required within 8 h, the infusion was increased by 0.15 to 0.25 mcg/kg/h.[3] Of note, less morphine was required by either of the dexmedetomidine groups than the midazolam comparator.[3] **Following cardiothoracic surgery:** An average infusion rate of 0.3 ± 0.05 mcg/kg/h (range, 0.2–0.75) for 14.7 ± 5.5 h (range 3–26) was used in 38 children for up to 26 h; a loading dose was not used.[4] Of the six children who developed hypotension, three responded to a dose reduction; however, three required drug discontinuation.[4] **Facilitate opioid weaning in cardiac transplant:** A 6-month-old infant and a 7-year-old child sedated for 8 weeks and 15 days prior to transplant and for 4 weeks and 3 days after, respectively, were given 1 mcg/kg over 10 min followed by 0.8–1 mcg/kg/h and 0.5–1 mcg/kg/h for 10 and 8 days, respectively.[5] Doses were then weaned as tolerated over 6 days and 24 h.[5] The manufacturer states that the infusion should not extend beyond 24 h.[6]
Dosage adjustment in organ dysfunction	Use with caution in patients with renal or hepatic impairment. Dose reduction should be considered.[6,7]
Maximum dosage	The maximum loading dose was 1.92 mcg/kg over 10 min and the maximum infusion rate reported was 1.14 mcg/kg/h. This was used for short-term (~45 min) procedural sedation.[1] In *adults*, a loading dose of 2.5 mcg/kg over 10 min was followed by a 2.5 mcg/kg/h infusion.[8]
IV push	A rapid rate of infusion is associated with increased adverse cardiovascular effects.[6]
Intermittent infusion	An initial loading dose of 0.92 ± 0.36 mcg/kg administered over 5 min or 1 mcg/kg over 10 min has been used.[1,2] This is followed by a continuous infusion.
Continuous infusion	Dilute to 1–4 mcg/mL with NS and infuse slowly via a controlled infusion pump.[1,6] Also compatible with D5W, R, RL, and mannitol 20%.[8]
Other routes of administration	No information available to support administration by other routes.
Maximum concentration	4 mcg/mL.[6,7]

Cautions related to IV administration	Because of known cardiovascular effects, including bradycardia, sinus arrest, and hypotension, patients should be continuously monitored.[1,6] Slowing the rate of the infusion may modify the cardiovascular effects.[6]
Other additives	Contains 9 mg sodium chloride/mL.[7]
Comments	The manufacturer states that the infusion should not extend beyond 24 h.[6] Withdrawal reactions including nervousness, hypertension, and agitation may occur with chronic administration and abrupt discontinuation.[6,7] Dexmedetomidine appears to have less effectiveness in infants <1 year.[3,4] Bradycardia (high 40s–low 50s) was reported in a 5-week-old girl with trisomy 21, who had a large atrioventricular septal defect and was also receiving digoxin.[9]

Dextrose

Brand names	Various manufacturers
Dosage	**Hypoglycemia:** (Neonatal hypoglycemia is a metabolic emergency. Serious neurological injury can occur if normal blood glucose is not established.) **Preterm neonates:** 0.1–0.2 g/kg bolus (1–2 mL/kg of 10% dextrose) followed by 6 mg/kg/min.[1,2] **Term neonates and infants >6 months:** 0.2–0.5 g/kg (2 mL/kg of 10% dextrose—2.5 mL/kg of 20%) bolus administered slowly followed by 6–12 mg/kg/min.[2-9] Neonates with persistent hypoglycemia may require >12–15 mg/kg/min.[2,8] **Infants <6 months and children:** 0.5–1 g/kg (2–4 mL/kg of 10% to 25% dextrose)[9] bolus administered slowly followed by 3–7.5 mg/kg/min. Titrate dose to serum glucose concentration >40[1,3,4] or >50 mg/dL.[2] **Hyperkalemia in neonates:** 0.2–1 g/kg (3.2–16 mg/kg/min) initially in combination with insulin. Dextrose (grams) to insulin (units) ratios should range from 1.3–3.9.[10] Hypertonic dextrose solutions are irritating to veins and may cause phlebitis if infused peripherally. Usually, the concentration infused peripherally is limited to 11.5% to 12.5% dextrose.[3,9,11] In emergencies, 25% dextrose has been infused peripherally.[9]
Dosage adjustment in organ dysfunction	Glucose requirement during liver failure may be increased due to depletion of glycogen stores.
Maximum dosage	1 g/kg not to exceed 0.8 g/kg/h in *adults*.[11] 15–25 mg/kg/min (0.9–1.5 g/kg/h) has been given to hyperinsulinemic neonates.[3,12,13]
IV push	0.2–0.5 g/kg over 1 min.[7,9] Too rapid infusion may result in hyperglycemia.[14] (See Comments section.)
Intermittent infusion	Over 30 min–2 h (treatment of hyperkalemia).[9]
Continuous infusion	≤30% dextrose, depending on indication and venous access.[5,7,15] 4.5–15 mg/kg/min.[3-7,12]
Other routes of administration	No information available to support administration by other routes.[14]
Maximum concentration	25% dextrose.[9] Concentrated dextrose should be infused through a central line; however, in emergencies 25% dextrose has been infused peripherally. (See Cautions related to IV administration section.) 12.5% dextrose for peripheral lines except for emergency situations. (See IV push section.) 30% dextrose infused through a central line.[15]

American Society of
Health-System Pharmacists
7272 Wisconsin Avenue
Bethesda, Maryland 20814
301-657-3000
Fax: 301-652-8278

P861-NOTICE2

October 2008

Important Correction Notice

Pediatric Injectable Drugs Eighth Edition (The Teddy Bear Book)

The publisher wishes to inform you of a correction in the monograph for Dextrose

Page 134 – Dextrose

"Dosage" section – Hypoglycemia should read as follows:

Term neonates and infants < 6 months

Infants ≥ 6 months and children

Dextrose

Cautions related to IV administration

Infusion of hypertonic dextrose solutions is irritating to veins.[3,9,11] The osmolality or tonicity of body fluids is about 310 mOsm/L. The osmolarity of 10% dextrose is 505 mOsm/L, and 25% dextrose is 1330 mOsm/L.[11]

Other additives

None.

Comments

Hyperglycemia causes osmotic fluid shifts that may result in rapid dehydration and intraventricular hemorrhage in neonates.[1,7]

Following hyperglycemia, rebound hypoglycemia can occur because of stimulation of insulin secretion.[1,3]

Diazepam

Brand names	Valium, Zetran

Dosage

Respiratory depression and arrest requiring mechanical ventilation may occur. Be prepared to provide respiratory support if necessary. Monitor oxygen saturation. Reversal agents should be readily available.

Procedural sedation: Midazolam is the preferred benzodiazepine because of its rapid onset and short duration.[1-3] (See Midazolam monograph.) The lowest effective dose should be used. In infants give 0.05–0.1 mg/kg slowly titrated q 15–30 min for desired effect (up to 0.25 mg/kg).[3] Children should receive 0.04–0.3 mg/kg q 2–4 h[4] up to a cumulative dose of 0.75 mg/kg[5] within 8 h.[4]

Status epilepticus (convulsive): Lorazepam is the preferred benzodiazepine for use in the pediatric population.[6-8] (See Lorazepam monograph.)

Neonates: Not recommended due to benzyl alcohol content in product, prolonged sedation, and decreased ability to metabolize.[6-8] (See Other additives and Comments sections.)

Infants and children: 0.1–0.4 mg/kg repeat q 15 min for two to three doses.[9-13] (See Maximum dosage section.) Although several studies have used continuous infusion diazepam, midazolam or lorazepam are the preferred benzodiazepine for continuous administration. (See Continuous infusion section and Midazolam and Lorazepam monographs.)

Tetanus (muscle spasms): Neonates should receive 0.83–1.67 mg/kg/h as continuous infusion[14] or 20–50 mg/kg/d divided q 2 h.[14,15] (See Comments section.) If >30 days to ≤5 years, give 1–2 mg q 3–4 h as necessary[16] or 15 mg/kg/d divided q 2 h.[15] If >5 years, give 5–10 mg q 3–4 h.[16]

Dosage adjustment in organ dysfunction

No dosage adjustment required in renal dysfunction[17]; however, one source recommends caution when giving multiple doses.[16] Adjust dosage in patients with hepatic dysfunction.[16]

Maximum dosage

1 mg/kg, not to exceed a total dose of 5 mg in children <5 years or 10 mg in children ≥5 years.[16] 2.7 mg/kg was given without adverse effects to a neonate[18] and 1.7 mg/kg/h was given via continuous infusion.[19] Doses should not exceed 1 mg/kg/h because they may be associated with benzyl alcohol toxicity.[20] (See Other additives section.)

IV push

5 mg/mL (available commercially)[16,21] infused over 3 min,[16] not to exceed 2 mg/min in infants and children[22] and 5 mg/min in older children and *adults*.[16] Diazepam is incompatible with most IV solutions.[23]

Intermittent infusion

No information available to support administration by this method.

Continuous infusion

0.2 mg/mL in D5W or NS has been used for continuous infusion.[24] Although a review on continuous infusion diazepam has been published,[24] this administration method is rarely used.

0.01 mg/kg/min increased by 0.005 mg/kg/min q 15 min to a maximum dosage of 0.03 mg/kg/min[25]; however, doses should not exceed 1 mg/kg/h because they may be associated with benzyl alcohol toxicity.[20]

Other routes of administration

Although undiluted (5 mg/mL) diazepam can be given deep into a muscle, it is not the preferred route in the treatment of status epilepticus.[23] The product is alkaline and prone to cause tissue damage,[26] and its bioavailability is erratic when given IM. For these reasons, midazolam is the benzodiazepine of choice for IM administration. (See Midazolam monograph.) No information available to support administration by other routes.

Maximum concentration

5 mg/mL for IV push.[16,21]

Cautions related to IV administration

Thrombophlebitis may occur,[16] and tissue necrosis may occur following infiltration.[26,27] To reduce the possibility of venous thrombosis, phlebitis, local irritation, and (rarely) vascular impairment, inject slowly (see IV push section), into a large vein.[16]

Other additives

Benzyl alcohol: Not the preferred benzodiazepine in neonates because of benzyl alcohol. Each 1 mL contains 1.5% benzyl alcohol as a preservative.[23] Benzyl alcohol in small doses as a preservative in drugs is considered safe in newborns.[28] However, a 3-week-old, very low birth weight (710 g) infant who received clindamycin experienced a profound desaturation that required resuscitation after the third and fourth doses, which was subsequently related to the benzyl alcohol preservative.[29] One report of benzyl alcohol poisoning occurred in a 5-year-old child receiving up to 2.4 mg/kg/h of diazepam by continuous infusion.[20] Administration of saline flushes containing benzyl alcohol (bacteriostatic water for injection) was associated with a fatal gasping syndrome, intraventricular hemorrhage, metabolic acidosis, and increased mortality in preterm infants.[30]

Hypersensitivity reactions to benzyl alcohol in parenteral products have been reported in *adults*.[31,32]

Propylene glycol: 2 mg/mL product contains 0.18 mg of propylene glycol.[23] Propylene glycol is added to parenteral drugs as a solubilizer. Rapid infusion of medications that contain propylene glycol has resulted in respiratory depression and cardiac dysrhythmias.[33] Its half-life is three times longer in neonates than in *adults*[28] and has caused hyperosmolality[34] and refractory seizures[35] in preterm neonates receiving 3 g/d.

Comments

Withdrawal symptoms (e.g., convulsions, tremor, abdominal and muscle cramps, vomiting, and sweats) have occurred following abrupt discontinuation.[16]

Dosing in neonates is controversial since benzodiazepines may decrease blood pressure and cerebral blood flow velocity.[36] Diazepam should be used cautiously in this population. Some recommend the initial dose should be reduced by 50% in infants <2 months of age.[37] Neonates may experience prolonged CNS depression because of an inability to biotransform diazepam to an inactive metabolite.[38]

Abnormal movements of limbs (e.g., myoclonus or seizures) have been described in premature and full-term neonates given benzodiazepines.[39-41] The movements began a few minutes after a bolus injection and continued for several hours.[40,41]

Flumazenil, a specific benzodiazepine-receptor antagonist, is indicated for complete or partial reversal of benzodiazepine toxicity (see Flumazenil monograph).[42] May precipitate seizures in someone with known epilepsy who is dependent on benzodiazepines.

Diazoxide

Brand names	Hyperstat I.V.
Dosage	Diazoxide is not the drug of choice in hypertensive emergencies.[1,2] 1–3 mg/kg to a maximum of 150 mg q 5–15 min (minibolus method) or in *adults* 50–100 mg q 5–15 min.[1-8] In children, 3–5 mg/kg infused over 30 min results in less hypotension and hyperglycemia.[5] In hypertensive emergencies, blood pressure should be frequently monitored to ensure that it does not decrease too quickly.[1,4,9] One group recommended that the blood pressure decrease by one-third of the desired total blood pressure decrease within 6–12 h, a further one-third decrease within the next 24 h, with the final one-third decrease achieved over the next 2 days.[3] Alternatively, a blood pressure decrease of <25% within minutes to 1 h, followed by further decreases over the next 2–6 h if the patient is stable, has been suggested.[1]
Dosage adjustment in organ dysfunction	None.[10]
Maximum dosage	3 mg/kg, not to exceed 150 mg if given IV push[1,4] or a maximum total initial dose of 5 mg/kg infused over 30 min.[5] Diazoxide is usually used for <4–5 days[1]; it should not be used >10 days.[4]
IV push	The manufacturer recommends infusion over <30 sec.[4] Others advocate infusion over a longer time period to reduce adverse effects.[3,5]
Intermittent infusion	In children, 3–5 mg/kg over 30 min.[5] In *adults*, 15 mg/min (undiluted) to a total dose of 5 mg/kg.[11-13]
Continuous infusion	0.25–5 mcg/kg/min for 8 to 24 h in children has been suggested.[3]
Other routes of administration	Not recommended.[4]
Maximum concentration	15 mg/mL (undiluted).
Cautions related to IV administration	Administer by peripheral vein.[4] Too rapid decrease in blood pressure can result in serious unwanted side effects.[1,2] Use with caution in patients with impaired cerebral or compensatory hypertension such as infants with arteriovenous shunt or coarctation of the aorta.[1,2] Patients should be in a supine position during and for 1 h after administration of the drug.[1,4] Extravasation may cause local inflammation and pain without necrosis.[4] Treatment is with warm compresses and rest.[4]

Other additives	None.
Comments	Do not use in patients with known hypersensitivity to diazoxide, other thiazides, or sulfonamide-derived drugs.[4] Hyperglycemia from diazoxide may require treatment with insulin or oral hypoglycemic agents.[1] On the other hand, diazoxide has been used to treat hypoglycemia due to a variety of causes including oral hypoglycemics.[15] In 36 children, transitory nausea, flushing, shoulder pain or burning following injection, tachycardia, and bitter taste in mouth were reported.[16] Some but not all of these children had hyperglycemia.[16] Sodium and water retention may occur after frequent injections. A diuretic may be required.[4] This drug is >90% protein bound and may displace other protein-bound drugs resulting in higher free serum concentrations of the displaced drug.[4] Protect from light.[1] Darkened solutions should not be used because they may be subpotent.[1] Diazoxide inhibits glucagon-stimulated insulin release resulting in a false-negative insulin response to glucagon.[4]

Digoxin

Brand names Lanoxin

Dosage

Dosage based on lean body weight and normal renal function.[1] Administer one-half of total digitalizing dose (TDD) initially, one-fourth 8–12 h after the first dose, and the remaining one-fourth 8–12 h after the second dose.[2-5] Assess clinical response before administering each dose.[1]

Age	TDD (mcg/kg)	Maintenance Dose (mcg/kg/d)
Premature neonates	15–30[1,3-10]	5–10 divided q 12 h[3-5,7-11]
Full-term neonates	10–30[1,3,5,6]	8–10 divided q 12 h[2,5,11]
Infants <2 y	30–50[2,5,6]	10–12 divided q 12 h[2,5,6,11]
Children 2–10 y	20–35[1,3,5]	8–10 divided q 12 h[5,11]
Children >10 y	8–12[1]	2–3 divided q 12 h[1,12] or given once daily[13]

Because large variability exists in patient response to initial and maintenance doses, individualize dosage based on serum concentration and clinical response.

Dosage adjustment in organ dysfunction

Adjust maintenance doses in patients with renal dysfunction.[8,14] If CrCl is 10–50 mL/min, give 25% to 75% of normal dose q 36 h, and if CrCl is <10 mL/min, give 10% to 25% of normal dose q 48 h.[14]

Decrease TDD by 50% in patients with end-stage renal disease.[14] Dosing should be optimized by measuring serum concentrations.

Maximum dosage

TDD should not exceed 1 mg.[15] Maintenance dose generally approximates 30% of TDD. Maximum maintenance doses rarely exceed 10 mcg/kg/d or 0.25 mg/d.[2-11,16]

IV push

Undiluted (100 mcg/mL) over at least 5 min or longer.[1,17] Rapid IV infusion causes systemic and coronary arteriolar vasoconstriction.[1]

Intermittent infusion

Dilute at least fourfold (25 mcg/mL) with D5W, NS, or SW[1,17] and infuse over >5 min.[1] Use of less than a fourfold volume of diluent may result in precipitation.[1] Compatible with LR and ½NS for 4–6 h at 23°C.[17] A 1:10 dilution may improve the accuracy of dose measurement.[7,18] (See Comments section.)

Continuous infusion

No information available to support administration by this method.

Other routes of administration

IM administration is not recommended because of local pain, irritation, and tissue damage.[17] If it must be given IM, it should be given by deep injection followed by massage of the area.[1,17] Inject no more than 2 mL (200 mcg) at any one site.[17]

Maximum concentration	100 mcg/mL for pediatric patients and 250 mcg/mL for *adults*.[1,19]
Cautions related to IV administration	Inadvertent over administration may occur if a tuberculin syringe is used to measure very small doses.[1,7,18,20] (See Comments section.) Do not aspirate fluid or blood into the syringe containing digoxin because administration of residual drug left in the syringe hub may cause an overdose.[7,18] For PN compatibility information, please see Appendix C.
Other additives	Pediatric (100 mcg/mL) and *adult* (250 mcg/mL) injection contains propylene glycol 40% and alcohol 10%.[17] Propylene glycol is added to parenteral drugs as a solubilizer. Rapid infusion of medications that contain propylene glycol has resulted in respiratory depression and cardiac dysrhythmias.[21] Its half-life is three times longer in neonates than in *adults*[22] and has caused hyperosmolality[23] and refractory seizures[24] in preterm neonates receiving 3 g/d.
Comments	For dose volumes <0.1 mL, prepare a 1:10 dilution to improve measurement accuracy. Dilute 0.1 mL of digoxin (100 mcg/mL) with 0.9 mL of saline to make a 10-mcg/mL concentration. Use the two-syringe technique to make the dilution: draw up the drug in one syringe and the diluent in another. Inject drug into diluent syringe and mix well. This technique avoids "syringe dead space overdose," which can occur when additional fluid is drawn into a drug-containing syringe. Failure to use the two-syringe technique causes drug in the dead space to be drawn up also, and it can result in a significantly larger dose than intended (5 mcg vs. 8–12 mcg for digoxin).[7,18,20] Serum digoxin concentrations will be falsely elevated if drawn during the predistribution phase (i.e., within 6 h of digoxin dose).[5,27] Depending on the assay used, serum digitalis concentrations may be falsely elevated because of endogenous digoxin-like immunoreactive substances in patients with renal or hepatic dysfunction, neonates, infants, and children.[28-33] Electrolytes should be monitored. Hypercalcemia may increase the risk of toxicity.[1] Toxicity may also occur with hypokalemia and hypomagnesemia despite serum drug concentrations within therapeutic range.[1] Monitoring EKG may assist in the diagnosis of digoxin-associated toxicity. In patients experiencing serious cardiac effects due to digitalis toxicity, the standard therapy is administration of digoxin-immune Fab using weight and serum drug concentrations to determine dose.[1]

Digoxin Immune Fab

Brand names Digibind

Dosage

For manifestations of severe digitalis toxicity unresponsive to other therapies. Anaphylaxis may occur. (See Comments section.)[1]

Dose should be based on amount of digoxin or digitoxin ingested or on serum digitalis concentration.[1-3] 38 mg (one vial) binds 0.5 mg of digoxin or digitoxin.[1] To calculate the total body load of digitalis, use either[1,3-10]:

Dosing method based on estimated amount ingested

For digoxin tablets, oral solution, or IM injection[10]

$$\text{Dose in mg} = \frac{(\text{dose ingested (mg)} \times 0.8)}{0.5} \times 38$$

For digitoxin tablets, digoxin capsules, IV digoxin, or IV digitoxin[10]

$$\text{Dose in mg} = \frac{\text{dose ingested (mg)}}{0.5} \times 38$$

Dosing method based on measured serum *digoxin* concentration[1,10]

Weight (kg)	SDC† 1 ng/mL	SDC† 2 ng/mL	SDC† 4 ng/mL	SDC† 8 ng/mL	SDC† 12 ng/mL	SDC† 16 ng/mL	SDC† 20 ng/mL
1	0.4 mg*	1 mg*	1.5 mg*	3 mg	5 mg	6 mg	8 mg
3	1 mg	2 mg	5 mg	9 mg	14 mg	18 mg	23 mg
5	2 mg	4 mg	8 mg	15 mg	23 mg	30 mg	38 mg
10	4 mg	8 mg	15 mg	30 mg	46 mg	61 mg	76 mg
20	8 mg	15 mg	30 mg	61 mg	91 mg	122 mg	152 mg
40	0.5 vial	1 vial	2 vials	3 vials	5 vials	7 vials	8 vials
60	0.5 vial	1 vial	3 vials	5 vials	7 vials	10 vials	12 vials
70	1 vial	2 vials	3 vials	6 vials	9 vials	11 vials	14 vials
80	1 vial	2 vials	3 vials	7 vials	10 vials	13 vials	16 vials
100	1 vial	2 vials	4 vials	8 vials	12 vials	16 vials	20 vials

*Dilution of reconstituted vial to 1 mg/mL may be desirable.
†SDC = serum digoxin concentration.

or

$$\text{Dose in mg} = \frac{\text{serum } digoxin \text{ concentration (ng/mL)} \times \text{weight (kg)}}{100} \times 38$$

Dosing method based on measured serum *digitoxin* concentration[10]

$$\text{Dose in mg} = \frac{\text{serum } digitoxin \text{ concentration (ng/mL)} \times \text{weight (kg)}}{1000} \times 38$$

Amount ingested unknown or SDC unavailable[1,10]**:** Give 760 mg (20 38-mg vials).

Dosage adjustment in organ dysfunction

Fab fragments may be eliminated more slowly in patients with renal failure.[1,9]

Maximum dosage

Not established. Following acute ingestion, 760 mg should be sufficient. For chronic ingestion, a single vial (38 mg) should be sufficient for infants and small children (<20 kg) and 228 mg (six vials) should be sufficient for children ≥20 kg and *adults*.[1]

Digoxin Immune Fab

IV push	In one study, an 1800-g infant received 160 mg over 5 min.[6] May give dose more rapidly in cases of impending cardiac arrest.[1]
Intermittent infusion	1–9.5 mg/mL over 20–60 min[1,5,8,11] through a 0.22-micron filter.[1] After reconstitution, no additional dilution is needed prior to administration.[9] Reconstituted solutions are stable for 4 h under refrigeration at 2°C to 8°C.[1] For very small doses, a reconstituted vial can be diluted to 1 mg/mL with 34 mL of NS.[1] May also be administered in D5W.[3]
Continuous infusion	No information available to support administration by this method.
Other routes of administration	No information available to support administration by other routes.
Maximum concentration	9.5 mg/mL.[1]
Cautions related to IV administration	Anaphylactoid, hypersensitivity, and febrile reactions have occurred.[1,9] Patients allergic to papain, chymopapain, or another papaya extract may be allergic to Fab.[1] Individuals at high risk for allergy should receive a test dose.[1] Give a 1:100 dilution by mixing 0.1 mL of reconstituted Fab (9.5 mg/mL) in 9.9 mL NS (95 mcg/mL). Inject 0.1 mL of the dilution through 0.22-micron filter intradermally or place one drop on skin and make a ¼″ scratch through drop with a sterile needle.[1] Evaluate test site for 20–30 min.[1,9] Epinephrine should be immediately available.
Other additives	None.
Comments	Indicated for the treatment of life-threatening digoxin- or digotoxin-induced ventricular arrhythmias or progressive bradyarrhythmias, ingestion of >10 mg of digoxin in previously healthy *adults* or 4 mg in previously healthy children, ingestion resulting in a serum concentration >10 ng/mL, and digoxin-associated progressive hyperkalemia (serum concentration >5 mEq/L).[1] Signs and symptoms of digitalis intoxications should improve within 30 min of Fab administration and most patients respond within 4 h.[9] If there is no response to normal doses, investigate other causes for clinical toxicity.[1,9] If no other cause is determined, a second dose of Fab (one-fourth to one-half of the initial dose) may be administered (monitor for hypersensitivity reaction).[9] Total serum digitalis concentrations increase dramatically following Fab administration[1,4,7,12,13] so total serum digitalis concentrations should not be measured for at least 5–7 days after treatment.[13] Monitoring free digoxin concentrations has been proposed to determine if additional Fab is needed, confirm possible rebound toxicity, or guide the reinitiation of digoxin therapy.[14-18] Redigitalization should not be done until all Fab has been eliminated (approximately 80–100 h).[9] Elimination will be prolonged in patients with renal insufficiency.[9] Patients receiving digoxin for atrial fibrillation may have a rapid ventricular response as Fab removes the digitalis.[19] Heart failure may be exacerbated as digoxin concentrations decrease.[1] May cause a rapid fall in serum potassium; patients should be monitored closely.[1,8,9]

Dihydroergotamine Methanesulfonate

Brand names	D.H.E 45, Migranal
Dosage	IV dihydroergotamine, given in conjunction with an antiemetic, is an appropriate choice for treatment of severe migraine; however, it should be reserved for patients who do not respond to any other drug therapy, including 5-HT_1 selective receptor agonists.[1] Safety and efficacy of dihydroergotamine not established in children.[1] **6–9 years:** 0.1–0.15 mg repeated q 20 min for three doses (up to 1 mg/d).[2-4] **9–12 years:** 0.15–0.2 mg repeated q 20 min for three doses (up to 1 mg/d).[2-4] **12–16 years:** 0.2–0.25 mg repeated q 20 min for three doses (up to 1 mg/d).[2-4] **Adolescents and adults (>16 years):** 1 mg at first sign of headache; repeat hourly to a maximum total dose of 2 mg in a 24-h period.[1] One report gave 0.1 mg q 8 h.[5] (See Other routes of administration section.)
Dosage adjustment in organ dysfunction	Contraindicated in patients with severe renal or hepatic dysfunction.[1]
Maximum dosage	1 mg/d in children[6] and 2 mg/d in *adults* if given IV.[1] If given IM or SC mg up to 3 g/d in *adults*.[1] Total weekly IM, subcutaneous, or IV dosage should not exceed 6 mg.[1]
IV push	Over 1–2 min.[1]
Intermittent infusion	No information.
Continuous infusion	3 mg of dihydroergotamine in 1000 mL NS has been administered at a constant rate over 24 h in *adults*.[6]
Other routes of administration	May be administered IM or SQ.[1,7] IM or subcutaneous dose of dihydroergotamine mesylate in *adults* is 1 mg initially,[7] followed by 1 mg at 1-h intervals until the attack has abated or until a total of 3 mg has been given in a 24-h period.[1]
Maximum concentration	1 mg/mL.[1]
Cautions related to IV administration	IV administration may lead to hypertension or vasospasm, possibly resulting in gangrene or death in patients with compromised circulation.[1]

Other additives	None.
Comments	Metoclopramide (0.2 mg/kg) may be administered 30 min prior to dihydroergotamine to reduce the incidence of abdominal discomfort.[1,2] Concomitant antiemetics may not be needed with IM administration.[8] Rarely, cases of acute myocardial infarction in *adults* and arrhythmias have occurred.[2] A 4-year-old with cyclic vomiting syndrome developed intestinal ischemia after receiving 0.1 mg q 8 h (total eight doses).[9]

Diltiazem HCl

Brand names	Cardizem injectable
Dosage	Intravenous diltiazem is not considered first line treatment of dysrhythmias or hypertension in children.[1] Only a few reports of IV diltiazem use in children have been published.[2-4] **Atrial tachycardias:** Seven children from 0.6–13 years old were given 0.25 mg/kg over 5 min followed by a continuous infusion of 0.5–0.15 mg/kg/h for up to 126 h as a bridge to definitive treatment.[2] Calcium gluconate and volume were readily available prior to initiation of diltiazem.[2] In *adults*, 0.25 mg/kg (≤20 mg) over 2 min. If the response is inadequate after 15 min, a second bolus of 0.35 mg/kg (≤25 mg) can be given.[5,6] This may be followed by a continuous infusion of 5 mg/h increased by 5 mg/h up to 15 mg/h until heart rate is controlled.[5] Blood pressure and continuous ECG monitoring is recommended.[6] **Pulmonary hypertension:** Five neonates on ECMO were given 1–2 mg twice daily that was titrated upwards to 3–7 mg given four times daily.[3]
Dosage adjustment in organ dysfunction	Cautious use is recommended in patients with renal or hepatic disease.[5]
Maximum dosage	In *adults*, a repeat bolus dose of 25 mg (0.35 mg/kg) and a continuous infusion of 15 mg/h for up to 24 h are suggested as reasonable.[5]
IV push	5 mg/mL (undiluted) over 2 min.[5,6]
Intermittent infusion	Not indicated.
Continuous infusion	1, 0.83, or 0.45 mg/mL in D5W, NS, or D5½NS.[5,6]
Other routes of administration	Not indicated.
Maximum concentration	5 mg/mL.[5,6]
Cautions related to IV administration	Monitor ECG and blood pressure during infusion.[5,6] Atropine is recommended for bradycardia.[5] Vasopressors are recommended to treat hypotension.[5] (See Comments section.)

Other additives

Cardizem Lyo-Ject® includes a diluent that contains benzyl alcohol.[5] Benzyl alcohol in small doses as a preservative in drugs is considered safe in newborns.[7] However, a 3-week-old, very low birth weight (710 g) infant who received clindamycin experienced a profound desaturation that required resuscitation after the third and fourth doses, which was subsequently related to the benzyl alcohol preservative.[8]

Administration of saline flushes containing benzyl alcohol (BW) was associated with a fatal gasping syndrome, intraventricular hemorrhage, metabolic acidosis, and increased mortality in preterm infants.[9] This should not be used in neonates.

Hypersensitivity reactions to benzyl alcohol in parenteral products have been reported in *adults*.[10,11]

Comments

While practitioners recommend having an IV dose of calcium available should hypotension occur,[2,12] the manufacturer states that the response to calcium is inconsistent.[5]

In those receiving cyclosporine, adding diltiazem may increase cyclosporine serum concentrations and increase the risk for nephrotoxicity.[6] Other drugs including carbamazepine and some benzodiazepines may also have their clearance decreased if diltiazem is added.[6]

Diphenhydramine HCl

Brand names	Benadryl
Dosage	**Acute hypersensitivity or dystonic reactions** **Neonates:** Contraindicated because of potential CNS effects.[1,2] **Infants and children:** 1–2 mg/kg/dose[3-8] up to 5 mg/kg/d or 150 mg/m²/d divided q 6–8 h.[1,2]
Dosage adjustment in organ dysfunction	No adjustment is necessary in patients with renal dysfunction.[9]
Maximum dosage	50 mg/dose,[3] not to exceed 300 mg/d.[1,2] In *adults*, the maximum is 100 mg/dose, not to exceed 400 mg/d.[1,2,10]
IV push	≤50 mg/mL[1,2] slowly over 5 min.[3,4,6,7]
Intermittent infusion	≤50 mg/mL in D5W, D10W, LR, NS, ½NS or R[11] not to exceed 25 mg/min.[1,2]
Continuous infusion	≤50 mg/mL in D5W, D10W, LR, NS, ½NS, or R.[1,2,11]
Other routes of administration	50 mg/mL may be given by deep muscular injection.[1,2]
Maximum concentration	50 mg/mL (available commercially).[1,2]
Cautions related to IV administration	Local necrosis has been associated with the administration of IV diphenhydramine by the subcutaneous or intradermal routes.[1,2] For PN compatibility information, please see Appendix C.
Other additives	The multidose vial contains 0.1 mg/mL benzethonium chloride.[1]
Comments	Overdose may result in hallucinations, convulsions, respiratory arrest, arrhythmias, or death.[1,12] Although antihistamines may diminish mental alertness, paradoxical hyperactivity may occur in pediatric patients.[1] One paper describes adjuvant analgesic therapy with diphenhydramine 25 mg IV q 4 h in addition to fentanyl PCA in an 8-year-old patient with end stage oncologic pain.[13]

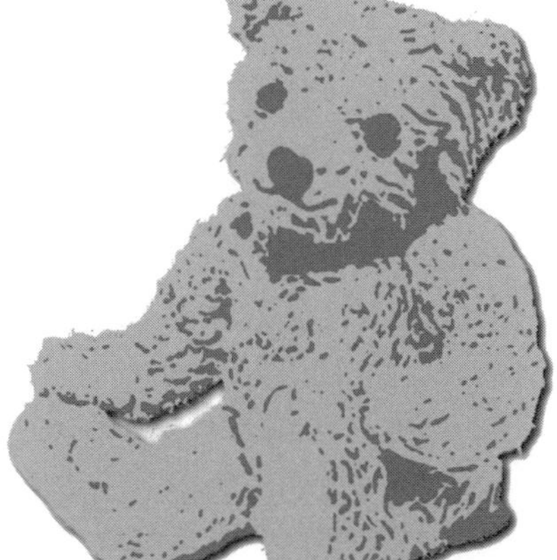

Dobutamine HCl

Brand names	Dobutrex, generic
Dosage	2.5–10 mcg/kg/min increased by 2.5–5 mcg/kg/min q 20–40 min up to 25 mcg/kg/min.[1-16] Given the wide variability in clearance, doses must be individualized.[11,17,18] (See Comments section.)
Dosage adjustment in organ dysfunction	No dosage adjustment required in renal dysfunction.[19]
Maximum dosage	40 mcg/kg/min has been used in *adults*[1,2]; however, this dose is associated with increased toxicity.[2]
IV push	Not indicated.
Intermittent infusion	Not indicated.
Continuous infusion	Usually, 0.25–1 mg/mL[7,20] in D5W, D5NS, D5½NS, D10W, Isolyte M with dextrose 5%, LR, D5LR, Normosol-M in D5W, 20% Osmitrol in Water for Injection, NS, or sodium lactate ⅙ M.[1] Not compatible with strongly alkaline solutions such as sodium bicarbonate or diluents containing both sodium bisulfite and ethanol.[1] The PALS guidelines and AAP recommend the following formula for preparation of the infusion: 6 × weight (kg) = mg of drug to be added to IV solution for a total volume of 100 mL. An infusion rate of 1 mL/h provides 1 mcg/kg/min.[15,16] This formula estimates initial concentration. Ultimately, the concentration of the drug should consider the patient's fluid requirements. Despite widespread use of the above formula, recent JCAHO® guidelines recommend the implementation of "standardized concentrations" of vasoactive medications."[21]
Other routes of administration	Not indicated. Intraosseous administration may be used in postresuscitation stabilization.[16]
Maximum concentration	5 mg/mL (361 mOsm/kg).[1,20] The concentration used depends on the patient size and/or fluid requirements. For example, a patient who requires a large amount of dobutamine or a fluid-restricted patient may require a more concentrated fluid.
Cautions related to IV administration	Infiltration or extravasation results in local inflammation and pain. Isolated cases of skin necrosis have been reported.[2] Tachycardia, arrhythmias (PVCs), and hypertension may occur, especially at greater infusion rates. For PN compatibility information, please see Appendix C.

Other additives

Some products contain sodium bisulfite.[1]

Sulfites may cause hypersensitivity reactions and these are more common in *adults* with asthma. Most reactions are mild but can include anaphylactic symptoms and life-threatening or less severe asthma episodes.[22-24] Epinephrine may be required in severe cases; and if the sulfite-free product is not available, the sulfite-preserved epinephrine should be used.[22]

Comments

Hemodynamic instability may be attributed to significant variability between the ordered dosage and the actual solution concentration of dobutamine.[25]

The tachycardia produced by dobutamine may make it unacceptable for use in children after cardiopulmonary bypass.[4]

Long-term infusion (i.e., 3–4 days) has produced tolerance to hemodynamic effects and necessitated dosage increases in *adults*.[26]

May be filtered through a 0.2-micron filter without significant dobutamine loss.[20]

Dolasetron Mesylate

Brand names	Anzemet
Dosage	Information is available in children 2 years of age and older.[1,2] **Prevention of chemotherapy induced nausea and vomiting:** 1.8 mg/kg with a maximum of 100 mg is a standard dose.[1-4] Escalating doses, administered 30 min before chemotherapy, have been studied.[3] Doses of 1.2 and 1.8 mg/kg were more effective than doses of 0.6 and 2.4 mg/kg.[3] **Prevention of postoperative nausea and vomiting:** 0.35 mg/kg up to 12.5 mg is a standard dose.[1,2,4] One study evaluated 0.35 mg/kg or 12.5 mg given 15 min prior to the end of strabismus surgery and found no difference between the antiemetic effects.[5] Another found that 0.5 mg/kg or 25 mg given at the time of intubation for tonsillectomy were effective.[6]
Dosage adjustment in organ dysfunction	None required.[1]
Maximum dosage	**Chemotherapy related nausea and vomiting:** 1.8 mg/kg up to 100 mg.[1,2] The 2.4-mg/kg dose with the total dose not stated was no more effective than the 1.8-mg/kg dose.[3] **Postoperative nausea and vomiting:** 12.5 mg/dose is the maximum recommended dose[1,2]; however, 25 mg have been used.[6]
IV push	100 mg over 30 sec in *adults* (undiluted).[1,2]
Intermittent infusion	May dilute to 0.25–2 mg/mL in NS, D5W, D5½NS, or D5LR and infuse over 15 min.[1]
Continuous infusion	Not indicated.[1]
Other routes of administration	No information to support administration by other routes.
Maximum concentration	20 mg/mL.
Cautions related to IV administration	The active metabolite of dolasetron (hydrodolasetron) may cause EKG changes (PR, QTc, QT prolongation, and QRS widening). Use with caution in children with congenital QT syndrome or in children receiving concomitant medications that prolong the QT interval.[1,2]
Other additives	Contains 38.2 mg of mannitol/mL.[1]
Comments	In moderate-to-severe emetogenic chemotherapy, efficacy can be enhanced with the addition of dexamethasone or methylprednisolone.[2,4]

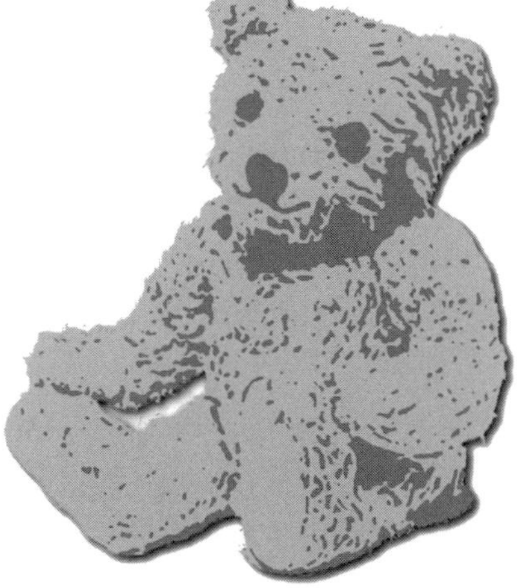

Dopamine HCl

Brand names	Generic
Dosage	0.5–10 mcg/kg/min[1-11] increased by 1–10 mcg/kg/min q 10–40 min up to 25 mcg/kg/min.[1-5,8,12,13] In certain cases, larger doses may be required. (See Maximum dosage section.) In hypotensive preterm neonates, doses of 5–20 mcg/kg/min are usual.[12-16] If doses >10–15 mcg/kg/min are required to maintain blood pressure or cardiac output then epinephrine, norepinephrine or dobutamine should be added.[2] Infusions >20 mcg/kg/min are associated with an increased risk for dysrhythmias.[17] The intravascular volume should be corrected before starting dopamine.[1-3,18]
Dosage adjustment in organ dysfunction	Dopamine clearance is decreased in critically ill children with renal or hepatic dysfunction.[19]
Maximum dosage	Usually 50 mcg/kg/min.[1] 75 mcg/kg/min has been used in children with advanced circulatory decompensation.[2,17] Doses as large as 125 mcg/kg/min have been given to neonates.[2]
IV push	Not indicated.
Intermittent infusion	Not indicated.
Continuous infusion	400–800 mcg/mL in D5LR, D5NS, D5½NS, D2.5W, D5W, D10W, LR, mannitol 20%, NS, or sodium lactate ⅙ M.[1,20] Not compatible with strongly alkaline solutions such as sodium bicarbonate.[1] The PALS guidelines and AAP recommend the following formula for preparation of the infusion: 6 × weight (kg) = mg of drug to be added to IV solution for a total volume of 100 mL. An infusion rate of 1 mL/h provides 1 mcg/kg/min.[3] This formula estimates an initial concentration. Ultimately, the concentration of the drug should consider the patient's fluid requirements or fluid limitations. Despite widespread use of the above formula, recent JCAHO® guidelines recommend the implementation of "standardized concentrations" of vasoactive medications.[21]
Other routes of administration	Not indicated. Intraosseous administration may be used in postresuscitation stabilization.[3]
Maximum concentration	3.2 mg/mL (295 mOsm/kg).[20] Concentrations up to 6 mg/mL have been infused into large veins (i.e., central vein) of extremely fluid-restricted patients.[22]

Dopamine HCl

Cautions related to IV administration

Extravasation may cause local ischemia and tissue necrosis.[1,23] Aliquots of phentolamine mesylate (5–10 mg in 10 mL NS) should be injected using a fine hypodermic needle into the ischemic area.[1] This should be done as soon as possible and within the first 12 h of noting the extravasation.[1] A 65-year-old patient receiving dopamine and dobutamine experienced swelling at the infusion site that resolved with local injection of 3 mL of terbutaline (1 mg in 10 mL NS) given SC.[24]

Two case reports of distal extremity gangrene have been related to dopamine infusion, and in one infant the catheter had good blood return and no signs of infiltration or extravasation were present.[25,26] Digital ischemia with sudden onset of extremity cyanosis (without evidence of infiltration) was observed in a 2-week-old neonate after infusing dopamine via a peripheral line into the left saphenous vein and right hand. The authors suggested that dopamine be infused through a central line.[27]

Infusion through an umbilical artery catheter is not recommended.[28]

For PN compatibility information, please see Appendix C.

Other additives

Sodium metabisulfite.[1,2] Sulfites may cause hypersensitivity reactions, and these are more common in *adults* with asthma. Most reactions are mild but can include anaphylactic symptoms and life-threatening or less severe asthma episodes.[29-31] Epinephrine may be required in severe cases; and if the sulfite-free product is not available, the sulfite-preserved epinephrine should be used.[29]

Comments

"Low-dose" dopamine (<5 mcg/kg/min) does not appear to prevent or reduce the incidence of acute oliguric renal failure in critically ill patients and is no longer recommended. Furthermore, low doses of dopamine may suppress respiratory drive, increase myocardial oxygen demand, worsen splanchnic oxygenation, impair GI function and impair endocrine and immunologic systems.[32]

Doses of 5–10 mcg/kg/min affect beta-receptors and are used for inotropic response; and doses >10 mcg/kg/min affect alpha-receptors and are used to increase blood pressure, heart rate, and peripheral vascular resistance.[33] Because doses >20 mcg/kg/min may decrease renal blood flow,[4] either epinephrine, norepinephrine, or dobutamine should be used concomitantly if continued ionotropic support is needed.[2]

Significant variability between the ordered dosage and the actual solution concentration of dopamine may occur and account for hemodynamic changes when infusates are replaced. Failure to consider the HCl salt in the stock drug accounts for some of the inaccuracy in preparation.[34]

A prospective study in 20 preterm infants with arterial hypotension refractory to volume therapy noted that dobutamine or dopamine (10 mcg/kg/min) increased MAP and decreased superior mesenteric artery resistance and proposed that the risk for developing necrotizing enterocolitis during infusion would be reduced.[7]

A 16-year-old patient with pulmonary vascular obstructive disease developed suprasystemic pressure in the right ventricle during dopamine infusion. It was suggested that dopamine may be contraindicated in patients with this underlying disease.[35] In a blinded, cross-over trial in 19 children (2–54 months of age) requiring inotropic support after cardiac surgery, dopamine in doses >7 mcg/kg/min caused pulmonary vasoconstriction. The authors concluded that dopamine should not be used in infants with increased PVR secondary to pulmonary hypertension.[36]

An evaluation of 629 children undergoing cardiovascular surgery found that a younger age, longer cardiopulmonary bypass time and infusion of dopamine or milrinone were associated with the development of junctional ectopic tachycardia.[37] The authors suggest that dopamine be discontinued in those who develop this condition.

Studies using a first-order kinetic model were unable to relate clearance to age.[19,38] Using a nonlinear model, clearance varied according to concentration, and increased weight (but not age) was related to a decreased clearance.[39] Still another study reported that clearance is almost two times greater in those <2 years old.[40]

May be filtered through a 0.2-micron filter without significant dopamine loss.[20]

Doxapram HCl

Brand names	Dopram

Dosage

Contraindicated in seizure disorders; possible pulmonary embolism; mechanical disorders of ventilation; evidence of head injury, cerebral vascular accident, or cerebral edema; and in cardiovascular disorders including those associated with hyperthyroidism.[1]

Neonates: Reserve for neonates unresponsive to theophylline or caffeine. (See Other additives and Comments sections.)

Apnea: Loading dose of 2.5–3 mg/kg[2,3] followed by continuous infusion of 0.2 mg/kg/h.[3-6] Increase dose in 0.5-mg/kg/h increments q 24–48 h until infant responds or has received 2.5 mg/kg/h for 48 h. Then decrease dose to lowest that controls apnea.[5] In one study, 0.2 mg/kg/h was as effective as 1–2.5 mg/kg/h when used with a methylxanthine.[3]

Weaning from ventilator: 2.5 mg/kg/h as continuous infusion in premature neonates.[7] Start with dose of 0.5–1 mg/kg/h and titrate to ≤2.5 mg/kg/h for 48 h.[7]

Older than 12 years[1]

Chronic obstructive pulmonary disease (COPD) with acute hypercapnia: 1–2 mg/min increased to 3 mg/min with arterial blood gas assessments q 30 min for 2 h duration of therapy.

Drug induced CNS depression: 2 mg/kg at 1–2 h intervals or follow bolus dose with continuous infusion of 1–3 mg/min until arousal. Daily dose should not exceed 3 g.

Postanesthetic use: 0.5–1 mg/kg at 5-min intervals to an accumulated dose of 2 mg/kg or 5 mg/min continuous infusion until adequate response, then decrease rate to 1–3 mg/min to a total dose of 4 mg/kg (usual maximum 300 mg).

Dosage adjustment in organ dysfunction

Use with caution in patients with significantly impaired renal or hepatic function.[1]

Maximum dosage

2.5 mg/kg/h for 48 h in neonates.[4-7] 3 g/d in *adults*.[1]

Maximum total dose for respiratory depression following anesthesia is 4 mg/kg not to exceed 3 g/d in *adults*.[1]

IV push

Not recommended. Rapid infusion may result in hemolysis.[1]

Intermittent infusion

For loading dose dilute in D5W, D10W, or NS (1 mg/mL) and infuse no faster than 5 mg/min in *adults*.[1]

Continuous infusion

Add 250 mg (12.5 mL) to 250 mL D5W, D10W, or NS (~1 mg/mL) and infuse 1–5 mg/min in *adults* for postanesthetic use or with drug-induced CNS depression. Add 400 mg (20-mL vial) to 180 mL D5W, D10W, or NS (2 mg/mL) and infuse 1–3 mg/min in *adults* with COPD.[1]

Other routes of administration

No information available to support administration by other routes.

Maximum concentration	2 mg/mL in D5W, D10W, or NS.[1,8]
Cautions related to IV administration	Monitor blood pressure closely for evidence of hypertension.[1,6,9] Extravasation should be avoided. Use of a single injection site over an extended period may result in thrombophlebitis or local skin irritation.[1]
Other additives	**Benzyl alcohol:** The only product available in the U.S. contains benzyl alcohol 0.9% as a preservative.[1] Benzyl alcohol in small doses as a preservative in drugs is considered safe in newborns.[10] However, a 3-week-old, very low birth weight (710 g) infant who received clindamycin experienced a profound desaturation that required resuscitation after the third and fourth doses, which was subsequently related to the benzyl alcohol preservative.[11] Hypersensitivity reactions to benzyl alcohol in parenteral products have been reported in *adults*.[12,13]
Comments	A group of preterm infants with mental delay was compared to a control group matched for gestational age, birth weight, sex, intraventricular hemorrhage grade, and socioeconomic status.[14] Analysis of their respiratory therapy showed that steroid use and methylxanthine use was similar. However, both oxygen supplementation and doxapram therapy were longer in the case group compared to controls.[14] A subsequent group of investigators evaluated 20 preterm neonates during escalating doxapram doses using cerebral Doppler ultrasonography and near-infrared spectroscopy.[15] They found that doxapram increased oxygen consumption and requirements and at the same time decreased oxygen delivery and proposed that these effects are caused by decreased cerebral blood flow.[15] QTc interval prolongation has been reported in premature infants receiving 0.5–1 mg/kg/h for 72 h.[16] Monitor heart rate, blood pressure, and deep tendon reflexes.[1]

Doxycycline Hyclate

Brand names	Doxy, Doxychel Hyclate, Vibramycin I.V.
Dosage	**Children <8 years of age:** (See Comments section.)[1] **Children ≥8 years of age** **≤100 lbs. (45 kg):** 4.4 mg/kg/d (given in one or two divided doses) on day 1 followed by 2.2–4.4 mg/kg/d given once daily or divided q 12 h.[2-4] **>100 lbs. (45 kg):** 200 mg/d (given in one or two divided doses) on day 1 followed by 100–200 mg/d given once daily or 200 mg/d divided q 12 h.[2,4,5]
Dosage adjustment in organ dysfunction	No dose adjustment necessary.[7] While one reference suggests doxycycline accumulates in renal failure,[6] others have found little to no accumulation in *adults*.[8,9]
Maximum dosage	300 mg/d for syphilis in children ≥8 years of age and >100 lbs. (45 kg).[2]
IV push	Not recommended.[10]
Intermittent infusion	0.1–1 mg/mL[2,10-13] in D5LR, D5W, LR, NS, or R[2,4,10] over 1–4 h or longer.[2,3,11-13]
Continuous infusion	No information available to support administration by this method.
Other routes of administration	May be administered via intrapleural infusion; dilute 500 mg of doxycycline with 25–30 mL of sterile NS. Instill via thoracostomy tube after drainage of pleural cavity by thoracentesis.[10]
Maximum concentration	1 mg/mL.[10]
Cautions related to IV administration	Phlebitis occurs frequently.[12,14] For PN compatibility information, please see Appendix C.
Other additives	100- and 200-mg vials contain 480 and 960 mg of ascorbic acid, respectively. Mannitol is also present in some preparations.[10]

Comments

Because tetracyclines may permanently discolor teeth, historically their use has been discouraged in children <8 years of age unless other drugs are ineffective or contraindicated.[1,4,15-17] However, recent concerns regarding both Rocky Mountain spotted fever and ehrlichiosis have caused the American Academy of Pediatrics to recommend doxycycline 4.4 mg/kg/d (maximum 100 mg/dose) divided q 12 h if either of the above infections are suspected.[18]

Protect from direct sunlight.[10]

Doxycycline may cause false-positive urinary glucose results when cupric sulfate solution–based tests (Clinitest, Benedict's, or Fehling's solution) are used.[19] Glucose oxidase methods (Clinistix) may be associated with false-negative test results.[19]

Doxycycline may be beneficial in rheumatoid arthritis, but one study in *adults* found no evidence of reduction in disease activity or collagen crosslink production.[20]

One study showed that oral administration of antacids might significantly enhance clearance of IV doxycycline.[21]

Nail discoloration has occurred in an 11-year-old receiving oral doxycycline 200 mg on day 1 followed by 100 mg daily for 10 days.[22]

Droperidol

Brand names	Inapsine

Dosage

A black box warning was added to prescribing information in 2001 because of reports of deaths associated with QT prolongation and torsades de pointes in patients treated with droperidol. Cases have occurred in patients with no known risk factors for QT prolongation and some have been fatal.[1]

Droperidol should only be used in patients who fail to respond to other therapies and risks of administration must be weighed against any potential benefit.[1] Prior to administration, all patients should have a 12 lead ECG to assess for QT interval prolongation.[1]

Contraindicated in those with known or suspected QT prolongation including those with congenital long QT syndrome.[1]

Maximum initial dose for children 2–12 years of age is 0.1 mg/kg. Additional doses should be administered with caution.[1]

Postoperative nausea/vomiting

Prophylaxis: 0.015–0.075 mg/kg/dose[2-9] concomitantly with anesthesia induction,[3,7,9] immediately after induction,[2,6] 30 min before end of procedure,[5] or at end of procedure.[4]

Treatment: 0.1 mg/kg/dose.[8] Administer additional doses with caution.[1]

Dosage adjustment in organ dysfunction

Use cautiously in patients with impaired hepatic or renal function.[10]

Maximum dosage

2.5 mg/dose.[3] 2.5 mg per 20–25 lbs. in *adults.*[11]

IV push

2.5 mg/mL given by slow IV injection, over 2–5 min.[10] (See Comments section.)

Intermittent infusion

No information is available to support administration by this method.

Continuous infusion

No information is available to support administration by this method.

Other routes of administration

2.5-mg/mL solutions may be given IM.[10]

Maximum concentration

2.5 mg/mL.[10]

Cautions related to IV administration

Elevated blood pressure has occurred when given concomitantly with fentanyl and other parenteral analgesics.[11]

For PN compatibility information, please see Appendix C.

Other additives

None.

Comments

Fluids and other measures should be readily available to manage hypotension.[11]

Acute dystonia has been reported in two patients (ages 14 and 16 years) receiving droperidol (0.04 and 0.08 mg/kg) with patient controlled analgesia.[12]

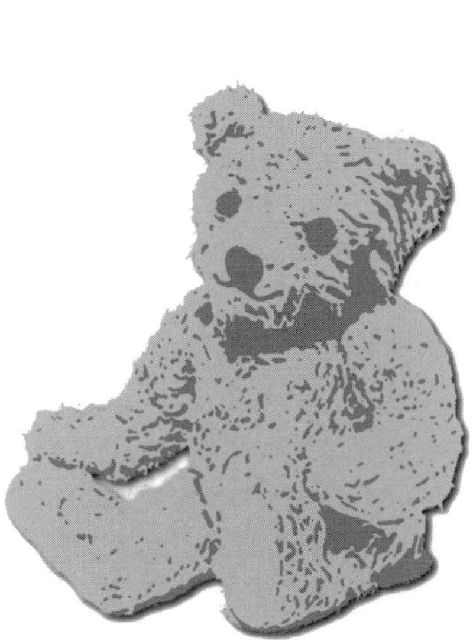

Edrophonium Chloride

Brand names	Enlon, Reversol, Tensilon

Dosage

Atropine sulfate injection should be available to reverse signs and symptoms of life-threatening cholinergic reaction.[1]

Antiarrhythmic: Edrophonium has been used to terminate supraventricular tachycardia but has generally been replaced by other antiarrhythmic agents.

Myasthenia gravis (diagnosis): Edrophonium establishes the diagnosis in 90% to 95% of patients suspected of having the disease.[1] If a cholinergic reaction occurs after the initial dose, the test should be discontinued.

Infants: 0.04 mg/kg over 1 min followed by 0.16 mg/kg if no response.[2]

Children: ≤34 kg and >34 kg should receive an initial dose of 1 mg and 2 mg over 1 min, respectively.[1] If no response within 45 sec, repeat dose q 30–45 sec up to a maximum cumulative dose of 5 mg for children ≤34 kg and up to 10 mg for heavier children and adolescents.[1]

Alternatively, some recommend that children receive a total of 0.2 mg/kg or 6 mg/m^2.[1] One-fifth of the dose should be given over 1 min. If no response occurs in 45 sec, the remainder should be given.

Myasthenia gravis (assessment of anticholinesterase therapy): Edrophonium is used to determine the adequacy of chronic dosing of another anticholinesterase medication in a patient with myasthenia gravis.

0.04 mg/kg given 1 h after administration of the oral drug being used to chronically treat myasthenia gravis.[1] If the patient's muscle strength or forced vital capacity improves following edrophonium, the dose of the chronic therapy should be increased.[2,3]

Because it requires several days for result to occur following changes in chronic oral dosage, the patient should be tested with edrophonium q 1–3 d after dosage adjustment of the chronic medication.[1]

Postsurgical reversal of nondepolarizing neuromuscular blocking agents: 0.4–1 mg/kg administered IV over 30–45 sec and repeated q 5–10 min as needed.[3-7] If a larger dose of edrophonium is required, it should be preceded by IV atropine sulfate (0.01 mg/kg; minimum 0.1 mg and maximum 2 mg).[1,2]

Dosage adjustment in organ dysfunction	No information available.
Maximum dosage	Maximum cumulative dose is 5 mg for children ≤34 kg and up to 10 mg for heavier children and *adults*.[1]
IV push	10 mg/mL given over 1 min.[1]
Intermittent infusion	Not recommended.
Continuous infusion	Not recommended.

Edrophonium Chloride

Other routes of administration	Edrophonium is usually given IV but may also be given 0.5–1 mg IM or SC.[1] Children weighing up to 34 kg should receive 2 mg IM for the diagnosis of myasthenia gravis, and children weighing more than 34 kg should receive 5 mg IM. There is a delay of 2–10 min before a reaction is noted following IM administration.[1]
Maximum concentration	10 mg/mL.[1]
Cautions related to IV administration	Hypersensitivity, arrhythmias, bronchospasm, and laryngospasm have been reported.[1]
Other additives	May contain sodium bisulfites. Sulfites may cause hypersensitivity reactions and these are more common in *adults* with asthma. Most reactions are mild but can include anaphylactic symptoms and life-threatening or less severe asthma episodes.[8-10] Epinephrine may be required in severe cases; and if the sulfite-free product is not available, the sulfite-preserved epinephrine should be used.[8]
Comments	While edrophonium reverses the effects of most nondepolarizing neuromuscular blocking agents, it is less effective in reversing depolarizing agents such as mivacurium, decamethonium, and succinylcholine.[1,7] Use with caution in patients with cardiovascular disease (especially those taking digoxin or quinidine) or asthma.[1] Administration of edrophonium may prolong the effect of succinylcholine.[1]

Enalaprilat

Brand names	Vasotec I.V.
Dosage	Enalapril maleate (orally administered) is a prodrug of enalaprilat. It is well-absorbed following oral administration; hence, dosage of the two medications is not comparable. Clinicians should pay attention to dosage when converting between dosage forms. **Hypertensive or congestive heart failure (left-right ventricular shunt)** **Neonates:** 10 mcg/kg/dose,[1] 5–30 mcg/kg/d divided q 8–24 h[2,3] or 100 mcg/kg/d divided q 6 h.[4] **Infants and children:** The fourth report on the diagnosis, evaluation, and treatment of high blood pressure in children and adolescents recommends doses of 50–100 mcg/kg up to 1.25 mg/dose.[5] Titrated according to blood pressure response. Doses have ranged from 5–100 mcg/kg.[6-10] Clinical response should occur in <15 min, and peak effect after first dose should occur by 4 h.[11] **Adolescents and adults:** 0.625–1.25 mg repeated q 6 h as needed.[12]
Dosage adjustment in organ dysfunction	Adjust dosage in patients with renal dysfunction.[11,13] If CrCl is 10–50 mL/min, administer 50% to 100% of a dose; if CrCl is <10 mL/min, administer 25% to 50% of the dose.[14] Premature infants may also require extended dosing intervals because of decreased glomerular filtration rates and prolonged duration of action.[2]
Maximum dosage	120 mcg/kg/d divided q 6 h[4] and 150 mcg/kg/d divided q 8 h[1] have been used. In hypertensive emergencies, 320 mcg/kg q 6 h has been used.[6] Dose of 5 mg[3] and 20 mg/d have been recommended.[10,15]
IV push	Not recommended. However, an infusion over 60 sec has been given without adverse effects.[2,7,8]
Intermittent infusion	Infuse undiluted or dilute in D5LR, D5NS, D5W, Isolyte E, or NS[12] (see Maximum concentration section) and infuse over 5 min.[11,12] For neonates, mix 1 mL (1.25 mg) in 49 mL D5W or NS for a 25-mcg/mL solution.[16]
Continuous infusion	Not recommended.[12]
Other routes of administration	Not recommended.[12]
Maximum concentration	1.25 mg/mL.[11]
Cautions related to IV administration	Anaphylactoid reactions have occurred.[11] Angioedema associated with laryngeal edema has been reported. Anaphylaxis requires immediate treatment with epinephrine, oxygen, IV steroids, and airway management. Monitor for hypotension, especially in volume-depleted patients,[11] for 1–3 h after the first dose or following an increase in dosage. For PN compatibility information, please see Appendix C.

Other additives

Benzyl alcohol: Contains benzyl alcohol 0.9% as a preservative.[11] Benzyl alcohol in small doses as a preservative in drugs is considered safe in newborns.[17] However, a 3-week-old, very low birth weight (710 g) infant who received clindamycin experienced a profound desaturation that required resuscitation after the third and fourth doses, which was subsequently related to the benzyl alcohol preservative.[18]

Administration of saline flushes containing benzyl alcohol (bacteriostatic water for injection) was associated with a fatal gasping syndrome, intraventricular hemorrhage, metabolic acidosis, and increased mortality in preterm infants.[19] This should not be used in neonates.

Hypersensitivity reactions to benzyl alcohol in parenteral products have been reported in *adults*.[20,21]

Comments

Transient hyperkalemia has been reported.[11]

Neonates have decreased elimination and extended duration of action; hence, they may experience prolonged hypotension and acute renal failure.[2,5]

Enoxaparin Sodium

Brand names Lovenox

Dosage

Prophylaxis[1,2]

<2 months of age: 0.75 mg/kg SC q 12 h.

>2 months of age: 0.5 mg/kg SC q 12 h.

Therapeutic anti-factor Xa (anti-Xa) concentrations for prophylaxis range from 0.1–0.4 units/mL.[1,3]

Treatment[1-6]

<2 months of age: 1.5 mg/kg SC q 12 h.

>2 months of age: 1 mg/kg SC q 12 h.

Theraputic anti-Xa concentrations for treatment range from 0.5–1 unit/mL.[3]

Compared to infants ≥37 weeks gestational age (GA), those <37 weeks GA required larger doses both to achieve target anti-Xa concentrations (1.9 ± 0.6 mg/kg q 12 h vs. 1.6 ± 0.3) and to maintain target anti-Xa concentrations (2.1 ± 0.6 mg/kg q 12 h vs. 1.7 ± 0.3).[7] In a retrospective chart review, 10 preterm infants (24–34 weeks GA) required a mean dose of 2.27 mg/kg (2–3.5) q 12 h to maintain a therapeutic anti-Xa concentration.[3] Similarly, doses from 0.94–2.36 mg/kg (mean 1.69) q 12 h in patients ≤2-months-old and from 0.56–1.6 mg/kg (mean 1.06) q 12 h in patients >2 months old were required to achieve therapeutic anti-Xa concentrations.[8]

Concentrations should be drawn 4–6 h after a SC dose.[9,10] The following recommendations are made for dosage adjustment[9,10]:

Anti-Xa (units/mL)	<0.35	0.35–0.49	0.5–1	1.1–1.5	1.6–2	>2
Dose adjust	Increase dose 25%	Increase dose 10%	No change	Decrease dose 20%	Decrease dose 30%	Decrease dose 40%
Re-dose	On time	On time	On time	On time	Delay dose 3 h	Delay dose until anti-Xa <0.5
Measure anti-Xa	4 h after next dose	4 h after next dose	Every other day	4 h after next dose	4 h after next dose	q 12 h until <0.5

Dosing in adults[11]

Abdominal surgery, thromboembolic prophylaxis: 40 mg SC once daily.

Hip or knee replacement surgery prophylaxis: 30 mg SC q 12 h.

Unstable angina or myocardial infarction: 1 mg/kg SC q 12 h.

Treatment of DVT with or without PE: 1 mg/kg SC q 12 h or 1.5 mg/kg SC once daily.

Dosage adjustment in organ dysfunction

Doses may need to be reduced in pediatric patients with cardiac conditions or impaired renal or liver function.[7,8] In *adults* with CrCl <30 mL/min, decrease dose to 30 mg SC once daily.[11]

Maximum dosage

1.5 mg/kg in *adults*.[1] One group reported that 3.5 mg/kg q 12 h was required to produce therapeutic anti-Xa concentrations in a preterm neonate.[3]

IV push	Not indicated. (See Comments section.)
Intermittent infusion	Not indicated.
Continuous infusion	Not indicated.
Other routes of administration	Administered SC, not IM.[11]
Maximum concentration	150 mg/mL (commercially available).[11,12]
Cautions related to IV administration	Not indicated for IV administration. (See Comments section.)
Other additives	Prefilled syringes and graduated prefilled syringes are preservative-free. Each multiple-dose vial (300 mg/mL) contains benzyl alcohol 15 mg/mL.[1] Benzyl alcohol in small doses as a preservative in drugs is considered safe in newborns.[13] However, a 3-week old, very low birth weight (710 g) infant who received clindamycin experienced a profound desaturation that required resuscitation after the third and fourth doses, which was subsequently related to the benzyl alcohol preservative.[14] Administration of saline flushes containing benzyl alcohol (BW) was associated with a fatal gasping syndrome, intraventricular hemorrhage, metabolic acidosis, and increased mortality in preterm infants.[15] This should not be used in neonates. Hypersensitivity reactions to benzyl alcohol in parenteral products have been reported in *adults*.[16,17]
Comments	Enoxaparin has been associated with the development of heparin-induced thrombocytopenia (HIT) in a pediatric patient.[18] Enoxaparin diluted with preservative-free sterile water for injection to 20 mg/mL did not lose significant anticoagulant activity for 4 weeks.[19] One 29-week, GA preterm infant (normal cranial ultrasound) with a suspected radial artery thrombus and discolored fingers was given 1 mg/kg IV q 8 h for 7 days.[20] The perfusion improved and only the tip of one finger was ultimately affected.[20] There was no bleeding associated and no future thromboses were noted.[20]

Epinephrine HCl

Brand names	Adrenalin Chloride

Dosage

Anaphylaxis: The airway should be maintained and oxygen should be administered.

Mild symptoms (e.g., pruritus, erythema, urticaria, angioedema): 0.01 mL/kg of the 1:1000 dilution (0.01 mg/kg) given IM. This may be followed by administration of antihistamines.[1,2] The epinephrine dose can be repeated q 10–20 min for up to three doses if symptoms continue or recur. The patient should be observed for 4 h.[2] SC administration is no longer recommended as higher concentrations are more rapidly achieved with IM administration.[2]

Life-threatening symptoms (e.g., severe bronchospasm, laryngeal edema, other airway compromise, shock, cardiovascular collapse): 0.01 mg/kg (0.1 mL/kg of the 1:10,000 dilution) by IV repeated q 10–20 min as required.[2,3] Continuous infusion should be started if repeated doses are required. Add 1 mL (1 mg) of 1:1000 to 250 mL of D5W (4 mcg/mL) and infuse at 0.1 mcg/kg/min that is increased gradually to 1.5 mcg/kg/min to maintain blood pressure.[2]

Patients previously on beta-adrenergic blocking agents may be less responsive to epinephrine and may require more aggressive therapy.[1] Likewise, some anaphylactic reactions (e.g., latex allergy) require large doses.[3]

Asthma: *The National Asthma Education and Prevention Program*[4] *Expert Panel Report 2: Update on Selected Topics 2002* states that there is no proven advantage of systemic beta-agonist therapy over aerosol. However, it lists a dose of 10 mcg/kg (0.01 mg/kg) administered SC (0.01 mL/kg of 1:1000 dilution) up to 0.3–0.5 mg.[4] May give q 20 min for three doses.[3-5]

Cardiopulmonary resuscitation (see Comments section)

Asystole: 0.01mg/kg (0.1 mL/kg of 1:10,000) up to 1 mg IV or intraosseously (IO) or 0.1 mg/kg endotracheally (ET) (0.1 mL/kg of 1:1000) up to 10 mg.[6] Repeat q 3–5 min as needed.[6]

No survival benefit from routine high-dose epinephrine 0.2 mg/kg (0.2 mL/kg of 1:1000) IV, IO, or ET has been found, and it may be harmful, particularly in asphyxia.[7-11] High-dose epinephrine may be considered in exceptional circumstances such as beta-blocker overdose.[7]

Bradycardia

Neonates: 0.01–0.03 mg/kg (0.1–0.3 mL/kg of 1:10,000) given IV or IO. Repeat q 3–5 min as needed.[12] Alternatively, 0.1 mg/kg through ET followed by 1 mL NS until IV/IO access established. Safety and efficacy of the ET route of administration have not been evaluated.[12]

Infants and children, initial doses: 0.01 mg/kg (0.1 mL/kg of 1:10,000) given IV or IO.[3,6] If given ET, administer 0.1 mg/kg (0.1 mL/kg of the 1:1000 dilution) followed by a 1–5 mL saline flush.[6] Repeat q 3–5 min as needed.[3,6]

Persistent shock after volume resuscitation: 0.1 mcg/kg/min increased by 0.1 mcg/kg/min to desired response (up to 3 mcg/kg/min).[3]

Dosage adjustment in organ dysfunction	No dosage adjustment required.

Maximum dosage

The recommended maximum IV/IO dose is 0.03 mg/kg for neonates[10] and 0.01 mg/kg for infants and children.[6] Continuous infusion of ≤3 mcg/kg/min may be used after resuscitation in children with persistent shock.[3]

Although IV/ET/IO doses of 0.2 mg/kg (0.2 mL/kg of 1:1000) were safely given as high-dose therapy to patients who failed standard therapy,[13-15] no survival benefit from routine high-dose epinephrine has been found, and it may be harmful.[7-11]

IV push

0.1 mg/mL (1:10,000) in NS over seconds.[3,16] The 1 mg/mL (1:1000) solution should be used for high-dose therapy only, not for initial therapy. Because standard and high-dose therapy require different dilutions, take caution to avoid errors in product selection and dosing.

Intermittent infusion

Not indicated.

Continuous infusion

Compatible in D–LR, D–R, D–S, D5LR, D5NS, D5W, D10W, LR, NS, or R.[17] (See Dosage and Maximum dosage sections.)

The PALS guidelines and the AAP recommend the following formula for preparation of the infusion: 0.6 × weight (kg) = mg of drug to add to IV solution for a total volume of 100 mL. An infusion rate of 1 mL/h provides 0.1 mcg/kg/min.[3] This formula estimates an initial concentration. Ultimately, the concentration of the drug should consider the patient's fluid requirements or fluid limitations.

Despite widespread use of the above formula, recent JCAHO® guidelines recommend the implementation of "standardized concentrations" of vasoactive medications.[18]

Other routes of administration

The IV and IM routes are the preferred methods of administration in pediatric patients. In children, the IM dose should be injected into the anterolateral aspect of the thigh; administration in the buttock should be avoided.[1,19] In life-threatening situations, may also be given IO (0.1 mL/kg of a 1:10,000 solution) or ET (0.1 mL/kg of a 1:1000 solution) route.[3,6] SC route has been used in asthma.[4,5]

Maximum concentration

0.1 mg/mL (1:10,000 solution) for IV push and IO or ET administration.[3,6] The EpiPen, Jr delivers a dose of 0.15 mg (0.3 mL of 0.5 mg/mL, 1:2000) and the EpiPen delivers a dose of 0.3 mg (0.3 mL of 1 mg/mL, 1:1000). For continuous infusion, 64 mcg/mL has been recommended as a maximum.[20]

Cautions related to IV administration

Bradycardia, tachycardia, dysrhythmias, myocardial ischemia, syncope, weakness, renal failure, and hypertension have occurred.[19,21-24]

Extravasation may cause local ischemia and tissue necrosis.[1] Therefore, infusion should be via a secure peripheral catheter or, preferably, a central route.[1] Aliquots of phentolamine mesylate, 5–10 mg in 10 mL of NS infiltrated with a fine hypodermic needle around and into the extravasation area, should reverse blanching immediately. Use this antidote within the first 12 h of extravasation.[25] A series of case reports on a 13-year-old, a 31-year-old, and a 39-year-old who accidentally discharged an epinephrine autoinjector into their thumbs reported that local injection of 1 or 3 mL of SC terbutaline (1 mg in 10 mL NS) was an effective alternative to phentolamine.[26]

For PN compatibility information, please see Appendix C.

Epinephrine HCl

Other additives

Some products contain metabisulfite. Sulfites may cause hypersensitivity reactions, and these are more common in *adults* with asthma. Most reactions are mild but can include anaphylactic symptoms and life-threatening or less severe asthma episodes.[27-29] Epinephrine may be required in severe cases; and if the sulfite-free product is not available, the sulfite containing epinephrine should be used.[21]

Comments

ET doses are two to two-and-a-half times larger than IV. The dose should be diluted in 1–5 mL saline, depending on patient size, prior to ET tube instillation.[1]

Epinephrine is easily destroyed by oxidants and in alkaline solutions; therefore, solutions should be protected from light.[19] Do not infuse if solution is pinkish, darker than slightly yellow, or if it contains a precipitate.[19]

Hemodynamic instability may be attributed to significant variability between the ordered dosage and the actual solution concentration of epinephrine. Failure to consider the HCl salt in the stock drug accounted for some, but not all, of the inaccuracy in preparation.[30]

A 13-month-old infant (8.6 kg) inadvertently given 327 mcg/kg of epinephrine IV developed metabolic acidosis and hypertension followed by tachycardia and pulmonary edema requiring mechanical ventilation.[31]

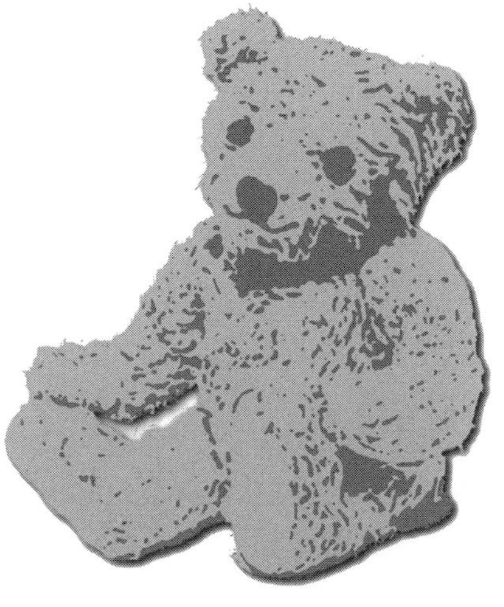

Epoetin Alfa

Brand names	Epogen, Procrit

Dosage

To ensure the erythropoietic response, iron status should be evaluated and supplemental iron prescribed if stores are low. Transferrin saturation should be ≥20% and ferritin should be ≥100 ng/mL.[1]

Anemias (a target hemoglobin (Hb) of 12 g/dL is usual)

End-stage renal disease: 10–150 units/kg three times weekly after dialysis through venous line in patients on hemodialysis.[2-7] In patients receiving continuous ambulatory or cycling peritoneal dialysis, SC injection is preferred, but 300 units/kg IV once a week have been used.[8]

HIV-infected children, zidovudine-treated: 40 and 90 units/kg three times weekly for 1 and 1.5 months were used in a 4- and 14-year-old child. Failure of adequate response in the 4-year-old child was attributed to use of a low dose for a short length of time.[9]

Children on chemotherapy: In children from 5–18 years of age, an initial dose of 600 units/kg (maximum 40,000 units) weekly for 16 weeks was used. If Hb did not increase by 1 g/dL after 4–5 weeks, the dose was increased to 900 units/kg (maximum 60,000 units). Sixty percent of patients required the increased dose.[1] In 37 children (1–18 years) with solid tumors, 300 units/kg was given three times weekly if the Hb was <12 g/dL, and 150 units/kg was given three times weekly if the Hb was ≥12 g/dL and ≤16 g/dL.[10] Epoetin was not given if the Hb was ≥16 g/dL.[10]

Prematurity: 100–400 units/kg either two to three times weekly up to 10 weeks,[11-15] daily for 10–14 days,[16-18] or five times a week for 2 weeks.[19] Generally, the initiation of treatment varies from within 72 h of life to 5 weeks of age.

Epidermolysis bullosa: 150 or 350 units/kg three times a week.[20]

Adjust dosage monthly to achieve and maintain a Hb concentration of ≤12 g/dL. If Hb has increased by <1 g/dL during initial 4 weeks of therapy (with adequate iron stores), then increase dose by 25% q 4 weeks until at target Hb. If the Hb increases by >1 g/dL in 2 weeks or the Hb is increasing and approaching 12 g/dL, then decrease dose by 25%.[1,21,22]

Preoperative cardiac surgery (to reduce the need for blood transfusion): 150 or 300 units/kg given two or three times approximately 1 week prior to surgery and postoperatively for two doses or until the hematocrit is increased to the preoperative value.[23,24]

Dosage adjustment in organ dysfunction	No dosage adjustment required.[1,21]
Maximum dosage	Not established. 900 units/kg/week have been given to children with cancer.[1] Doses of 1200[12] and 5000[25] units/kg/week have been given to neonates.
IV push	Rapid.
Intermittent infusion	Dilute dose in 2 mL of protein-containing parenteral nutrition fluid or 2 mL of 5% albumin and infuse over 4 h (to mimic the pharmacokinetics of SC dosing).[15]
Continuous infusion	Can be mixed in IV fluids containing at least 0.05% protein (amino acids).[16,26,27]

Other routes of administration

SC route is preferred except in patients on hemodialysis when IV administration is preferred.[1] For SC administration the dose can be diluted 1:1 with bacteriostatic 0.9% sodium chloride injection, USP, with benzyl alcohol 0.9%. Bacteriostatic saline decreases the discomfort from SC injection. This is not necessary when using the product that contains benzyl alcohol.[1,22] (See Other additives section.) IM is not indicated.

Maximum concentration

40,000 units/mL.[1,21]

Cautions related to IV administration

Do not administer through same IV line as other drugs.[22]

For PN compatibility information, please see Appendix C.

Other additives

1 mL single-use vials (2000, 3000, 4000, and 10,000 units/mL) also contain 2.5 mg human albumin, 5.8 mg sodium citrate, 5.8 mg NaCl, and 0.06 mg citric acid in SW.[1,21]

1-mL single-use vials (40,000 units/mL) also contain 2.5 mg human albumin, 1.2 mg sodium phosphate monobasic monohydrate, 1.8 mg sodium phosphate dibasic anhydrate, 0.7 mg sodium citrate, 5.8 mg NaCl, and 6.8 mg citric acid in SW.[1,21,22]

2-mL multidose vials (10,000 units/mL) and 1-mL multidose vials (20,000 units/mL) also contain 2.5 mg human albumin, 1.3 mg sodium citrate, 8.2 mg NaCl, 0.11 mg citric acid, and benzyl alcohol 1% in SW.[1,21,22]

Benzyl alcohol in small doses as a preservative in drugs is considered safe in newborns.[28] However, a 3-week-old, very low birth weight (710 g) infant who received clindamycin experienced a profound desaturation that required resuscitation after the third and fourth doses, which was subsequently related to the benzyl alcohol preservative.[29]

Administration of saline flushes containing benzyl alcohol (BW) was associated with a fatal gasping syndrome, intraventricular hemorrhage, metabolic acidosis, and increased mortality in preterm infants.[30] This should not be used in neonates.

Hypersensitivity reactions to benzyl alcohol in parenteral products have been reported in *adults*.[31,32]

Comments

Failure to respond may be a result of iron deficiency.[1,11,12,21,22] Following the erythropoietin infusion, IV ferrous gluconate[5] or iron dextran[15,33] may be given to patients who have inadequate iron stores and who are unable to tolerate oral iron.

Hypertension[1,3,5,8] and blood vessel[4] or vascular access occlusion[2,5] have occurred in children with renal failure. A 12-year-old boy with end stage renal disease developed hypertension with encephalopathy that resolved with discontinuation of phenytoin and erythropoietin.[34]

Transient neutropenia was associated with larger erythropoietin doses in preterm neonates.[35]

Pure red cell aplasia, in association with neutralizing antibodies to erythropoietin (anti-EPO antibodies), has been reported as a rare yet important reaction in *adults* and children, particularly those with chronic renal failure.[21,36] Any child with a loss of response to erythropoietin should be evaluated.

Ertapenem

Brand names	Invanz
Dosage	Because ertapenem has been administered to a limited number of pediatric patients, the doses and side effects have not been established in this age group.[1] **3 months to 12 years:** 30 mg/kg/d divided q 12 h up to 1 g/d.[1-3] **13 to 17 years of age:** 20 mg/kg q 24 h up to 1 g.[1-3]
Dosage adjustment in organ dysfunction	Adjust dosage in patients with renal dysfunction. Although there are no data in pediatric patients with renal insufficiency, it is recommended that the dose be decreased by 50% in *adults* with CrCl ≤30 mL/min.[1,4,5]
Maximum dosage	1 g/d.[1]
IV push	Not given via this method.
Intermittent infusion	20 mg/mL in NS given over 30 min.[1] Do not dilute in dextrose containing solutions.[1]
Continuous infusion	No information to support administration via this method.
Other routes of administration	May be administered IM following reconstitution with 1% lidocaine HCl injection, USP (in saline without epinephrine).[1,6] No information available to support administration by other routes.
Maximum concentration	20 mg/mL.[1]
Cautions related to IV administration	Ertapenem is contraindicated in patients who have demonstrated anaphylactic reactions to beta-lactams.[1] If a decision is made to give ertapenem to a patient with known beta-lactam hypersensitivity, the patient should be closely observed for allergenicity.
Other additives	Contains approximately 137 mg (6 mEq) of sodium/g of ertapenem.[1]
Comments	Neurotoxicity of the carbapenem antibiotics has been reported.[7,8] In *adults*, seizures most often occur after 7 days and appear to be related to an underlying CNS disorder, impaired renal function, and/or large doses.[8] Because of the risk of seizures, the drug should be used cautiously in patients with CNS infections or renal dysfunction, patients with history of seizure disorders, and when used in combination with drugs that lower the seizure threshold.[9] If seizures occur, the patient should undergo a neurological assessment and anticonvulsants should be initiated.[1] The dosage of and need for ertapenem should be assessed.[1]

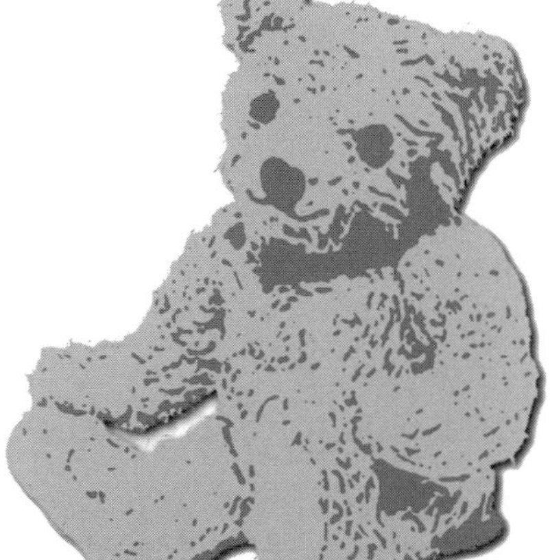

Erythromycin Gluceptate/Lactobionate

Brand names	Erythrocin Lactobionate-I.V., Ilotycin Gluceptate

Dosage

Neonates

PNA	<1200–2000 g	≥2000 g
<7 d	20 mg/kg/d divided q 12 h[1,2]	20 mg/kg/d divided q 12 h[1,2]
≥7 d	30 mg/kg/d divided q 8 h[1,2]*	40 mg/kg/d divided q 8 h[1,2]

*Until 4 weeks of age.

Infants and children

Mild-to-moderate infections: Not appropriate.[2]

Severe infections: 15–50 mg/kg/d divided q 6 h up to 4 g/d.[2]

Biologic warfare or bioterrorism: The CDC and other experts recommend that treatment of inhalational anthrax spores due to biologic warfare or bioterrorism should be started on a multiple-drug parenteral regimen that includes ciprofloxacin or doxycycline and one or two additional anti-infective agents (i.e., chloramphenicol, clindamycin, rifampin, vancomycin, clarithromycin, imipenem, penicillin, or ampicillin).[3,4]

Pelvic inflammatory disease: The 2006 CDC guidelines do not include erythromycin as first-line therapy for PID due to N. gonorrhoeae.[5] However, the manufacturer recommends 500 mg q 6 h for at least 3 days followed by an additional 7 days of oral therapy.[1,6] Some recommend intravenous therapy (500 mg q 6 h) for 7–10 days due to concerns that oral dosage is inadequate.[1,6]

Prokinetic agent: Although studies have yielded conflicting results,[7,8] doses of 45–48 mg/kg/d divided q 6–8 h,[9] 3 mg/kg/h continuous infusion,[10] and 1 mg/kg infused over 30 min followed by octreotide[11] have been used in children.

Dosage adjustment in organ dysfunction

Adjust dosage in patients with renal dysfunction.[12] (See Comments section.) If CrCl is <10 mL/min, administer 50% to 75% of normal dose.[12] Use cautiously in persons with hepatic dysfunction.[1,13]

Maximum dosage

50 mg/kg/d, not to exceed 4 g/d for severe infections.[2]

IV push

Not recommended due to local irritation and risk of cardiovascular effects.[1,14]

Intermittent infusion

1–5 mg/mL in NS, LR, or Normosol® over 20–120 min.[1,14] (See Cautions related to IV administration and Comments sections.)

Alternatively, after vials of lyophilized powder are reconstituted with preservative-free SW, the drug can be diluted in D5W, D5LR, or D5NS if first buffered with 1 mL of Neut® (4% sodium bicarbonate) for each 100 mL of diluent.[14]

Continuous infusion

Preferred to intermittent delivery.[1] Significant cardiovascular effects (i.e., bradycardia, hypotension, cardiac arrest, arrhythmias) may depend on serum concentration and/or infusion rate. Delivery over ≥60 min may reduce the likelihood of the cardiac effects; however, the effects may or may not be eliminated. Concentration ≤1 mg/mL is recommended.[14]

Erythromycin Gluceptate/Lactobionate

Other routes of administration

No information available to support administration by other routes.

Maximum concentration

5 mg/mL.[1] The osmolality of 5 mg/mL in D5W and NS is 265 and 291 mOsm/kg, respectively.[14] 10 mg/mL has been recommended for administration via a central venous line.[15]

Cautions related to IV administration

Thrombophlebitis frequently occurs.[16]

Ventricular arrhythmias (in individuals with pre-existing myocardial disease), nausea, vomiting, and abdominal cramps have occurred.[16-19]

Bradycardia and hypotension have been reported in neonates[19-21] and in a child.[22] Prolonging the infusion to ≥60 min has been recommended to decrease potential direct cardiotoxicity.[21,22] However, hypotension resulted following a change to oral erythromycin, leading the authors to speculate that a hypersensitivity reaction had occurred.[22]

For PN compatibility information, please see Appendix C.

Other additives

Vials containing the equivalent of 1 g of erythromycin have 180 mg of benzyl alcohol as a preservative; vials containing the equivalent of 500 mg of erythromycin have 90 mg of benzyl alcohol.[1] Benzyl alcohol in small doses as a preservative in drugs is considered safe in newborns.[23] However, a 3-week-old, very low birth weight (710 g) infant who received clindamycin experienced a profound desaturation that required resuscitation after the third and fourth doses, which was subsequently related to the benzyl alcohol preservative.[24]

Administration of saline flushes containing benzyl alcohol (bacteriostatic water for injection) was associated with a fatal gasping syndrome, intraventricular hemorrhage, metabolic acidosis, and increased mortality in preterm infants.[25] This should not be used in neonates.

Hypersensitivity reactions to benzyl alcohol in parenteral products have been reported in *adults*.[26,27]

Comments

Although high-frequency sensorineural deafness occurred in a 17-year-old with renal failure,[28] this complication usually occurs in older patients.[29-31]

Because erythromycin inhibits the CYP3A4 isozyme and is associated with numerous drug interactions, consult appropriate resources for dosing recommendations before combining any drug with erythromycin.

Esmolol HCl

Brand names	Brevibloc
Dosage	Esmolol should be used with caution in patients with bradycardia, poor left ventricular function, high-degree heart block, congenital heart defects with right-to-left shunting, chronic airway disease (e.g., asthma), or other peripheral vascular disease.[1] **Antiarrhythmic (tachyarrhythmias):** Initiate dose of 600 mcg/kg over 2 min followed by 200 mcg/kg/min.[2] Dose should be increased by 50–100 mcg/kg/min q 5–10 min until >10% decrease in heart rate or blood pressure occurs.[2] A continuous infusion of 1000 mcg/kg/min has been used safely.[2] Studies have evaluated infants as young as 6 months.[3] An 8-day-old with severe tachycardia secondary to neonatal tetanus received a loading dose of 1000 mcg/kg over 1 min followed by a continuous infusion of 120 mcg/kg/min.[4] **Hypertensive crisis** (see Cautions related to IV administration section) **Loading dose:** 500–600 mcg/kg over 1 min.[3,5-7] Doses of 750,[8] 1000,[4] and 200[8] mcg/kg were used in a 15-year old, a neonate, and an 18-month-old, respectively. **Maintenance dose:** 100–500 mcg/kg/min initially.[2-4,7-9] Increase rate by 25,[3] 50–100 mcg/kg/min[5,9] q 5–10 min until heart rate or mean blood pressure decreases by at least 10%. One study reported that postoperative cardiac patients required a mean dose of 700 mcg/kg/min to normalize blood pressure.[1] In patients having coarctation repair, a larger dose may be required (mean = 830 mcg/kg/min).[1]
Dosage adjustment in organ dysfunction	No dosage adjustment required in renal dysfunction.[11]
Maximum dosage	1000 mcg/kg as a single dose[4] and 1000 mcg/kg/min.[2]
IV push	10 mg/mL given over 1–2 min.[2,3,8,12]
Intermittent infusion	Not administered by other routes.
Continuous infusion	10 mg/mL in D5LR, D5NS, D5½NS, D5R, D5W, LR, NS, ½NS, or R prior to infusion.[12-14]
Other routes of administration	Not administered by other routes.
Maximum concentration	20 mg/mL[1,2,12,14] The 2500-mg ampul is not for direct injection. Concentrations >10 mg/mL are associated with more severe vein irritation and phlebitis. Extravasation may result in serious local reactions, including tissue necrosis.[12,15]
Cautions related to IV administration	Monitor heart rate, blood pressure, EKG, and respiratory rate continuously during therapy.[15] Titrate doses to achieve beta blockade (usually defined as a 10% decrease in heart rate or mean blood pressure).[2,3,12,15] If hypotension occurs, decrease the infusion rate or discontinue esmolol.[12] Once esmolol is discontinued, effects last approximately 2–16 min.[2,3] Extravasation may result in serious local reactions, including tissue necrosis.[12,15]

Other additives	Each mL of the remixed injection (2500 mg/250 mL contains 5.9 mg NaCl and 2.8 mg sodium acetate trihydrate and each mL of the injection (100 mg/10 mL) contains 2.8 mg sodium acetate trihydrate.
	Propylene glycol: Each mL of the concentrate (2500 mg/10 mL) product contains 25% propylene glycol. Propylene glycol is added to parenteral drugs as a solubilizer. Rapid infusion of medications that contain propylene glycol has resulted in respiratory depression and cardiac dysrhythmias.[16] Its half-life is three times longer in neonates than in *adults*[17] and has caused hyperosmolality[18] and refractory seizures[19] in preterm neonates receiving 3 g/d.
Comments	Concomitant use of morphine may increase esmolol serum concentration up to 50%.[20]

Ethacrynate Sodium

Brand names	Edecrin Sodium
Dosage	0.5–1 mg/kg, repeat if needed q 8–12 h.[1-9]
Dosage adjustment in organ dysfunction	Should not be given if the patient is anuric.[1,2]
Maximum dosage	2 mg/kg,[6] not to exceed 100 mg in *adults*.[1,2]
IV push	Not recommended.[1,2,10] (See Cautions related to IV administration section.)
Intermittent infusion	1 mg/mL in D5W or NS, infused over 20–30 min or over several minutes through a running IV infusion solution.[13] A concentration of 2 mg/mL infused over 5–10 min was used in 22 children from 2 months–17 years of age[6] and suggested by others.[11]
Continuous infusion	1 mg/mL in D5W or NS[2,10] or 2 mg/mL in D5W.[6] (See Comments section.)
Other routes of administration	Should not be given IM or SC because of local pain and irritation.[1,2,10]
Maximum concentration	2 mg/mL.[6]
Cautions related to IV administration	In *adults*, irreversible deafness[12] and upper GI bleeding[13] have occurred following infusion. Rapid administration has been associated with reversible deafness, acute vertigo, and tinnitus.[14] (See Comments section.)
Other additives	Contains 0.165 mEq sodium/50 mg of ethacrynic acid equivalent.[10,15] Contains 62.5 mg mannitol/50 mg ethacrynate.[2,10]
Comments	Local pain and irritation at the infusion site have occurred.[1,2] Alternating doses of ethacrynic acid with furosemide may not overcome diuretic resistance.[7] The duration of treatment is directly related to the development of sensorineural hearing loss in neonates with persistent pulmonary hypertension.[11] Investigators point out that this may be transient; however, they suggest that infusion over at least 5–10 min may be protective.[11] Reconstitution with D5W products that have a pH <5 results in hazy or opalescent solutions. These should not be used.[2,10]

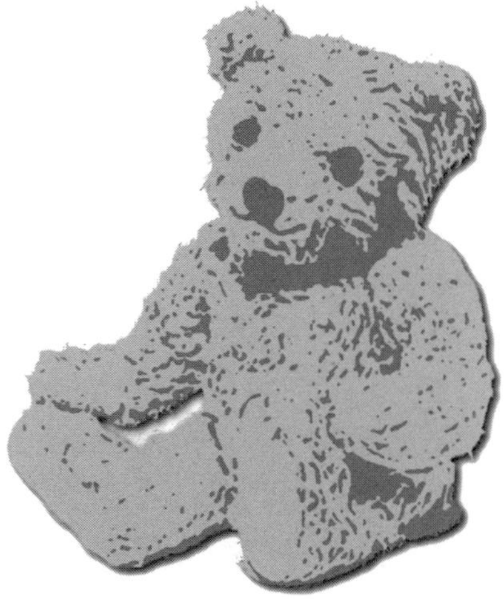

Etomidate

Brand names	Amidate
Dosage	Etomidate should not be used in children <10 years of age because of lack of sufficient safety and efficacy data.[1] 0.3 mg/kg given over 30–60 sec; however, usual doses range between 0.1–0.6 mg/kg.[1-4] Loss of consciousness generally occurs in about 60 sec of administration.[1] Etomidate has been given via continuous infusion (0.02 mg/kg/min); however, prolonged infusions should be avoided due to the potential for propylene glycol toxicity.[1]
Dosage adjustment in organ dysfunction	No dosage adjustment is necessary in renal or hepatic dysfunction; however, renal dysfunction may increase likelihood of propylene glycol toxicity. (See Other additives section.)
Maximum dosage	1.1 mg/kg.[6]
IV push	Over 30–60 sec.[1,7]
Intermittent infusion	No information available to support administration by this method.
Continuous infusion	Etomidate has also been administered as a continuous infusion, 0.02 mg/kg/min; however, it should not be given for prolonged periods.[5] (See Comments section.)
Other routes of administration	No information available to support administration by other routes.
Maximum concentration	Should be administered undiluted, 2 mg/mL.[7,8]
Cautions related to IV administration	Transient pain at the injection site.
Other additives	**Propylene glycol:** Contains propylene glycol 35% (v/v).[1] Propylene glycol is added to parenteral drugs as a solubilizer. Rapid infusion of medications that contain propylene glycol has resulted in respiratory depression and cardiac dysrhythmias.[8] Its half-life is three times longer in neonates than in *adults*[9] and has caused hyperosmolality[10] and refractory seizures[11] in preterm neonates receiving 3 g/d. Propylene glycol toxicity has been reported following infusion of etomidate.[12]
Comments	Because of the risk of prolonged suppression of endogenous cortisol and aldosterone secretion in certain patients (e.g., septic shock, head trauma), the manufacturer recommends against administering etomidate for prolonged periods as a continuous intravenous infusion.[1] Transient skeletal muscle movements occur in about ⅓ to ½ of patients.[1] The movements are predominately Myoclonic, but tonic, ocular, and averting movements have been noted. Movements are normally bilateral, but unilateral activity has also been reported. Administration of fentanyl may decrease movements that are deemed disturbing.[1]

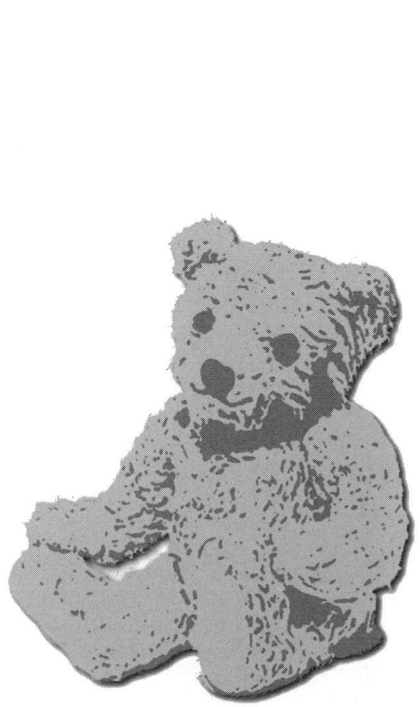

Etoposide

Brand names	VePsid, Toposar

Dosage

Consult institutional protocol for complete dosing information.

Etoposide is used as a component of combination therapy or as single agent therapy in multiple pediatric and hematologic neoplasms.

A general dosage regimen has included 60–150 mg/m²/d IV for 2–5 days q 3–6 weeks.[1,2]

Specific regimens include the following:

AML remission induction: 150 mg/m² for 2–3 days starting with course 2.[1-3]

Brain tumor: 150 mg/m² on days 1–3 or days 2–3 of treatment course.[1,4]

Neuroblastoma or osteosarcoma: 100 mg/m² over 1 h on days 1–5 of cycle.[1,5,6]

High dose conditioning regimen for BMT: 60 mg/kg as a single dose in combination chemotherapy.[1,7,8]

Dosage adjustment in organ dysfunction

The dose of etoposide should be reduced by 25% in patients with a CrCl of 15–50 mL/min.[9] The manufacturer states that no data exists on patients with a CrCl <15 mL/min and further dosage reductions are likely to be necessary. Other sources suggest a 50% dosage reduction for patients with a CrCl <15 mL/min.[1,10]

Use caution in patients with hepatic dysfunction.[11] Specifically, a 50% dosage reduction is recommended for patients with a serum bilirubin of 1.5–3 mg/dL and a 75% dosage reduction for a serum bilirubin >3 mg/dL.[1] Another source recommends that if the serum bilirubin is 1.5–3 mg/dL or the AST is 60–180 units, the dosage should be reduced by 50%; if the bilirubin is 3–5 mg/dL or AST >180, reduce the dosage by 75%; and if bilirubin is >5 mg/dL, do not administer.[12]

Maximum dosage

Not established.

IV push

Not recommended.[9,13] Rapid administration has been associated with the development of hypotension.

Intermittent infusion

Dilute to 0.2–0.4 mg/mL with D5W or NS and infuse over at least 30–60 min.[9,13] If volume is a concern, it may be infused over a longer time period, up to 210 min.[9,11]

Continuous infusion

Has been administered as a continuous infusion over 5 days.[11] No therapeutic benefit exists and use is not established. High-dose etoposide administered as a continuous infusion has been associated with more nonhematological toxicities compared to intermittent infusions.[14]

Other routes of administration

IT, intraperitoneal, and intrapleural administration not recommended.

Etoposide

Maximum concentration

0.2–0.4 mg/mL.[9,13] A precipitate has developed with concentrations >0.4 mg/mL.

Cautions related to IV administration

Hypotension has been reported with rapid administration of etoposide.[9,11] Stop or slow the rate of the infusion, and administer IV fluids if necessary.[11] Infusing etoposide at a rate slower than 100 mg/m²/h (or 3.3 mg/kg/h) has been shown to minimize hypotensive effects.[1]

Anaphylactic reactions have been seen with etoposide administration, manifesting as bronchospasm, tachycardia, dyspnea, and hypotension. Higher rates of anaphylaxis have been seen in children that receive higher than recommended concentrations of etoposide.[9]

Other additives

Each mL contains 30 mg benzyl alcohol, 80 mg modified polysorbate 80/tween 80, 650 mg polyethylene glycol, and 30.5% ethyl alcohol.[9,13]

Life-threatening renal and liver failure have been seen in pediatric patients that received a vitamin E product containing polysorbate 80.[9]

Benzyl alcohol in small doses as a preservative in drugs is considered safe in newborns.[15] However, a 3-week-old, very low birth weight (710 g) infant who received clindamycin experienced a profound desaturation that required resuscitation after the third and fourth doses, which was subsequently related to the benzyl alcohol preservative.[16]

Administration of saline flushes containing benzyl alcohol (bacteriostatic water for injection) was associated with a fatal gasping syndrome, intraventricular hemorrhage, metabolic acidosis, and increased mortality in preterm infants.[17] This should not be used in neonates.

Hypersensitivity reactions to benzyl alcohol in parenteral products have been reported in *adults*.[18,19]

Comments

The surfactant component may alter drop size. Administration with infusion devices that do not operate via drop size is recommended.[13]

Administration devices made up of acrylic or acrylonitrile, butadiene, and styrene (ABC) should be avoided, as they have cracked and leaked when used with etoposide.[9]

Etoposide is associated with a low (10% to 30%) risk of emesis.[20] Patients should receive antiemetic therapy to prevent acute and delayed nausea and vomiting. The recommended therapy is a corticosteroid on every day chemotherapy is administered; alternatives are a phenothiazine (e.g., prochlorperazine) or a butyrophenone (e.g., droperidol).[20,21] Therapy for delayed nausea and vomiting is generally not needed. Breakthrough medications should also be offered, such as a phenothiazine (e.g., prochlorperazine), a butyrophenone (e.g., droperidol), a substituted benzamide (e.g., metoclopramide), or a benzodiazepine (e.g., lorazepam). Selection should be based on what the patient is currently receiving for acute emesis prophylaxis.

Famotidine

Brand names	Pepcid
Dosage	**Neonates:** 0.5 mg/kg q 24 h.[1] **Infants and children:** 0.8–2.4 mg/kg/d divided q 8–12 h.[2-9]
Dosage adjustment in organ dysfunction	Adjust dosage in patients with severe renal dysfunction.[10-12] If CrCl is >50 mL/min, administer normal dose q 12–24 h.[10] If CrCl is 10-50 mL/min, administer normal dose q 36–48 h.[10] If CrCl is <10 mL/min, administer normal dose q 72–96 h or give 50% of a normal dose q 36–48 h.[10] Another source suggests that if CrCl is >50 mL/min, give 50% to 75% of a normal dose; if CrCl is 10–50 mL/min, give 10% to 50% of a normal dose; and if CrCl is <10 mL/min, give 10% of a normal dose.[11]
Maximum dosage	Usually 40 mg/d.[12] In one study, children who failed to respond to lower doses were given two 1.6-mg/kg doses (≤40 mg) 8 h apart.[4] 160 mg q 6 h orally has been given with no serious adverse effects to *adults* with hypersecretory conditions.[12]
IV push	2–4 mg/mL in NS, D5W, D10W, LR, or SW[12-14] and infused over ≥2 min[12] and ≤10 mg/min.[13]
Intermittent infusion	0.2 mg/mL in NS, D5W, D10W, LR, sodium bicarbonate 5%, or SW[12] infused over 15–30 min.[12,13]
Continuous infusion	In *adults*, the total daily dose has been added to a compatible fluid and infused over 24 h.[15] Stable in PN[16] and TNA[17] solutions for 24 h at room temperature.
Other routes of administration	No information available to support administration by other routes.
Maximum concentration	4 mg/mL.[12,13]
Cautions related to IV administration	None known. For PN compatibility information, please see Appendix C.
Other additives	Each mL of the concentrated injection contains 4 mg L-aspartic acid and 20 mg mannitol; each 50 mL of the premixed injection contains 6.8 mg L-aspartic acid and 450 mg sodium chloride.[12,13] Multidose vials contain benzyl alcohol 0.9% as a preservative.[12,13] Benzyl alcohol in small doses as a preservative in drugs is considered safe in newborns.[18] However, a 3-week-old, very low birth weight (710 g) infant who received clindamycin experienced a profound desaturation that required resuscitation after the third and fourth doses, which was subsequently related to the benzyl alcohol preservative.[19]

Other additives (cont.)

Administration of saline flushes containing benzyl alcohol (bacteriostatic water for injection) was associated with a fatal gasping syndrome, intraventricular hemorrhage, metabolic acidosis, and increased mortality in preterm infants.[20] This should not be used in neonates.

Hypersensitivity reactions to benzyl alcohol in parenteral products have been reported in *adults*.[21,22]

Comments

Two of 18 critically ill children failed to respond to two 1.6-mg/kg doses (≤40 mg) given 8 h apart.[4]

Prolonged dosing decreased the duration of effect.[4]

Cardiovascular adverse effects (negative inotropic effect) have occurred in *adults* on famotidine.[23]

The use of H2-blocker therapy has been associated with the incidence of necrotizing enterocolitis in very low birth weight infants.[24]

Fenoldopam

Brand names	Corlopam
Dosage	**Controlled hypotension during surgery (children <12 years)[1]:** 0.8 mcg/kg/min (range 0.2–3.2 mcg/kg/min) was the most effective dose; larger doses (>1–1.2 mcg/kg/min) produced no additional benefit in decreasing blood pressure; heart rate was significantly elevated at 3.2 mcg/kg/min. **Diuresis unresponsive to conventional therapy after cardiopulmonary bypass in neonates[2]:** 0.05–0.3 mcg/kg/min titrated over 24 h to a maximum dose of 1 mcg/kg/min has been given for 1–15 days. Urine output increased from 3.6 to 5.8 mL/kg/h resulting in an additional 158 mL/d urine. **Severe hypertension (children 1–17 years)[3]:** 0.2–0.8 mcg/kg/min.
Dosage adjustment in organ dysfunction	No dosage adjustment necessary for renal or hepatic dysfunction.[4,5]
Maximum dosage	Doses up to 4 mcg/kg/min have been given to children.[6] The manufacturer recommends a maximum dose of 1.6 mcg/kg/min in *adults.*[4,6]
IV push	Not recommended.[7]
Intermittent infusion	Not recommended.[7]
Continuous infusion	Dilute in D5W or NS to a concentration of 40 mcg/mL.[7] Infuse via continuous infusion pump appropriate for delivery of low infusion rates.[6] May begin at 0.1 mcg/kg/min with increases of 0.3 mcg/kg/min q 10–20 min. Titrate to desired effect.[6] In volume-restricted patients, fenoldopam may be diluted in D5W or NS to a final concentration of 60 mcg/mL.[6]
Other routes of administration	No information available to support other routes of administration.
Maximum concentration	60 mcg/mL.[6]
Cautions related to IV administration	Rapid titration of dose may cause hypotension.[4] Reflex tachycardia occurs with larger doses.[1]
Other additives	Each ampule contains 1 mg sodium metabisulfite/mL.[4,7] Sulfites may cause hypersensitivity reactions and these are more common in *adults* with asthma. Most reactions are mild but can include anaphylactic symptoms and life-threatening or less severe asthma episodes.[8-10] Epinephrine may be required in severe cases; and if the sulfite-free product is not available, the sulfite-preserved epinephrine should be used.[8]

Comments

Tachycardia and hypotension are the most commonly observed adverse events in pediatric patients.[6] Increased intraocular pressure and hypokalemia have also been reported in *adults*.[4]

One neonate receiving fenoldopam for 48 h after Norwood procedure acutely clotted the Blalock-Taussig shunt and required ECMO therapy for resuscitation; this event was thought to be potentially related to the brisk diuresis achieved (451 mL).[2]

A 3-year-old with glomerulonephritis status postrenal transplantation who developed severe hypertension secondary to renal failure/renal graft rejection failed to respond to 1.5 mcg/kg/min.[11]

Blood pressure should be monitored continuously during therapy with fenoldopam.[6]

Fentanyl Citrate

Brand names	Sublimaze, generic

Dosage

Anesthesia: 10–50 mcg/kg/dose.[1-7]

Sedation/analgesia

Intermittent dosing

Neonates: 1–4 mcg/kg q 2–4 h.[9]

Infants and children: 1–3 mcg/kg q 30–60 min.[9]

Continuous infusion: Loading dose of 1–5 mcg/kg[10,11] followed by continuous infusion of 1–20 mcg/kg/h (normal starting dose of 1 mcg/kg/h)[9-12]; titrate the infusion rate by 0.5-mcg/kg/h increments until desired effect occurs (usually 1–3 mcg/kg/h).[13] For adequate sedation in the intensive care setting, larger doses may be required.[14] Tolerance to sedation may develop with continuous infusion.[12] Premature neonates with hyaline membrane disease have been given 0.5–2 mcg/kg/h (mean, 1.1 mcg/kg/h) during mechanical ventilation.[15]

Dosage adjustment in organ dysfunction

The elimination of fentanyl is prolonged in both hepatic and renal dysfunction; therefore, lower initial doses are recommended.[9] In all cases, fentanyl doses should be titrated to clinical effect.

During ECMO, fentanyl is sequestered by the circuit, primarily the membrane oxygenator, that may become saturated over time.[16] Therefore, much larger doses may be required during early ECMO.[16]

Maximum dosage

75–100 mcg/kg/dose for anesthesia.[4,17] Do not use larger doses outside of the operating room or intensive care setting because of the potential for severe respiratory depression and need for intubation.[1,18]

IV push

50 mcg/mL given over 1–3 min.[2,4,5,9,19,20] Apnea may occur with rapid injection.[18] (See Cautions related to IV administration section.)

Intermittent infusion

Usual IV administration is via push over 1–3 min or continuous infusion.

Continuous infusion

Undiluted or diluted in D5W or NS to a concentration that achieves desired flow rates and dose for continuous infusion.[9,13,18,21]

Other routes of administration

May be given IM.[9] Has been given as a continuous infusion by the SC route.[22]

Maximum concentration

50 mcg/mL.[9,22]

Cautions related to IV administration

Apnea may occur with rapid bolus injection. Peak respiratory depression occurs 5–15 min after dosing.[18,22]

Chest wall rigidity is related to high doses and rapid escalation to moderate doses. (See Comments section.) A nondepolarizing skeletal muscle relaxant or naloxone may be required for reversal.[5,23-25]

For PN compatibility information, please see Appendix C.

Other additives	NaOH or HCl may be added to adjust the pH to 4–7.5.[21]
Comments	Respiratory depression is reversible with naloxone.[9,18] Neonates may be more sensitive to respiratory depressant effects and chest wall rigidity than *adults*.[2,20,25] Withdrawal syndrome is associated with both dose and duration of therapy.[26,27] SC fentanyl (5–9 mcg/kg/h for 3–7 days) has been used to wean children from sedation after prolonged exposure.[22] Acute dystonia has occurred following combined treatment with fentanyl and propofol.[28] Emergence agitation following sevoflurane or desflurane anaesthesia was greater with fentanyl than with use of a preoperative caudal block or preoperative midazolam with thiopental induction.[29,30]

Ferric Gluconate

Brand names	Ferrlecit
Dosage	**Iron deficiency in hemodialysis patients (chronic renal failure):** 1.5 mg/kg (≤125 mg/dose) × eight dialysis sessions is recommended by manufacturer.[2,3] Doses of 1–5 mg/kg have been evaluated and shown limited additional efficacy with doses >3 mg/kg and potential added toxicity.[4-7] (See Cautions related to IV administration section.) The *National Kidney Foundation Guidelines for Chronic Anemia* do not provide specific recommendations for ferric gluconate in pediatric patients; however, it suggests an equivalent dose for *adults* of 100 mg iron dextran or 125 mg ferric gluconate × eight dialysis sessions.[8] **Test dosing:** The manufacturer previously recommended a 25-mg *adult* test dose (diluted in 50 mL NS over 1 h); however, this is no longer recommended since reactions to 25-mg doses are no more frequent or severe than to usual doses in *adults*.[1]
Dosage adjustment in organ dysfunction	No information available; however, considering the distribution characteristics of iron, there should be no dose adjustment necessary relative to liver or kidney function.
Maximum dosage	While doses >3 mg/kg have been used, they are associated with increased adverse effects.[5,6] Maximum total dose is 125 mg.[2,3]
IV push	May be administered undiluted (12.5 mg/mL) at a rate up to 12.5 mg/min. Higher infusion rates may be associated with increased adverse effects.[2,3] (See Cautions related to IV administration section.)
Intermittent infusion	Dilute in 25 mL NS and administer over 1 h.[2,3] Stability in other solutions has not been evaluated and is not recommended.[2,3] If adverse effects occur during infusion (see Cautions related to IV administration section), reducing the dose and/or infusion rate may reduce the likelihood of their occurrence.[1]
Continuous infusion	No information available to support administration by continuous infusion.
Other routes of administration	No information available to support administration by other routes.
Maximum concentration	12.5 mg/mL.[2,3]
Cautions related to IV administration	Acute and delayed hypersensitivity reactions have been reported at a much lower rate with ferric gluconate than with iron dextran products.[9-13] Typical reactions during infusions include flushing, hypotension, nausea, vomiting, and diarrhea,[9-13] which may be related to release of free iron. Premedication may not decrease the incidence of reactions[14]; however, reductions in dose and/or infusion rates have been effective in preventing reactions in *adults*.[1]

Other additives

Each mL contains 9 mg of benzyl alcohol, 20% w/v sucrose, in water for injection at a pH of 7.7–9.7.[3] Benzyl alcohol in small doses as a preservative in drugs is considered safe in newborns.[16] However, a 3-week-old, very low birth weight (710 g) infant who received clindamycin experienced a profound desaturation that required resuscitation after the third and fourth doses, which was subsequently related to the benzyl alcohol preservative.[17]

Administration of saline flushes containing benzyl alcohol (BW) was associated with a fatal gasping syndrome, intraventricular hemorrhage, metabolic acidosis, and increased mortality in preterm infants.[18] This should not be used in neonates.

Hypersensitivity reactions to benzyl alcohol in parenteral products have been reported in *adults*.[18,19]

Comments

A reaction to one parenteral iron product does not predict a similar response to a different product.[1]

Filgrastim

Brand names	Neupogen, Granulocyte Colony-Stimulating Factor (G-CSF)

Dosage

Aplastic anemia: 400–1200 mcg/m²/d for 2 weeks; neutrophil counts decreased to baseline in 2–10 days after treatment was discontinued.[1] 400 mcg/m²/d for 1–90 days was used in conjunction with immunosuppressive therapy and effects were found to be transient.[2]

Bone marrow transplantation: 5–10 mcg/kg/d administered ≥24 h after chemotherapy and ≥24 h after bone marrow infusion.[3] The table depicts dosing based on neutrophil response.[4]

Absolute Neutrophil Count (ANC)	Filgrastim Adjustment
If ANC >1000/mm³ × 3 d	Reduce dose to 5 mcg/kg/d
If ANC remains >1000/mm³ for 3 more d	Discontinue filgrastim
If ANC decreases to <1000/mm³	Resume dose at 5 mcg/kg/d

Cancers (acute lymphocytic leukemia, non-Hodgkin's lymphoma, Wilm's tumor, neuroblastoma (advanced-stage), rhabdomyosarcoma, CNS tumors, acute myelogenous leukemia): 5–17 mcg/kg/d.[5-9]

Congenital neutropenia or agranulocytosis: 3–15 mcg/kg/d SC as a single dose or divided and given twice a day[10] or 10–30 mcg/kg/d as an intermittent infusion up to 60 mcg/kg/d as a continuous infusion.[11]

Postchemotherapy neutropenia (acute lymphocytic leukemia, Wilm's tumor, neuroblastoma (advanced-stage), rhabdomyosarcoma, CNS tumors, metastatic sarcoma): 5–17 mcg/kg/d.[7-9]

Neutropenia and sepsis in neonates: 5–10 mcg/kg once[11-14] or twice[12,15] a day for 3–6 d.

Neutropenia/neutrophil dysfunction due to glycogen storage disease type 1b: 3–8 mcg/kg/d for up to 290 days[16] or 3–7.5 mcg/kg/d (SC) for 6–12 months.[17]

Mobilization of peripheral blood progenitor cells (PBPCs): 10–24 mcg/kg/d SC for 3 to 5 days before PBPC apheresis.[18-20]

Dosage adjustment in organ dysfunction	No information available to support the need for dosage adjustment.
Maximum dosage	Not established. 120 mcg/kg/d has been given as continuous infusion.[21] Children with severe chronic neutropenia (19 months–14 years) have received 3–8 mcg/kg/d for up to 290 days.[3,16]
IV push	Not indicated.
Intermittent infusion	≥5 mcg/mL in D5W.[22,23] Dilute in 50–100 mL of D5W and infuse over 15–60 min.[1,3,10-13,23] Solutions that are 5–15 mcg/mL should contain a final albumin concentration of 2 mg/mL before the filgrastim is added.[3,22,23] (See Comments section.)

Continuous infusion

Concentrations ≤5 mcg/mL are not recommended.[22,23] If concentration is 5–15 mcg/mL, normal human serum albumin should be added at a final concentration of 0.2% (2 mg/mL).[23] The total daily dose may be diluted in 10–50 mL and infused continuously over 24 h by SC infusion at a rate not to exceed 10 mL/24 h.[3,11,22,23] (See Comments section.)

Other routes of administration

SC administration either as a bolus injection or continuous infusion is recommended.[22] Not administered IM.[3]

Maximum concentration

300 mcg/mL for SC administration[22] or ≥5 mcg/mL for SC or IV infusion.[23]

Cautions related to IV administration

Anaphylaxis occurs more frequently with IV infusion and usually occurs within 30 min of infusion.[3,22] Epinephrine, antihistamines, corticosteroids, and/or bronchodilators are usually effective in alleviating symptoms.[3,22]

Other additives

Additive	300 mcg per 1-mL Vial	480 mcg per 1.6-mL Vial	300 mcg per 0.5-mL Syringe	480 mcg per 0.8-mL Syringe
Acetate	0.59 mg	0.94 mg	0.295 mg	0.472 mg
Sorbitol	50 mg	80 mg	25 mg	40 mg
Tween 80	0.004%	0.004%	0.004%	0.004%
Sodium	0.035 mg	0.056 mg	0.0175 mg	0.028 mg

Comments

Dilution in NS may cause precipitation.[22]

Albumin is added to concentrations from 5–15 mcg/mL to prevent adsorption of filgrastim to glass or plastic administration sets.[23]

Rare cases of splenic rupture have been reported; some were fatal. Abdominal pain or shoulder tip pain that occurs during infusion should be evaluated.[22]

Allergic reactions, typically occurring within 30 min from the onset of the infusion, have been reported and may occur more frequently with IV therapy.

A CBC including a platelet count should be obtained before initiation therapy with filgrastim and should be repeated at least twice a week during treatment.[22]

Fluconazole

Brand names Diflucan

Dosage

Daily dose varies according to infecting organism and response to therapy. Duration of therapy is generally 4 weeks for systemic infections and 10–12 weeks following sterilization of cerebrospinal fluid in patients with cryptococcal meningitis.[1]

Neonates

Treatment: 5–6 mg/kg/dose, per following schedule for dosing interval.[1-11]

≤7 days: q 72 h.

7–14 days: q 48 h.

>14 days: q 24 h.

Although one study reported doses as large as 12 mg/kg/d given as a single dose in 20 patients (0–17 years of age), the authors did not specify whether any neonates received this dose.[8]

Prophylaxis: 3–6 mg/kg/dose (per schedule above for dosing interval).[12,13]

Infants and children

Cryptococcal meningitis: Initial dose of 12 mg/kg (400 mg) followed by 6–12 mg/kg (200–400 mg) given once daily.[1,4,14-18]

Immunocompromised (e.g., leukemia, bone marrow transplant): 6–12 mg/kg given once daily.[14,15,17]

Oropharyngeal/esophageal candidiasis: Initial dose of 6 mg/kg followed by 3 mg/kg given once daily.[1,17]

Systemic candidiasis: Initial dose of 12 mg/kg (400 mg) followed by 6–12 mg/kg (200–400 mg) given once daily.[1,4,14-17]

To maintain therapeutic serum concentrations, children may require more frequent dosing than *adults*.[15,19]

Dosage adjustment in organ dysfunction

Adjust dosage in patients with renal dysfunction.[1,11,20,21] If CrCl is 21–50 mL/min, administer 50% of normal dose; and if CrCl is <20 mL/min, administer 25% of normal dose.[1,22]

Following hemodialysis, patients should be given the recommended dose.[1,22] During continuous arteriovenous hemodiafiltration in an *adult*, total body clearance was similar to normal healthy volunteers.[23]

Maximum dosage

12 mg/kg/d[1,14] not to exceed 600 mg/d in older children and *adults*.[1]

A 6-month-old with hydrocephalus and mycotic ventriculitis received 22 mg/kg/d with concomitant intraventricular administration (4 mg/24 h).[24]

IV push

Not recommended.[1]

Intermittent infusion

≤2 mg/mL in D5W or LR.[25] Doses ≤6 mg/kg may be given over 1 h[7,9,19] while doses >6 mg/kg should be given over 2 h in pediatric patients.[9,15] Not to exceed 200 mg/h in *adults*.[1]

Continuous infusion	No information available to support administration by this method.
Other routes of administration	Has been administered intraventricularly (4 mg/24 h in an infant and 5 or 7.5 mg/24 h and 7.5 or 10 mg/12 h in an 18-year-old).[24]
Maximum concentration	2 mg/mL.[1,25]
Cautions related to IV administration	None known. For PN compatibility information, please see Appendix C.
Other additives	Available in glass or plastic containers in either sodium chloride or dextrose. Each mL of solution contains either 9-mg NaCl or 56-mg dextrose, depending on the diluent.[1,25] The plastic containers contain DEHP.[1]
Comments	Because fluconazole's effects on CYP2C9/10 and CYP3A3/4, it is associated with numerous drug interactions.[1,26] Consult appropriate resources for dosing recommendations before combining any drug with fluconazole.

Flumazenil

Brand names	Romazicon

Dosage

Little information is available concerning flumazenil in pediatric patients. The doses listed may come from case reports on a single patient.[1] Be prepared to manage seizures. Do not use flumazenil until neuromuscular blockade has been fully reversed.[2] Not indicated for ethanol, barbiturate, tricyclic, general anesthetic, or narcotic overdose.[2]

IV dosing is individualized according to the desired level of consciousness.

Reversal of

Benzodiazepine-induced anesthesia or conscious sedation: 0.01 mg/kg (up to 0.2 mg) over 15 sec (0.2 mg/min).[1,3-8] The maximum cumulative dose is 0.05 mg/kg or 1 mg, whichever is smaller.[1,6,8] Most patients require five doses.[2,6] If the patient does not respond within 5 min, sedation is probably not related to a benzodiazepine.[2] A single, large dose of 0.1–0.2 mg has been used successfully.[9,10] Conversely, one study used low doses (0.002 mg/kg).[11] Another study used a 10-mcg/kg loading dose followed by 5 mcg/kg/min until the patient awoke or until a maximum of 1 mg had been infused.[3] Some patients who regain complete consciousness may develop sedation within 19–50 min.[2]

Benzodiazepine overdose or ingestion: 0.01 mg/kg; if no effect in 1–2 min, repeat dose q 2 min until patient responds or a total of 1 mg is given. A single dose of 0.2 mg (0.017 mg/kg) was used in a 12-kg child.[13] Initial doses may be followed by 0.004–0.005 mg/kg/h for 2–6 h to prevent resedation.[14,15]

Neonatal apnea due to prenatal benzodiazepine exposure: 0.02 mg/kg followed by 0.05 mg/kg/h.[16]

Dosage adjustment in organ dysfunction	No dosage adjustment required in renal dysfunction.[17] Flumazenil clearance is reduced to 40% to 60% in mild-to-moderate hepatic disease and to 25% in severe hepatic dysfunction. Although the initial dose should not be reduced, repeat doses should be reduced or the interval prolonged in patients with hepatic dysfunction.[2]
Maximum dosage	0.2 mg/dose up to cumulative dose of 1 mg in infants and children.[2,9] Seventy-five percent of *adults* respond to 3 mg.[2] Doses above 3 mg do not produce additional effects.[2] If resedation occurs, may administer up to 3 mg in 1 h.[2]
IV push	0.1 mg/mL over 15–30 sec.[2,18] Tachycardia and hypertension occurred in *adults* receiving rapid infusions or excessive doses.[19]
Intermittent infusion	0.05 mg/mL in D5W, LR, or NS is stable for 24 h.[2,18,20]
Continuous infusion	Has been given by this method; however, the final concentration and solution type was not provided.[3]
Other routes of administration	Because of the risk of local irritation, the drug is recommended for IV use only.[2]
Maximum concentration	0.1 mg/mL (commercially available).[2]

Cautions related to IV administration

To minimize pain or local inflammation, the manufacturer recommends infusion through a freely running injection site into a large vein.[2] Extravasation may cause local irritation.[2]

Monitor patient for return of sedation or respiratory depression for 2 h after administration of last dose of flumazenil.[2,6,9] Due to the short duration of flumazenil, compared to some benzodiazepines, resedation may occur. This is especially true in the pediatric population. Patients experiencing resedation may require repeat bolus doses or continuous infusion.

Other additives

Parabens: Contains 1.8 mg methylparabens, 0.2 mg propylparabens/mL.[2] Paraben preservatives may cause hypersensitivity reactions that are more common with cutaneous exposure.[21] However, one case of pruritus and bronchospasm that occurred following infusion of hydrocortisone, which contained parabens, has been reported.[22]

Comments

Contraindicated in those receiving a benzodiazepine for control of life-threatening condition (e.g., ICP or status epilepticus) or those who are allergic to benzodiazepines.[2]

Flumazenil should not be used in those with symptoms of serious concurrent tricyclic antidepressant overdosage.[2] These symptoms include motor abnormalities (e.g., twitching, rigidity, focal seizures), arrhythmias (e.g., wide QRS complexes, ventricular arrhythmias, heart block), anticholinergic effects (e.g., mydriasis, dry mucosa, hypoperistalsis), or cardiovascular collapse.[2]

Although rare (1% to 2%), seizures may occur in patients who have a dependence on benzodiazepines for seizure control.[2]

Fomepizole

Brand names	Antizol
Dosage	Unknown if the pharmacokinetics in infants and children differs from *adults* due to insufficient studies; hence, safety and efficacy in children has not been established.[1] Currently, fomepizole is safer than ethanol or hemodialysis for the treatment of suspected or confirmed ethylene glycol or methanol poisoning and should be used as first-line therapy.[2-4] Loading dose of 15 mg/kg over 30 min[1,5-8] followed by 10 mg/kg q 12 h for four doses.[1,6] Because fomepizole induces its own metabolism, the dose should be increased to 15 mg/kg q 12 h after five doses have been given.[1] If used concurrently with hemodialysis, the interval should be decreased to q 4 h (see Comments section).[1,6] Some advocate a continuous infusion of 1–1.5 mg/kg/h during hemodialysis.[2,9,10] Some recommend concurrent administration of thiamine,[8,11] pyridoxine,[8,11] and folic acid.[4,7] (See Comments section.) Fomepizole should be continued until ethylene glycol or methanol concentrations are undetectable or have decreased below 20 mg/dL and the patient is asymptomatic with a normal pH.[1]
Dosage adjustment in organ dysfunction	Fomepizole is extensively metabolized and metabolites are primarily excreted renally.[1] Dosage adjustments for renal or hepatic insufficiency not studied.
Maximum dosage	15 mg/kg/dose.[1]
IV push	Not recommended.[1]
Intermittent infusion	Dilute appropriate dose with at least 100 mL of NS or D5W and infuse loading and maintenance doses over 30 min.[1]
Continuous infusion	Continuous infusions of 1–1.5 mg/kg/h during hemodialysis have also been suggested.[2,9,10]
Other routes of administration	No information available to support administration by other routes.
Maximum concentration	<25 mg/mL. Venous irritation and phlebosclerosis occurred in volunteers who received concentrations of 25 mg/mL.[1]
Cautions related to IV administration	Do not give undiluted or by bolus injections.[1] Venous irritation and phlebosclerosis can occur with bolus injections (over 5 min) using a concentration of 25 mg/mL.[1]

Other additives	None.

Comments

Fomepizole does not affect existing acid but works by halting further acid production. It promotes the breakdown of formic acid (metabolite of methanol); therefore, supplemental intravenous folate (1 mg/kg) should be considered in those poisoned with methanol.[4,7]

Thiamine (100 mg q 6 h) and pyridoxine (1 mg/kg up to 50 mg q 6 h) may be administered to prevent the formation of oxalic acid in those who have ingested ethylene glycol.[8,11]

If a dose was given at the beginning of a hemodialysis session and it has been ≥6 h, the next scheduled dose of fomepizole should be given.[1] If it has been <6 h, do not administer a dose.[1]

If the time between the last dose of fomepizole and the end of a hemodialysis session has been >3 h, the next scheduled dose should be given.[1] Fifty percent of the dose should be administered if the time is between 1–3 h.[1] If it has been <1 h, do not give a dose at the end of the dialysis session.[1]

Vertical nystagmus, lasting 60 min, has been reported within 2 h of a single 15-mg/kg dose of fomepizole in a 6-year-old child.[8] This adverse effect has not been reported in any other patient.

Foscarnet, Trisodium Phosphonoformate

Brand names	Foscavir
Dosage	**CMV Retinitis:** 180 mg/kg/d in two to three divided doses for 14–21 days, followed by 90–120 mg/kg once daily as maintenance.[1-5] **HSV infection resistant to acyclovir:** 80–120 mg/kg/d in two to three divided doses until the infection has resolved.[1,2,6,7] **Varicella infection resistant to acyclovir:** 80–120 mg/kg/d in two to three divided doses until the infection has resolved.[8,9]
Dosage adjustment in organ dysfunction	Dosage adjustments are recommended for renal dysfunction.[1,2] Data is limited regarding use in patients with baseline CrCl <50 mL/min or SCr >2.8 mg/dL, or in patients receiving hemodialysis or peritoneal dialysis; use is not recommended in these patients.[2] One reference suggests administering 28 mg/kg for CrCl >50 mL/min; 15 mg/kg for CrCl 10–50 mL/min; and 6 mg/kg for CrCl <10 mL/min.[10] Much more in-depth dosing recommendations may be found in the tertiary literature.[2]
Maximum dosage	180 mg/kg/d during induction therapy.[1,3-5]
IV push	Not recommended.[11]
Intermittent infusion	For peripheral administration, dilute with D5W or NS to a concentration of 12 mg/mL. For infusion via a central line, no dilution required. Infuse at a rate not to exceed 60 mg/kg over 1 h or 120 mg/kg over 2 h.[11]
Continuous infusion	No information.
Other routes of administration	Not recommended.
Maximum concentration	12 mg/mL in NS or D5W for peripheral infusion and 24 mg/mL for central administration.[11]
Cautions related to IV administration	Patients should be adequately hydrated prior to receiving foscarnet. Diuresis should be established prior to the first dose by administering NS or D5W; administer fluid concurrently with subsequent doses of foscarnet.[2] To avoid local irritation, administer via a vein that provides adequate blood flow for rapid dilution and distribution.[2] For PN compatibility information, please see Appendix C.
Other additives	None.
Comments	Foscarnet carries a boxed warning describing renal impairment as its major toxicity and the potential for seizure development due to electrolyte disturbances.[2] Foscarnet deposits in teeth and bone have been documented in animal studies, especially during early growth and development; deposits in bone in humans.[2] One report described successful HIV rescue therapy over 4 weeks in a 4-year-old with 90 mg/kg IV q 12h foscarnet in combination with IV zidovudine and oral nelfinavir and nevirapine.[12]

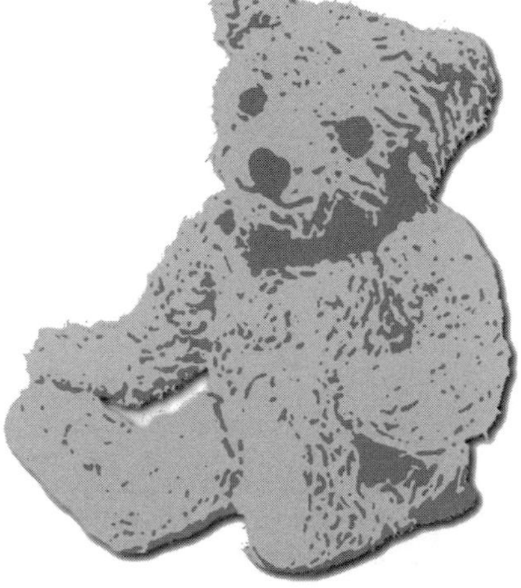

Fosphenytoin

Brand names	Cerebyx

Dosage

Doses of fosphenytoin are expressed in phenytoin sodium equivalents (PEs); therefore, fosphenytoin and phenytoin products can be converted directly (1 PE = 1 mg phenytoin).[1]

In obese patients the loading doses should be calculated on adjusted body weight using the following equation[2]:

Dosing weight (kg) = ideal body weight (IBW) + 1.33 (measured weight - IBW). (See Appendix B.)

Acute seizure or status epilepticus

Loading doses (assumes no previous fosphenytoin/phenytoin)

Neonates (few published reports in newborns; may prefer to use phenobarbital or a benzodiazepine): 15–24 mg PE/kg has been used in the treatment of acute seizures and results in total phenytoin concentrations of 10.5–34.5 mg/L (mean 21.6 mg/L) 8–12 h after a dose.[3,4]

Infants and children: 15–20 mg PE/kg.[1,5-7] Some reports have noted a failure to obtain "therapeutic" serum concentration after adequate doses.[7-9]

Maintenance doses: 4–8 mg PE/kg/d given as two to three doses.[5-7] Final maintenance dose needs to be individualized. In most cases, doses are comparable to that used with phenytoin. Some reports have noted a failure to obtain "therapeutic" serum concentration despite adequate doses.[7-9]

Post-traumatic epilepsy (see status epilepticus for dosing): Although prophylactic phenytoin for the prevention of epilepsy following head trauma is controversial, some have reported that it reduces early post-traumatic epilepsy.[10-12] It should not be used for the prevention of late epilepsy.[12] Children with severe, acute neurotrauma have markedly altered protein binding and phenytoin metabolism and may require larger doses and more frequent dosing.[13] Free serum phenytoin concentration should be monitored.

Dosage adjustment in organ dysfunction

Dosage adjustment may be required in patients with hepatic or renal dysfunction.[1] Free phenytoin serum concentrations should be measured in newborns, in patients with renal dysfunction, or in those who are hypoalbuminemic because of decreases in protein binding, increases in volume of distribution, and altered clearance.[14,15] Although several equations have been used to predict free phenytoin serum concentrations in those with low albumin or renal failure, they may overpredict concentrations and are not recommended for use in children.[16] Larger does may be required in obese patients.[2]

Maximum dosage

Typically patients require <8 mg PE/kg/d from chronic dosing. Patients receiving medications known to increase the metabolism of phenytoin may require larger doses. One study in infants suggests that larger fosphenytoin maintenance doses (10 mg PE/kg/d) and more frequent dosing may be required.[8,13]

IV push

Not recommended.[1] (See Cautions related to IV administration section.)

Intermittent infusion

≤25 mg PE/mL in D5W or NS[1,9] at a rate of 1–3 PE/kg/min (maximum of 150 mg PE/min).[1,5]

Continuous infusion

Not given via this method.

Other routes of administration

Rapidly absorbed via the IM route.[17] Doses of 15–18.7 mg PE/mg have been given to patients >6 months. Total injection volumes: infants 1–6.1 mL, children 2.6–8.7 mL, adolescents 5–12 mL.[6] Maintenance doses have been given IM for up to 4 days in volumes of 0.3–6 mL.[6] For IM administration, the quadriceps have been recommended. Although irritation may occur at the site of injection, the incidence is less than that noted with phenytoin sodium.[18] To minimize irritation, rotate the injection site and use multiple injection sites for large medication volumes. Has been given intraosseously.

Maximum concentration

25 PE/mL in D5W or NS.[1]

Cautions related to IV administration

Administration of >3 mg PE/kg/min (150 mg PE/min) may lead to hypotension, bradycardia, and/or arrhythmias.[1] Vomiting and pruritus (groin and neck areas) have also occurred in children with faster rates of IV administration.[5,19]

Other additives

There are approximately 0.0037 mmoL of phosphate in 1 PE of fosphenytoin.[1] (See Comments section, formaldehyde.)

Comments

Because large variability exists in patient response to initial and maintenance doses, individualize dosage based on serum concentration and clinical response. It is recommended that phenytoin concentrations not be measured until at least 2 h after an IV dose and for 4 h after an IM dose of fosphenytoin.[4,9,19]

Because phenytoin induces the CYP2C19 and CYP3A families and UGT, it can be associated with numerous drug interactions.[20] Phenytoin may also serve as a substrate and can be inhibited or induced by other drugs. Consult appropriate resources for dosing recommendations before combining any drug with fosphenytoin or phenytoin.

Formaldehyde is produced on conversion to phenytoin. No accumulation has been noted in *adults* and children during short-term use; however, caution is warranted in those with renal impairment.

Fosphenytoin may cross react with phenytoin in fluorescence polarization immunoassay and EMIT assays giving falsely elevated fosphenytoin concentrations if measured too soon after a dose of fosphenytoin. It is recommended that phenytoin concentrations not be measured until at least 2 h after an IV dose of fosphenytoin and for 4 h after an IM dose of fosphenytoin.[21]

Hyperphosphatemia has been attributed to fosphenytoin in a 17-year-old patient with renal failure.[22]

Furosemide

Brand names	Lasix
Dosage	**Diuresis**[1,2] **Intermittent dosing** **Neonates** **<29 weeks postconceptional age:** 1 mg/kg q 24 h.[3] **>32 weeks postconceptional age:** 1 mg/kg q 12 h.[3] **Infants and children:** 0.5–2 mg/kg q 4,[4,5] 6,[6] or 24 h.[4,7-19] Dose may be increased by 1 mg/kg to achieve desired response.[7-9,11] **Continuous infusion dosing:** 0.1 mg/kg bolus (≥1 mg) followed by continuous infusion of 0.05–0.4 mg/kg/h.[4-6,19] Continuous infusion of 2.5 ± 0.3 mg/kg/d in 11 infants resulted in similar urine output to 15 infants who received 6.8 ± 1.2 intermittent bolus dosing.[20] Resistance to diuretics may develop. Alternating doses of furosemide with ethacrynic acid may not overcome diuretic resistance.[21] **Nephrotic syndrome:** 0.5–2 mg/kg after albumin 25% infusion.[22-27]
Dosage adjustment in organ dysfunction	Larger doses may be required in patients with renal dysfunction.[1] Contraindicated in patients with anuria.[1] During ECMO, 63% to 87% of the dose was adsorbed to the circuit and saturation occurred by 30 min.[28]
Maximum dosage	6 mg/kg.[7,9]
IV push	10 mg/mL slowly over 1–2 min, not to exceed 4 mg/min.[1,29] Doses of 0.5–1 mg/kg have been given over 1–2 min in infants and children (0.5 mg/kg/min).[8-10] (See Cautions related to IV administration section.)
Intermittent infusion	Dilute in an equal volume of D5W, LR, or NS[1] and infuse at ≤4 mg/min not to exceed 0.5 mg/kg/min.[8,9,12]
Continuous infusion	Dilute to 1–2 mg/mL[2] in D5W, LR, or NS for continuous infusion.[1,29]
Other routes of administration	May be given IM at same doses as IV; however, the pH of the product (i.e., 8–9.3) will likely produce irritation on administration.[29]
Maximum concentration	10 mg/mL.[29]
Cautions related to IV administration	Transient and permanent ototoxicity has been associated with administration rates >4 mg/min or >0.5 mg/kg/min.[30,31] Aminoglycosides potentiate the ototoxicity of loop diuretics.[32-35] For PN compatibility information, please see Appendix C.

Other additives	Contains 0.162 mEq sodium/mL.[29]

Comments

Electrolyte abnormalities including hypokalemia can occur; therefore, monitoring serum potassium concentration is important.[1]

Premature neonates with respiratory distress syndrome may have an increased risk of persistent patent ductus arteriosus secondary to furosemide stimulation of renal production of prostaglandin E2.[36]

Up to 65% of premature infants develop nephrocalcinosis following prolonged therapy.[2,37] About 50% experience resolution within 5–6 months of drug discontinuation[39]; however, obstructive nephrolithiasis can occur.[40] High urinary calcium excretion rates, low urinary calcium citrate to creatinine ratios, and an alkaline urinary pH may increase the likelihood of developing renal calcifications.[2] Renal ultrasonography is warranted a few months after initiation of therapy.[38]

Use cautiously in jaundiced neonates at risk for kernicterus. *In vitro* studies have shown bilirubin displacement in pooled cord blood samples from critically ill neonates receiving furosemide.[41]

Numerous drug interactions are known.[1] Consult appropriate resources for dosing recommendations before combining any drug with furosemide.

Ganciclovir Sodium

Brand names Cytovene

Dosage

CMV prophylaxis in high-risk hosts

Bone marrow, liver, kidney transplantation: 10 mg/kg/d divided q 12 h for 1 week, then 5 mg/kg given once daily or 6 mg/kg/d for 5 days/week for 100 days.[1-7] Maintenance doses of 5 mg/kg/d for 3–5 days per week were well-tolerated but did not prevent reactivation of CMV.[8]

One reference recommends 6 mg/kg/d for 1 month, followed by 6 mg/kg/d for 5 weeks for a total of 100 mg/d for liver transplantation patients.[9]

Cardiac transplantation: One reference recommends 10 mg/kg/d divided q 12 h for 2 weeks followed by 6 mg/kg/d for 2 weeks, combined with CMV-IgG therapy at 0, 2, 4, 6, 8, 12, and 16 weeks.[10]

Lung transplantation: One reference gave 10 mg/kg/d divided q 12 h for 2 weeks followed by 5 mg/kg/d for up to 5 months.[11]

CMV retinitis: 10 mg/kg/d divided q 12 h for 14–21 days, then 5 mg/kg/d given 7 days/week or 6 mg/kg/d given 5 days/week.[5,12]

CMV infection in allograft recipients: 7.5–10 mg/kg/d divided q 8–12 h for 14–47 days.[13-16]

Symptomatic congenital CMV infections: 5–15 mg/kg/d divided q 12 h in neonates and infants.[17-25]

CMV/HIV coinfection (use not established): One infant received 10 mg/kg/d divided q 12 h for 2 weeks, then 5 mg/kg/d as maintenance.[26]

Human herpesvirus-6 in bone marrow transplantation (use not established)

Prophylaxis: 10 mg/kg/d divided q 12 h for 1 week prior to transplantation followed by 5 mg/kg/d for 120 days after transplant.[27]

Treatment: 10 mg/kg/d divided q 12 h for 2 weeks followed by 5 mg/kg given daily or three times/week for 4 weeks.[27]

Dosage adjustment in organ dysfunction

Adjust dosage in patients with renal dysfunction.[12] If CrCl is between 10 and 50 mL/min, give normal dose q 24–48 h; if CrCl is <10 mL/min, give normal dose q 48–96 h.[28]

Other references suggest the following dose adjustments[12,15]:

CrCl (mL/min)	Induction	Maintenance
50–69	2.5 mg/kg q 12h	2.5 mg/kg q 24 h
25–49	2.5 mg/kg q 24h	1.25 mg/kg q 24 h
10–24	1.25 mg/kg q 24h	0.625 mg/kg q 24 h
<10	1.25 mg/kg three times/week following hemodialysis	0.625 mg/kg three times/week following hemodialysis

Dose adjustments should also be considered in patients with hematologic toxicity. No dose adjustment is necessary with hepatic dysfunction.

Maximum dosage

15 mg/kg/d has been given to infants[23]; recommended maximum dose per labeling is 10 mg/kg/d.[12]

Ganciclovir Sodium

IV push	Contraindicated.[12,29] (See Cautions related to IV administration section.)
Intermittent infusion	Reconstitute 500 mg in 10 mL of SW and then dilute to ≤10 mg/mL in D5W, LR, NS, or R and infuse over 1 h.[12,29] (See Comments section.) BW (containing parabens) is incompatible with ganciclovir; reconstitution with BW may cause precipitation.[12]
Continuous infusion	No information available to support administration by this method.
Other routes of administration	IM or SC injection not recommended and may result in severe tissue irritation due to high pH.[12,29]
Maximum concentration	10 mg/mL.[12,29]
Cautions related to IV administration	Use safe handling techniques (latex gloves, protective eyewear, and other protective equipment); ganciclovir is carcinogenic and mutagenic.[12] Has a pH of 11. Therefore, avoid direct contact with skin or mucous membranes. If contact occurs, wash skin thoroughly with soap and water and rinse eyes thoroughly with plain water. For PN compatibility information, please see Appendix C.
Other additives	Contains 46 mg sodium/500 mg vial of ganciclovir.[12]
Comments	Ganciclovir labeling includes a boxed warning for hematologic toxicity (granulocytopenia, anemia, and thrombocytopenia).[12] It should not be administered to patients with an absolute neutrophil count <500 cells/mm^3 or a platelet count <25,000 cells/mm^3.[12] Morphological changes to the neutrophils of a 13-year-old allogeneic BMT patient were attributed to twice-daily infusions of ganciclovir. The changes resolved within 48 h of discontinuing the drug.[30] Adequate hydration is recommended during therapy.[12] Decreased renal function and myelosuppression have been reported in children; renal function improved with a dose decrease.[15] IV ganciclovir may be beneficial in infants with CMV associated cholestasis.[31] Ganciclovir has been used to treat CMV enterocolitis in an 8-week-old and protein-losing enteropathy and retinitis in a 6-week-old infant.[32,33] *In vivo* placental transfer of ganciclovir has occurred in a premature neonate born to a woman with AIDS receiving ganciclovir therapy for CMV retinitis and pneumonitis.[34] Because ganciclovir is associated with numerous drug interactions,[12] consult appropriate resources for dosing recommendations before combining any drug with ganciclovir.

Gentamicin Sulfate

Brand names Garamycin, Jenamicin

Dosage

Except in neonates, dosage should be based on the following equation[1]:

Dosing weight = IBW + 0.4 (TBW – IBW). (See Appendix B.)

Loading dose: Although limited data are available, some researchers advocate an initial 3–5 mg/kg dose in neonates and infants.[2-4]

Maintenance dose

Neonates: Dose is estimated using age and weight,[5-7] gestational age,[8-20] or postmenstrual plus neonatal age.[21]

Based on age and weight[5-7]:

PNA	<1200 g	1200-2000 g	≥2000 g
<7 d	2.5 mg/kg q 18–24 h[5,6]*	2.5 mg/kg q 12 h[6,7]	2.5 mg/kg q 12 h[6,7]
≥7 d		2.5 mg/kg q 8–12 h[6,7]	2.5 mg/kg q 8 h[6,7]

*Until 4 weeks of age.

Based on gestational age[8-20]:

Gestational Age	Dose
≤7 d	
<28 weeks	2.5 mg/kg q 24 h[8-20]
28–34 weeks	2.5 mg/kg q 18 h[8-20]
>7 days	
<28 weeks	2.5 mg/kg q 18 h[8-20]
28–34 weeks	2.5 mg/kg q 12 h[8-20]

Based on postmenstrual and postnatal age[21]:

Postmenstrual Age	Postnatal Age	Dose
≤29 weeks or significant asphyxia, PDA, or treatment with indomethacin	≤7 d	5 mg/kg q 48 h
	8–28 d	4 mg/kg q 36 h
	≥29 d	4 mg/kg q 24 h
30–34 weeks	≤7 d	4.5 mg/kg q 36 h
	≥8 d	4 mg/kg q 24 h
≥35 weeks	ALL*	4 mg/kg q 24 h

*Until 4 weeks of age.

Although the above *NeoFax* dosing is used by some practitioners, the most recent edition of the *American Academy of Pediatrics Red Book: Report of the Committee on Infectious Diseases* continues to recommend 2.5 mg/kg/dose administered in multiple daily doses for newborns of all gestational ages.[6]

Infants and children

Mild-to-moderate infections: Not appropriate.[6]

Severe infections: 2.5 mg/kg q 8 h.[4,6,10,22-25]

Once-daily dosing: Several investigators have reported that once-daily dosing has comparable efficacy and perhaps less toxicity than classical 8–12 h dosing.[26-36] A single dose of *aminoglycoside* has been given once daily (over 20–30 min) in critically ill infants and children with severe gram-negative infections,[27-29] bone marrow transplantation,[30] or in febrile neutropenic patients with cancer.[31-35] At this time, the use of once-daily dosing in infants and children is controversial.[36,37] The most recent edition of the *American*

Dosage (cont.)

Academy of Pediatrics Red Book: Report of the Committee on Infectious Diseases continues to recommend 2.5 mg/kg/dose administered in multiple daily doses in all age groups.[6] Once-daily dosing should only be done in combination with appropriate beta-lactam antibiotics in neutropenic patients and in those with *Pseudomonas aeruginosa* or *Serratia marcescens*.[38]

Bacterial endocarditis (prophylaxis): Patients undergoing genitourinary and gastrointestinal procedures should be given ampicillin 50 mg/kg up to 2 g within 30 min of starting a procedure.[6] High-risk patients should also be given 1.5 mg/kg of gentamicin plus another 25 mg/kg dose of ampicillin in 6 h.[6]

Bacterial endocarditis (treatment): Patients with enterococcal endocarditis that are sensitive to penicillin, gentamicin, and vancomycin should receive gentamicin 3 mg/kg/d divided q 8 h plus ampicillin (300 mg/k/d divided q 4–6 h).[39] If symptoms have been present for ≤3 months, treat for 4 weeks; and if longer than 3 months, treat for 6 weeks.[39]

Dosage adjustment in organ dysfunction

Adjust dosage in patients with renal dysfunction.[40] If CrCl is between 10–50 mL/min, give a normal dose q 24–48 h; if CrCl is <10 mL/min, give a normal dose q 48–72 h.[40] Dosage adjustment should be based on serum concentrations, pharmacokinetic parameters, and pharmacodynamic response.

Maximum dosage

Larger doses or shorter dosing intervals of aminoglycosides are sometimes required in patients with cystic fibrosis,[41-44] major thermal burns or dermal loss,[45] ascites, or in patients with febrile granulocytopenia.[31-35] Based on similarities between aminoglycosides, prolonged dosing interval may be required in those receiving ECMO.[47] As with other aminoglycosides, individualize dosage based on serum concentrations.

IV push

Not recommended. Aminoglycosides have been safely administered by rapid IV push (over 3–5 min).[48-50] However, ototoxicity has been associated with elevated peak serum concentrations following bolus administration in *adults*.[51]

Intermittent infusion

10 mg/mL or 40 mg/mL (undiluted as provided by manufacturer)[7] or dilute dose in appropriate volume of D5W or NS and infuse over 20–30 min using a constant-rate volumetric infusion device.[52]

Continuous infusion

Not recommended. Toxicity occurs more frequently, and the value of this administration method compared to intermittent infusion has not been established.[51,53,54]

Other routes of administration

May be administered IM.[52]

Maximum concentration

40 mg/mL[7]; however, the volume must allow for accurate measurement and administration over 30–60 min.

Cautions related to IV administration

Chills, fever, tachycardia, and decreased systolic blood pressure have been associated with a pyrogenic, endotoxin-like reaction following once-daily administration of gentamicin.[55,56]

For PN compatibility information, please see Appendix C.

Gentamicin Sulfate

Other additives	**Sulfites:** May cause hypersensitivity reactions and these are more common in *adults* with asthma. Most reactions are mild but can include anaphylactic symptoms and life-threatening or less severe asthma episodes.[57-59] Epinephrine may be required in severe cases; and if the sulfite-free product is not available, the sulfite-preserved epinephrine should be used.[57] **Parabens:** May cause hypersensitivity reactions that are more common with cutaneous exposure.[60] However, one case of pruritus and bronchospasm occurred following infusion of hydrocortisone, which contained parabens.[61]

Comments

Because large variability exists in patient response to therapy, individualize dosage based on serum concentrations, clinical response, and renal function. Recommended peak and trough serum gentamicin concentration are 4–12 mg/L and <2 mg/L, respectively.[62] Desired peak concentrations are dependent on the site of infection.

Although serum concentration monitoring has become routine practice in many institutions, not all patients require monitoring.[63,64] Monitoring is indicated if the patient is not clinically responding, is ≤3 months of age, has disease that requires large doses or high concentrations (CNS infections, endocarditis, pneumonia, ascites, burns), has decreased or unstable renal function, or will be treated more than 10 days.

Serum concentrations may be falsely elevated when blood samples are collected through central venous Silastic catheters.[65]

The beta-lactam ring of penicillins can link with an amino sugar of the aminoglycoside and inactivate the aminoglycoside.[66-68] To avoid this potential interaction, administer penicillins 1 h before or after an aminoglycoside, adequately flush the infusion line between each infusion, or infuse them through separate lines. *In vivo* inactivation that is dose-dependent can also occur, particularly in patients with renal failure.[68-70] In patients with end-stage renal failure, gentamicin half-life was decreased by 22–31 h after carbenicillin or ticarcillin was added to the drug regimen.[69]

Cochlear and/or vestibular ototoxicity has been associated with all aminoglycoside antibiotics.[38] Total AUC is a better indicator of ototoxic risk than either peak or trough serum concentration.[71,72] Use with caution in other drugs (e.g., macrolide antibiotics, loop diuretics, platinum-based chemotherapeutic agents) known to cause ototoxicity.

Aminoglycosides accumulate in renal cortical tissue and may damage proximal tubule cells leading to oliguric renal failure. This has been associated with elevated trough serum concentrations. Risk of nephrotoxicity may increase if aminoglycosides are combined with other potentially nephrotoxic drugs.[38]

Aminoglycosides may cause neuromuscular blockade that is pronounced in patients with renal insufficiency, neuromuscular disease, and hypocalcemia.[68,73] The effects of nondepolarizing neuromuscular blockers may be prolonged during aminoglycoside use.[68]

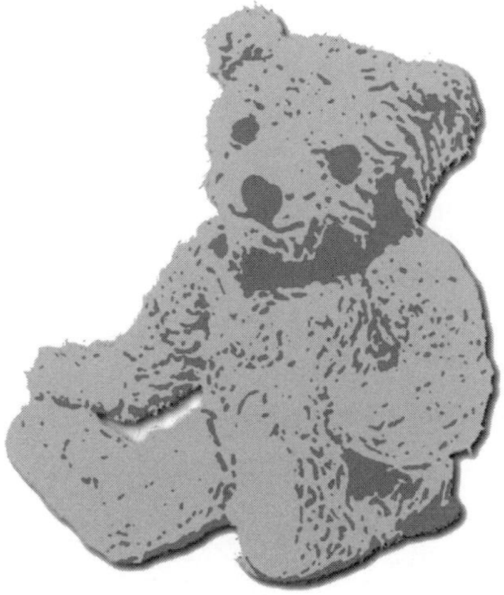

Glycopyrrolate

Brand names	Robinul, generic
Dosage	**Intraoperative (arrhythmias secondary to drugs or vagal traction reflexes)** **Infants and children:** 4 mcg/kg[1-4] but ≤0.1 mg as a single dose.[2] May be repeated at 2- to 3-min intervals as needed.[1] **Preanesthetic:** Single dose 30–60 min prior to the induction of anesthesia or at the time of preanesthetic narcotic and/or sedative administration.[1-6] **Neonates:** 3–5 mcg/kg (for intubation).[5] **Infants and children:** 4 mcg/kg for children >2 years old; up to 9 mcg/kg may be needed for infants 1 month–2 years old.[1] **Reversal of neuromuscular blockade** **Neonates:** 10 mcg/kg.[7] **Infants and children:** 5–10 mcg/kg.[8,9] One manufacturer recommends up to 0.4 mg/kg glycopyrrolate for every 1 mg neostigmine or 5 mg pyridostigmine for children.[1] A second recommends 0.2 mg of glycopyrrolate for every 1 mg of neostigmine or 5 mg of pyridostigmine for most patients.[10] Alternatively, 10 mcg/kg of glycopyrrolate for every 50[11] mcg/kg of neostigmine has been used. To minimize adverse muscarinic effects, it should be administered in the same syringe with the neostigmine or pyridostigmine, anticholinesterase agents.[12]
Dosage adjustment in organ dysfunction	Patients with renal impairment have delayed elimination; thus, glycopyrrolate should be used with caution in this group.[1]
Maximum dosage	The maximum intraoperative dose is 0.1 mg.[1,12]
IV push	0.2 mg/mL (undiluted)[12] given over 5–10 sec for reversal of neuromuscular blockade.[8]
Intermittent infusion	Can be administered via Y-site injection with a compatible IV fluid such as D5½NS, D5W, D10W, NS, or R.[10-12]
Continuous infusion	No information available to support administration by this method.
Other routes of administration	Given IM at same doses as IV.[2,13]
Maximum concentration	0.2 mg/mL.[2]
Cautions related to IV administration	Dysrhythmias have been reported in children.[1]

Other additives

Contains benzyl alcohol 0.9% as a preservative.[2] Benzyl alcohol in small doses as a preservative in drugs is considered safe in newborns.[14] However, a 3-week-old, very low birth weight (710 g) infant who received clindamycin experienced a profound desaturation that required resuscitation after the third and fourth doses, which was subsequently related to the benzyl alcohol preservative.[15]

Administration of saline flushes containing benzyl alcohol (BW) was associated with a fatal gasping syndrome, intraventricular hemorrhage, metabolic acidosis, and increased mortality in preterm infants.[16] This should not be used in neonates.

Hypersensitivity reactions to benzyl alcohol in parenteral products have been reported in *adults*.[17,18]

Comments

Pretreatment with glycopyrrolate did not alter the incidence of ventricular arrhythmias during halothane anesthesia.[2]

Granisetron HCl

Brand names	Kytril
Dosage	**Prevention of chemotherapy-induced nausea and vomiting:** 10, 20, or 40 mcg/kg,[1-10] given 5[5,6]–30[1-4,7,8,11] min prior to chemotherapy. Granisetron is not approved for use in children <2 years of age[1]; however, it has been used in an 11-month-old infant.[2] For breakthrough nausea and vomiting in the first 24 h of chemotherapy, the dose can be repeated.[12] In *adults*, a 0.05-mg dose was given 30 min prior to chemotherapy, followed by a 0.04-mg/h continuous infusion.[13] **Prevention of postoperative nausea and vomiting:** 10, 20, 40, 80, or 100 mcg/kg doses have been given.[14-17] The 40-mcg/kg dose was more effective than the 10-mcg/kg dose.[14] There was no difference in effectiveness between doses of 40 mcg/kg and 80 or 100 mcg/kg.[15,17] The combination of granisetron and dexamethasone is more effective than granisetron alone.[18,19]
Dosage adjustment in organ dysfunction	The manufacturer recommends no dosage adjustment in renal or hepatic dysfunction.[1] Clearance is significantly decreased in hepatic impairment; however, the pharmacokinetics of granisetron are highly variable and larger doses are well-tolerated.[1]
Maximum dosage	Although doses of 100 mcg/kg have been safely used,[17] 40 mcg/kg is the usual maximum dose.[1-3]
IV push	1 mg/mL (undiluted) has been given over 30 sec in *adults*.[1,20,21] A 40-mcg/kg dose (concentration unspecified) has been infused over 30 sec in children.[22] (See Cautions related to IV administration section.)
Intermittent infusion	20–50 mcg/mL in D5W, D5¼ NS , D5½ NS , or NS[1,20] infused over 2–5 min[1,5,6,16,20] or 30 min.[3,4,7]
Continuous infusion	Although continuous infusion has been used in *adults*,[13] its use has not been reported in pediatric patients.
Other routes of administration	Has been given IM in *adults*.[23,24]
Maximum concentration	Undiluted. 0.1 mg/mL (preservative free) or 1 mg/mL (multidose vial).
Cautions related to IV administration	The data on the effect of granisetron on electrocardiography (ECG) is inconsistent. One pediatric study in 22 children receiving chemotherapy for acute leukemia demonstrated transient changes on ECG but no clinical symptoms after 40 mcg/kg was infused over 30 sec.[22] In *adults*, a 30-sec or 5-min infusion of 10 mcg/kg resulted in a statistically significant prolongation in the QTc interval; however, no clinical symptoms were reported.[21] In four of 12 *adults*, bradycardia, integral change of P-waves, junctional escape beat, and atrioventricular block occurred.[25] Doses of 80 mcg/kg or 120 mcg/kg, in single or split doses, produced no clinically significant effects on ECG, pulse rate or blood pressure in *adults*.[26] For PN compatibility information, please see Appendix C.

Other additives

Single-dose, 1-mL vials contain 9 mg NaCl.[1]

The 4-mL multidose vials (1 mg/mL) contain 9 mg NaCl, 2 mg citric acid, and 10 mg benzyl alcohol per mL.[1] Benzyl alcohol in small doses as a preservative in drugs is considered safe in newborns.[27] However, a 3-week old, very low birth weight (710 g) infant who received clindamycin experienced a profound desaturation that required resuscitation after the third and fourth doses, which was subsequently related to the benzyl alcohol preservative.[28]

Administration of saline flushes containing benzyl alcohol (BW) was associated with a fatal gasping syndrome, intraventricular hemorrhage, metabolic acidosis, and increased mortality in preterm infants.[29] This should not be used in neonates.

Hypersensitivity reactions to benzyl alcohol in parenteral products have been reported in *adults*.[29,30]

Comments

A decrease in effectiveness has been noted with prolonged use.[8] Response appears to be best in children <6 years of age[7] and is least in girls.[8]

Pharmacokinetic parameters were significantly more variable in children with ALL who were given 1–3 mg (48.6–85.7 mcg/kg) compared to *adults* with lung cancer who were given 3 mg (41.7–53.6 mcg/kg).[32]

Haloperidol Lactate

Brand names	Haldol
Dosage	**Agitation in critically ill children and pediatric burn patients:** Doses have ranged from 0.013–0.28 mg/kg.[1-3] One report described a loading dose of 0.09 and 0.1 mg/kg followed by 0.015 and 0.025 mg/kg q 6 h in a 9-month and 11-month old, respectively, and a loading dose of 0.2 or 0.25 mg/kg followed by 0.05–0.15 mg/kg q 8 h in three adolescents.[3] The usual *adult* dose is 1–2 mg IV q 2–4 h or 2–5 mg IM q 4–8 h.[4] In patients requiring multiple doses (e.g., eight 10-mg doses in 24 h or >10 mg/h for more than 5 h) a continuous infusion of 5–10 mg/h has been suggested.[4]
Dosage adjustment in organ dysfunction	No dosage adjustment required in renal dysfunction.[5]
Maximum dosage	50 mg up to 500 mg/d has been used in *adults*.[6]
IV push	May be administered by slow IV push.[7]
Intermittent infusion	5 mg/mL or diluted in D5W. No information available for rate of administration.
Continuous infusion	1 mg/mL in D5W.[8]
Other routes of administration	IM is the preferred route of administration.[1,6,9]
Maximum concentration	5 mg/mL (undiluted).
Cautions related to IV administration	QT prolongation and torsades de pointes have been reported with IV administration in *adults*.[10] ECG should be monitored at baseline and periodically during treatment, and the dosage should be reduced or drug should be discontinued if prolongation of the QT interval occurs.[3] (See Comments section.) Hypotension and dystonic reactions may occur.[6] Care should be taken to avoid skin contact with haloperidol, since contact dermatitis may occur.[4] For PN compatibility information, please see Appendix C.
Other additives	Contains methylparaben and propylparaben.[11] Paraben preservatives may cause hypersensitivity reactions that are more common with cutaneous exposure.[12] However, one case of pruritus and bronchospasm that occurred following infusion of hydrocortisone, which contained a paraben, has been reported.[13]
Comments	Haloperidol may lower the seizure threshold.[4] Use cautiously in patients with a history of epilepsy or in those receiving antiepileptic medications.[4] In children, cardiac effects after ingestion are rare.[11] However, a 29-month-old girl developed bradycardia and arrhythmia and an 11-month-old boy developed bradycardia and hypotension after ingestion of 265 mg.[14]

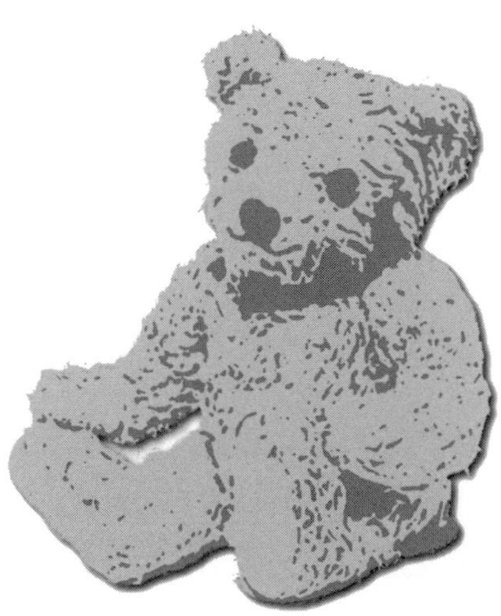

Heparin Sodium

Brand names Various manufacturers

Dosage

Cardiac catheterization: 100–150 units/kg bolus to achieve activated clotting times (ACT) >200 sec.[1,2] Monitor ACT q 1–2 h and administer additional heparin as needed.[1]

Catheter patency

Arterial lines: 0.5–2 units/mL.[3] 0.5 unit/mL in premature or low birth weight infants and patients with multiple lines.[3]

Peripheral IV catheter infusing parenteral nutrition: 0.5–1 unit/mL (final concentration).[15-19] May need to decrease to 0.5 unit/mL in small neonates receiving large volumes. (See Comments section.)

Peripheral IV lock irrigation: Usually 1 mL of 10 units/mL instilled q 8 h.[4-6] However, concentrations (10–100 units/mL), volumes (2–5 mL), and dosing intervals may vary widely depending on institutional protocols.[3,6] Some studies suggest there is no clinical difference between 2 units/mL, 10 units/mL, and saline.[7,8]

Umbilical artery catheter patency: 0.5–2 units/mL of infusate as continuous infusion.[9-14] (See Comments section.)

Continuous arteriovenous hemofiltration: Loading dose of 100 units/kg followed by 5–7 units/kg/h was successfully used in neonates.[20]

Extra corporeal membrane oxygenation: 75–100 units/kg followed by 25–35 units/kg/h usually titrated to ACT of 180–225 sec.[21] (See Dosage adjustment in organ dysfunction section.)

Promotion of fat emulsion clearance: 1 unit/mL of infusate as continuous infusion.[22,23]

Systemic heparinization for thromboembolic disease (see Cautions related to IV administration section)

Neonates: Loading dose of 50 units/kg of preservative-free heparin followed by 20–35 units/kg/h, titrated to desired aPTT.[2,3,24,25]

Infants and children: Loading dose of 50–100 units/kg followed by 10–25 units/kg/h, titrated to desired aPTT.[20,24,28,29]

Protocol for Systemic Heparin Administration and Adjustment for Pediatric Patients*

Stage	Description	aPTT, s	Bolus, units/kg	Hold, min	Rate Change, %	Repeat aPTT
I	Loading dose		75 IV over 10 min			
II	Initial maintenance dose					
	Infants <1 y Infants >1 y		28/h 20/h			
III	Adjustment*	<50	50	0	+10%	4 h
		50–59	0	0	+10%	4 h
		60–85	0	0	0	next day
		86–95	0	0	-10%	4 h
		96–120	0	30	-10%	4 h
		>120	0	60	-15%	4 h
IV	Obtain blood for aPTT check 4 h after loading dose and 4 h after every change in rate					
V	When aPTT values are in therapeutic range, perform daily CBC and aPTT measurement					

*Reproduced with permission from *Chest*.[2]

Heparin Sodium

Dosage adjustment in organ dysfunction	No dosage adjustment is recommended; dosage should be titrated to the appropriate aPTT.[3,30] Patients with renal dysfunction may be at greater risk for hemorrhage. During ECMO, heparin adsorbs onto the circuit. Up to one-half of the heparin administered may be inactivated by the circuit.[31]
Maximum dosage	Individualize dosage based on aPTT,[2,30,32,33] or in some neonatal cases, ACT.[28] ≤35 units/kg/h have been used in neonates with major vessel thrombosis.[28]
IV push	The only time heparin is given by this method is for catheter lock purposes.
Intermittent infusion	Loading dose should be given over 10 min.[2] Continuous infusion is the preferred method of administration.
Continuous infusion	Undiluted or dilute to desired concentration (usually ≤40 units/mL) in D-LR, D-R, D-S, D5NS, D5½NS, D5W, D10W, fat emulsion 10%, LR, NS, ½NS, PN, or R.[32]
Other routes of administration	Not for IM use[30,32]; however, deep SC administration of low dose heparin may be used for postoperative thromboembolism prophylaxis.[30,32]
Maximum concentration	Undiluted (1000–40,000 units/mL).[32]
Cautions related to IV administration	Bleeding may result from overdosage.[33] Neonates may be at increased risk for intracranial hemorrhage.[34] Very low birth weight infants may receive pharmacologic doses with frequent IV line flushes.[3] Heparin-induced thrombocytopenia (HIT), a potentially serious side effect, may occur and is not dose related.[35,36] For PN compatibility information, please see Appendix C.
Other additives	The preservative-free premixed heparin sodium and 0.9% sodium chloride injection in plastic container in 500 and 1000 mL bags by Baxter contains 186 mEq sodium/L, 154 mEq chloride/L, 6 mEq citrate/L, and 16 mmol phosphate/L.[30] While some products are preservative- and antioxidant-free, many heparin products contain sodium metabisulfite, benzyl alcohol, or parabens. **Sulfites:** Sulfites may cause hypersensitivity reactions and these are more common in *adults* with asthma. Most reactions are mild but can include anaphylactic symptoms and life-threatening or less severe asthma episodes.[37-39] Epinephrine may be required in severe cases; and if the sulfite-free product is not available, the sulfite-preserved epinephrine should be used.[40]

Other additives (cont.)

Benzyl alcohol: Benzyl alcohol in small doses as a preservative in drugs is considered safe in newborns.[37] However, a 3-week-old, very low birth weight (710 g) infant who received clindamycin experienced a profound desaturation that required resuscitation after the third and fourth doses, which was subsequently related to the benzyl alcohol preservative.[41]

Administration of saline flushes containing benzyl alcohol (bacteriostatic water for injection) was associated with a fatal gasping syndrome, intraventricular hemorrhage, metabolic acidosis, and increased mortality in preterm infants.[42] This should not be used in neonates.

Hypersensitivity reactions to benzyl alcohol in parenteral products have been reported in *adults*.[43,44]

Paraben: Paraben preservatives may cause hypersensitivity reactions that are more common with cutaneous exposure.[45] However, one case of pruritus and bronchospasm that occurred following infusion of hydrocortisone, which contained a paraben, has been reported.[46]

Comments

Neonates have demonstrated both resistance and sensitivity to heparin.[15] Protamine sulfate reverses the effects of heparin. (See Protamine Sulfate monograph.)

One group of investigators concluded that the addition of heparin to fluids infused to neonates peripherally did not affect catheter life significantly.[19] Similarly, a systematic review of 10 studies that met review criteria could not support the use of heparin in neonates receiving peripheral infusions.[47]

There have been anecdotal reports of precipitation when certain heparin premixed products that contain phosphate are coinfused with calcium chloride.

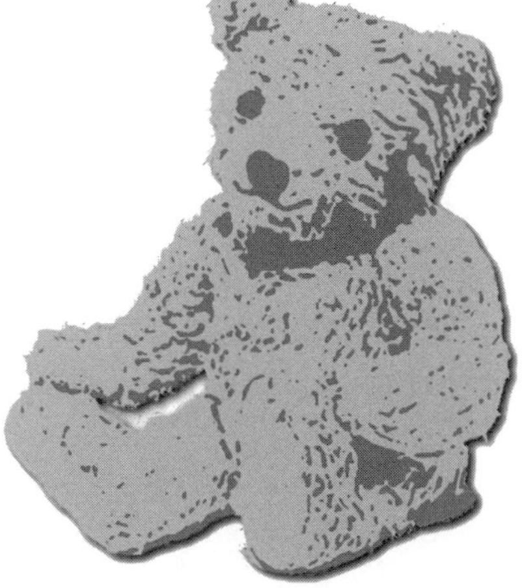

Hydralazine HCl

Brand names	Apresoline
Dosage	**Hypertension/heart failure:** 0.1–0.5 mg/kg q 3–6 h[1-12], 1.7–3.5 mg/kg/d divided q 4–6 h,[13,14] or 500–100 mg/m²/d divided q 4–6 h.[14] **Hypertensive emergency:** 0.2–0.6 mg/kg q 4 h.[14,15] In hypertensive emergencies, blood pressure should be frequently monitored to ensure that it does not decrease too quickly.[14-16] One group recommended that the blood pressure decrease by one-third of the desired total blood pressure decrease within 6–12 h, a further one-third decrease within the next 24 h, with the final one-third decrease achieved over the next 2 days.[17] Alternatively, a blood pressure decrease of <25% within minutes to 1 h followed by further decreases over the next 2–6 h if the patient is stable has been suggested.[14]
Dosage adjustment in organ dysfunction	Adjust dosage in patients with renal dysfunction.[14,19] If CrCl is 10–50 mL/min, administer a normal dose q 8 h.[19] If CrCl is <10 mL/min, administer a normal dose q 8–16 h.[19]
Maximum dosage	1.5 mcg/kg/min,[2,6] 2 mg/kg q 3–6 h[2,6,11] up to 9 mg/kg/d[20] or a 20[21]–25[8,10]mg dose.
IV push	20 mg/mL over 1–2 min in infants.[1,7,22] A 12-year-old child received 0.32 mg/kg over 2 min.[3]
Intermittent infusion	No information to support administration by this method.
Continuous infusion	The manufacturer does not recommend adding to infusion solutions.[22]
Other routes of administration	0.2–0.6 mg/kg/dose may be given IM.[15,23]
Maximum concentration	20 mg/mL.[22]
Cautions related to IV administration	Monitor blood pressure and heart rate for 30–60 min after infusion.[24,25] Tachycardia and fluid retention are common.[15] May use adjuvant beta-blocker and/or diuretic to combat these effects.[14,26] Combination with beta-blocker may reduce hydralazine dose requirements.[26]
Other additives	Contains 103.6 mg propylene glycol/mL.[22] Propylene glycol is added to parenteral drugs as a solubilizer. Rapid infusion of medications that contain propylene glycol has resulted in respiratory depression and cardiac dysrhythmias.[27] Its half-life is three times longer in neonates than in *adults*[28] and has caused hyperosmolality[29] and refractory seizures[30] in preterm neonates receiving 3 g/d.

Other additives (cont.)

Contains 0.65 mg methylparaben and 0.35 mg polyparaben/mL.[22]

Paraben preservatives may cause hypersensitivity reactions that are more common with cutaneous exposure.[31] However, one case of pruritus and bronchospasm that occurred following infusion of hydrocortisone, which contained parabens, has been reported.[32]

Comments

Acetylation is a major route of elimination. The metabolism of hydralazine will be variable in fast and slow acetylators.[14]

Hydralazine should not be diluted in dextrose or other sugar-containing solutions because of the formation of hydrazones, which are associated with toxicity (e.g., headache, nausea, vomiting).[33]

Reduce dosage when converting from oral to IV therapy. One study established that 20–25 mg of IV hydralazine hydrochloride was estimated to equal 75–100 mg of oral hydralazine.[14]

May paradoxically reduce pressor response to epinephrine.[14]

If peripheral neuritis develops (paresthesias, numbness, tingling), use concomitantly with pyridoxine.[14]

May cause SLE or rheumatoid arthritis. Most patients developing symptoms will be slow acetylators.[14] If symptoms occur, consider performing appropriate laboratory studies. If tests confirmatory, discontinue use of hydralazine unless potential benefit outweighs risk.[14]

Color change occurs after dilution with most IV solutions. Color changes within 8–12 h after admixture do not indicate loss of potency when stored at ≤30°C.[22]

Hydrochloric Acid (HCl)

Brand names	Various manufacturers

Dosage

Central venous catheter clearance: Using a 3-mL or larger syringe, instill a volume of 0.1 N HCl equal to the catheter volume (0.2–2 mL) and allow it to dwell for at least 20 min.[1-4] (See Comments section.) Then withdraw and discard HCl, and flush the catheter with an appropriate solution. If unsuccessful, this procedure can be repeated.[1-3]

Severe metabolic alkalosis (not first line therapy; see Comments section): 0.1–0.2 mEq/kg/h until alkalosis is corrected.[5] A 16-day-old infant with refractory metabolic alkalosis received 0.5 mmol/kg/h for 5.5 h, then 0.75 mmol/kg/h for 4.5 h, and 1 mmol/kg/h for 4 h.[6]

The amount of HCl to correct the alkalosis can be calculated using[7]:

Chloride deficit
mEq HCl = 0.2 L/kg x weight (kg) x [103 – observed serum Cl (mEq/L)]

Bicarbonate excess
mEq HCl = 0.5 L/kg x weight (kg) x [observed serum HCO_3 (mEq/L) – 24]

Base-excess
mEq HCl = 0.3 L/kg x weight (kg) x measured base excess (mEq/L)

The chloride-deficit method usually results in a lower dose than the other two. The dose calculated using the chloride deficit should be infused over ≥12 h, and the dose calculated using the bicarbonate excess or base-excess method over ≥24 h.[7] Arterial blood gas and electrolytes should be measured q 4 h during the infusion and therapy adjusted as needed.[7]

Dosage adjustment in organ dysfunction	No information available.
Maximum dosage	Not established. Rates up to 25 mEq/h have been reported.[8] Monitor arterial pH closely during therapy and discontinue HCl when alkalosis has been corrected.
IV push	Contraindicated.
Intermittent infusion	Not indicated.
Continuous infusion	Deficits are replaced by continuous infusion with frequent (q 4 h) monitoring of arterial blood gas.[7] Correction of alkalosis usually occurs within 12–24 h.[7] Because of the sclerosing potential, the rate of infusion should not exceed 0.2 mmol/kg/h.[9]
Other routes of administration	Contraindicated.
Maximum concentration	Usually 0.2 N[8,9]; however, a 0.5 N solution has been used via central line.[6] (See Comments section.) One study reported use of a 1% (10 mg/mL) solution for chemically occluded catheters.[10]

Hydrochloric Acid (HCl)

Cautions related to IV administration

Administer through a central venous catheter whose proper placement has been radiographically confirmed.[5,8]

Although 0.1 N HCl has been given through a peripheral line, it always results in pain at the injection site and may cause thrombophlebitis. It has also been added to an amino acid and lipid solution and infused peripherally in infants with alkalosis.[11]

For PN compatibility information, please see Appendix C.

Other additives

None.

Comments

The diameter of the syringe tip is inversely related to the pressure generated when pushing fluid through. Therefore, larger syringes are used to instill dwell therapies to avoid catheter rupture.[3]

Concentrated HCl diluted to 0.1 N HCl in D5W, NS, or SW provides 0.1 mEq/mL of hydrogen and chloride ion and has a pH of 1–1.5.

HCl is indicated for hypochloremic metabolic alkalosis if NaCl or KCl are contraindicated or if correction is required immediately (e.g., arterial pH >7.55, hepatic encephalopathy, arrhythmia, digitalis cardiotoxicity).[8]

In an *in vitro* study, the surface and interior of pulmonary artery catheters infused with 0.2, 0.3, or 0.4 N HCl showed degenerative changes.[12]

Hydrocortisone Sodium Phosphate/Succinate

Brand names	Hydrocortone Phosphate, A-HydroCort, Solu-Cortef

Dosage

Doses are based on severity of disease and patient response.[1-3] The lowest dose that results in the desired effect should be used.[1-3] (See Comments section.)

Adrenal insufficiency

Acute

Infants and young children: 1–2-mg/kg IV bolus followed by 25–150 mg/d divided q 6–8 h.[4]

Older children: 1–2-mg/kg IV bolus followed by 150–250 mg/d divided q 6–8 h.[5]

Physiologic replacement: 0.25–0.35 mg/kg/d IM as a single dose.[4]

Anti-inflammatory/immunosuppressive therapy: 1–5 mg/kg/d[4] up to 2 g/d[5] or 30–150 mg/m^2 given once a day or divided q 12 h.[4]

Asthma: Hydrocortisone has been used for asthma treatment[6]; however, the National Asthma Education Program Expert Panel (NAEEP) Report lists methylprednisolone sodium succinate for treating status asthmaticus.[7] The NAEEP recommends that asthmatics (*adult*) who have received systemic corticosteroids in the past 6 months and who will undergo surgery be given 100 mg hydrocortisone q 8 h during surgery with rapid weaning postoperatively.[7] (See Comments section.)

Congenital adrenal hyperplasia (emergency treatment): 1–2 mg/kg followed by 2 mg/kg q 8 h until oral therapy can be resumed.[8] Oral replacement therapy is usual.[9,10]

Cystic fibrosis (use not established): 10 mg/kg/d divided q 6 h for 10 days added to standard treatment of infants hospitalized for lower respiratory illness resulted in a greater and more sustained improvement in lung function following hospitalization.[11]

Neonatal uses (preservative-free): (See Other additives section.)

Hypoglycemia: 5 mg/kg/d divided q 12 h.[9]

Hypotension: 2–6 mg/kg/d divided q 6, 12, or 24 h depending on response.[12,13]

Dosage adjustment in organ dysfunction	Use with caution in renal dysfunction.[1] Those with cirrhosis of the liver or who are hypothyroid may have an exaggerated response.[2]
Maximum dosage	Not established. Use of high doses for >48–72 h may result in hypernatremia.[3]
IV push	Over ≥30 sec.[2,3]
Intermittent infusion	Dilute hydrocortisone sodium phosphate in D5W or NS.[1,2] Over 10 min[3] up to 30 min.[5] Dilute hydrocortisone sodium succinate to 0.1–1 mg/mL in D5NS, D5W, or NS for IV infusion.[3] However, 5 mg/mL in D5W was administered to 19 children without apparent adverse effects.[5]
Continuous infusion	Both salts have been given by continuous infusion in D5NS, D5W, or NS; however, the solution concentrations were not specified.[14]
Other routes of administration	Both hydrocortisone sodium phosphate and succinate may be given IM.[1] Hydrocortisone sodium phosphate may be given SC.[1,2]

Hydrocortisone Sodium Phosphate/Succinate

Maximum concentration

Hydrocortisone phosphate 50 mg/mL (undiluted).[2]

Hydrocortisone sodium succinate 60 mg/mL (3000 mg/50 mL diluent).[3]

Cautions related to IV administration

Anaphylaxis has occurred with both salt forms.[15,16]

For PN compatibility information, please see Appendix C.

Other additives

Hydrocortisone sodium phosphate: Contains sodium bisulfite and parabens.[2] Sulfites may cause hypersensitivity reactions and these are more common in *adults* with asthma. Most reactions are mild but can include anaphylactic symptoms and life-threatening or less severe asthma episodes.[17-19] Epinephrine may be required in severe cases; and if the sulfite-free product is not available, the sulfite-preserved epinephrine should be used.[17]

Paraben preservatives may cause hypersensitivity reactions that are more common with cutaneous exposure.[20] However, one case of pruritus and bronchospasm that occurred following infusion of hydrocortisone, which contained a paraben, has been reported.[21]

Hydrocortisone sodium succinate: Contains 2.066 mEq of sodium/g.[3] One product is preservative-free, but most contain benzyl alcohol.[3] Benzyl alcohol in small doses as a preservative in drugs is considered safe in newborns.[17] However, a 3-week-old, very low birth weight (710 g) infant who received clindamycin experienced a profound desaturation that required resuscitation after the third and fourth doses, which was subsequently related to the benzyl alcohol preservative.[22]

Administration of saline flushes containing benzyl alcohol (bacteriostatic water for injection) was associated with a fatal gasping syndrome, intraventricular hemorrhage, metabolic acidosis, and increased mortality in preterm infants.[23] This should not be used in neonates.

Hypersensitivity reactions to benzyl alcohol in parenteral products have been reported in *adults*.[24,25]

Comments

Patients on chronic steroid therapy may require increased doses during stress.[3]

Supraphysiologic doses may result in suppressed pituitary adrenal function. Symptoms of corticosteroid withdrawal syndrome include fever, myalgia, arthralgia, and malaise.[1] Therapy of more than a few days should be decreased gradually.[26,27]

Important adverse effects include increased risk for immunosuppression and infection.[1] In one report, neonates who received IV hydrocortisone for refractory hypotension were more likely to develop disseminated candidal infection than those who did not.[30]

Other adverse effects include musculoskeletal effects, fluid and electrolyte abnormalities, cataracts, and hyperglycemia.[1]

One study in 26 stable asthmatic children reported that 30 mcg/m^2 infused over 24 h increased FEV1 values in those with nocturnal asthma by blunting the diurnal nadir in endogenous cortisol secretion.[28]

H2 antagonists (e.g., ranitidine) may be used as prophylaxis against steroid-induced gastric ulcer, especially in nonenterally-fed patients.

In a study to evaluate hydrocortisone in preventing bronchopulmonary dysplasia associated with adrenal insufficiency, extremely low birth weight neonates (500 to 999 g) were randomized to placebo or 0.5 mg/kg q 12 h for 12 days followed by 0.5 mg/kg/d for 3 days. Compared to the placebo group also receiving indomethacin, the treated group also receiving indomethacin had a higher incidence of gastrointestinal perforation leading to early study termination.[29]

Drugs that enhance hepatic clearance (e.g., phenytoin, phenobarbital, ephedrine, rifampin) may decrease blood levels and lessen physiologic activity.[1,3]

Ifosfamide

Brand names	Ifex
Dosage	Consult institutional protocols for complete dosing information. Ifosfamide is used for pediatric bone and soft tissue sarcomas, as well as Wilms' tumor, neuroblastoma, and germ cell tumors. Common pediatric regimens include 1200–1800 mg/m^2/d for 5 d q 21–28 d or 5 g/m^2/d as a single 24-h infusion or 3 g/m^2/d for 2 days.[1-4] High-dose therapy with 3500 mg/m^2/d for 5 days has also been used.[5]
Dosage adjustment in organ dysfunction	The dose of etoposide should be reduced by 25% in patients with a CrCl <10 mL/min.[6] No specific guidelines exist on ifosfamide use in patients with hepatic insufficiency. However, one investigator recommended a decrease in the ifosfamide normal dosage by 75% in patients with an AST >300 or a bilirubin >3.0 mg/dL.[7]
Maximum dosage	Not established.
IV push	Not recommended.
Intermittent infusion	Dilute with SW to 50 mg/mL, then further dilute solution to a final concentration of 0.6–20 mg/mL with D5W, LR, or NS and infuse over a minimum of 30 min.[8]
Continuous infusion	Ifosfamide has been administered as a continuous infusion.[9] Compared to intermittent administration, this route is associated with greater nephrotoxicity.[10] One paper suggested no mechanistic reason for this effect.[9]
Other routes of administration	No information available to support administration by other routes.
Maximum concentration	50 mg/mL.[8]
Cautions related to IV administration	See Comments section. For PN compatibility information, please see Appendix C.
Other additives	None.

Comments

Ifosfamide is a known bladder irritant. Clinical trials have shown the development of hemorrhagic cystitis in 50% of patients receiving 1.2 g/m^2 of ifosfamide.[8] Therefore, vigorous hydration (i.e., a minimum of 2 L of IV or PO fluids per day) and the uroprotectant, Mesna, are recommended in conjunction with ifosfamide administration.

Ifosfamide has been associated with severe nephrotoxicity.[1,11] Risk factors include age <5 years, history of cisplatin therapy, nephrectomy, renal impairment, or cumulative doses of ifosfamide >50–60 g/m^2.

Ifosfamide is associated with a moderate (30% to 90%) risk of emesis.[12] Patients should receive antiemetic therapy to prevent acute and delayed nausea and vomiting. The recommended therapy is a 5HT3 receptor antagonist in combination with dexamethasone every day chemotherapy is administered.[12,13] These agents may be continued for up to 4 days after chemotherapy administration for the prevention of delayed nausea and vomiting. Breakthrough medications should also be offered, such as a phenothiazine (e.g., prochlorperazine), a butyrophenone (e.g., droperidol), a substituted benzamide (e.g., metoclopramide), or a benzodiazepine (e.g., lorazepam).

Imipenem–Cilastatin Sodium

Brand names

Primaxin I.M., Primaxin I.V.

Dosage

Suspensions of either formulation should not be given intravenously.[1]

Neonates

PNA	<1200 g	1200–2000 g	≥2000 g
<7 d	25 mg/kg q 12 h[1,2]*	25 mg/kg q 12 h[1-3]	25 mg/kg q 12 h[1-3]
≥7 d		25 mg/kg q 8 h[1,2]	25 mg/kg q 6 h[1-3]

*Until 4 weeks of age.

Infants and children

Mild-to-moderate infections: 40–60 mg/kg/d divided q 6 h up to 2 g/d.[3]

Severe infections: 60–100 mg/kg/d divided q 6 h up to 4 g/d.[1,3-9]

Smaller doses may be administered over 20–30 min; however, doses larger than 500 mg should be infused over 40–60 min.[1]

Biologic warfare or bioterrorism: The CDC and other experts recommend that treatment of inhalational anthrax spores due to biologic warfare or bioterrorism should be started on a multiple-drug parenteral regimen that includes ciprofloxacin or doxycycline and one or two additional anti-infective agents (e.g., chloramphenicol, clindamycin, rifampin, vancomycin, clarithromycin, imipenem, penicillin, or ampicillin).[10,11]

Dosage adjustment in organ dysfunction

Adjust dosage in patients with renal dysfunction.[1,12] If CrCl is 10–50 mL/min, give 50% of a normal dose of imipenem; if CrCl is <10 mL/min, give 25% of a normal dose of imipenem.[12]

Maximum dosage

100 mg/kg/d.[1,3] Up to 2 g/d in mild-to-moderate infections[1,3,5,13] and 4 g/d in severe infections.[1,3,13,14] IM dosages >1500 mg/d are not recommended.[1]

IV push

Not recommended.[1]

Intermittent infusion

2.5–5 mg/mL in D5NS, D5¼NS, D5½NS, D5W, D10W, or NS given over 20–60 min.[1] The manufacturer recommends that smaller doses be infused over 20–30 min and that doses >500 mg be infused over 40–60 min.[1] Doses ≤500 mg have been infused over 15 min in children.[13] (See Cautions related to IV administration section.)

Continuous infusion

Not recommended.[1]

Other routes of administration

Suspension for IM administration should be reconstituted with 1% lidocaine HCl without epinephrine.[1] IM administration should not be used for severe or life-threatening infections (e.g., sepsis, endocarditis).[1] Administer by deep injection into a large muscle.[1] To avoid accidental injection into a blood vessel, verify needle placement via aspiration.[1]

Maximum concentration	5 mg/mL.[1]
Cautions related to IV administration	If a decision is made to give this medication to a patient with known hypersensitivity to penicillins, cephalosporins, other beta-lactams, the patient should be closely observed for allergenicity. Epinephrine, oxygen, intravenous steroids, and airway management may be required. Decrease administration rate in those who develop nausea during infusion.[1] May cause pain at the injection site, phlebitis/thrombophlebitis, and erythema.[1] For PN compatibility information, please see Appendix C.
Other additives	The 250- and 500-mg intravenous vials contain 0.8 mEq (18.8 mg) and 1.6 mEq (37.5 mg) of sodium, respectively. The 500- and 750-mg intramuscular vials contain 1.4 mEq (32 mg) and 2.1 mEq (48 mg) of sodium, respectively.[15]
Comments	Neurotoxicity of the carbapenem antibiotics has been reported.[16,17] Two neonates who received 20 mg/kg/d and 80 mg/kg/d of imipenem experienced seizures.[18] Seizures as early as the first day of therapy or after 3 days have been reported in children with meningitis. Three of 82 pediatric patients with cancer developed seizures attributed to imipenem/cilastatin.[19] In *adults*, seizures most often occur after 7 days and appear to be related to an underlying CNS disorder, impaired renal function, and/or large doses.[20] Because of the risk of seizures, the drug should not be used in patients with CNS infections and in patients with a history of seizure disorders.[1] Use cautiously in combination with drugs that lower the seizure threshold and in patients with renal dysfunction. May cause false-positive urinary glucose results when cupric sulfate solution-based tests (Clinitest or Benedict's or Fehling's solutions) are used.[21] Glucose oxidase methods (Clinistix) are not associated with false-positive test results.[21] Because imipenem is associated with numerous drug interactions, consult appropriate resources for dosing recommendations before combining any drug with imipenem.

Immune Globulin Intravenous

Brand names Carimune NF; Gammagard Liquid; Gammagard S/D; Gamunex; Iveegam EN; Octagam; Sandoglobulin; Panglobulin NF; Polygam S/D

Dosage

400–2000 mg immune globulin intravenous (IGIV)/kg depending on indication.[1-31]

Advanced HIV infection: 300–400 mg/kg/d q 4 weeks.[2,3]

Bone marrow transplant: 100–500 mg/kg/d q 7 d for 3 months and then monthly for 9 months with or without one dose before transplantation,[4,5] or beginning 8 days before transplantation and q 7 d for 4 months.[6]

Guillain-Barré syndrome (use not established): 1000 mg/kg/d for 2 days or 400 mg/kg/d for 5–7 days resulted in modest benefits.[7,8]

Hemolytic disease of the newborn (use not established): 500 mg/kg/d for 1–3 days was associated with a decreased need for exchange transfusion and a shorter duration of phototherapy in neonates with blood group incompatibility.[9,10]

HIV-associated thrombocytopenia: 500–1000 mg/kg/d for 3–5 days.[2]

Idiopathic thrombocytopenic purpura: 250–1000 mg/kg/d for 1–7 days initially and then as needed to maintain platelet count >30,000/mm^3.[1,11-13]

Kawasaki disease: A single 2000 mg/kg/d given over 10–12 h[2,14-19] is recommended over 400 mg/kg/d for 4 consecutive days.[15,17,20] Patients who have persistent fever or who have recrudescent fever after treatment may be retreated.[2,19,21] Some advocate pulse steroid rather than a repeat dose of IVIG; however, corticosteroid use may be associated with coronary artery abnormalities[2,22] and, therefore, should be reserved for children in whom ≥ two courses of IVIG have been ineffective.[19]

Obsessive-compulsive and tic disorder associated with pediatric autoimmune neuropsychiatric disorders associated with streptococcal infection (PANDAS) (use not established): Children randomized to receive 1000 mg/kg/d for 2 days experienced significant improvements in neuropsychiatric symptoms within 1 month compared to placebo.[30]

Primary immunodeficiency: 200–400 mg/kg/d q 3–4 weeks to maintain serum IgG trough concentrations ≥400–500 mg/dL.[1,2,11] High-dose (800 mg/kg q 4 weeks) reduced the number of infections from 3.5 to 2.5 in 230 days and decreased the infection duration from 29 to 22 days.[23]

Sepsis prevention in premature neonates: 500[24-26]–1000[24-28] mg/kg/d at varying intervals to achieve an IgG concentration ≥700 mg/dL.[27,28]

Sydenham's chorea (use not established): In four children who received 1000 mg/kg/d for 2 days, a 72% improvement in chorea severity scores was noted 1 month after treatment. The long-term response was similar to that seen with prednisone, but the response occurred more rapidly with IVIG.[29]

Toxic epidermal necrolysis/Stevens-Johnson syndrome (use not established): A report presented seven children and reviewed case reports for 28 other children who received an average of 2500 mg/kg/d (range 1500–5800 mg/kg) for 1–7 days. The majority of patients did have a positive response; however, disease reactivation did occur infrequently.[31]

Dosage adjustment in organ dysfunction

IVIG infusion has resulted in renal failure in certain individuals. Therefore, it is recommended that patients be adequately hydrated prior to infusion, serum creatinine and BUN should be measured, and urine output followed.

No dosage adjustment may be required in renal dysfunction; however, in patients with pre-existing renal insufficiency or at risk for renal insufficiency, recommended doses should not be exceeded, the dilution should be at the minimum concentration possible, and the rate of infusion should be as slow as is practical.[1] Products containing sucrose have been associated with renal dysfunction more often than those without; this should be considered when choosing a product.

Maximum dosage	2000 mg/kg.[14,15]
IV push	Not recommended.[1]
Intermittent infusion	Initial and maximum infusion rates vary according to product selected. Usual initial rate is 0.01–0.02 mL/kg/min. If no adverse effects occur within 15–30 min, rate may be increased.[1] (Consult manufacturer's guidelines for appropriate infusion rates.) Doses of 400 mg/kg may be infused over 2 h[2,17,24]; however, doses of 2000 mg/kg should be infused over 8–12 h.[17]
Continuous infusion	No information available to support administration by this method.
Other routes of administration	IVIG is only given IV. Immune globulin IM is administered intramuscularly. (See Comments section.)
Maximum concentration	3% to 12% (product specific).[1] Dilute according to manufacturer's directions.[1]
Cautions related to IV administration	Infusion reactions including facial flushing, chest tightness, chills, fever, dizziness, nausea, vomiting, diaphoresis, and hypotension may occur within 30–60 min of start of the infusion. If any of these reactions occurs, decrease the infusion rate or stop the infusion until the reaction subsides; then restart at a slower rate.[1] Epinephrine should be available if needed. One large British study found that infusion reactions occurred at a rate of 0.7% in children <10 years, which is not significantly different from the *adult* rate (0.8%).[32] Renal dysfunction and failure have been reported, especially in patients with pre-existing renal disease, at risk for renal dysfunction, or with volume depletion. In these patients, the minimum concentration and the slowest infusion rate should be used. The risk may be higher in brands containing sucrose as a stabilizer.[1] For PN compatibility information, please see Appendix C.

Other additives

Carimune NF:	1.67 g sucrose and <20 mg NaCl/g protein.[33]
Gammagard Liquid:	0.25 M glycine.[1]
Gamunex:	0.16–0.24 M glycine and ≤0.216 g/L of caprylate.[1]
Gammagard S/D:	Each mL (5%) contains 8.5 mg NaCl, 3 mg albumin, 22.5 mg glycine, 20 mg glucose, 2 mg polyethylene glycol, 1 mcg tri(n-butyl) phosphate, 1 mcg octoxynol 9, and 100 mcg polysorbate 80.[1]
Iveegam EN:	Each mL (5%) contains 50 mg glucose and 3 mg NaCl Polyethylene glycol may be present in the final product at concentrations <0.5 g/dL.[1]
Octagam:	Each mL contains 50 mg protein (≥96% IgG), 100 mg maltose, ≤5 mcg of Triton X-100, ≤1 mcg of TNBP, ≤0.2 mg of IgA, ≤0.1 mg IgM, and ≤0.03 mmol of sodium.[34]
Panglobulin:	1.67 g sucrose, <20 mg NaCl/g protein.[1]

Immune Globulin Intravenous

Other additives *(cont.)*	**Polygam S/D:**	Each mL (5%) contains 8.5 mg NaCl, 3 mg albumin, 22.5 mg glycine, 20 mg glucose, 2 mg polyethylene glycol, 1 mcg tri(n-butyl) phosphate, 1 mcg octoxynol 9, and 100 mcg polysorbate 80.[1]
	Sandoglobulin:	1.67 g sucrose, <20 mg NaCl/g protein.[35]

Comments

Filtration requirements for constitution and administration vary among products. Refer to manufacturer's recommendations for specific requirements and filter information.[1,11,17]

Aseptic meningitis syndrome has been reported following administration of IVIG to patients with idiopathic thrombocytopenia purpura or Kawasaki syndrome.[36-40]

Considerations in choosing a product should include carbohydrate and IgA content, IgG subclass distribution and amounts, product concentration, and osmolality.

The manufacturing process of the two products associated with hepatitis C development has been revised to eliminate possible contamination with this virus.[41]

Transient neutropenia can occur after immune globulin infusion in children with idiopathic thrombocytopenic purpura.[42]

A severe hemolytic anemia has been reported following infusion of high-dose IGIV for Kawasaki disease.[43]

Although infrequent, renal insufficiency and failure have been reported within 7 days of infusion in patients from 3–91 years of age.[44]

Administration of products containing maltose may result in false interpretations of blood glucose readings when glycose dehydrogenase pyrroloquinolinequinone- or glycose-dye-oxidoreductase-based testing methods are used.[34]

The length of time between immune globulin intravenous administration and vaccination with measles, mumps, and rubella (MMR) vaccine varies according to dose as follows[2]:

IVIG Dose	Interval before Vaccination
300–400 mg/kg	8 mo
1000 mg/kg	10 mo
1600–2000 mg/kg	11 mo

Immune globulin IM (not IVIG) is administered IM at doses of 0.02–1.2 mL/kg for postexposure prophylaxis of hepatitis A, measles, rubella, and varicella-zoster.[1] 1.3 mL/kg is administered for the prophylactic treatment of infection in patients with IgG-deficiency or other antibody-deficiency disease, then maintenance doses of 0.66 mL/kg (≥100 mg/kg) are administered q 3–4 weeks. The maximum single IM dose is 30–50 mL in *adults* and 20–30 mL in infants and small children. If the IM dose exceeds 10 mL, it should be divided and injected into several sites to reduce local pain and discomfort.

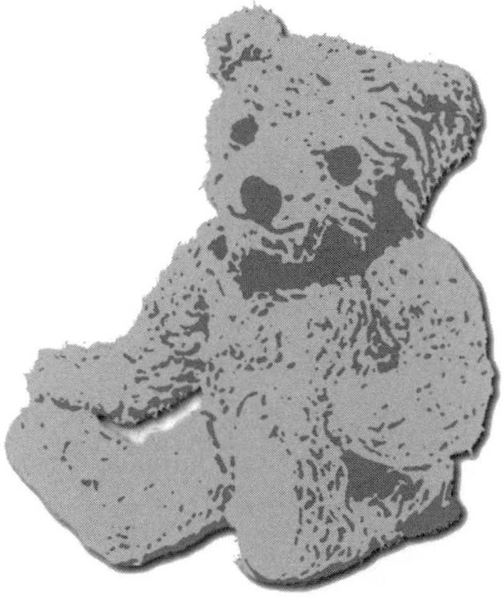

Inamrinone Lactate*

Brand names	Inocor
Dosage	Because inamrinone lactate has been administered to only a limited number of pediatric patients, the doses and side effects have not been established.[1] Although it has been used successfully to treat myocardial dysfunction and increased systemic or pulmonary vascular resistance, it has generally been replaced by milrinone. **Loading dose:** Usually 0.75–1 mg/kg over 2–3 min.[2-7] May repeat two to four times q 15 min to a total loading dose of 3 mg/kg.[1-6] One group gave 1.5 mg/kg as a single dose[8]; another group administered 4.5 mg/kg over 2 h.[9] Total loading doses have ranged from 0.75–4.5 mg/kg.[4,10] **Maintenance infusion:** It is difficult to predict the optimal infusion rate due to as much as a sixfold variation in the pharmacokinetics of inamrinone lactate in children[1]; hence, dose should be titrated to effect. **Neonates:** 3–7.5 mcg/kg/min.[10,11] **Infants and children:** 2–20 mcg/kg/min.[2]
Dosage adjustment in organ dysfunction	Adjust dosage in renal dysfunction.[1,12] If CrCl is <10 mL/min, give 50% to 75% of a normal dose.[12]
Maximum dosage	Not established. The PALS guidelines recommends up to 20 mcg/kg/min.[2] One group administered doses up to 40 mcg/kg/min for 30 min in seven children who had undergone cardiac surgery.[13] This study did not show statistically significant increases in stroke volume or cardiac index at the larger doses. Total dosage (initial, supplemental doses and cumulative infused dose) should not generally exceed 10 mg/kg/d in *adults*,[1] but doses up to 18 mg/kg/d have been infused for short periods in *adults*.[1] A 2.5-month-old infant died from accidental infusion of 180–198 mcg/kg/min.[14]
IV push	5 mg/mL (commercially available) given over 2–3 min.[1] One group of investigators infused 0.75 mg/kg over 30 sec.[7] Another group noted that hypotension was related to the infusion rate and recommended dividing any loading dose larger than 0.75 mg/kg into two or three smaller doses.[3]
Intermittent infusion	Although concentration and solution type were not specified, a loading dose of 4.5 mg/kg has been infused over 2 h.[9]
Continuous infusion	1–3 mg/mL in ½NS or NS.[1] Do not dilute inamrinone lactate with dextrose solutions prior to infusion because an interaction can result in loss of potency. However, it can be infused through a Y-connector into an infusing solution that contains dextrose.[1]
Other routes of administration	May be given IO.[2] No information available to support administration by other routes.
Maximum concentration	5 mg/mL for IV bolus.[1]

*Previously amrinone.

Cautions related to IV administration

May cause hypotension and arrhythmias.[1]

Other additives

Sulfites: Each 5-mg dose contains 0.25 mg sodium metabisulfite. Sulfites may cause hypersensitivity reactions and these are more common in *adults* with asthma. Most reactions are mild but can include anaphylactic symptoms and life-threatening or less severe asthma episodes.[16-18] Epinephrine may be required in severe cases; and if the sulfite-free product is not available, the sulfite-preserved epinephrine should be used.[16]

Comments

Thrombocytopenia has been reported. In one study involving 16 children (1–134 months of age), eight developed thrombocytopenia within 19–71 h after initiation of inamrinone lactate. When inamrinone lactate was discontinued, thrombocytopenia resolved after 54 ± 15 h.[6]

Because inamrinone lactate is associated with several drug-drug interactions, consult appropriate resources for dosing recommendations before combining any drug with inamrinone lactate.

Indomethacin Sodium Trihydrate

Brand names Indocin I.V.

Dosage

Patent Ductus Arteriosus, (PDA—closure of the ductus arteriosus)

Prophylaxis (used for subclinical PDA and routine prophylaxis during the first day of life in very low birth weight newborns): 0.1 mg/kg/d for 5 d.[1-4] Continuous infusion has been used (0.004 mg/kg/h) from 6–12 h postnatal age until ductus closure.[4] Routine prophylaxis has not been found to improve survival without neurosensory impairment at 18 months of age.[5,6]

Treatment

Conventional dosing[1,7-14]

PNA at First Dose	Dose 1	Dose 2	Dose 3
<2 d	0.2 mg/kg	0.1 mg/kg	0.1 mg/kg
2–7 d	0.2 mg/kg	0.2 mg/kg	0.2 mg/kg
>7 d	0.2 mg/kg	0.25 mg/kg	0.25 mg/kg

Doses are given over 20–30 min at 8,[14] 12,[1,7-11] 18,[10] or 24[1,7,12] h intervals. (See Cautions related to IV administration section.) If a second course of indomethacin is necessary, one to three doses may be administered at 12–24 h intervals.[7]

Nonconventional dosing

Continuous infusion: A 36-h infusion of indomethacin (0.011 mg/kg/h) for closure of a PDA has been reported to reduce alterations in cerebral, renal, and mesenteric blood flow compared to bolus administration.[15,16] Reports of the use of continuous infusions of indomethacin for prophylaxis and closure of PDAs have been reported at rates of 0.004–0.011 mg/kg/h, respectively.[4,15,16]

Prolonged dosing: Various prolonged low dose (0.1 mg/kg/dose q 24 h for six doses)[2,3,17-19] and dose escalating regimens (increasing doses by 0.1 mg/kg/dose q 12 h)[20] have been evaluated with variable success in PDA closure rates and incidence of adverse reactions.

Prevention of intraventricular hemorrhage: 0.1 mg/kg q 24 h for three doses, beginning at 6–12 h of age.[9,21]

Dosage adjustment in organ dysfunction

Contraindicated in neonates with significant renal dysfunction.[7] The manufacturer recommends withholding additional doses if oliguria (urine output <0.6 mL/kg/h) occurs at the time of a scheduled dose.[7] Additional doses should be given only when renal function returns to normal. Most practitioners would administer a normal dose of indomethacin q 24 h if urine output is above 0.6 mL/kg/h. (See Comments section.)

Maximum dosage

0.25–0.4 mg/kg[8,22] or cumulative 0.9–1 mg/kg in 3 d.[20,23]

IV push

Although indomethacin has been given over 5–10 sec,[7,24,25] rapid administration causes a significant decrease in mesenteric artery[26] and cerebral[23-28] blood flow, which may contribute to development of necrotizing enterocolitis [26] or cerebral ischemia.[24,27,28] Should be given over 20–30 min.[29]

Intermittent infusion

0.5–1 mg/mL in preservative-free NS or SW[7] infused over 20–35 min.[7,26]

Indomethacin Sodium Trihydrate

Continuous infusion	Admixed in D5W or NS to deliver 0.011 mg/kg/h for 36 h (solution expires in 24 h).[20]
Other routes of administration	IM administration not recommended due to severe extravasation injuries.[7]
Maximum concentration	1 mg/mL.[7,29]
Cautions related to IV administration	Urine output may transiently decrease.[7,8] If it is <0.6 mL/kg/h at the time of the second or third scheduled dose, do not give that dose until laboratory studies indicate that renal function is normal.[7,8] Low dose infusions of dopamine to prevent indomethacin-induced renal dysfunction may be used.[30] Avoid extravasation.[7] Because indomethacin may cause vasoconstriction and decrease blood flow to the intestines, it should not be infused via an umbilical catheter into vessels near the superior mesenteric artery. For PN compatibility information, please see Appendix C.
Other additives	None.
Comments	A second course of one to three doses may be given using above guidelines.[7,31] In one study, the serum indomethacin concentrations varied 20-fold, 24 h after a 0.2-mg/kg dose. The relationship between serum concentrations and ductus closure is unclear. Indomethacin concentrations 24 h after a dose correlated with constriction of the ductus and the time of subsequent reopening was also related to the plasma concentration.[31] Exceeding 0.25 mcg/mL may not be predictive of permanent closure of the ductus.[8] Acute renal failure may occur.[7] Monitor urine output and renal function in patient receiving indomethacin for PDA. Bleeding has occurred in premature infants receiving indomethacin orally.[32] Monitor platelets in patient receiving indomethacin for PDA. Hypoglycemia developed during indomethacin therapy and persisted for up to 72 h. Close monitoring of serum glucose concentrations and adjustment of glucose infusion rates is recommended.[33-35] Because indomethacin is associated with numerous drug interactions consult appropriate resources for dosing recommendations before combining any drug with indomethacin.

Infliximab

Brand names	Remicade
Dosage	**Crohn's disease:** 5 mg/kg/dose repeated as needed,[1-5] 5 mg/kg every 8 weeks for a year if showing a favorable response[6] or 5 mg/kg at 0, 2, and 6 weeks with continuation for recurrence of clinical symptoms.[6,7] Another study reported benefits with 5 mg/kg administered on days 0, 15, and 45.[8] Doses of 1 mg/kg are less effective.[9] **Refractory juvenile idiopathic arthritis (JIA):** 3–4 mg/kg initially or at weeks 0, 2, and 6 weeks followed by maintenance therapy up to 10 mg/kg every 4–8 weeks.[10,11] **JIA uveitis:** 5–10 mg/kg at weeks 0, 2, and 4 followed by infusions every 6–8 weeks with a more rapid infusion rate based on tolerance (stable vital signs).[12] In a case series of pediatric uveitis patients with or without associated JIA, all patients responded to infliximab at 5–10 mg/kg at 2–8 week intervals.[13] **Refractory Kawasaki syndrome:** Limited data suggests that a single infusion of 5–10 mg/kg may be beneficial in patients who have not responded to two doses of IVIG and daily high-dose aspirin therapy.[14] **Ulcerative colitis:** 5 mg/kg[15-18] initially followed by 5–10 mg/kg in 2 weeks[16] or 5 mg/kg as induction therapy at 0, 2, and 6 weeks with maintenance treatment every 6–8 weeks.[3,17,18]
Dosage adjustment in organ dysfunction	Information not available.
Maximum dosage	Doses up to 20 mg/kg have been used in *adults*[19] and one case series reported successful treatment of a 15-year-old patient receiving an 18-mg/kg dose.[13]
IV push	Not recommended.[19]
Intermittent infusion	In pediatric studies, once infusions were prepared according to the package insert, the infliximab infusion rate was increased after 15 min from 15 mL/h to 30 mL/h for 15 min to 60 mL/h for 30 min to 90 mL/h to complete the infusion[12] or was increased q 15 min from 10 mL/h to 20 mL/h to 40 mL/h to 80 mL/h to a maximum of 125 mL/h based on the stability of vital signs.[20] The maximum infusion rate in *adults* is 250 mL/h. The infusion should be administered over ≥2 h.[19]
Continuous infusion	Not indicated.
Other routes of administration	No information available to support administration by other routes.
Maximum concentration	4 mg/mL.[21]

Cautions related to IV administration

Infusion reactions following administration of infliximab have occurred in 8.1% to 38.6% of pediatric patients and commonly include flushing, chest pain, and shortness of breath.[20,22-24] These are believed to be caused by the production of antibodies to infliximab. The concomitant administration of immunomodulating medications (or use within the preceding 4 months) is believed to be protective. Although premedication with hydrocortisone, diphenhydramine and antipyretics is common, efficacy in preventing infusion-associated reactions has not been established.[23] Infusion reactions can occur after the first or any subsequent dose[22] but are most likely to occur after the second or third infusion.[20] A history of an infusion reaction does not automatically predict future infusion-related reactions. Infusion reactions can be managed with the use of diphenhydramine, acetaminophen, and prednisone or by slowing down the rate of infusion.[19] The infusion should be stopped indefinitely if this regimen does not improve symptoms or if the use of epinephrine is required.

Three to 12 days after an infusion, a delayed infusion reaction may be experienced. Treatment is similar to an acute infusion reaction and may resolve with 1 to 3 days. Longer intervals between treatments (more than a year) increase the risk of delayed infusion reactions.

Other additives

Contains no preservatives.[21]

Comments

Administer the infusion using an in-line, low-protein-binding filter with a pore diameter ≤1.2 microns.[19]

Before initiating infliximab, it is recommended that patients are screened for tuberculosis (TB) due to a concern about reactivating latent TB; however, a negative skin test does not rule out the possibility of disease since patients with immune diseases may exhibit cutaneous anergy.[25]

Serious infections have occurred in patients receiving infliximab and other TNF-blocking medications. In addition, caution should be exercised when administering infliximab to patients with active or chronic infection.[21] The combination of infliximab with other TNF-blocking medications is not recommended. A patient information sheet supplied by the manufacturer should be given to the patient before administering infliximab.

Live virus vaccines (measles-mumps-rubella, varicella, ratavirus) should be avoided during treatment.[19]

Insulin

Brand names	Humulin R, Novolin R, Humulin R (concentrated U-500)

Dosage

Glucose intolerance in low birth weight infants: 0.03–1 unit/kg/h initially as continuous infusion with the dose titrated to desired blood glucose concentration.[12-17] The average requirements during parenteral nutrition in infants 1000 g or less was 0.45 unit/kg/h (range 0.05–1) and in those >1000 g was 0.3 unit/kg/h (range 0.05–0.5).[16] Similarly, very low birth weight neonates (750 ± 211 g) who were receiving parenteral nutrition, required 0.07–4.2 units/kg/h for hyperglycemia to resolve.[17] (See Comments section.)

Hyperglycemic crises in diabetes (diabetic ketoacidosis [DKA] and hyperosmolar hyperglycemic state [HHS]): Patients should be hydrated with NS and baseline electrolytes obtained prior to beginning insulin.[1]

A continuous infusion of 0.05–0.1 unit/kg/h[1,2] may be preceded by a loading dose of 0.1–0.15 unit/kg.[1,3-11] Blood glucose should be measured q 1–4 h and the dose titrated to glucose concentration.[1-11] DKA resolution has occurred when HCO_3 is >18, anion gap is ≤12, and pH is >7.3. HHS has resolved when the osmolality is <315 mOsm/kg and the individual is alert.[1] The blood glucose should decrease by 50–70 mg/dL/h.[1] Too rapid a decrease may cause cerebral edema. When blood glucose is 250–300 mg/dL, the continuous infusion should be decreased to 0.05–0.1 unit/kg/h. In newly-diagnosed patients, SC dosing can be started using 0.1–0.25 unit/kg q 6 h when the blood glucose is <200 mg/dL.[11] (See Comments section.)

Hyperkalemia (after therapy with $NaHCO_3$ and calcium gluconate): 0.05–0.01 unit/kg/h infused with 400 mg dextrose/kg.[2] A ratio of 1 unit of insulin for every 1.2–3.1 (2.2 ± 0.6) g of dextrose has been used to treat hyperkalemic, premature neonates.[18] One unit of insulin for every 4 g of dextrose has been used in infants and children.[2] Titrate dose to maintain desired serum glucose concentration. Measure serum potassium q 6 h and discontinue therapy when potassium concentrations are ≤6 mEq/L.[19]

Dosage adjustment in organ dysfunction

In *adults*, if CrCl is 10–50 mL/min, give 75% of the normal dose; if CrCl is <10 mL/min, give 50% of normal dose.[20]

Maximum dosage

Doses up to 4.2 units/h have been required occasionally in very low birth weight neonates (<1000 g) during first 2 weeks of life.[16,17] It has been speculated that the increased requirement in very low birth weight neonates is due to insulin resistance, inappropriate insulin secretion, or decreased sensitivity of the liver to insulin effects.[21] In DKA, some endocrinologists do not use more than 3 units/h in children.[1] (See Comments section.)

IV push

Rapid for loading dose in DKA[3-5,10,22] or HHS.[1] It has been recommended that children <20 years not be given a loading dose.[23]

Intermittent infusion

Not indicated.

Continuous infusion

0.1–1 unit/mL in NS.[9,24] (See Dosage section.)

Other routes of administration

IM and SC are alternative routes of administration. IM administration results in faster absorption than SC.[11] However, in DKA and HHS these routes of administration may require hourly dosing of insulin. Neither IM nor SC dosing should be used in patients with hypovolemic shock, hyperosmolar hyperglycemia, or hyperkalemia.[23]

Maximum concentration	100 units/mL for IM or SC dosing.[23]
Cautions related to IV administration	Serum glucose concentrations should be monitored closely for early detection of hypoglycemia.[1,3,4,11,23] Only regular insulin products can be infused IV.[23,25] For PN compatibility information, please see Appendix C.
Other additives	Each mL of the concentrated Humulin R product (500 units/mL) contains 16 mg glycerin, 2.5 mg *m*-cresol, and zinc oxide to a total Zn content of 0.017 mg/100 units.[26]
Comments	Insulin binds to glass bottles, plastic IV bags, syringes, and tubing and results in decreased delivery of insulin. IV tubing has been primed with an insulin solution to saturate insulin-binding sites and prevent further absorption.[3,4,15,22,24,27] Alternatively, human serum albumin occupies binding sites on glass[28] and plastic and has been added to insulin-containing solutions[6,19,22] to increase insulin delivery. In low birth weight infants, a 12–14 h delay in response was noted when IV tubing was not primed with insulin.[15] Whether this was due to lack of priming or insulin resistance was not evaluated. Because insulin is associated with numerous drug interactions, consult appropriate resources for dosing recommendations before combining any drug with insulin.

Interferon Alfa-2a

Brand names	Roferon-A
Dosage	**Childhood angiomatous disease (hemangiomas):** 1–3 million units/m² SC for up to 33 months.[6-11] **Chronic hepatitis B or C:** 3–10 million units/m² IM or SC three times per week.[3-5] **Craniopharyngiomas:** 8 million units/m² SC followed by 8 million units/m² SC three times per week have been used with limited success in a small number of patients >4 years old.[12] **Philadelphia chromosome-positive chronic myelogenous leukemia (CML):** Usually, 2.5–10 million units/m² IM or SC.[1,2] One child was increased to 20 million units/m² and this dose was continued for >110 weeks.[2] In another child, therapy was continued for >168 weeks.[2] However, deaths have been reported in children with Philadelphia chromosome-negative CML who received doses of 30 million units/m².[2] **Subacute sclerosing panencephalitis:** Limited research suggests that 10 million units/m² three times a week SC in combination with lamivudine and isoprinosine may be beneficial.[14]
Dosage adjustment in organ dysfunction	Caution is recommended in patients with creatinine clearance < 50 mL/min.[1] Limited data suggests that dose adjustment is not needed in patients receiving hemodialysis.[14]
Maximum dosage	Dependent on the specific indication for use. The maximum dose for *adults* with Kaposi's sarcoma or cutaneous T-cell lymphoma is 36 million units/d SC for 10–12 weeks.[1] Doses in pediatric patients typically do not exceed 10 million units/m².
IV push	Not indicated.
Intermittent infusion	Not indicated.
Continuous infusion	Not indicated.
Other routes of administration	Prefilled, single-dose syringes are to be administered SC only.[1]
Maximum concentration	36 million international units/mL.[1]
Cautions related to IV administration	IV administration not indicated.

Other additives

While the amount of interferon alfa-2a varies, the specific additives are the same. Each mL contains 7.21 mg NaCl, 0.2 mg polysorbate 80, 10 mg benzyl alcohol, and 0.77 mg ammonium acetate.[1] Tetracycline is used in the manufacturing process but is below detectable levels in the final product.[1]

Benzyl alcohol in small doses as a preservative in drugs is considered safe in newborns.[15] However, a 3-week-old, very low birth weight (710 g) infant who received clindamycin experienced a profound desaturation that required resuscitation after the third and fourth doses, which was subsequently related to the benzyl alcohol preservative.[16]

Administration of saline flushes containing benzyl alcohol (bacteriostatic water for injection) was associated with a fatal gasping syndrome, intraventricular hemorrhage, metabolic acidosis, and increased mortality in preterm infants.[17] This should not be used in neonates.

Hypersensitivity reactions to benzyl alcohol in parenteral products have been reported in *adults*.[18,19]

Comments

Alpha interferons cause or aggravate fatal or life-threatening neuropsychiatric, autoimmune, ischemic, and infectious disorders. Patients should be monitored closely, and periodic clinical and laboratory valuations should be performed. Patients with persistently severe or worsening signs or symptoms of these conditions should be withdrawn from therapy. In many cases, but not all, these disorders resolve after therapy is discontinued.[1]

Common side effects in pediatric patients include flu-like symptoms, fever, weight loss, elevation of transaminases, and neutropenia.[4,7,10-12] Dosing at night may decrease the flu-like adverse effects.[20]A sharp, febrile response with rigors and other constitutional symptoms including peripheral cyanosis, nausea, vomiting, and severe myalgias may occur with doses of 50–120 million units.[20]

Alpha interferons suppress bone marrow function and may result in severe cytopenias, including very rare events of aplastic anemia. Obtain complete blood counts (CBC) pretreatment and monitor routinely during therapy. Alpha interferon therapy should be discontinued in patients who develop severe decreases in neutrophil ($<0.5 \times 10^9/L$) or platelet counts ($<25 \times 10^9/L$).[1]

Use with caution in patients with cardiac disease, renal or hepatic disease, autoimmune disease, transplanted organs, psychiatric disorders, or seizure disorders.[1,25]

Injection site reactions include burning, pruritus, erythema, pain, rash, edema, and vesiculation.[20] Rotating injection sites may help to minimize local reactions.

Rare cases of spastic diplegia and other neurological abnormalities have been reported in infants who have received interferon alfa-2a for hemangiomas.[11] This side effect is not believed to be dose related; therapy should be discontinued if signs consistent with spastic diplegia develop.[20]

One child had a grand-mal seizure while receiving 10 million units/m^2 and the interferon was discontinued.[11]

Patients receiving interferon alfa for massive hemangiomas are at increased risk for hemodynamic changes following initiation of therapy. This patient population should receive close monitoring at the start of therapy.[20]

Interferon may interfere with the clearance of theophylline. Patients receiving concurrent interferon alfa and theophylline should be monitored closely for possible theophylline toxicity.[22]

Growth was temporarily disrupted in children with chronic hepatitis B who were treated with interferon alfa.[23] Some clinicians feel that children ≤2 years old should not receive interferon alfa because growth retardation during early life may hinder overall development.[24]

Interferon Alfa-2b

Brand names Intron A for Injection

Dosage

Chronic hepatitis B with compensated liver disease: The manufacturer recommends 3 million units/m² SC three times/week for 1 week, then increased to 6 million units/m² three times/week for 16–24 weeks in children from 1–17 years of age.[1] Children from 3–15 years of age have been treated with 3–10 million units/m² SC or IM[2-8] for up to 1 year, alone or in combination with lamivudine.[9,10] Larger doses are associated with higher rates of viral clearance.[3]

Chronic hepatitis C: Children ≥2 years of age have received 3–5 million units/m² SC three times/week[11-14] or 0.1 million units/kg/d for 2 weeks then three times/week for 26 weeks.[15]

Cutaneous melanoma[16]: In a small tolerability study, 15 children from 1.5 to 17 years old received induction therapy with 20 million units/m² IV five times/week for 4 weeks. This was followed by 10 million units/m² SC 3 days/week for 48 weeks.

Hemangiomas or Kasabach-Merritt syndrome: 100,000–6 million units/m²/d SC for ≥9 weeks.[17-20] One group treated 39 children from 1.5 to 158 months of age with 3 million units/m²/d SC for 6 months.[20] Treatment continued for another 6 months, and in those who responded the interval was changed to three times/week; however, in those without hemangioma regression, the dose was increased to 6 million units/m²/d SC.[20] In Kasabach-Merritt syndrome (an aggressive vascular tumor), six of eight children responded to 3 million units/d that was given for up to 12 months.[21]

Relapsed T-cell acute lymphoblastic leukemia (ALL) or non-Hodgkin's lymphoma (NHL): Twenty children from 3–18 years of age were given 30 million units/m²/d to three times/week IV or SC; two of these developed congestive heart failure.[22] Doses from 3–50 million units/m² were used in pediatric ALL, NHL, and Philadelphia chromosome-positive CML in a limited number of patients.[23]

Dosage adjustment in organ dysfunction

Recommendations for dosage decreases are according to hematologic indices and liver function. In addition, recommended dosage changes vary according to disease being treated.

Chronic hepatitis B

Dose	WBC	Granulocytes	Platelets
Decrease 50%	$<1.5 \times 10^9$/L	$<0.75 \times 10^9$/L	$<50 \times 10^9$/L
Discontinue	$<1 \times 10^9$/L	$<0.5 \times 10^9$/L	$<25 \times 10^9$/L

Malignant melanoma (abnormalities during induction or maintenance therapy)

Withhold doses: granulocytes <500 mm³ but >250 mm³; SGPT/SGOT >5–≤10 × upper limit of normal (restart at 50% of initial dose once normal).

Permanently discontinue: Granulocytes <250 mm³ or SGPT/SGOT >10 x upper limit of normal.

Follicular lymphoma: Permanently discontinue if serum creatinine >2 mg/dL.

Maximum dosage Chronic hepatitis B maximum *adult* dose is 35 million units IM or SC/week for 16 weeks.[1]

IV push Not indicated.

Intermittent infusion After reconstitution with the provided diluent, the appropriate dose to be given IV should be injected into a 100-mL bag of NS to a concentration that is >10 million units/100 mL (or 0.1 million international units/mL).[1]

Interferon Alfa-2b

Continuous infusion	Not indicated.
Other routes of administration	Both SC and IM permitted in most indications; however, IM administration is not recommended in patients with platelet counts <50,000/mm^2.[1]
Maximum concentration	50 million units/mL for IM or SC; ≥0.1 million units/mL for IV infusion; 10 million units/mL for interlesional injection.[1]
Cautions related to IV administration	The solution vials for injection and the multidose pens for injection are not indicated for IV use or for malignant melanoma induction therapy.[1] Transient hypotension and syncope have occurred especially with IV interferon.[1,24]
Other additives	When the powder is reconstituted with the provided diluent, each mL contains 20 mg glycine, 2.3 mg sodium phosphate dibasic, 0.55 mg sodium phosphate monobasic, and 1 mg albumin (human).[1] The provided diluent no longer contains a preservative. Each mL of the solution vials for injection (given IM, SC, intralesional) and the multidose pens for injection (given SC) contain 7.5 mg sodium chloride, 1.8 mg sodium phosphate dibasic, 1.3 mg sodium phosphate monobasic, 0.1 mg edetate disodium, 0.1 mg polysorbate 80, and 1.5 mg *m*-cresol. Tetracycline is used in the manufacturing process but is below detectable levels in the final product.[1]

Comments

Alfa interferons cause or aggravate fatal or life threatening neuropsychiatric, autoimmune, ischemic, and infectious disorders. Patients should be monitored closely, and periodic clinical and laboratory evaluations should be performed. Patients with persistently severe or worsening signs or symptoms of these conditions should be withdrawn from therapy. In many cases, but not all, these disorders resolve after therapy is discontinued.[1]

A flu-like syndrome of fever, fatigue, malaise, myalgia, chills, headache, arthralgia, and rigors occurs frequently. Severity of this increases with higher dosages.[1,2,6,17,24,25] Fevers peak within 6 h and may persist for up to 12 h. Pretreatment with antipyretics (e.g., APAP or NSAIDs) may be beneficial. Dosing at night may decrease the flu-like adverse effects.[1,24]

A sharp, febrile response with rigors and other constitutional symptoms including peripheral cyanosis, nausea, vomiting, and severe myalgias may occur with doses of 50–120 million units.[24]

Alfa interferons suppress bone marrow function and may result in severe cytopenias, including very rare events of aplastic anemia. Obtain complete blood counts (CBC) pretreatment and monitor routinely during therapy. Alfa interferon therapy should be discontinued in patients who develop severe decreases in neutrophil (<0.5 x 10^9/L) or platelet counts (<25 x 10^9/L).[1]

Although infrequent, serious acute hypersensitivity reactions have been reported in patients receiving interferon alfa.[1,24] If such a reaction should occur, therapy should be discontinued immediately and appropriate medical management provided.

In addition to the flu-like syndrome, children may experience anorexia, somnolence, agitation, alopecia, weight loss, neutropenia, thrombocytopenia, anemia, and growth retardation.[1-3,6,12,14,16,22,23,25]

Interferon alfa-2b should be used with caution in patients with renal transplants, psoriasis, sarcoidosis,[1] or autoimmune diseases.[25,27]

Injection site reactions include burning, pruritus, erythema, pain, rash, edema, and vesiculation.[24] Rotating injection sites may minimize local reactions.

Interferon may interfere with the clearance of theophylline. Patients receiving concurrent interferon alfa and theophylline should be monitored closely for possible theophylline toxicity.[26]

As in *adults*, children may be at risk for the development of CHF[23] or retinal vascular complications[28] although only a few cases have been documented.

Irinotecan HCl

Brand names	Camptosar
Dosage	Consult institutional protocol for complete dosing information. Irinotecan is used as a component of combination therapy or as a single agent to treat multiple pediatric tumors, including neuroblastoma, hepatocellular tumors, Wilms' tumor, osteosarcoma, rhabdomyosarcoma, and CNS tumors, including medulloblastoma, ependymomas, brain stem gliomas, and astrocytomas.[1] **Refractory solid tumors (low-dose, protracted schedule):** 20 mg/m^2/d for 5 days for 2 consecutive weeks repeated q 21 d.[1-3] **Refractory solid tumors or CNS tumors:** 50 mg/m^2/d for 5 days repeated q 21 d.[1,4] **Heavily pretreated refractory solid tumors or CNS tumors:** 125 mg/m^2/dose once weekly for 4 weeks, repeated q 6 weeks.[1,5] **Less heavily pretreated refractory solid tumors or CNS tumors:** 160 mg/m^2/dose once weekly for 4 weeks, repeated q 6 weeks.[1,5]
Dosage adjustment in organ dysfunction	No information to guide administration of irinotecan in patients with hepatic (i.e., serum bilirubin >2 mg/dL) or renal dysfunction.[6] Some studies suggest that patients with moderate hepatic dysfunction (i.e., serum bilirubin of 1–2 mg/dL) and a prior history of abdominal or pelvic radiation may be at increased risk of developing neutropenia.[7] Some clinicians reduce dose in this scenario.
Maximum dosage	Not established. In clinical trials, single dosages up to 345–750 mg/m^2 have been administered to *adult* cancer patients.[6] No antidotes for overdosages are known. Patients should receive supportive care to prevent neutropenia and diarrhea.
IV push	Not recommended.
Intermittent infusion	Dilute with either NS or D5W to a final concentration of 0.12–2.8 mg/mL and infuse over 60–90 min.[6] Most clinical trials used 250–500 mL of D5W as diluent, as the relatively acidic pH of irinotecan favors dilution with D5W over NS.[7]
Continuous infusion	Not established. Currently under investigation.[8] Hepatic arterial continuous infusions have been explored in *adult* colorectal cancer patients with metastases to the liver.[9]
Other routes of administration	No information available to support administration by other routes.
Maximum concentration	2.8 mg/mL.[6]
Cautions related to IV administration	A higher incidence of cholinergic side effects has been reported with shorter infusion times.[1] Refrigeration of admixtures containing NS is not recommended due to the development of visible particulates.[6]

Other additives	None.

Comments

Irinotecan is associated with both acute (within first several hours) and delayed (24 h after drug administration) diarrhea, both of which can be dose-limiting.[6] Patients should be premedicated with 0.01 mg/kg of IV atropine (maximum dose: 0.4 mg) to prevent acute diarrhea and should receive a prescription for loperamide to prevent delayed diarrhea. Acute diarrhea is usually transient and patients may develop cholinergic symptoms such as rhinitis, miosis, flushing, or lacrimation. However, delayed diarrhea can have life-threatening consequences, such as dehydration, electrolyte disturbances, fever, or severe neutropenia.[6] If patients develop late diarrhea, loperamide should be administered q 3 h while the patient is awake and q 4 h while the patient is asleep for up to 24 h after complete resolution of loose stools. Please note that this loperamide regimen differs from what is listed on the package insert for OTC cases of diarrhea. The table below lists the suggested doses based on weight of the child.[1]

Dose of Loperamide Based on Weight of Patient

Weight (kg)	Immediate Dose	Daytime Dose (q 3 h)*	Nighttime Dose (q 4 h)
8–10	1 mg	0.5 mg	0.75 mg
10.1–20	1 mg	1 mg	1 mg
20.1–30	2 mg	1 mg	2 mg
30.1–43	2 mg	1 mg q 2 h	2 mg
>43	4 mg	2 mg q 2 h	4 mg

*Unless noted.

Patients that develop severe neutropenia and/or diarrhea while on normal dosages of irinotecan may need pharmacogenetic testing to evaluate if they are homozygous for the UGT1A1 allele that has been associated with increased irinotecan side effects.[6] Homozygous patients may require a dosage reduction.

Patients should have a baseline absolute neutrophil count >1500 cells/mm^3 and a platelet count >100,000 cells/mm^3 before drug administration.[6] The manufacturer has outlined dosage reductions for diarrhea, neutropenia, and neutropenic fever in the package insert.[6]

Irinotecan is associated with a moderate (30% to 90%) risk of emesis.[10] Patients should receive antiemetic therapy to prevent acute and delayed nausea and vomiting. The recommended therapy is a 5HT3 receptor antagonist in combination with dexamethasone on every day chemotherapy is administered.[10,11] These agents may be continued for up to 4 days after chemotherapy administration for the prevention of delayed nausea and vomiting. Breakthrough medications should also be offered, such as a phenothiazine (e.g., prochlorperazine), a butyrophenone (e.g., droperidol), a substituted benzamide (e.g., metoclopramide), or a benzodiazepine (e.g., lorazepam).

Iron Dextran

Brand names	INFeD, DexFerrum

Dosage

Test dosing: A one-time test dose should be administered prior to initiating therapy. Guidelines for the use of parenteral iron for children with renal disease recommend a weight adjusted test regimen of [1]:

Weight	Test Dose
<10 kg	10 mg
10–20 kg	15 mg
>20 kg	25 mg

Others have recommended the use of the standard *adult* test dose of 25 mg.[2-6] Test doses should be administered slowly over ≤50 mg/min followed by the administration of the remainder of the initial dose 1 h after the test dosing is complete.[1,2] Anaphylactic reactions occur with the first few minutes of infusion; therefore, immediate access to emergency medications (i.e., epinephrine) and trained personnel should be available.[1]

Some practitioners suggest that the daily dose be added to PN solutions, and heart rate, blood pressure, respiration, and temperature can be monitored q 15 min for the first hour of the initial dose.[4] (See Cautions related to IV administration section.)

Anemia of prematurity: In conjunction with erythropoietin therapy, 0.2–1 mg/kg/d[7,8] or 5 mg/kg/week has been added to PN solutions or infused over 4–6 h.[9] Doses up to 10 mg/kg/week[9] of iron dextran have been used to maintain serum ferritin levels.

Studies utilizing alternative forms of parenteral iron (iron sucrose) with erythropoietin have utilized doses of 2 mg/kg/d and up to 20 mg/kg/week.[10-12]

Iron-deficiency anemia: The deficit (mL of iron dextran) can be calculated based on hemoglobin (Hgb)[2]:

5–15 kg

$$\text{Total iron dose (mL)}^* = 0.0442\,(\text{Desired Hgb}^\dagger - \text{Observed Hgb}) \times \text{wt (kg)} + (0.26 \times \text{wt [kg]})$$

*50 mg/mL, undiluted product.
†Desired Hgb for children is usually 12 g/dL.

>15 kg

The same equation is used. However, the individual's lean body mass (LBM) in kg is substituted for weight in obese individuals. LBM can be calculated in those >5 feet tall as follows:

LBM (males): 50 kg + 2.3 kg for each inch over 5 feet.

LBM (females): 45.5 kg + 2.3 kg for each inch over 5 feet.

≤100 mg (up to 2 mL) may be administered daily until the calculated amount to correct the deficit is achieved.[13]

Correction secondary to blood loss[14]**:** The deficit can be calculated based on hematocrit (Hct).

$$\text{Total iron dose (mL)}^* = 0.02 \times \text{Blood loss (mL)} \times \text{Hct (as decimal fraction)}$$

*50 mg/mL, undiluted product.

Dosage (cont.)

Long-term PN: Maintenance dose of 0.11–0.15 mg/kg/d[15-17] or monthly infusion of estimated requirements. (See Continuous infusion section.)

Iron deficiency in hemodialysis (HD) patients (chronic renal failure): *The National Kidney Foundation Guidelines for Chronic Anemia* recommend weight adjusted dosing of iron dextran in children[1,18]:

Patient Weight	<10 kg	10–20 kg	>20 kg
Each dose or dialysis × 10 doses	0.5 mL (25 mg)	1 mL (50 mg)	2 mL (100 mg)

Alternatively, 2–4 mg/kg (≤100 mg) three × week for 10 doses during erythropoietin therapy.[6,19]

Iron deficiency in peritoneal dialysis patients (chronic renal failure): *The National Kidney Foundation Guidelines for Chronic Anemia* recommend weight adjusted dosing of iron dextran in children.[1] This dose can be repeated to maintain adequate iron stores.

Patient Weight	<10 kg	10–20 kg	>20 kg
Iron dose	125 mg	250 mg	500 mg
Volume of saline for infusion	75 mL	125 mL	250 mL

Dosage adjustment in organ dysfunction

No information available; however, considering the distribution characteristics of iron, there should be no dose adjustment necessary relative to liver or kidney function.

Maximum dosage

In most cases, daily doses should not exceed the following weight based doses.[2,14]

Patient Weight	Dose (mg)
<5 kg	25 mg
≥5–≤10 kg	50 mg
>10 kg	100 mg

IV push

May be administered undiluted (50 mg/mL) at a rate of <50 mg/min.[2,14,20] Administration by this method is not recommended. (See Cautions related to IV administration section.)

Intermittent infusion

Dilution is not recommended by the manufacturer since product was originally developed for IM use. However, IV administration is preferred via dilution in 50–1000 mL NS and infusion over 4–6 h.[3,6,14,20] Dextrose solutions may be employed but may increase the incidence of phlebitis.[14,20]

Continuous infusion

The iron deficit can be replaced over several days by adding iron to PN solutions in daily amounts not exceeding maximum daily recommendations.[21] As an alternative, the daily iron requirement can be added to each day's PN solution.[15-17] (See Maximum dosage and Comments sections.) 10 mg iron dextran/L was visually compatible in neonatal PN solutions containing at least 2% amino acids.[22]

Other routes of administration

Although the IV route is preferred, iron dextran has been administered IM using Z-track technique into upper quadrant of buttock.[1,13,20] May be associated with pain, staining of skin, tissue necrosis or abscess, and sarcoma development at the injection site.[23]

Iron Dextran

Maximum concentration	50 mg/mL.[1,14,22]
Cautions related to IV administration	Acute and delayed hypersensitivity reactions have been reported at a higher rate with iron dextran than other parenteral iron products in large *adult* studies.[24-27] One study reported a higher rate of hypersensitivity reactions with the high molecular weight dextran (Dexferrum) than the lower molecular weight (InFed).[25] Use particular caution in patients with multiple drug allergies.[1] Successful receipt of test doses or prior therapeutic doses does not ensure safety. Most patients who develop severe reactions have received prior doses without incident.[1] Acute reactions include hypotension, bronchospasm, pharyngeal/angioedema, urticaria, and pruritus.[13,24-27] Premedication does not appear to decrease the incidence of acute reactions. Delayed reactions such as arthralgias, myalgias, headache, fever, and lymphadenopathy may appear 24–48 h after infusion. For PN compatibility information, please see Appendix C.
Other additives	Each mL contains NS.[1]
Comments	A hypersensitivity reaction to one parenteral iron product does not predict a similar response to a different product. Serum ferritin monitoring is recommended to prevent potential iron overload.[1,13,14] Although not recommended by the manufacturer, iron dextran has been administered in PN formulations. Results of studies evaluating iron dextran stability and compatibility in PN solutions are inconsistent.[28,29] To ensure compatibility, the PN solution should contain at least 2% amino acids.[22]

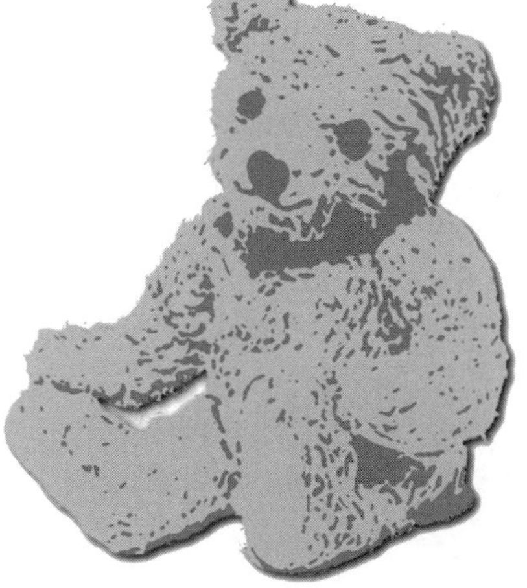

Isoproterenol HCl

Brand names	Isuprel
Dosage	Doses in children range from 0.03–2 mcg/kg/min, usually starting at a lower dose and titrated up to desired response.[1-10] In *adults*, IV bolus doses range from 0.02–0.06 mg and increase to 0.01–0.2 mg; continuous infusion starts at 5 mcg/min and is titrated up to 20 mcg/min.[1,11] EKG monitoring during infusion is essential.[1,11] Adequate oxygenation and fluid status should be maintained during infusion to minimize risk of ventricular arrhythmias and myocardial ischemia.[12] In *adults*, heart rate >110 beats/min or EKG changes warrant a decrease in dose or discontinuation.[1,11] **Asthma:** Not recommended.[13] Newer therapies have largely replaced its use in the treatment of shock and pulmonary hypertension.[14,15] **Cardiac arrhythmias and CPR**: Not considered the drug of choice. However, the 2005 PALS guidelines state that a continuous infusion of epinephrine or isoproterenol may be used for persistent bradycardia with continued hemodynamic compromise during CPR.[16]
Dosage adjustment in organ dysfunction	Administer with caution to patients with renal insufficiency.[11]
Maximum dosage	Critically ill children from 2 days to 14 years of age received doses ≤5.5 mcg/kg/min.[7] (See Comments section.) In *adults* with advanced shock, >30 mcg/min adjusted according to heart rate, blood pressure, urine output, and central venous pressure has been used.[1]
IV push	0.2 mg in *adults*.[11]
Intermittent infusion	Not indicated.
Continuous infusion	Usually 0.4–4 mcg/mL in D-LR, D-R, D-S, D5LR, D5NS, D5W, D10W, LR, or NS for IV infusion.[11,17] The PALS guidelines and AAP recommend the following formula for preparation of the infusion: 0.6 × weight (kg) = mg of drug to add to IV solution for a total volume of 100 mL. An infusion rate of 1 mL/h provides 0.1 mcg/kg/min.[12] This formula estimates an initial concentration. Ultimately, the concentration of the drug should consider the patient's fluid requirements or fluid limitations. Despite widespread use of the above formula, recent JCAHO® guidelines recommend the implementation of "standardized concentrations" of vasoactive medications.[18]
Other routes of administration	In *adults*, IM or SC administration is recommended as initial therapy if time is not critical.[1,11]
Maximum concentration	20 mcg/mL in D5W or NS.[1,5,11]

Cautions related to IV administration

Patients with cardiac glycoside toxicity and tachycardia must not be given isoproterenol.[1,11]

Cardiac dysrhythmias,[5,19] EKG changes suggestive of transient myocardial ischemia,[20] and abnormal echocardiographic and enzymatic findings suggestive of myocardial dysfunction have been reported in pediatric patients.[6,8] Although rare in pediatric patients, myocardial ischemia may occur.[6,8,21,22] Two adolescents with severe asthma who were treated with isoproterenol had myocardial necrosis at autopsy.[21,22]

For PN compatibility information, please see Appendix C.

Other additives

Each mL contains 7 mg sodium chloride, 1.8 mg sodium lactate, 0.12 mg lactic acid, and 1 mg sodium metabisulfite.[1,11]

Sulfites may cause hypersensitivity reactions and these are more common in *adults* with asthma. Most reactions are mild but can include anaphylactic symptoms and life-threatening or less severe asthma episodes.[23-25] Epinephrine may be required in severe cases; and if the sulfite-free product is not available, the sulfite-preserved epinephrine should be used.[23]

Comments

Ten postoperative cardiac pediatric patients received doses of 0.029 ± 0.002 mcg/kg/min while nine with reactive airway disease received 0.5 ± 0.1 mcg/kg/min. Clearance was lower in the postoperative cardiac patients compared to those with reactive airway disease.[7]

Risk factors for the development of arrhythmias include severe asthma, acidosis, and concomitant use of theophylline or corticosteroids.[11]

Tolerance may occur following prolonged use.[11]

Itraconazole

Brand names	Sporanox
Dosage	Experience with itraconazole in children is limited[1]; currently there is no established dosage range for pediatric patients. **Children:** 5–10 mg/kg/d given as a single dose or divided into two doses.[1,2] **Adults:** 200–400 mg/d given as a single dose or divided into two doses.[1]
Dosage adjustment in organ dysfunction	Contains cyclodextrin as a solubilizer; cyclodextrin is rapidly eliminated via glomerular filtration.[3] Therefore, itraconazole should not be used in patients with CrCl <30 mL/min and should be used with caution in patients with CrCl between 30 and 50 mL/min or in patients receiving renal replacement therapy.[4-6] Use with caution in patients with hepatic impairment.[4]
Maximum dosage	400 mg/d in *adults*.[1,4]
IV push	Not recommended.[4]
Intermittent infusion	Dilute to a 3.33 mg/mL concentration in NS to be infused over 1 h.[4]
Continuous infusion	No information available to support administration by this method.
Other routes of administration	No information available to support administration by other routes.
Maximum concentration	3.33 mg/mL in NS.[4]
Cautions related to IV administration	Dilute only with NS; incompatible with D5W or LR.[4] A dedicated infusion line should be used for administration; do not introduce concomitant medications in the same bag or same line.[4]
Other additives	Each mL contains 400 mg hydroxypropyl-beta-cyclodextrin and 25 microliters of propylene glycol.[4] Hydroxypropyl-beta-cyclodextrin has produced pancreatic adenocarcinomas in rats.[4] The clinical significance to humans is unknown. Propylene glycol is added to parenteral drugs as a solubilizer. Rapid infusion of medications that contain propylene glycol has resulted in respiratory depression and cardiac dysrhythmias.[7] Its half-life is three times longer in neonates than in *adults*[8] and has caused hyperosmolality[9] and refractory seizures[10] in preterm neonates receiving 3 g/d.

Comments

Itraconazole labeling includes a boxed warning describing the potential risk for negative inotropic effects and congestive heart failure.[4] It should not be used in patients with underlying ventricular dysfunction unless the benefits outweigh the risks of therapy.

Has been associated with rare cases of hepatotoxicity, including liver failure and death.[4]

Itraconazole is a potent inhibitor of CYP3A4. Serious cardiac events, including QT prolongation, torsades de pointes, ventricular tachycardia, cardiac arrest, and/or sudden death have occurred in patients using cisapride, pimozide, or quinidine concomitantly with itraconazole and/or other CYP3A4 agents.[4] Several drugs are contraindicated per itraconazole's boxed warning.[4] Consult appropriate resources for dosing recommendations before combining any drug with itraconazole.

Bone defects have occurred in rats receiving itraconazole.[4]

Anaphylaxis and Stevens-Johnson syndrome have been reported very rarely.[4]

Kanamycin Sulfate

Brand names	Kantrex

Dosage

Inappropriate for use in mild-to-moderate infections.[1]

Except in neonates, dosage for the aminoglycosides should be based on the following equation[2,3]: Dosing weight = IBW + 0.4 (TBW – IBW). (See Appendix B.)

Neonates

PNA	<1200 g	1200–2000 g	≥2000 g
<7 d	7.5 mg/kg q 12 h[4]	7.5 mg/kg q 12 h[5-7]	7.5–10 mg/kg q 12 h[5-7]
≥7 d	7.5 mg/kg q 12 h[4]*	7.5–10 mg/kg q 8–12 h[5-7]	10 mg/kg q 8 h[5-8]

*Until 4 weeks of age.

Infants and children: 15–30 mg/kg/d divided q 8–12 h.[1,5,8] No information exists for once- daily kanamycin dosing.

Dosage adjustment in organ dysfunction

Adjust dosage in patients with renal dysfunction.[9] If CrCl is 10–50 mL/min, give normal dose q 24–72 h; if CrCl is <10 mL/min, give normal dose q 48–72 h.[9]

Maximum dosage

40–50 mg/kg/d, 500 mg/kg per course of therapy.[10] Daily *adult* dose is 1–1.5 g/d.[1,8] Larger doses or shorter dosing intervals of aminoglycosides are sometimes required in patients with cystic fibrosis, major thermal burns or dermal loss, ascites, or in patients with febrile granulocytopenia.[11-13] As with other aminoglycosides, individualize dosage based on serum concentrations.[14]

IV push

Although aminoglycosides have been safely administered over 15 sec,[15] 1 min,[16] and 3–5 min,[17] rapid infusion is not used.

Intermittent infusion

2.5–5 mg/mL in D5NS, D5W, D10W, LR, or NS[18] infused over 20–30 min using a constant-rate volumetric infusion device.[14,18]

Continuous infusion

Although aminoglycosides have been given by continuous infusion,[19-21] this method of administration is not recommended.[8] Administration of a normal daily dose over 24 h results in low serum concentrations[20] and nephrotoxicity may occur more frequently.[21]

Other routes of administration

May be given IM.[1,8,22,23] No information available for administration by other routes.

Maximum concentration

5 mg/mL.[14] The amount of diluent should be sufficient to infuse the drug over 20–30 min.[14] The osmolality of 250-mg/mL solution ranged from 858 to 952 mOsm/kg depending on the testing method used.[18]

Cautions related to IV administration

None.

For PN compatibility information, please see Appendix C.

Other additives

Sulfites: Contains 0.45% sodium bisulfite.[18] Sulfites may cause hypersensitivity reactions, which are more common in *adults* with asthma. Most reactions are mild but can include anaphylactic symptoms and life-threatening or less severe asthma episodes.[24,25] Epinephrine may be required in severe cases; and if the sulfite-free product is not available, the sulfite-preserved epinephrine should be used.[24]

Comments

Because large variability exists in patient response to therapy, individualize dosage based on serum concentrations, clinical response, and renal function. Recommended peak and trough serum kanamycin concentrations are 15–30 mg/L and 5–10 mg/L, respectively.[14]

Serum concentrations may be falsely elevated when samples are collected through central venous Silastic catheters.[26]

Although serum concentration monitoring has become routine practice in many institutions, not all patients require monitoring.[27,28] Monitoring is indicated if the patient is not clinically responding, is ≤3 months of age, has disease that requires large doses or high concentrations (CNS infections, endocarditis, pneumonia, ascites, burns), has decreased or unstable renal function, or will be treated more than 10 days.

The beta-lactam ring of penicillins can link with an amino sugar of the aminoglycoside and inactivate the aminoglycoside.[18] This is dose-dependent and particularly problematic in patients with renal failure. To avoid this potential interaction, administer penicillins 1 h before or after an aminoglycoside, adequately flush the infusion line between each infusion, or infuse them through separate lines.

Cochlear and/or vestibular ototoxicity has been associated with all aminoglycoside antibiotics.[8] Either total dose (>500 mg/kg)[10] or total AUC are better indicators of ototoxic risk than either peak or trough.[29,30] Use with caution in other drugs (e.g., macrolide antibiotics, loop diuretics, platinum-based chemotherapeutic agents) known to cause ototoxicity.

Aminoglycosides accumulate in renal cortical tissue and may damage proximal tubule cells leading to oliguric renal failure. This has been associated with elevated trough serum concentrations. Risk of nephrotoxicity may increase if aminoglycosides are combined with other potentially nephrotoxic drugs.[8]

Aminoglycosides may cause neuromuscular blockade that is pronounced in patients with renal insufficiency, neuromuscular disease, and hypocalcemia.[31,32] The effects of nondepolarizing neuromuscular blockers may be prolonged during aminoglycoside use.[31]

Ketamine HCl

Brand names Ketalar, generic

Dosage

Oxygen saturation should be monitored, and resuscitation and intubation equipment should be readily available for respiratory support.[1-3]

Pretreatment with atropine or other drying agent prevents vagal-mediated bradycardia and decreases secretions.[1-4]

Emergence reactions (e.g., dream-like states, hallucinations, delirium) occur in ~12% of *adults*.[1] Of children who were premedicated with midazolam prior to ketamine, 1% of those <10 years of age and 4.2% of those ≥10 years of age experienced a severe emergence reaction.[5] Minimizing verbal, tactile, and visual stimulation after dosing decreases the likelihood of these reactions.[1] Short- or ultra-short acting barbiturates may be used as treatment.[1]

Infants ≤3 months have a higher incidence of airway complications, and some recommend that ketamine be avoided in this age group.[6]

Anesthesia

Induction

IV: 1–4.5 mg/kg.[1]

IM: 5–13 mg/kg.[1,7]

Maintenance: One-half to full induction dose repeated as needed[1] or 1–5 mg/kg/h by continuous infusion.[8]

Adjunct to intubation: 1–2 mg/kg IV.[2]

Procedural sedation/analgesia: Usually IV doses of 0.25–5 mg/kg and IM doses of 0.5–13 mg/kg are used for nonsurgical procedures.[2,6] In 32 children undergoing muscle biopsy, 2 mg/kg IV that was repeated in 10 min if needed or 10 mg/kg IM was used.[9] In the emergency department, 3–4 mg/kg IM has been used.[4,10-12] For emergencies, the AAP recommends 1–2 mg/kg IM or 0.5–1 mg/kg IV.[2] One group reported using a 1 mg/kg IV bolus followed by 51.4 ± 3.54 mcg/kg/min for the procedure's duration.[13]

Sedation in the intensive care unit (use not established): After cardiac surgery, 10 children were given 1 or 2 mg/kg/h for 24 h.[14] Others report doses of 0.5–1 mg/kg followed by 10 mcg/kg/min for 48–72 h.[15]

Severe bronchospasm (use not established): A case report of an 8-month-old who received two doses of 1.4 mg/kg 10 min apart followed by 0.2 mg/kg/h that was weaned over 40 h included a review of 11 cases.[16] The reviewed cases also improved with bolus doses of 0.5–4.8 mg/kg and three of these also received a continuous infusion of 1 or 2.5 mg/kg/h for 8–24 h.[16] A separate retrospective review identified 17 mechanically ventilated children who improved with bolus doses of 2 mg/kg followed by a continuous infusion of 20–60 mcg/kg/min (1.2–3.6 mg/kg/h) for 12–96 h.[17] Mechanical ventilation was avoided in two children with severe asthma who were given 2 mg/kg followed by 2–3 mg/kg/h.[18]

Opioid withdrawal (use not established): A 9.5-kg toddler who failed traditional fentanyl weaning strategies was started on ketamine at 10 mg/h. The fentanyl was successfully weaned off and then the ketamine was weaned.[19]

Dosage adjustment in organ dysfunction

Prolonged effects may be observed in patients with liver disease. Consider dose reductions in patients with hepatic impairment.[4]

Maximum dosage

Not established. Large doses prolong recovery and increase the risk of adverse events. IV doses up to 11 mg/kg and IM doses up to 17 mg/kg have been used during surgery.[6]

IV push	Over 60 sec not to exceed 2 mg/min in *adults.*[1] The 100-mg/mL solution must be diluted prior to administration.[20]
Intermittent infusion	1 or 2 mg/mL in SW, D5W, or NS.[1,20]
Continuous infusion	1 or 2 mg/mL.[1,20]
Other routes of administration	May be given by the IM route.[10,11,21]
Maximum concentration	50 mg/mL for IV push.[1] The 100-mg/mL vial must be diluted prior to IV infusion.[20]
Cautions related to IV administration	Rapid administration (<60 sec) may result in increased pressor response and/or increased apnea and respiratory depression.[1] Incompatible with barbiturates and diazepam. If used concomitantly with ketamine, barbiturates and diazepam must be infused separately.[1]
Other additives	None.
Comments	Does not impair laryngeal reflexes or independent airway maintenance; however, transient laryngospasm, apnea, and respiratory arrest have occurred.[6,13,22] A 12-year-old female with severe pain due to a cervical spinal tumor received a 7.5-mg test dose of ketamine followed by a continuous infusion ranging from 26–410 mg/24 h. She received long-term therapy for 67 days in a home-care setting.[23] A previously healthy 8-year-old female developed severe neurogenic pulmonary edema following a 6.25-mg/kg IM dose for dressing changes for first-degree burns.[24] Use with caution in patients at risk for increasing intracranial pressure.[1]

Ketorolac Tromethamine

Brand names Toradol

Dosage

The FDA announced June 2005 that revised labeling and the distribution of medication guides is necessary for all COX-2 selective and nonselective nonsteroidal anti-inflammatory drugs (NSAIDs), including ketorolac. At the time of publication, the labeling for ketorolac had not yet been revised.[1]

Note box warnings on current labeling[2]

Gastrointestinal: Contraindicated in patients with active peptic ulcer disease, recent GI bleeding/perforation, or history of peptic ulcer disease or GI bleeding.

Renal: Contraindicated in patients with advanced renal impairment and in patients with risk for renal impairment due to hypovolemia.

Bleeding: Contraindicated in patients with suspected/confirmed cerebrovascular bleeding, hemorrhagic diathesis, incomplete hemostasis, before any major surgery and intraoperatively, and others at high risk of bleeding.

Hypersensitivity: Contraindicated in patients with previous hypersensitivity to ketorolac or aspirin or other NSAID.

Other contraindications: IT or epidural administration (alcohol content), labor and delivery, nursing mothers, concomitant aspirin, or other NSAID use.

Combined duration of therapy (IV and oral) should not exceed 5 days.

Daily dosing significantly lower for oral (40 mg) compared to IV/IM (120 mg) administration.

Adjust dosage (do not exceed 60 mg/d) in patients ≥65 years of age, <50 kg, or with moderately elevated SCr.

Indicated as a single-dose therapy for pediatric patients not to exceed 30 mg (IM) and 15 mg (IV).

Antipyretic: 0.5–1 mg/kg as a single dose.[3,4]

Bladder spasms (postoperative after ureteral reimplantation) (use not established): 0.5 mg/kg given q 6 h for 48 h.[5]

Analgesia/pain management

Surgery/procedures: The use of a lower, single dose of 0.5 mg/kg has been recommended.[6-8] Single doses of 0.5–1.5 mg/kg have been given to infants ≥1 month and children after induction of general anesthesia or at beginning of procedure, 30 min before the end of surgery/procedure, or immediately postoperative.[6-20] One study in neonates gave 1 mg/kg.[21]

Multidose therapy: 0.5 mg/kg q 6 h.[3,7,16] May give a loading dose of 1 mg/kg prior to beginning maintenance dosing.[3,22] Some patients have also received a loading dose followed by 0.17 mg/kg/h as a continuous infusion.[22] One study in neonates, infants, and children supports the use of 0.5 mg/kg q 8 h for 1–2 days postsurgery.[23]

While the manufacturer's labeling prohibits therapy beyond 5 days,[2] an early report of clinical experience with ketorolac in children documents the use of 0.17–1 mg/kg q 4–6 h for an average length of 3.4 days (range 1–12) and up to 31 doses.[3]

Maintenance dose requirements of ketorolac are similar in children, adolescents, and *adults*.[24]

Dosage adjustment in organ dysfunction

Contraindicated in advanced renal impairment and in patients at risk for renal failure due to volume depletion.[2] If CrCl is 10–50 mL/min, give 50% of the normal dose; if CrCl is <10 mL/min, give 25% to 50% of the normal dose.[25]

Ketorolac Tromethamine

Maximum dosage	30 mg IM or 15 mg IV in children.[2] A single 60-mg loading dose was administered to a 16-year-old adolescent.[3]
IV push	15 and 30 mg/mL given over ≥15 sec.[2] Has been given over 1–5 min in children.[26] The 60-mg/2 mL product is intended for IM use only.[2]
Intermittent infusion	Not generally administered by this method.
Continuous infusion	Although solution type and concentration were not specified, it has been given by this method.[22] Compatible in D5NS, D5W, LR, R, and NS.[27]
Other routes of administration	Can be given IM (15 mg/mL or 30 mg/mL undiluted or 60 mg/2 mL single-use vial for IM use only) deep into the muscle by slow administration.[2] Bioavailability and efficacy of IV and IM routes of administration are comparable.[28] Because of pain associated with IM administration, IV is preferred in children.[3]
Maximum concentration	30 mg/mL.[2]
Cautions related to IV administration	Anaphylactic reactions may occur in patients with a history of hypersensitivity to other nonsteroidal anti-inflammatory agents, including aspirin, or in patients with nasal polyps, asthma, angioedema, or bronchospastic reactions of the histamine-dependent type.[2,22]
Other additives	**15 mg/mL contains per mL:** 10% (w/v) ethanol and 6.68 mg NaCl.[2] **30 mg/mL contains per mL:** 10% (w/v) ethanol and 4.35 mg NaCl.[2] **60 mg/2 mL contains per mL:** 10% (w/v) ethanol and 8.7 mg NaCl.[2]
Comments	Ketorolac (0.5 mg/kg) has been used for pediatric migraine headaches.[29] Ketorolac (0.9 mg/kg) has been used in pediatric sickle cell vaso-occlusive pain crisis.[30] Ketorolac (0.5 mg/kg) has been used for IV regional anesthesia with lidocaine (2 mg/kg) in an 11-year-old and 15-year-old with complex regional pain syndrome.[31] Ketorolac was considered a contributing factor to hematuria in a 16-year-old adolescent and to incision-site bleeding in an 11-year-old child.[3] While post-tonsillectomy patients receiving 1 mg/kg ketorolac had fewer emetic episodes than those given 0.1 mg/kg/dose of morphine, they had more major bleeding.[19] More measures to control bleeding were also noted post-tonsillectomy in children receiving ketorolac (1 mg/kg) compared to those receiving 35 mg acetaminophen/kg rectally.[20] A pharmacokinetic study in 36 children found that a 0.5 mg/kg dose IV resulted in similar concentrations over a 6-h period as that reported for *adults*.[6] The pharmacokinetic parameters were not different among ages 1–3 years, 4–7 years, 8–11 years, and 12–16 years.[6]

L-Cysteine HCl

Brand names	Various manufacturers
Dosage	30–40 mg/g pediatric amino acid[1-3] or 0.4–1 mmol/kg (~48–121 mg/kg).[4,5]
Dosage adjustment in organ dysfunction	In hepatic and renal dysfunction, the overall dose of amino acids should be decreased. In these cases, using mg/g pediatric amino acids would be appropriate because this dosage is based on the grams of amino acids provided and not on patient weight.
Maximum dosage	Based on mg/g pediatric amino acids: 30 mg/g in those prescribed 3 g/kg and 40 mg/g in those prescribed 2.5 g/kg results in a 90- or 100-mg/kg dose, respectively.[1-3] Doses of 121 mg/kg have also been used.[4,5]
IV push	Not administered by this method.
Intermittent infusion	Not administered by this method. However, parenteral nutrition regimens may infuse via cycling regimens over periods of time <24 h.
Continuous infusion	Given via PN solution.
Other routes of administration	Not indicated.
Maximum concentration	Dependent on volume of parenteral nutrition solution.
Cautions related to IV administration	Peripheral infusion of amino acids may result in local reactions and phlebitis.[1]
Other additives	None. However, contaminant aluminum is present.[1]
Comments	L-cysteine HCl addition to PN solutions formulated with pediatric amino acids results in normalization of plasma amino acid patterns in infants.[2,4] Acidosis, primarily in neonates, has been reported.[4,5] The pH of L-cysteine HCl is about 1–2.5.[1] It has been added to solutions formulated with standard amino acid solutions to acidify the solution and enhance calcium and phosphorous solubility.[6] L-cysteine exists in equilibrium with its dimer, cystine, and the extent of dimerization depends on pH. 1 mmol = 121 mg of cysteine/cystine. L-cysteine hydrochloride monohydrate contains 5.7 mEq Cl/g of L-cysteine HCl.

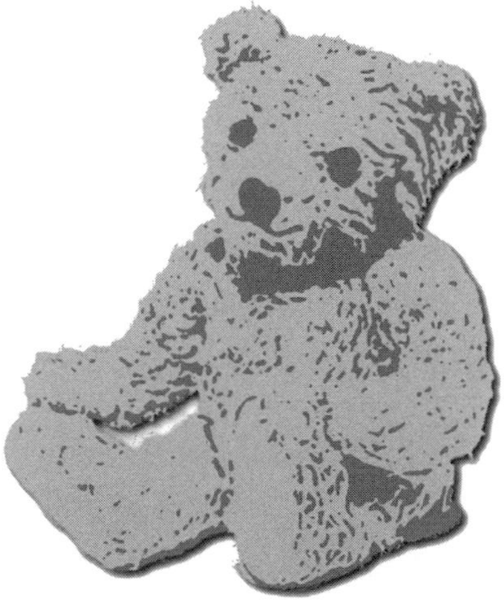

Labetalol HCl

Brand names	Normodyne, Trandate
Dosage	Little information is available on the dosing or dosing frequency of labetalol in pediatric patients. (See Comments section.) **Intermittent infusion:** 0.25–1 mg/kg[1-3] over 2 min up to 40 mg.[2] The dose can be repeated at 10-min intervals to a maximum of 3–4 mg/kg up to a total dose of 300 mg.[1] The maximum hypotensive effect usually occurs within 5–15 min after injection.[4] **Continuous infusion:** 0.5–3 mg/kg/h titrated to patient's blood pressure.[1-5] In a study of 13 children (3.6–15.3 years of age), the mean initial dose was 0.55 mg/kg (range of 0.2–1 mg/kg) and was followed by 0.78 mg/kg/h (range of 0.25–1.5 mg/kg/h).[3] In a retrospective study involving 25 children with hypertensive emergencies, doses of 1–3 mg/kg/h were used safely and effectively.[5]
Dosage adjustment in organ dysfunction	Use with caution in patients with severe hepatic dysfunction.[4] If CrCl is <10 mL/min, adequate blood-pressure control may be achieved with once-daily dosing.[4] While it is effective in severe renal dysfunction, it may have limited efficacy if mean arterial pressure is significantly elevated.[6,7]
Maximum dosage	1 mg/kg/dose[1-3] up to 40 mg.[2] A cumulative dose of 3–4 mg/kg per event and up to 300 mg per event.[1] Continuous infusion doses up to 3 mg/kg/h have been used.[5]
IV push	5 mg/mL (commercially available) not to exceed 2 mg/min.[8]
Intermittent infusion	No information available to support administration by this method.
Continuous infusion	1 mg/mL in D5LR, D2.5½NS, D5NS, D5¼NS, D5⅓NS, D5½NS, D5W, LR, or NS.[8]
Other routes of administration	No information available to support administration by other routes.
Maximum concentration	5 mg/mL for IV injection and 1 mg/mL for continuous infusion.[8]
Cautions related to IV administration	Patients must be kept in a supine position during administration because a substantial fall in blood pressure may occur upon standing.[4]
Other additives	**Parabens:** Some products contain methyl and/or propyl parabens.[8] Paraben preservatives may cause hypersensitivity reactions that are more common with cutaneous exposure.[9] However, one case of pruritus and bronchospasm occurred following infusion of hydrocortisone, which contained parabens, has been reported.[10]

Comments

Because labetalol has negative inotropic and dromotropic activity, it is contraindicated in patients with asthma, chronic lung disease, overt cardiac failure, greater than first degree heart block, cardiogenic shock, or severe bradycardia.[4]

Labetalol metabolites in the urine may cause falsely elevated concentrations of urinary catecholamines (e.g., metanephrine, normetanephrine, vanillylmandelic acid) when measured by fluorimetric or photometric methods.[4] When screening labetalol-treated patients suspected of having pheochromocytoma or when evaluating those with the tumor, specific assay methods such as high-performance liquid chromatography (HPLC) with solid phase extraction should be used.[4]

Labetalol may produce a false-positive amphetamine test when urine is screened using the Toxi-Lab A or Emit-d.a.u. assays.[4]

Lansoprazole

Brand names	Prevacid
Dosage	In *adults*, oral and IV dosage have been found to be similar in gastric acid suppression.[1] No studies of IV lansoprazole have been published to date in pediatric patients. General ranges from pediatric oral dosing studies are as follows: **Gastroesophageal reflux and esophagitis:** 0.7–1.5 mg/kg every day.[2-4] Optimal starting dose of 1.4–1.5 mg/kg/d has been suggested.[2-3] **Neonates and infants:** 14.3–23.8 mg/m² every day for up to 14 days.[5] **Children 1–11 years** **≤10 kg**: 7.5 mg every day for up to 8 weeks.[6] **10–30 kg:** 15 mg every day for 8–12 weeks.[7-13] **>30 kg:** 30 mg every day for 8–12 weeks; may increase up to 30 mg bid if symptomatic after ≥2 weeks.[7-13] **Children 12–17 years of age**[7,11,14] **Nonerosive gastroesophageal reflux**: 15 mg every day for 8–12 weeks. **Erosive esophagitis:** 30 mg every day for 8–12 weeks.
Dosage adjustment in organ dysfunction	No dosage adjustment necessary with renal dysfunction[7,15]; however, should consider dose adjustment in patients with severe hepatic dysfunction.[7]
Maximum dosage	60 mg/d.[7,16]
IV push	No information available to support administration by this method.
Intermittent infusion	Dilute reconstituted drug (6 mg/mL) in 50 mL of D5W, LR, or NS and infuse over 30 min using in-line filter provided.[7]
Continuous infusion	90–120 mg IV load followed by 6–9 mg/h has been given for 24 h in *adults*.[17]
Other routes of administration	No information available to support administration by other routes.
Maximum concentration	Reconstituted drug (6 mg/mL) in a minimum of 50 mL of diluent.[7]
Cautions related to IV administration	Use in-line filter provided and observe closely for precipitation which may form when reconstituted drug is mixed with IV solutions. While holding filter below the level of the solution, connect luer adapter of administration set to filter using a twisting motion. Open the administration set clamp and slowly prime filter (0.7 mL), then close the administration set clamp and check for air bubbles.[7]

Other additives	None.
Comments	Common adverse effects include headache, constipation, and elevated serum gastrin levels.[9] An 8½-year-old patient developed skin flushing and transient hypertension with oral lansoprazole.[5] Administration of proton pump inhibitors has been associated with increased risk of developing gastroenteritis and pneumonia in children.[18] Lansoprazole is metabolized by CYP3A4 and CYP2C19. Lansoprazole does not have clinically significant drug interactions with most drugs metabolized through the CYP system.[7] Dosage adjustments may be necessary with concomitant administration of theophylline or warfarin.[7]

Levocarnitine

Brand names	Carnitor
Dosage	**Hemodialysis:** 10–40 mg/kg/dose following dialysis.[1-3] Other papers support the use of considerably lower doses of 2–5 mg/kg/dose following dialysis.[4-6] The clinical practice recommendations for anemia in chronic kidney disease in children state there is no firm evidence to support its use.[7] **Primary carnitine deficiency/metabolic disorders:** A loading dose of 50 mg/kg followed by 50–60 mg/kg/d divided q 3–6 h or given continuously.[1,8,9] **PN supplementation in neonates/infants with little or no enteral intake:** 10–30 mg/kg/d.[10-17] **Valproate-associated hepatotoxicity** **Active hepatotoxicity/overdose:** 150–500 mg/kg/d, up to 3 g/d.[18,19] **Prophylaxis against valproate or other anticonvulsant-associated hepatotoxicity:** 15–100 mg/kg/d has been used in children with or without hyperammonemia.[19] Decreased ammonia levels were seen after 9 days of treatment with 1000 mg/m^2/d divided in two equal doses.[20]
Dosage adjustment in organ dysfunction	No dose adjustment recommended. However, carnitine is excreted renally and renal insufficiency may lead to the accumulation of potentially toxic metabolites.[1,7]
Maximum dosage	**PN supplementation:** 48 mg/kg/d has been given (see Comments section).[21] **Metabolic disorders:** 300 mg/kg/dose (age not specified).[1] **Valproate induced hepatotoxicity:** 3 g/d.[18,19] **VPA/anticonvulsant therapy:** 100 mg/kg/d or 1000 mg/m^2/d.[19]
IV push	200 mg/mL over 2–3 min.[1]
Intermittent Infusion	0.5–8 mg/mL in NS or LR. May be given for up to 24 h in PVC plastic bags.[1]
Continuous infusion	May be added to PN solutions and infused over 24 h or during a PN cycling schedule.[10-12,14,15,17] One study documented stability of carnitine via PN and TNA with Y-site administration of 20% fat emulsion at all study points (IV bag, distal to filter, after mixing with fat emulsion) for up to 24 h at room temperature and up to 30 days when stored at 4°C to 5°C.[22] Another study evaluated stability with carnitine in TNA and observed creaming.[23]
Other routes of administration	No information available to support administration by other routes.
Maximum concentration	1 g/5 mL (200 mg/mL).[1]
Cautions related to IV administration	None known.

Other additives	None.
Comments	Higher metabolic rate, greater nitrogen excretion, and lower weight gain were associated with 48 mg/kg/d given via PN in 12 preterm neonates.[21] L-carnitine (oral and IV) has been noted to cause seizures in patients with and without pre-existing seizure disorder.[1] Children and infants experiencing reported seizures have had other risk factors, including microcephaly, large doses of carnitine, and metabolic acidosis.[24] IV carnitine has been shown to be beneficial in childhood cardiomyopathy.[25] Life-threatening lactic acidosis associated with reverse transcriptase inhibitors was corrected in an HIV-positive 10-year-old patient with 12–50 mg/kg/d L-carnitine.[26]

Levothyroxine Sodium

Brand names	Synthroid, Levothroid

Dosage

Congenital or acquired hypothyroidism: 5–8 mcg/kg q 24 h[1] or[2]

Age	IV Dose is 50% to 75% of the Oral Doses Listed Below
0–3 mo	10–15 mcg/kg/d
0–6 mo	8–10 mcg/kg/d
6–12 mo	6–8 mcg/kg/d
1–5 y	5–6 mcg/kg/d
6–12 y	4–5 mcg/kg/d
>12 y	2–3 mcg/kg/d
Growth and puberty complete	1.6–1.7 mcg/kg/d

The AAP recommends an initial oral dosage of 10–15 mcg/kg/d for infants with hypothyroidism.[3] IV dose should be 50% to 75% of oral doses.[2]

The goal of therapy is to normalize T4 within 2 weeks and TSH within 1 month.[3] Neonates and infants with very low or undetectable serum T4 concentrations (<5 mcg/dL) should be started at the higher end of the dosage range.[3] Patients with evidence of cardiac disease or long-standing or severe hypothyroidism should receive a lower starting dose.[2,4,5] Adjust dosage based on clinical response and serum FT4 and TSH.[3,4]

Dosage adjustment in organ dysfunction	No information available.
Maximum dosage	Not established. In *adults* with myxedema coma or stupor, without concomitant severe heart disease, may give doses of 200–500 mcg.[4]
IV push	40–100 mcg/mL in NS[4] over 2–3 min.[6] Use only NS for reconstitution.[4]
Intermittent infusion	No information available to support administration by this method. Should not be mixed with IV infusion solutions.[2]
Continuous infusion	No information available to support administration by this method. Should not be mixed with IV infusion solutions.[2]
Other routes of administration	May be administered by IM injection; however, because absorption is variable following IM administration, IV is preferred.[2]
Maximum concentration	100 mcg/mL[4]; however, one reference recommends a final concentration of 20 mcg/mL.[1]

Cautions related to IV administration

Large, sudden doses of IV levothyroxine may have cardiovascular risks.[4]

Other additives

None.

Comments

The aim of therapy is to ensure normal growth and development.[3]

Excessive doses should be avoided since they may result in craniosynostosis and accelerate bone age, resulting in premature epiphyseal closure and short stature.[2,5]

Early, high-dose levothyroxine therapy has been shown to eliminate the negative impact that congenital hypothyroidism has on IQ and CNS development.[3,7,8]

Pseudotumor cerebri has been reported to follow levothyroxine therapy in both *adults* and infants and children.[9]

One study documented improved hemodynamic stability, which may translate into improved donor organ viability, with thyroxine (loading dose followed by continuous infusion) in critically ill children with documented brain death.[10]

Because levothyroxine is associated with numerous drug interactions,[2] consult appropriate resources for dosing recommendations before combining any drug with levothyroxine.

Lidocaine HCl

Brand names	Xylocaine
Dosage	**Arrhythmias (ventricular-resistant to electrical cardioversion or in pulseless ventricular tachycardia)** Lidocaine solutions that contain epinephrine must not be used to treat arrhythmias. See Other routes of administration section for information related to endotracheal and intraosseous administration in those without IV access. **Initial:** 0.5–1 mg/kg (maximum single dose 100 mg) q 5–10 min until desired effect or maximum total dose of 3–5 mg/kg.[1-4] Decrease loading dose by 50% in patients with moderate to severe congestive heart failure. **Maintenance:** 0.5–3 mg/kg/h (10–50 mcg/kg/min).[1-4] If more than 15 min has lapsed between initial dose and start of infusion, give 0.5–1 mg/kg.[3] **Epilepsy (refractory status):** Initial dose of 1–3 mg/kg over 2 min.[3,5-12] If seizures do not stop in 2 min give an additional dose of 0.5 mg/kg.[3] A continuous infusion of 2–6 mg/kg/h effectively controlled severe intractable seizures in neonates,[7,8] infants,[9,10] and children.[11] A dose of 1.5–3.5 mg/kg/h has been used in *adults*.[12] (See Comments section.) **Intracranial pressure (acute increases due to procedures):** 1–1.5 mg/kg given 30 sec prior to intubation or endotracheal suctioning to reduce airway reflexes.[2,13,14] **Pain associated with Anti-GD2 antibody therapy (use not established):** A loading dose of 2 mg/kg infused over 30 min before antibody therapy, followed by a continuous infusion of 1 mg/kg/h.[15] The infusion should be discontinued 2 h after antibody therapy is stopped.
Dosage adjustment in organ dysfunction	Decrease dose in patients with shock, congestive heart failure, liver failure, or decreased liver blood flow.[3,16,17] Doses should not exceed 20 mcg/kg/min.[3] No dosage adjustment required in renal dysfunction.[18]
Maximum dosage	1 mg/kg (maximum single dose 100 mg) until desired effect or maximum total dose of 5 mg/kg[1-4] or <300 mg in 1 h.[19] Administration of ≤88 mcg/kg/min (50 mg/min) by continuous infusion has been proposed.[20] Dosage should be titrated using serum concentration monitoring. (See Comments section.)
IV push	10–20 mg/mL.[3,21] Generally over 2–3 min, not to exceed 0.7 mg/kg/min or 50 mg/min, whichever is less.[19]
Intermittent infusion	Not recommended due to short half-life.
Continuous infusion	Usually 1–2 mg/mL; however, 8 mg/mL in D5W has been used in fluid-restricted patients.[3]

Other routes of administration

Generally not given via other methods. Can be given IM into the deltoid muscle provided bradycardia is not present.[2] A formulation specific for IM delivery is no longer available in the United States. For endotracheal administration give 2–3 mg[1] and for IO administration give 1 mg/kg.[3]

Maximum concentration

20 mg/mL for IV push[3,21] and 8 mg/mL for infusion in fluid-restricted patients.[21]

Cautions related to IV administration

Excessive serum concentrations may produce myocardial depression with widened QRS interval as well as CNS symptoms of drowsiness, nausea, vomiting, disorientation, seizures, and muscle twitching.[3,4] Therefore, cardiac monitoring is essential and serum concentration monitoring is suggested. (See Comments section.)

For PN compatibility information, please see Appendix C.

Other additives

Sulfites: Some multidose vials may contain sulfites. Sulfites may cause hypersensitivity reactions and these are more common in *adults* with asthma. Most reactions are mild but can include anaphylactic symptoms and life-threatening or less severe asthma episodes.[22,23] Epinephrine may be required in severe cases; and if the sulfite-free product is not available, the sulfite-preserved epinephrine should be used.[22]

Parabens: Some multidose vials may contain methylparabens. Paraben preservatives may cause hypersensitivity reactions that are more common with cutaneous exposure.[24] However, one case of pruritus and bronchospasm, which occurred following infusion of hydrocortisone, which contained parabens, has been reported.[25]

Comments

Contraindicated in infants with congenital heart disease and in those with severe heart block.[7] Monitor for bradycardia and hypotension. Widening of the QRS interval by >0.02 sec or significant ventricular slowing suggests toxicity.[2] Because large variability exists in patient response to initial and maintenance doses, individualize dosage based on serum concentration and clinical response.

Transient neonatal mydriasis has been reported in a neonate treated with lidocaine for seizures.[26]

Reference range: 1.5–5 mg/L for antiarrhythmic effect and toxicity.[3] The reference range for the management of status epilepticus has not been established.

Linezolid

Brand names	Zyvox

Dosage

Neonates

PNA	<1200 g	1200–2000 g	≥2000 g
<7 d	20–30 mg/kg/d divided q 8–12 h[1-3]*	20–30 mg/kg/d divided q 8–12 h[1-3]	20–30 mg/kg/d divided q 8–12 h[1-3]
≥7 d		30 mg/kg/d divided q 8 h[1,2,4]	30 mg/kg/d divided q 8 h[1,2,4]

*Until 4 weeks of age.

Infants and children: 30 mg/kg/d divided q 8 h up to 1200 mg/d.[1,2,4-8] A 4½-month-old infant with endocarditis was given 45 mg/kg/d divided q 8 h for 7 weeks.[9]

Adolescents and adults: 1200 mg/d divided q 12 h.[1,2]

Central line infection: 2mg/mL plus 100 units of heparin as an 8-h catheter lock.[10] Used in combination with 30 mg/kg/d divided q 8 h given systemically.

Dosage adjustment in organ dysfunction

No adjustment recommended in renal impairment. Metabolites may accumulate in renal impairment although the clinical significance is unknown.[1] No adjustment in mild-to-moderate hepatic impairment; caution should be used in severe hepatic impairment.[1]

Maximum dosage

15 mg/kg q 8 h was administered for 7 weeks to an infant.[9] 1200 mg/d in those older than 12 years of age.[1,2]

IV push

Not recommended.[1]

Intermittent infusion

2 mg/mL over 30–120 min.[1,11]

Continuous infusion

No information on administration by continuous infusion.

Other routes of administration

No information available to support administration by other routes.

Maximum concentration

2 mg/mL (commercially available).[1]

Cautions related to IV administration

None.

For PN compatibility information, please see Appendix C.

Other additives

Contains 0.38 mg of sodium/mL.[11]

Comments

Serotonin syndrome has been reported in patients given linezolid concurrent with a serotonergic agent (e.g., SSRI).[12,14] One report involved a 4-year-old child given *oral* linezolid and fluoxetine.[12]

Elevations in serum transaminase have been reported.[1,15]

Although reversible thrombocytopenia may occur,[1] one study in children (median age 1.65 years) found no difference in platelet count for linezolid (n=215) vs. vancomycin (n=101) treated patients.[7]

An 11-year-old girl with HIV developed tooth discoloration after receiving linezolid *orally* (600 mg twice daily) for 28 days.[16] Her teeth returned to normal color after discontinuation of linezolid and manual removal of the brown discoloration by a dentist.

Lorazepam

Brand names	Ativan
Dosage	Respiratory depression and arrest requiring mechanical ventilation may occur. Be prepared to provide respiratory support if necessary. Monitor oxygen saturation. Reversal agents should be readily available. (See Comments Section.) **Adjunct to antiemetic therapy:** Single doses of 0.01 mg/kg have been used preoperatively for nausea associated with strabismus surgery[1]; however, single doses of at least 0.04 mg/kg (maximum dose 3 mg) were required for emesis associated with chemotherapy.[2,3] Multiple doses of 0.04–0.08 mg/kg (maximum dose 2 mg) may be given q 6 h as needed.[1,2,4] **Adjunct for intubation:** 0.05–0.1 mg/kg.[5] **Procedural sedation[6]:** Many consider midazolam the benzodiazepine of choice for procedural sedation.[7-9] (See Midazolam monograph.) 0.05 mg/kg (0.01–0.1 mg/kg) q 4–8 h[4,6,10] not to exceed 2 mg/dose.[5] For premedication therapy, give first *intravenous* dose 15–20 min before procedure and first *intramuscular* dose 2 h before procedure.[11] **Sedation with mechanical ventilation:** Use lowest effective dose. 0.025–0.05 mg/kg (maximum initial dose of 2 mg) given as intermittent infusion q 2–4 h or by continuous infusion, at a rate of 0.025 mg/kg/h (up to 2 mg/h).[12] (See Other additives section.) **Seizures** **Neonates:** 0.05–0.1 mg/kg.[13-17] If seizures continue after 10–15 min, repeat 0.05 mg/kg; if no response after 10–15 min, repeat 0.05 mg/kg to a maximum of 0.15 mg/kg.[4,15] (See Comments section.) **Infants and children:** 0.1 mg/kg[8-21] up to 4 mg.[19] If seizures continue after 10–15 min, repeat 0.05 mg/kg; if no response after 10–15 min, repeat 0.05 mg/kg.[4,19,20]
Dosage adjustment in organ dysfunction	No dosage adjustment required in renal dysfunction[22]; however, one source recommends caution when giving multiple doses.[11] Adjust dosage in patients with hepatic dysfunction.[11] Larger doses may be required in patients on ECMO since 50% of a dose may be extracted by the PVC tubing and the membrane oxygenator during bypass.[23]
Maximum dosage	4 mg/dose.[9,19] A 14-year-old with refractory seizures who had been on chronic clonazepam was given 0.25 mg/kg/dose to a cumulative dose of 186 mg (4.3 mg/kg) over 24 h.[24] Doses as large as 0.4 mg/kg have been safely administered.[1,25]
IV push	Not to exceed 2 mg/min[11,18,26] or 0.05 mg/kg over 2–5 min.[14] Although the manufacturer recommends diluting the commercially available solution 1:1 in D5W, NS, or SW,[26] undiluted 2-[18] and 4-mg/mL[19] solutions have been given.
Intermittent infusion	Not administered by this method.
Continuous infusion	0.2 mg/mL in D5W or NS has been administered in *adults*[27-30]; however, little information is available in pediatric patients.[12]

Other routes of administration

Although undiluted lorazepam can be given deep into a muscle, it is not the preferred route in the treatment of status epilepticus.[26] Midazolam is the benzodiazepine of choice for IM administration. (See Midazolam monograph.)

Maximum concentration

4 mg/mL.[31] To decrease the amount of benzyl alcohol administered (see Comments section) to neonates, add 1 mL of the 4-mg/mL product to 9 mL of preservative-free SW and use this preparation (0.4-mg/mL product) for dosing.[13]

Cautions related to IV administration

Inadvertent intra-arterial injection can cause vasospasm. This may produce gangrene and subsequent amputation.[26] If a patient complains of pain during injection, the infusion should be stopped and the site should be inspected.

For PN compatibility information, please see Appendix C.

Other additives

Benzyl alcohol: Contains benzyl alcohol 2% as a preservative.[26] Benzyl alcohol in small doses as a preservative in drugs is considered safe in newborns.[32] However, a 3-week-old, very low birth weight (710 g) infant who received clindamycin experienced a profound desaturation that required resuscitation after the third and fourth doses, which was subsequently related to the benzyl alcohol preservative.[33]

Administration of saline flushes containing benzyl alcohol (bacteriostatic water for injection) was associated with a fatal gasping syndrome, intraventricular hemorrhage, metabolic acidosis, and increased mortality in preterm infants.[34] This should not be used in neonates.

Hypersensitivity reactions to benzyl alcohol in parenteral products have been reported in *adults*.[35,36]

Propylene glycol: 2-mg/mL product contains 0.18 mg of propylene glycol.[26] Propylene glycol is added to parenteral drugs as a solubilizer. Rapid infusion of medications that contain propylene glycol has resulted in respiratory depression and cardiac dysrhythmias.[33] Its half-life is three times longer in neonates than in *adults*[37] and has caused hyperosmolality[38] and refractory seizures[36] in preterm neonates receiving 3 g/d. Accumulation of propylene glycol has been reported following administration by continuous infusion.[40,41]

Comments

An *adult* patient developed severe lactic acidosis as a result of propylene glycol from high-dose, continous infusion of lorazepam.[42] Continuous infusions of lorazepam have also been correlated with propylene glycol-associated renal toxicity in *adults* (increase in SCr).[43]

Dosing in neonates is controversial since benzodiazepines may decrease blood pressure and cerebral blood flow velocity.[44] Lorazepam should be used cautiously in this population. Some recommend the initial dose should be reduced by 50% in infants <2 months of age.[13]

Flumazenil, a specific benzodiazepine-receptor antagonist, is indicated for complete or partial reversal of benzodiazepine toxicity (see Flumazenil monograph).[26,45]

Abnormal movements of limbs (e.g., myoclonus or seizures) have been described in premature and full-term neonates.[46-48] The movements began a few minutes after a bolus injection and continued for several hours.[47,48]

Paradoxical reactions (i.e., anxiety, excitation, hostility, aggression, rage, etc.) may occur in children and have been reported in 10% to 30% of children <8 years of age.[11]

Lymphocyte Immune Globulin–Antithymocyte Globulin (equine)

Brand names	Atgam
Dosage	Used for induction of immunosuppression[1-7] and prevention of graft rejection in transplant patients.[8,9] Regimens vary according to indication and institution. (See Cautions related to IV administration section.) **Aplastic anemia:** 15 mg/kg/d for 10 days,[5] 10 mg/kg/d for 5 days,[10] or 40 mg/kg/d over 4 h for 4 days[11,12] followed by 10–30 mg/kg as a single dose every other day for seven additional doses.[13] **Bone marrow transplant:** 30–40 mg/kg/d over 12 h for 3–4 days prior to transplantation[7,14-16] or 20 mg/kg every other day for eight doses beginning the day before transplantation.[17] **Cardiac/lung transplant:** 25 mg/kg/d for 3 days.[3,20] **Cardiac transplant:** 15–20 mg/kg/d for 7 days.[4,20] **Cord blood transplant**: 30 mg/kg/d for 3 days before transplantation.[18] **Graft-versus-host disease:** 15 mg/kg over 3 h twice a day for 10 days for steroid-resistant disease.[19] **Renal transplant:** 2 mg/kg preoperatively and then 2 mg/kg/d for 9 days[2] or 5–25 mg/kg/d for 5–14 days[1,6,8,9,21,22] followed by 10–20 mg/kg as a single dose every other day for ≤2 weeks after transplant.[1] Adjust dose to maintain total rosette-forming cells at 10% of baseline and/or >50/mm^3. Duration of therapy may be longer in cadaveric allograft recipients.[9]
Dosage adjustment in organ dysfunction	With treatment, the drug should be discontinued in renal transplant patients who develop severe and unremitting thrombocytopenia or leukopenia.[22]
Maximum dosage	Not established. The largest reported dose is 7 g.[22]
IV push	Not given by this method.[22,23]
Intermittent infusion	≤4 mg/mL (preferably 1 mg/mL) in D5¼NS, D5½NS, or NS[22] given over 6 h for the first infusion and then ≥4 h for subsequent infusions.[8,22] Addition to dextrose injection is not recommended because low-salt concentrations can cause precipitation.[22]
Continuous infusion	Not indicated.
Other routes of administration	No information available to support administration by other routes.
Maximum concentration	4 mg/mL.[23]

Lymphocyte Immune Globulin–Antithymocyte Globulin (equine)

Cautions related to IV administration

Anaphylactic reactions have occurred.[8] Epinephrine should be available and the drug should only be given in facilities in which intensive life support equipment and trained staff are present.[23]

Before the first infusion, an intradermal test dose should be administered. Intradermal injection of 0.1 mL of 1:1000 dilution and a saline control on a contralateral extremity should be observed q 15 min for 1 h. A wheal or erythema ≥10 mm or marked local swelling should be considered a positive test. However, a negative test dose does not preclude an anaphylactic reaction.[22] Further administration of Atgam should not be attempted if there is a history of systemic reactions, such as a generalized rash, tachycardia, dyspnea, hypotension, or anaphylaxis.[22] Chills, fever, itching, and erythema can be controlled with antipyretics, antihistamines or corticosteroids.[9,22] Many centers have developed premedication protocols to minimize these reactions.

Administer through an in-line, 0.2–1 micron filter into a high-flow vein.[22,23] Phlebitis occurs in 46% of children given the drug through a peripheral vein.[8] One study (n = 83), including six pediatric patients, reported that concurrent infusion of Atgam (15 mg/kg) plus 1000 units heparin and 20-mg Solu-Cortef per 250–500 mL of ½NS was associated with a IV site complication rate of 3.2%.[24] Hence, the study concluded that Atgam could be safely administered via a peripheral vein. Administration into a vascular shunt or arterial venous fistula has been suggested[22]; however, thrombosis may result.

Other additives

Each mL contains 50-mg horse gamma globulin stabilized in 0.3 M glycine. Air in the commercially available ampules has been replaced with nitrogen.[22,23]

Comments

Thrombocytopenia, neutropenia,[8,25] and serum sickness[5,25] have occurred.[8]

This product is made using both human and equine blood components; thus, there is a risk of the transmission of infectious agents, including viruses and the prion that causes Creutzfeldt-Jakob disease.[22]

Monitoring for bacterial and viral infections during therapy is important.[3] Antimicrobial prophylaxis may be included as a part of the treatment regimen.[2,3,9] Antibiotics can be discontinued if fever persists <48 h and cultures are negative.[26]

Lymphocyte Immune Globulin–Antithymocyte Globulin (rabbit)

Brand names	Thymoglobulin
Dosage	**Aplastic anemia:** 2.5–3.5 mg/kg/d infused over 6–8 h for 5 days either as initial treatment or following relapse.[1,2] **Bone marrow transplant:** 2–2.5 mg/kg/d infused over 1 h for 3 to 5 days before transplantation (cumulative dose up to 10 mg/kg).[5,6] **Cardiac transplant:** 1–2 mg/kg/d or every other day infused over 12 h as induction therapy for a total of five doses.[3] 1–2.5 mg/kg/d for 1 to 7 days as induction therapy has also been used.[4] **Liver and/or intestinal transplant:** 5 mg/kg infused over 6–8 h divided in two doses during and after transplantation.[7-9] **Renal transplant:** 1.5 mg/kg intra-operatively followed by 1.5 mg/kg/d for 4 to 6 days[10] or 1.5–2 mg/kg/d for up to 15 days during induction therapy.[11,12] Others reported administering 0.5–2.5 mg/kg/d for up to 14 doses.[13] More recently, 5 mg/kg was given q 24 h for two doses followed by 2.5 mg/kg/d for six to 10 doses.[14]
Dosage adjustment in organ dysfunction	With treatment, the dose should be decreased by half if the WBC is ≥2000–3000/mm³ or if platelets are ≥50,000–75,000/mm³. The drug should be stopped if the WBC is <2000/mm³ or platelets are <50,000/mm³.[15]
Maximum dosage	150 mg/d.[13]
IV push	Not indicated.
Intermittent infusion	Product labeling recommends infusing over ≥6 h into a high-flow vein through a 0.22-micron filter.[15] However, some suggest infusion over 4 h for any subsequent infusions.[16]
Continuous infusion	Not indicated.
Other routes of administration	No information available to support administration by other routes.
Maximum concentration	0.5 mg/mL.[15]
Cautions related to IV administration	Rarely, anaphylaxis has been reported.[15] If anaphylaxis should occur, the infusion should be immediately stopped and resuscitative support potentially including the use of subcutaneous epinephrine should be provided as clinically indicated. These patients should not be given antithymocyte globulin (rabbit) again. Patients commonly experience fever and chills. Decreasing the infusion rate or premedication with corticosteroids, acetaminophen, and an antihistamine within 1 h of the infusion may ameliorate these effects.[15,16]

Lymphocyte Immune Globulin–Antithymocyte Globulin (rabbit)

Other additives	Each 7-mL vial contains 50 mg of glycine, 50 mg of mannitol and 10 mg of sodium chloride[15]; this product contains no preservative.[16] Human red blood cells are used in the manufacturing process.[15]
Comments	Patients are at an increased risk for malignancies and infectious complications. The use of anti-infective prophylaxis is recommended.[15]

Magnesium Sulfate

Brand names	Various manufacturers, concentrations of 50%, 12.5%, 10%, 8%, 4%, 2%, and 1% are available.

Dosage

1 g $MgSO_4$ = 8.12 mEq Mg = 98.6 mg elemental Mg.[1] Doses are listed as $MgSO_4$.

Hypomagnesemia

Neonates: 25–50 mg/kg of $MgSO_4$ q 8–12 h for two or three doses.[2,3] (See Comments section.)

Infants and children: 25–50 mg/kg up to 2 g/dose q 6 h for three or four doses.[1] One 9-year-old child receiving tobramycin developed tetany and hypocalcemia and was treated with 950 mg $MgSO_4$ and 2 g calcium gluconate with symptom improvement within hours.[4]

Pediatric advanced life support (torsades de pointes or suspected hypomagnesemia): 25–50 mg/kg over 10–20 min up to a maximum of 2 g. More rapid infusion may be needed in torsades de pointes.[5,6]

Epilepsy (use not established): 20–100 mg/kg q 4–6 h.[5] Doses as large as 200 mg/kg may be used in children with acute nephritis who have severe seizures and encephalopathy.[5]

Arrhythmias, perioperative and postoperative (use not established): In one study, 30 mg/kg were infused over 10 min at the end of cardiopulmonary bypass. If serum Mg concentration decreased to <1.6–2.3 mg/dL at any time during the ICU stay, 10 mg/kg was given.[7]

Asthma (use not established): 25–75 mg/kg over 20 min.[8-13] Two *adults* with impending respiratory failure responded to a rapid infusion (2 min) of 2 g.[14]

Persistent pulmonary hypertension of newborn (use not established): Seven of nine infants who received 200 mg/kg followed by 20–50 mg/kg/h for up to 8 h survived.[15] Predicted mortality in these patients was 100%.

Dosage adjustment in organ dysfunction	Although no specific recommendations are available, serum concentration monitoring should guide dosing in patients with renal insufficiency who require ongoing supplementation such as occurs in patients receiving PN.[16] Should not be administered to patients with heart block or myocardial damage.[1]
Maximum dosage	In *adults*, 5 g (approximately 40 mEq) of $MgSO_4$ over 3 h.[1] In neonates, 250 mg/kg of $MgSO_4$ infused over 10 min were associated with respiratory depression and 400 mg/kg infused over 10–30 min were associated with an unacceptable rate of hypotension.[17]
IV push	50 mg/kg over 10–20 min during resuscitation.[6] Can be infused more quickly in torsades de pointes.[6]
Intermittent Infusion	Usually, ≤150 mg/min in *adults*.[5] Slower infusion results in a more sustained response in serum concentration.
Continuous infusion	May be added to PN solutions.[18]
Other routes of administration	Can be administered IM. Dilute to 200 mg/mL (20%) in infants and children. 250–500 mg/mL (25% to 50%) in *adults*.[18]

Magnesium Sulfate

Maximum concentration	200 mg/mL or 1.6 mEq/mL (20%) for IV administration.[1]
Cautions related to IV administration	Contraindicated in patients with heart block or with myocardial damage.[1] During IV push administration, monitor for cardiac dysrhythmias, hypotension, respiratory depression, and CNS depression.[1,2] Calcium gluconate is an antidote to hypermagnesemia.[5] For PN compatibility information, please see Appendix C.
Other additives	None.
Comments	Calcium salts (e.g., calcium gluconate) should be available as an antidote if respiratory depression or heart block occurs.[1,6] Magnesium replacement in a magnesium-deficient patient leads to an increase in parathyroid hormone production and a subsequent increase in serum calcium. In magnesium-replete patients, magnesium administration inhibits parathyroid hormone production and results in a decrease in serum calcium. Some have advocated administration of a 6 mg/kg/dose of elemental magnesium to distinguish between the two conditions.[3] Magnesium is associated with drug interactions between central nervous system depressants, neuromuscular blockers, and digoxin.[1,6]

Mannitol

Brand names	Osmitrol
Dosage	**Oliguria** **Test dose (renal function assessment):** 0.2 g/kg (6 g/m^2) to a maximum of 12.5 g over 3–5 min to produce a urine output of ≥1 mL/kg/h or 30–50 mL/h in *adults* for 1–3 h.[1-3] **Treatment:** 0.25–0.5 g/kg q 4–6 h.[3] **Cerebral edema/elevated intracranial pressure (ICP):** 0.25–1 g/kg over 15 min.[4-7] The AAP recommends 0.25 g/kg given over 5–15 min repeated as needed and 0.5 g/kg given over 15 min for an acute increase in ICP.[5] (See Comments section.) **Nephrotic syndrome:** Three children (ages 4, 7, and 9 years) with nephrotic syndrome and diuretic-resistant edema responded to furosemide (2 mg/kg) and 5 mL/kg of 20% mannitol infused over 1 h given daily for 5–7 days.[8]
Dosage adjustment in organ dysfunction	Mannitol should not be used in patients with anuria or severe renal disease.[2]
Maximum dosage	2 g/kg in 2–6 h[6] or 6 g/kg in 24 h.[2] However, there does not appear to be a therapeutic advantage to doses >1 g/kg.[7,9]
IV push	3–5 min in oliguria.[1-3] Rapid administration can result in hypotension, hyperosmolality, and elevations in ICP.[5,7]
Intermittent infusion	Over 15–60 min for cerebral edema, elevated ICP, or preoperative in neurosurgery.[2,9]
Continuous infusion	Sixty patients from age 1–73 were given a continuous infusion over 6–100 h (total dose 2–20 g/kg).[7]
Other routes of administration	Not indicated.[1]
Maximum concentration	25% solution.[10]
Cautions related to IV administration	To avoid infusion of mannitol crystals, warm the vial (and then cool it to body temperature) prior to administration. Use an IV set with an in-line filter for solutions containing ≥20% mannitol.[1,10] For PN compatibility information, please see Appendix C.
Other additives	None.

Comments

A variety of dosing strategies have been described, but the optimal dose for decreasing ICP without adverse effects is unknown.[2,4-7,9]

Mannitol increases the intravascular volume and can worsen hyponatremia. In addition, the resultant diuresis can lead to sodium and potassium losses. Electrolytes should be monitored.[1]

Monitor serum osmolality during mannitol therapy for elevated ICP. An osmotic gradient of >10 mOsm has resulted in adequate decreases in ICP.[9]

A 16-year-old and a 28-year-old with increased ICP and normal renal function developed reversible acute renal failure after receiving 2 and 4 days of doses ranging from 50 and 900 g/d.[11]

Whether saline or mannitol is more beneficial in treating increased ICP is not established.[4]

Use furosemide for elevated ICP in patients with pre-existing cardiac disease because mannitol increases the intravascular volume and may exacerbate congestive heart failure and pulmonary edema.[12]

Meperidine HCl

Brand names	Demerol, generic
Dosage	Because of the potential for adverse effects, meperidine has largely been replaced by other analgesics.[1] Respiratory depression and arrest requiring mechanical ventilation may occur.[2,3] Respiratory depression is reversible with an opiate antagonist (i.e., naloxone).[2,3] **Analgesia:** 0.5–2 mg/kg q 3–4 h as needed[2,4-6] or a loading dose of 0.3–1 mg/kg[2,7] followed by continuous infusion, beginning at 0.35 mg/kg/h and titrating to desired response up to 1.5 mg/kg/h.[2,7] (See Comments section.) **Preoperative sedation:** 0.25–1.5 mg/kg (usually IM or SC) and ≤100 mg given 30–90 min prior to procedure.[2,8-10] 2 mg/kg and ≤100 mg has been used IV.[11]
Dosage adjustment in organ dysfunction	Avoid repeated or high doses in patients with renal impairment.[2] The dose or frequency of dosing should be decreased in hepatic disease.[2] Those with renal and hepatic disease are at risk for accumulation of normeperidine, an active metabolite.[2,12] (See Comments section.)
Maximum dosage	2 mg/kg[7,9,11] and ≤100 mg/dose.[2,11] A continuous infusion of 1.5 mg/kg/h has been used in children with sickle-cell disease.[7] (See Comments section.)
IV push	Rapid injection increases risk for adverse reactions (e.g., respiratory depression, apnea, hypotension, cardiac arrest).[1] One group reported that five of 154 children undergoing endoscopy required supplemental oxygen for a short time after receiving 2 mg/kg infused over 1–2 min.[11]
Intermittent infusion	≤10 mg/mL infused slowly.[2,3]
Continuous infusion	1–10 mg/mL in D-LR, D-R, D-S, D5W, D10W, LR, NS, or ½NS.[2,14]
Other routes of administration	Usually given IM or SC for preoperative sedation.[2,8,10] Local tissue irritation and induration are more common with SC administration.[2] IM administration into or near nerve trunks may cause sensory-motor paralysis that may or may not be temporary.[2]
Maximum concentration	Not established. The manufacturer recommends dilution for IV administration.[2,3]
Cautions related to IV administration	Anaphylaxis has been reported.[13] For PN compatibility information, please see Appendix C.

Other additives

Products may contain sodium metabisulfite and/or phenol and *m*-cresol as preservatives.[2,3,14] Sulfites may cause hypersensitivity reactions and these are more common in *adults* with asthma. Most reactions are mild but can include anaphylactic symptoms and life-threatening or less severe asthma episodes.[15-17] Epinephrine may be required in severe cases; and if the sulfite-free product is not available, the sulfite-preserved epinephrine should be used.[15]

Comments

Meperidine is incompatible with heparin.[14,18] To avoid precipitation with heparin, flush heparinized IV catheters with NS before and after meperidine injection.[14,18]

The meperidine metabolite, normeperidine, may cause a variety of CNS effects including excitability, twitches, tremors, or seizures.[2,19,20]

The pharmacokinetics of meperidine are highly variable in neonates and infants. Half-life ranged from 3.3–59.4 h in 21 infants.[4] Clearance increased with increasing BSA; however, half-life was not different among those term infants <1 week of age, term infants >3 weeks of age (26–150 days of age), and preterm neonates (3.6–65 days of age).

When pain management was inadequate with morphine, a 32-month-old febrile and hyponatremic boy with 90% BSA burns was changed to a meperidine infusion.[21] One h after the dose had been gradually increased to 25 mg/kg/h, he began having intermittent seizures and became comatose. The meperidine was stopped, phenobarbital was started, and the seizures stopped after 6 h. While there were confounding factors, it was felt that the seizures were due to the large dose of meperidine.

A 6-week-old infant received two 1-mg/kg doses of IV meperidine during rigid bronchoscopy and developed acute orofacial dyskinesias (e.g., tongue thrusting, pursing or puckering, facial grimacing) that were unresponsive to 0.1 mg/kg of naloxone.[22] This lasted about 36 h; he had no residual effects.

Demerol, Phenergan, Thorazine [DPT] cocktail has been used to sedate children.[23-25] However, safer and more effective agents are available,[10,23,25] and this combination is no longer recommended.[26]

Contraindicated in those on MAO inhibitors.[2,3]

Meropenem

Brand names	Merrem
Dosage	If a decision is made to give meropenem to a patient with known beta-lactam hypersensitivity, the patient should be closely observed for allergenicity. Meropenem is contraindicated in patients who have demonstrated anaphylactic reactions to beta-lactams.[5] Epinephrine and oxygen should be readily available. **Neonates:** 15[1]–20 mg/kg q 12 h over 15–30 min.[2-4] A 15-day-old premature neonate (33 weeks gestational age; 1.59 kg) was given 120 mg/kg/d (interval not reported) for 8 weeks as treatment for a brain abscess.[4] **Infants and children** **Mild and moderate infections:** 60 mg/kg/d divided q 8 h up to 4 g.[2,5-8] **Serious infections:** 60–120 mg/kg/d divided q 8 h up to 6 g.[2,5-9] **Meningitis:** 120 mg/kg/d divided q 8 h up to 6 g.[2,9-11]
Dosage adjustment in organ dysfunction	Adjust dosage in patients with renal dysfunction.[5] If CrCl is 10–50 mL/min, give 50% of normal dose at normal intervals; if CrCl is <10 mL/min, give 50% of normal dose q 24 h.[5]
Maximum dosage	120 mg/kg/d up to 6 g/d.[2,5,11]
IV push	50 mg/mL in NS, D5, D10, D5NS, D5½NS, D5LR, or LR is given over 3–5 min.[5,12]
Intermittent infusion	50 mg/mL in NS, D5, D10, D5NS, D5½NS, D5LR, or LR and infused over 15–30 min.[5,12]
Continuous infusion	Not generally administered by this method.[5] Meropenem has been administered as a 3-h infusion for the treatment of CNS infections.[13] Additionally, a 24-h continuous infusion, divided into three 8-h infusions has been used in the treatment of critically ill *adults.*[14]
Other routes of administration	Intramuscular meropenem has been used in the treatment of urinary tract infections and pneumonia in *adults.*[15]
Maximum concentration	50 mg/mL.[5]
Cautions related to IV administration	May cause phlebitis at the injection site.[5] For PN compatibility information, please see Appendix C.
Other additives	Contains 3.92 mEq sodium/g of meropenem.[5]
Comments	Neurotoxicity of the carbapenem antibiotics has been reported.[16,17] In *adults*, seizures most often occur after 7 days and appear to be related to an underlying CNS disorder, impaired renal function, and/or large doses.[18] Because of the risk of seizures, the drug should be used cautiously in patients with CNS infections or renal dysfunction, patients with history of seizure disorders, and when used in combination with drugs that lower the seizure threshold.[19]

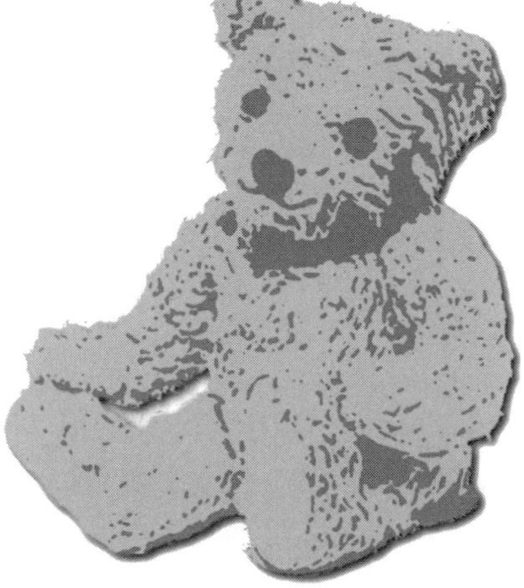

Methotrexate

Brand names Methotrexate, Folex, Methotrexate LPF, Folex PFS

Dosage

Consult protocol for complete information regarding methotrexate (MTX) and leucovorin dosages, hydration, and alkalinization.

Methotrexate is used for a variety of neoplastic disease states.

Cancer

Acute lymphocytic leukemia

High-dose therapy: Loading dose of 200 mg/m^2.[1,2] This is generally followed by 0.8–5 g/m^2/d infused over 2–24 h for 2–3 weeks.[1-4] Although doses as large as 33.6 g/m^2 have been infused over 4–48 h,[5-7] outcomes were not substantially improved over those noted with lower doses (1.2 g/m^2).[1]

Maintenance therapy: 20–50 mg/m^2 IV weekly.[1,8] Adjust dose to maintain a specific WBC count.

Lymphoma: 30 mg/m^2 IV push,[9] 300 mg/m^2 IV infusion over 4 h,[10] 1 g/m^2[11] up to 10 g/m^2 administered over 3–24 h,[12] 3–30 mg/kg[10] up to 50–200 mg/kg/dose infused over 3–6 h.[13]

Meningeal leukemia: Doses administered q 2–5 d until CSF normal, followed by weekly dose for 2 weeks, followed by monthly dose. IT doses in pediatric patients should be based on age (not BSA) as follows[14]:

Age (years)	IT Dose (mg)
<1	6
1	8
2	10
≥3	12

Only preservative-free methotrexate should be used for IT administration.[15]

Osteosarcoma: 1.25–15 g/m^2 infused over 4–6 h.[16-19]

Juvenile rheumatoid arthritis: 0.8–1.1 mg/kg/week,[20] 15 mg/m^2/week,[21] up to 40 mg/m^2/week.[22] Generally given orally or IM.

Dosage adjustment in organ dysfunction

Adjust dosage in patients with renal dysfunction. If CrCl is 10–50 mL/min, give 50% of a normal dose; if CrCl is <10 mL/min, do not administer.[23]

Patients with renal dysfunction or those demonstrating toxicity with previous doses of IT MTX may require leucovorin rescue in small doses.[24,25] Hemodialysis has limited usefulness in lowering plasma MTX in patients with renal failure,[26] but hemodialysis in combination with charcoal hemoperfusion has been successful in managing a patient with severe renal failure following high-dose MTX.[27] Oral administration of activated charcoal may be effective in lowering plasma MTX concentrations.[28]

Maximum dosage

Doses >100 mg/m^2 should be administered with leucovorin.[29] When given with leucovorin rescue, MTX may be escalated to the dosage that yields the best therapeutic effect.[29] Maximum IT dosage is 15 mg.[14]

IV push

<25 mg/mL. May be administered by this method.[15,30]

Intermittent infusion

<25 mg/mL. May be administered by this method.[10-12,15,30]

Continuous infusion	<25 mg/mL. Doses >100–300 mg/m² are generally administered by continuous infusion.[5-7,12,15,30]
Other routes of administration	May be administered IM, intra-arterial, and IT.[15,30] IT doses should be with a preservative-free product diluted to 1 mg/mL using an appropriate sterile preservative-free diluent such as sodium chloride injection.[15]
Maximum concentration	<25 mg/mL for IV or IM administration; 1 mg/mL for IT administration.[15]
Cautions related to IV administration	Two patients experienced anaphylactoid reactions to high-dose methotrexate and BCG injections for osteosarcoma.[31] For PN compatibility information, please see Appendix C.
Other additives	Methotrexate sodium for injection, lyophilized, preservative-free (single-use only) contains 7 mEq sodium/1 g vial.[15,32] Methotrexate sodium injection, isotonic liquid contains NaCl 0.215 mEq/mL. Available with preservatives and preservative free. The isotonic liquid product with preservatives contains benzyl alcohol.[15,32] Benzyl alcohol in small doses as a preservative in drugs is considered safe in newborns.[33] However, a 3-week-old, very low birth weight (710 g) infant who received clindamycin experienced a profound desaturation that required resuscitation after the third and fourth doses, which was subsequently related to the benzyl alcohol preservative.[34] Administration of saline flushes containing benzyl alcohol (bacteriostatic water for injection) was associated with a fatal gasping syndrome, intraventricular hemorrhage, metabolic acidosis, and increased mortality in preterm infants.[35] This should not be used in neonates. Hypersensitivity reactions to benzyl alcohol in parenteral products have been reported in *adults*.[36,37]
Comments	The administration of MTX has been associated with fatal pulmonary toxicity,[38] erythema and desquamation,[39] and death related to high doses.[19,40] Pulmonary toxicity may occur with low doses and be rapidly progressive.[30] Aggressive hydration from 100 mL/m²/h to 200 mL/m²/h during and after MTX must be administered in patients receiving intermediate to high doses of MTX to improve clearance and minimize toxicity.[3,7,29,41-45] Urinary alkalinization (pH >6.5) should be maintained during high-dose infusions of MTX and for 48 h after infusion.[3,29,41,42] Leucovorin should be administered with MTX when doses are ≥100 mg/m² and should be dosed according to the patient's protocol and the amount of MTX given.[29,41] Leucovorin dosages should be modified if MTX clearance is delayed.[29,41] MTX serum concentrations should be monitored when administering large doses of drug. The relationship between serum concentration and toxicity is well-established.[19,29,42,46,47] Recommended procedure is to monitor concentrations at 23 h and 44 h, and until concentrations decrease to <0.05 micromol/L.

Comments *(cont.)*

Clinical features known to place patients at risk for increased MTX toxicity include renal dysfunction,[43] dehydration,[19] vomiting,[7,43,48] diarrhea,[48] decreased urine flow,[49] urine pH below 6.5,[7,43,49] pleural effusions,[50,51] GI obstruction,[52] ascites,[50,51] concomitant use of nephrotoxic medications (e.g., amphotericin B and acyclovir),[7] previous history of cisplatin use,[53] Down's syndrome,[54] and drug interactions decreasing elimination of MTX (e.g., salicylates,[55] omeprazole,[56] NSAIDs,[57-59] sulfamethoxazole/trimethoprim,[60] probenecid,[55,61] and penicillins[62]).

Because MTX is associated with numerous drug interactions,[32] consult appropriate resources for dosing recommendations before combining any drug with MTX.

Methotrexate (250–1000 mg/m^2) is associated with a moderate (30% to 90%) risk of emesis.[63] Patients should receive antiemetic therapy to prevent acute and delayed nausea and vomiting. The recommended therapy is a 5HT3 receptor antagonist in combination with dexamethasone on every day chemotherapy is administered.[63,64] These agents may be continued for up to 4 days after chemotherapy for the prevention of delayed nausea and vomiting.

Methotrexate (50 mg/m^2 to <250 mg/m^2) is associated with a low (10% to 30%) risk of emesis.[63] Patients should receive antiemetic therapy to prevent acute nausea and vomiting. The recommended therapy is a corticosteroid on every day chemotherapy is administered; alternatives are a phenothiazine (e.g., prochlorperazine) or a butyrophenone (e.g., droperidol).[63,64] Therapy for delayed nausea and vomiting is generally not needed.

Methotrexate (<50 mg/m^2) is associated with a minimal (<10%) risk of emesis.[63] Generally, prophylaxis for acute and delayed emesis is not needed. Patients may receive one-time prophylaxis with a phenothiazine (e.g., prochlorperazine) or a butyrophenone (e.g., droperidol).[63,64]

Breakthrough medications for nausea and vomiting should be offered to patients receiving any dose of methotrexate. Appropriate medications include a phenothiazine (e.g., prochlorperazine), a butyrophenone (e.g., droperidol), a substituted benzamide (e.g., metoclopramide), or a benzodiazepine (e.g., lorazepam). Selection should be based on what the patient is currently receiving for acute antiemesis prophylaxis.[63,64]

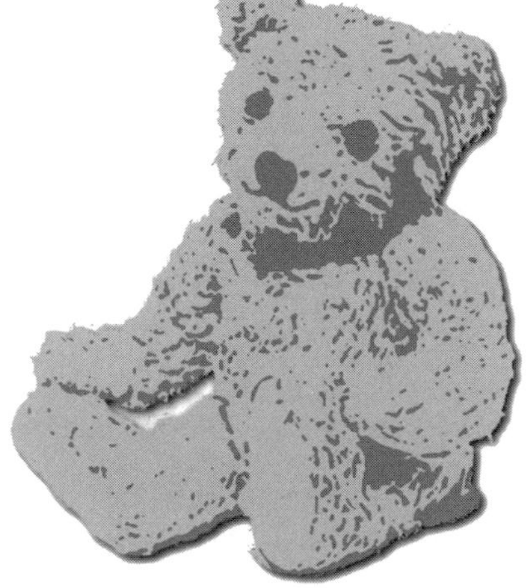

Methyldopate HCl

Brand names	Aldomet
Dosage	**Hypertensive crisis or emergency** **Initial dose:** 2–4 mg/kg/dose; if no effect is observed within 4–6 h, double the dose.[1] **Maintenance dose:** 5–50 mg/kg/d (usually 20–40 mg/kg/d) divided q 6 h[2,3] or 0.6–1.2 g/m²/d divided q 6 h.[2] In hypertensive emergencies, blood pressure should be frequently monitored to ensure that it does not decrease too quickly.[2,4,5] One group recommended that the blood pressure decrease by one-third of the desired total blood pressure decrease within 6–12 h, a further one-third decrease within the next 24 h, with the final one-third decrease achieved over the next 2 days.[6] Alternatively, a blood pressure decrease of <25% within minutes to 1 h followed by further decreases over the next 2–6 h if the patient is stable has been suggested.[2]
Dosage adjustment in organ dysfunction	Adjust dosage in patients with renal or hepatic dysfunction.[2,7] Active metabolite may accumulate in uremia.[2] If CrCl is 10–50 mL/min, administer normal dose q 8–12 h; if CrCl is <10 mL/min, give normal dose q 12–24 h.[7]
Maximum dosage	65 mg/kg/d, not to exceed 3 g/d or 2 g/m²[2] or 1 g/dose.[8] The maximum *adult* dose recommended by the manufacturer is 1 g q 6 h.[2]
IV push	Not recommended.[2]
Intermittent infusion	To avoid a paradoxical pressor effect, dilute in 50–100 mL D5W (≤10 mg/mL) and infuse slowly over 30–60 min.[1,2,9]
Continuous infusion	No information available to support administration by this method.
Other routes of administration	IM and SQ administration are not recommended due to erratic absorption.[2,9]
Maximum concentration	10 mg/mL.[2,9]
Cautions related to IV administration	The injectable product contains sodium bisulfite[9] and anaphylaxis may occur. (See Other additives section.) For PN compatibility information, please see Appendix C.
Other additives	Each mL contains 3.2 mg sodium bisulfite.[9] Sulfites may cause hypersensitivity reactions and these are more common in *adults* with asthma. Most reactions are mild but can include anaphylactic symptoms and life-threatening or less severe asthma episodes.[10-12] Epinephrine may be required in severe cases; and if the sulfite-free product is not available, the sulfite-preserved epinephrine should be used.[10]

Other additives (cont.)

Each mL contains 1.5 mg methylparaben and 0.2 mg propylparaben.[9]

Paraben preservatives may cause hypersensitivity reactions that are more common with cutaneous exposure.[13] However, one case of pruritus and bronchospasm that occurred following infusion of hydrocortisone, which contained parabens, has been reported.[14]

Comments

A decrease in blood pressure generally occurs within 4–6 h and lasts 10–16 h.[2]

A paradoxical pressor response has been reported.[1]

May cause urine to be discolored (pink/red to darkened).[2]

May cause positive Coombs' test; if evidence of hemolytic anemia, the drug should be discontinued.[2]

May cause hemolysis in patients with glucose-6-phosphate dehydrogenase deficiency.[2]

Methylprednisolone Sodium Succinate

Brand names	A-METHAPRED, Solu-Medrol, generic
Dosage	**Anti-inflammatory/immunosuppressive "pulse" therapy:** 30 mg/kg[1] followed by 10 mg/kg for 6 days,[2] 15–30 mg/kg on day 1 for 3–4 days,[3-6] or 600 mg/m² for 3 days.[7] **Asthma (status):** 1–2 mg/kg as a loading dose, followed by 2–4 mg/kg/d divided q 6 h.[8,9] Alternatively, 4 mg/kg/d divided q 6 h for 48 h, then 1–2 mg/kg/d (not to exceed 60 mg/d) divided q 12 h.[10] **Idiopathic thrombocytopenic purpura:** 30 mg/kg/d for 3 days.[11] **Pneumocystis carinii pneumonia** **≤13 years:** 4–8 mg/kg/d divided q 6–12 h for 5–7 days followed by oral prednisone.[12-14] **>13 years:** 30 mg q 12 h for 5 days, then 30 mg as single dose for 5 days,[15,16] and then 15 mg as single dose for 7 days,[15] to 11 days (or until antibiotic therapy is complete).[16] Begin within 24-72 h of initiating antipneumocystis therapy.[16] **Spinal-cord injury:** A loading dose of 30 mg/kg over 15 min followed in 45 min by a continuous infusion of 5.4 mg/kg/h.[17] Patients who receive methylprednisolone within 3 h of injury should be maintained on the regimen for 23 h. If methylprednisolone is not initiated until 3–8 h after injury, the patient should be maintained on the infusion for 48 h.[18] Although the National Acute Spinal Cord Injury trial did not include any patients <13 years old,[17,18] many pediatric clinicians have adopted this practice.[20,21] **Ventricular tachycardia/silent lymphocytic myocarditis (use not established):** 30 mg/kg as a single dose for 3 days.[21] **Chronic interstitial lung disease (use not established):** 300 mg/m² as a single dose for 3 days, repeated q 4–6 weeks.[22] **Lupus nephritis (use not established):** 30 mg/kg every other day for six doses.[17] **Periocular hemangiomas of infancy (use not established):** 2 mg/kg divided q 12 h for 2 days, then transition to oral corticosteroid to taper resulted in rapid hemangioma shrinkage and visual improvement in 15 infants.[23]
Dosage adjustment in organ dysfunction	No dosage adjustment required in patients with renal dysfunction.[24]
Maximum dosage	30 mg/kg,[1,3,4] up to 3 g/dose,[3] has been used as pulse therapy for severe glomerulonephritis, systemic lupus erythematosus, and renal transplant rejection.
IV push	Over 1 to several min.[25,26] High-dose (15 mg/kg; 500 mg) therapy should be infused over ≥30 min.[25,26] (See Cautions related to IV administration section.)
Intermittent infusion	Over 20–60 min.[1,4,5,25]
Continuous infusion	Has been administered by this method.[26] However, compatibility in D5NS, D5W, NS, and PN solutions is concentration dependent.[26] Consult appropriate resources before infusing methylprednisolone with these solutions.
Other routes of administration	May be administered IM.[26] IM not recommended in conditions prone to bleeding (i.e., idiopathic thrombocytopenic purpura).[16]

Methylprednisolone Sodium Succinate

Maximum concentration	125 mg/mL for IV push and 2.5 mg/mL for intermittent infusion.[25]
Cautions related to IV administration	Intractable hiccups, palpitations, and anaphylaxis have been reported.[8,9,27-30] Sudden unexpected death has occurred within minutes or hours of infusion in *adults* receiving ≥500 mg over <10 min.[31,32] For PN compatibility information, please see Appendix C.
Other additives	**Benzyl alcohol:** Contains benzyl alcohol.[25] Benzyl alcohol in small doses as a preservative in drugs is considered safe in newborns.[33] However, a 3-week-old, very low birth weight (710 g) infant who received clindamycin experienced a profound desaturation that required resuscitation after the third and fourth doses, which was subsequently related to the benzyl alcohol preservative.[34] Administration of saline flushes containing benzyl alcohol (BW) was associated with a fatal gasping syndrome, intraventricular hemorrhage, metabolic acidosis, and increased mortality in preterm infants.[35] This should not be used in neonates. Hypersensitivity reactions to benzyl alcohol in parenteral products have been reported in *adults*.[36,37] Contains 2.01 mEq sodium/g of methylprednisolone sodium succinate.[38]
Comments	Supraphysiologic doses of corticosteroids may result in suppressed pituitary-adrenal function, so therapy of more than a few days should be decreased gradually.[39] Children with a history of drug-induced cutaneous reactions are more likely to have an adverse reaction to IV corticosteroids.[40] A recent case was reported of a 14-year-old male with nephrotic syndrome being treated with oral prednisolone and developed Stevens-Johnson syndrome. The boy was changed to IV methylprednisolone 20 mg/kg/dose every other day. By day 2 of treatment, fever subsided and by day 4 the bullae began to subside.[41] Corticosteroid-induced bronchospasm with methylprednisolone in an *adult* with severe asthma was recently reported. The author recommends to consider corticosteroids as contributing factor in asthmatics who do not improve on IV steroids (especially if aspirin allergy also present), and skin testing may help guide safe alternative corticosteroids.[42] Based on multicenter placebo-controlled trials in *adults,* corticosteroids are contraindicated in the treatment of sepsis syndrome and septic shock.[43,44] Although there is no primary literature to support the practice, some neonatal and pediatric intensive care centers administer steroids to a subset of pediatric patients who are unresponsive to conventional therapies (fluids, pressors, antibiotics). Atrial fibrillation,[45] seizures, transient blindness,[46] and fatal varicella[47] have occurred after methylprednisolone administration. A pediatric study looking at effects of short-term (3 days) IV corticosteroids (i.e., methylprednisolone 2 mg/kg/d) on bone metabolism in infants and children reported significant, but reversible, inhibition of bone formation markers. This may be important in children who require multiple short courses of therapy.[48] A prospective, randomized trial looked at pulse-dosed methylprednisolone in initial treatment of Kawasaki disease (in combination with IVIG and aspirin) and noted faster resolution of fever, improvement in inflammatory markers, and shorter hospital stay.[49] Methylprednisolone 10–30 mg/kg as a single dose has also been used in treatment of refractory Kawasaki disease. A recent retrospective review concluded that corticosteroids are effective in treatment of fever in most patients who refractory to IVIG therapy. However, safety and efficacy of corticosteroids on coronary artery outcome could not be determined.[50]

Metoclopramide HCl

Brand names	Octamide PFS, Reglan
Dosage	**Emetogenic cancer chemotherapy:** 1–3 mg/kg 30 min prior to chemotherapy, with repeat doses q 2–3 h for 8–12 h.[1-3] Pretreatment with diphenhydramine may decrease the likelihood of extrapyramidal side effects seen with this dose.[4] One study used 0.4 mg/kg/h for 6 h in a 2-year-old boy.[5] (See Comments section.) In *adults,* a 0.6–3.5-mg/kg bolus 30 min prior to cisplatin infusion followed by 0.5 mg/kg/h for 8 h has been used.[6,7] **Gastroesophageal reflux:** 0.4–0.8 mg/kg/d divided q 6 h.[4,8] **Hypomotility:** 0.1 mg/kg q 4–6 h up to 0.5 mg/kg/d.[9] **Postsurgical nausea and vomiting prophylaxis:** 0.15–0.5 mg/kg up to 10 mg as a single dose infused after anesthesia induction or on arrival in the recovery room.[10-12] Repeat q 6–8 h as needed. Studies comparing metoclopramide to ondansetron for postoperative emesis after strabismus surgery[13,14] and post-tonsillectomy/adenotonsillectomy[15] have found ondansetron to be more effective. **Small bowel intubation (single dose only)[1]** **<6 years:** 0.1 mg/kg. **6–14 years:** 2.5–5 mg. **>14 years:** 10 mg.[1]
Dosage adjustment in organ dysfunction	The labeling recommends a 50% decrease in dose if CrCl <40 mL/min.[1] Another reference recommends adjustment of dose in patients with renal dysfunction as follows: if CrCl 10–50 mL/min, give 75% of a normal dose; if CrCl <10 mL/min, give 50% of a normal dose.[16]
Maximum dosage	**Emetogenic cancer chemotherapy:** 2 mg/kg when chemotherapy is started followed by 2-mg/kg doses 2, 6, and 12 h later.[2] In *adults,* 4 mg/kg as single dose[17] or 2 mg/kg q 2–3 h for a total of 10 mg/kg over 8.5 h[18] has been used for emetogenic cancer chemotherapy. **Reflux/motility:** 0.8 mg/kg/d.[19]
IV push	5 mg/mL[1,20] over 1–2 min in *adults* receiving a 10-mg dose.[1,20]
Intermittent infusion	Dilute doses >10 mg in 50 mL of a compatible fluid (e.g., D5W, D5½NS, NS, LR, R) and infuse over ≥15 min.[1,20]
Continuous infusion	Dilute doses >10 mg in at least 50 mL of a compatible fluid (e.g., D5W, D5½NS, NS, LR, R).[1,20] NS is the preferred diluent due to the stability of the solution.[1]
Other routes of administration	5-mg/mL solution may be given via IM administration.[1]

Metoclopramide HCl

Maximum concentration	5 mg/mL.[20] The osmolality of this solution is 280 mOsm/kg.[20]
Cautions related to IV administration	Rapid administration may result in anxiety, restlessness, and drowsiness.[1] For PN compatibility information, please see Appendix C.
Other additives	Each mL contains 8.5 mg NaCl.[20]
Comments	Neonates are more susceptible to methemoglobinemia during metoclopramide use.[1,8] Children are also more likely than *adults* to experience acute dystonic reactions; these reactions occur more frequently at larger doses.[1,3,21,22] 2.5 mg/kg as a bolus followed by 0.4-mg/kg/h continuous infusion resulted in a dystonic reaction (urinary retention) after 6 h in a child receiving chemotherapy.[5] Diphenhydramine (0.5–1 mg/kg) has been used to treat these reactions.[18,22,23] Gynecomastia related to metoclopramide use has been reported in pediatric patients.[24] Metoclopramide has been used for bedside transpyloric tube placement in pediatric ICU patients[25] and more recently to ease discomfort while placing nasogastric tubes in *adults*.[26]

Metronidazole/Metronidazole HCl

Brand names

Flagyl I.V. RTU (metronidazole), Metronidazole Injection (metronizadole), Flagyl I.V. (metronidazole HCl)

Dosage

Neonates: One report advocates a 15-mg/kg loading dose.[1]

PNA	<1200 g	1200–2000 g	≥2000 g
<7 d	7.5 mg/kg/d q 24–48[2-4]*	7.5 mg/kg/d q 24 h[2-4]	15 mg/kg/d divided q 12 h[1-4]
≥7 d		15 mg/kg/d divided q 12 h[2-4]*	30 mg/kg/d divided q 12 h[2-4]

*Until 4 weeks of age.

Although doses of 22.5 mg/kg/d divided q 8 h have been given for 5 days without problems, the authors suggested that less frequent dosing would be appropriate in newborns.[5,6]

Infants and children: For mild-to-moderate infections, give 30–45 mg/kg/d divided q 6 h up to 4 g/d.[3,4,7,8] Not indicated for severe infections.[4]

Clostridium difficile infection: 30 mg/kg/d divided q 6 h for 7–10 days.[4,9,10]

Surgical prophylaxis: 15 mg/kg over 30–60 min. Infusion should be completed 1 h before surgery and followed by 7.5 mg/kg at 6 and 12 h after the initial dose.[11,12]

Dosage adjustment in organ dysfunction

Adjust dosage in renal and hepatic dysfunction. If CrCl is <10 mL/min, give 50% of the normal dose.[13] Decrease dose by 50% to 67% in patients with hepatic impairment.[12]

Maximum dosage

4 g/d.[3]

IV push

Not recommended.[14]

Intermittent infusion

≤8 mg/mL in D5W, LR, or NS over 60 min.[12]

Continuous infusion

Although solution concentration and type were not provided, Metronidazole/Metronidazole HCl has been administered by this method.[14]

Other routes of administration

No information available to support administration by other routes.

Maximum concentration

8 mg/mL.[12]

Cautions related to IV administration

None.

For PN compatibility information, please see Appendix C.

Other additives	14 mEq of sodium/500 mg of metronidazole.[14]
Comments	An interaction between aluminum hub needles and the initial reconstituted solution of Flagyl I.V. results in an orange, reddish-brown, or rust discoloration after ≥6 h of contact.[14] Metronidazole inhibits alcohol dehydrogenase and other alcohol oxidizing enzymes to produce a disulfiram-type reaction (e.g., flushing, sweating, headache, and tachycardia) in patients who are concurrently given ethanol.[12] Metronidazole may interfere with specific assays to decrease values for AST, ALT, LDH, triglycerides, or glucose.[12]

Micafungin

Brand names	Mycamine
Dosage	Experience with micafungin in children, particularly neonates, is limited[1]; currently there is no established dose range for pediatric patients. **Treatment:** Reported doses have ranged from 0.5–6 mg/kg given once daily.[2-5] Larger doses may be necessary for children <8 years of age secondary to increased clearance.[2,6] **Prophylaxis:** 1 mg/kg given once daily (studies in transplant patients).[7,8] One study initiated therapy at 2–3 mg/kg/d for severe deep mycosis.[3] One study dosed micafungin based on patient weight and fungal species as follows. The dose was increased by 1 mg/kg increments at 5 days if disease was stable or progressive[4]: **<40 kg:** 1 mg/kg/d (*Candida albicans*) or 2 mg/kg/d (nonalbicans or germ-tube negative). **≥40 kg:** 50 mg/d (*Candida albicans*) or 100 mg/d (nonalbicans or germ-tube negative).
Dosage adjustment in organ dysfunction	No dosage adjustment necessary for renal dysfunction or moderate liver disease.[9-11] CVVH has little effect on micafungin kinetics; no dose adjustment or modification recommended.[8]
Maximum dosage	150 mg/d in *adults*.[1,9] One study reported the use of up to 200 mg/d in three patients.[4]
IV push	Not recommended.[9]
Intermittent infusion	Dilute dose of reconstituted micafungin (10 mg/mL) in 100 mL NS or D5W to a final concentration of 0.5–1.5 mg/mL and infuse over 1 h.[9]
Continuous infusion	No information available to support administration by this method.
Other routes of administration	No information available to support administration by other routes.
Maximum concentration	1.5 mg/mL.[9]
Cautions related to IV administration	Phlebitis and thrombophlebitis have been reported and occur more frequently with administration via a peripheral line.[9] Rapid infusions may result in histamine mediated reactions.[9] Isolated cases of serious hypersensitivity/anaphylaxis have also occurred.[9] Flush an existing line with NS prior to micafungin infusion.[9]

Other additives	None.
Comments	Possible development/exacerbation of arrhythmias, hypotension, and/or shock.[9] Possible abnormalities in liver function tests, renal dysfunction, and hematologic effects.[9] One neonatal study compared three dosing regimens (0.75, 1.5, and 3 mg/kg/d) in two infant weight groups (500–1000 g, and >1000 g). The smaller infants had decreased serum concentrations and increased clearance when compared to the larger infants.[12]

Midazolam HCl

Brand names Versed

Dosage

Respiratory depression and arrest requiring mechanical ventilation may occur, especially when used in conjunction with opiates and other sedatives.[1] Be prepared to provide respiratory support, if necessary. Monitor oxygen saturation. Reversal agents should be readily available.

The dose should be calculated on ideal body weight in obese patients.[2] (See Appendix B.)

Anesthesia induction: For children, 0.15 mg/kg initially followed by up to three doses of 0.05 mg/kg at 2-min intervals.[3] The time to induction was noted to be better with a dose of 0.3 mg/kg[4]; however, doses of 0.6 mg/kg did not reliably induce anesthesia in children given atropine and meperidine.[5]

Procedural sedation: Midazolam is the preferred benzodiazepine because of its rapid onset and short duration.[6-9] It does not possess analgesic activity and must be combined with other agents (i.e., fentanyl) when analgesia is needed.[6]

0.05–0.4 mg/kg immediately before the procedure then q 2–5 min to effect.[8-13] Onset 2–5 min (IM 10–20 min) duration 30–60 min (IM 45–120 min)[6,7] up to 2 mg/dose[10,11] and a total of 10 mg.[10] Some recommend age dependent dosing. (0.5–5 years: 0.05–0.1 mg/kg titrating to a max of 0.6 mg/kg).[7,8] (6–12 years: 0.025–0.05 mg/kg titrating to a max of 0.4 mg/kg).[7,8]

Sedation with mechanical ventilation: Bolus of 0.1–0.2 mg/kg over 2–5 min.[14-16] Do not administer a bolus dose to neonates.[15] Followed by 0.03–0.4 mg/kg/h.[14-18] Some recommend age dependent dosing in newborns <32 weeks gestation receiving 0.03 mg/kg/h and those >32 weeks receiving 0.06 mg/kg/h.[18]

Status epilepticus (refractory status epilepticus)[20-26]: A loading dose of 0.15–0.38 mg/kg[20-24] followed by a continuous infusion of 0.06–2 mg/kg/h.[20,24-27] Titrate by 0.06 mg/kg/h q 15 min.[23] The range of mean maintenance infusion was 0.14–0.84 mg/kg/h.[20,23,24] When weaning off midazolam, decrease dose by 0.06–0.12 mg/kg/h q 15 min.[23] Most patients regained full consciousness by an averaged 4 h after discontinuation of midazolam.[20]

Tachyphylaxis may require progressively larger dose within the first 24–48 h.[26]

Dosage adjustment in organ dysfunction

No dosage adjustment required in renal dysfunction.[28] Adjust dosage in patients with hepatic dysfunction.[1,2]

Maximum dosage

For anesthesia induction, single doses of ≤0.6 mg/kg have been used.[3,4] Total doses >5 mg are not usually necessary for conscious sedation in *adults*.[1] The largest dose given by continuous infusion was 0.7 mg/kg/h.[22]

IV push

1 or 5 mg/mL given over 20–30 sec for anesthesia induction.[1,4] Generally, given over 5 min in neonates.[29]

Intermittent infusion

Dilute to desired volume in D5W, LR, or NS and give over ≥2 min.[1,11]

Continuous infusion

Dilute to desired volume in D5W, LR, or NS.[1,11,14,17,19] (See Comments section.)

Other routes of administration

1 mg/mL.[1] IM doses of 0.15–0.5 mg/kg (maximum total dose 10 mg) have been administered safely in children requiring sedation or in patients in status epilepticus.[29-31] A 20% failure rate was noted following IM administration when midazolam was given prehospitalization.[31]

Has been given by buccal administration.

Maximum concentration

5 mg/mL for IV push[1,3] and 1 mg/mL for IM administration.[1]

Cautions related to IV administration

Respiratory depression and arrest requiring mechanical ventilation may occur following excessive dosing, rapid administration,[1,3,32] or use with fentanyl.[32,33]

For PN compatibility, please see Appendix C.

Other additives

Benzyl alcohol: Each 1 mL contains 1% benzyl alcohol as a preservative.[34] Benzyl alcohol in small doses as a preservative in drugs is considered safe in newborns.[35] However, a 3-week-old, very low birth weight (710 g) infant who received clindamycin experienced a profound desaturation that required resuscitation after the third and fourth doses, which was subsequently related to the benzyl alcohol preservative.[36] Administration of saline flushes containing benzyl alcohol (bacteriostatic water for injection) was associated with a fatal gasping syndrome, intraventricular hemorrhage, metabolic acidosis, and increased mortality in preterm infants.[37]

Hypersensitivity reactions to benzyl alcohol in parenteral products have been reported in *adults*.[38,39]

Comments

Dosing in neonates is controversial since benzodiazepines may decrease blood pressure and cerebral blood flow velocity.[40] Neonates may experience prolonged CNS depression because of an inability to biotransform diazepam to an inactive metabolite.[10] Midazolam should be used cautiously in this population.

Involuntary epileptiform movements were reported in preterm infants <32-weeks-old.[41,42] A withdrawal syndrome may begin 24 h after cessation of prolonged continuous infusion; however, it is typically observed 5–10 days after continual use.[32,42-45] Other investigators have shown that cumulative doses >60 mg/kg are highly correlated with withdrawal syndromes.[46]

Some practitioners recommend weaning a patient from midazolam to oral lorazepam.[47]

Midazolam Rate	Equivalent Oral Dose of Lorazepam
1 mcg/kg/min = 1.44 mg/kg/d	0.3 mg/kg/d = 0.1 mg/kg q 8 h
2 mcg/kg/min = 2.88 mg/kg/d	0.6 mg/kg/d = 0.1–0.15 mg/kg q 6 h
3 mcg/kg/min = 4.32 mg/kg/d	0.9 mg/kg/d = 0.1–0.15 mg/kg q 4–6 h
4 mcg/kg/min = 5.76 mg/kg/d	0.3 mg/kg/d = 0.15 mg/kg q 4 h

Source: From Cyndi Reid, Pharm.D., Department of Pharmaceutical Services, Children's Hospital of Michigan, Detroit, MI.

Flumazenil, a specific benzodiazepine-receptor antagonist, is indicated for complete or partial reversal of benzodiazepine toxicity (see Flumazenil monograph).[48] May precipitate seizures in someone with known epilepsy who is dependent on benzodiazepines.

Milrinone Lactate

Brand names	Primacor
Dosage	Because milrinone has been administered to a limited number of pediatric patients, the doses and side effects have not been established. (See Comments section.) **Hemodynamic support:** 50–100 mcg/kg as a loading dose[1-8] followed by a maintenance dose ranging from 0.2–1.2 mcg/kg/min.[1-9] Titrate dose to effect. One group of investigators recommends that for every increase of 0.25 mcg/kg/min, a 25-mcg/kg bolus be given.[3] **Ischemic injury due to meningococcal sepsis:** 25 mcg/kg bolus over 10 min followed by doses up to 0.75 mcg/kg/min.[10]
Dosage adjustment in organ dysfunction	Adjust dosage in renal dysfunction.[11] If CrCl is <10 mL/min, administer 50% to 75% of a normal dose.[11,12] Impaired milrinone clearance may result in significant hypotension.[3]
Maximum dosage	A loading dose of 100 mcg/kg[4,5] and a maintenance dose of 1.2 mcg/kg/min[9] in infants and children. Doses as large as 1.13 mg/kg/d have been given to *adults*.[1]
IV push	Although milrinone has been given over 30 sec,[6] most references suggest infusing over 10 min.[13,14]
Intermittent infusion	1 mg/mL or diluted in D5W, ½NS, or NS.[13] Although milrinone has been given over 30 sec–5 min,[6] most references suggest that the loading dose should be given over 10 min.[13,14]
Continuous infusion	≤200 mcg/mL in D5W, ½NS, or NS.[13,14] One study noted stability of a 400-mcg/mL solution in RL, D5W, ½NS, and NS.[15]
Other routes of administration	No information available to support administration by other routes.
Maximum concentration	1 mg/mL for loading dose[1] and 250 mcg/mL for continuous infusion.[2,3,14]
Cautions related to IV administration	EKG should be monitored during infusion for supraventricular and ventricular arrhythmias.[13] Blood pressure and heart rate should be monitored during the infusion. If the patient develops excessive hypotension, the infusion should be decreased or stopped.[13] Spontaneous bronchospasm has been reported.[13] A precipitate will form when furosemide is injected into an IV line infusing milrinone.[13,14] For PN compatibility information, please see Appendix C.
Other additives	None.

Comments

Milrinone is a positive inotrope and vasodilator that has little chronotropic activity.[13] It should not be used in patients with severe obstructive aortic or pulmonic valvular disease.[13] Milrinone may aggravate outflow tract obstruction in patients with hypertrophic subaortic stenosis.[13]

There is no experience in controlled studies with infusion ≥48 h.[8] In *adults* with Class III and IV CHF, long-term treatment did not improve symptoms and increased the risk of hospitalization and death.[13]

The total concentration of lactic acid varies from 0.95 mg/mL to 1.29 mg/mL.[13]

Mivacurium

Brand names	Mivacron
Dosage	Respiratory function must be supported and concurrent administration of a sedative is necessary. Monitoring of neuromuscular transmission with a peripheral nerve stimulator is recommended during continuous infusion or with repeated dosing.[1,2] Obese patients (≥30% of ideal body weight) should be dosed on ideal body weight.[2,3] (See Appendix B.) **Children 2–12 years of age:** 0.2 mg/kg repeated as needed to maintain pharmacological paralysis.[1-7] May follow initial dose by continuous infusion of 10–14 mcg/kg/min.[1-7]
Dosage adjustment in organ dysfunction	Standard doses may be used in patients with renal or hepatic dysfunction. Compared to healthy patients, the duration of neuromuscular blockade with mivacurium will be approximately one-and-a-half times longer in severe renal impairment and three times longer in end-stage liver disease. Infusion rates should be decreased by 50% in patients with hepatic disease. No adjustment is necessary in patients with renal dysfunction.[2,3]
Maximum dosage	Infusion rates as large as 31 mcg/kg/min have been used.[2]
IV push	2 mg/mL over 5–10 sec.[1,2]
Intermittent infusion	Not administered by this method.
Continuous infusion	≤0.5 mg/mL in D5W, D5NS, D5LR, LR, or NS.[1,8]
Other routes of administration	Not administered via other routes.
Maximum concentration	2 mg/mL for IV push and 0.5 mg/mL for continuous infusion.[2]
Cautions related to IV administration	Hypersensitivity reactions, hypotension, arrhythmias, and bronchospasm have been reported but appear to be rare.[2]
Other additives	May contain benzyl alcohol,[2,8] which in small doses as a preservative is considered safe in newborns.[9] However, a 3-week-old, very low birth weight (710 g) infant who received clindamycin experienced a profound desaturation that required resuscitation after the third and fourth doses, which was subsequently related to the benzyl alcohol preservative.[10] Administration of saline flushes containing benzyl alcohol (BW) was associated with a fatal gasping syndrome, intraventricular hemorrhage, metabolic acidosis, and increased mortality in preterm infants.[11] This should not be used in neonates. Hypersensitivity reactions to benzyl alcohol in parenteral products have been reported in *adults.*[12,13]

Comments

Prolonged paralysis has been reported after mivacurium administration in pediatric and *adult* patients with reduced plasma cholinesterase activity.[2,3,14,15]

Concomitant administration of other drugs (e.g., aminoglycosides, clindamycin, inhalational anesthetics, ketamine, magnesium, quinidine, or succinylcholine) may prolong neuromuscular blockade.[2,3] Consult appropriate resources for additional information on drug interactions.

Morphine Sulfate

Brand names	Astramorph PF, Duramorph, various generic; Infumorph (for microinfusion devices only)
Dosage	Respiratory depression and arrest requiring mechanical ventilation may occur.[1,2] Respiratory depression is reversible with an opiate antagonist (i.e., naloxone).[1,2] **Analgesia** **Infants <6 months:** 0.05–0.1 mg/kg followed by continuous infusion of 0.005–0.03 mg/kg/h.[3-8] (See Comments section.) Some suggest the maximum dose should not exceed 0.015–0.02 mg/kg/h.[3,5] Of note, gestational age and postconceptional age are directly related to clearance; thus, dosing requirements in preterm neonates are decreased.[6,8] **Infants ≥6 months/children:** 0.05–0.2 mg/kg q 2–4 h as needed[7,9,10] or 0.05–0.2 mg/kg followed by continuous infusion of 0.02–0.15 mg/kg/h.[7,9,11-15] (See Maximum dosage and Comments sections.) **Premedication for procedures in neonates/infants/children:** 0.1–0.2 mg/kg and ≤15 mg total dose.[1,9,16,17]
Dosage adjustment in organ dysfunction	Decrease dose in severe renal impairment. Use with caution in severe liver disease.[1] During ECMO, dosage requirements are increased even though studies have shown that clearance is decreased.[18] One study showed that up to 40% of the morphine dose may be bound to the membrane oxygenator or polyvinyl chloride tubing.[19]
Maximum dosage	The recommended initial maximum *adult* dose is 10 mg.[1,2] The maximum pediatric dose is 0.1–0.2 mg/kg not to exceed 15 mg.[1] With repeated dosing, tolerance can develop resulting in increased dosage requirements. (See Comments section.)
IV push	Over 4–5 min.[1,2] (See Cautions related to IV administration section.)
Intermittent infusion	Over 15–30 min.[1,2]
Continuous infusion	0.1–1 mg/mL in D5W, D10W, or NS.[1,20] (See Dosage and Comments sections.)
Other routes of administration	May be given IM or SC using 0.5, 1, 2, 3, 4, or 5 mg/mL.[3] IM is preferred when repeat doses are needed since SC dosing causes local tissue irritation and pain.[1] However, some believe that IV or SC gives better comfort and reliability and that IM dosing should not be used routinely.[1]
Maximum concentration	Usually 1 mg/mL for continuous infusion; however, more concentrated solutions have been used in fluid restricted patients or in those who have high dosage requirements.[2]
Cautions related to IV administration	Respiratory depression, hypotension, and chest wall rigidity may occur with rapid administration.[1,2] For PN compatibility information, please see Appendix C.

Other additives

Some morphine products contain chlorobutanol, phenol, sodium bisulfite, sodium metabisulfite, sodium phosphates, and/or sodium formaldehyde sulfoxylate.[20] Sulfites may cause hypersensitivity reactions and these are more common in *adults* with asthma. Most reactions are mild but can include anaphylactic symptoms and life-threatening or less severe asthma episodes.[21-23] Epinephrine may be required in severe cases; and if the sulfite-free product is not available, the sulfite-preserved epinephrine should be used.[21]

Comments

Tolerance to chronic dosing occurs and can significantly increase dose requirements.[1,2]

Continuous infusion provides better analgesia with fewer adverse effects than intermittent (PRN) dosing.[24]

Larger doses may be needed in cancer, burn, or other patients with severe pain. A continuous infusion of 2.6 mg/kg/h was given without adverse effects to a child with terminal malignancy.[12]

Patients with sickle-cell disease have higher plasma clearance of morphine than patients with other diseases and generally require larger doses to achieve adequate pain control.[10] This may be due to anemia-related changes in hepatic blood flow that accelerate renal or hepatic clearance. However, death from cardiopulmonary arrest due to high-dose morphine has been reported in a child with sickle-cell crisis.[25]

Neonates are less able than older children to conjugate morphine to morphine-6-glucuronide. This metabolite is 20 times more potent than morphine; hence, larger doses may be required in neonates.[26-30] Neonates do conjugate morphine to morphine-3-glucuronide, a respiratory stimulant and as a result intubated neonates may fight the ventilator despite high doses of morphine.[27,31]

Infants <6 months of age have significantly prolonged clearance compared to older children and *adults*.[3,4,7,26,32] Infants <6 months of age who are not on ventilators may experience irregular breathing patterns. Use morphine cautiously in these patients.[9,11]

A wide range of concentrations are available including 0.5, 1, 2, 4, 5, 8, 10, 15, and 25 mg/mL products for IV, IM, and SC administration. Errors in programming PCA pumps, including the substitution of a more concentrated product than the pump was programmed to infuse, have resulted in deaths.[33]

Multivitamins (Adult)

Brand names	M.V.I. Adult, M.V.I. Adult Unit Vial, MVI-12, Infuvite Adult
Dosage	**Daily for children ≥11 years and adults:** 5 mL from vial 1 and 5 mL from vial 2 of M.V.I. Adult or Infuvite Adult or 10 mL of mixed M.V.I.–12 Unit Vial.[1,2] **During pediatric vitamin shortages the adult products have been used[3]:** The A.S.P.E.N. 2006 Pediatric Multivitamin Task Force recommended that when a shortage is recognized, the pediatric multivitamins should be reserved for infants <2.5 kg or <36 weeks gestation. Infants who are able to ingest 50% of their nutrient needs should be switched to oral vitamins. For those who must receive the parenteral product, the following doses of the *adult* parenteral multivitamins were recommended. **2.5 kg up to 11 years of age:** Use half the *adult* dose (5 mL) and supplement vitamin K to a total dose of 200 mcg. (M.V.I. Adult and Infuvite Adult contain 150 mcg of vitamin K; M.V.I.-12 does not contain vitamin K.) **<2.5 kg or <36 weeks gestation:** 1 mL/kg of an *adult* product. *Adult* multivitamins contain excipients that are known to be toxic in preterm infants. (See Other additives section.)
Dosage adjustment in organ dysfunction	The possibility of hypervitaminosis A or D should be kept in mind in patients with renal failure.[1,2]
Maximum dosage	One-and-a-half to three times the usual daily dosage for 2 days for patients with multiple vitamin deficiencies or markedly increased requirements.[1,2,45] (See Comments section.)
IV push	Contraindicated.[6]
Intermittent infusion	Over ≥2 h.[4] However, the contents of M.V.I.-12 vials 1 and 2 (5 mL each) were diluted in 50 mL D5W and administered over 20 min without adverse effects in normal *adult* volunteers.[7]
Continuous infusion	Add to at least 500 mL (preferably 1000 mL) of IV fluid.[1,3,6]
Other routes of administration	No information available to support administration by other routes.
Maximum concentration	Dilute dose in ≥500 mL of a compatible IV fluid.[6]
Cautions related to IV administration	Rapid administration may result in dizziness, faintness, and tissue irritation.[1,3,6]

Other additives

M.V.I. Adult Dual Vial

Vial 1: Contains 30% propylene glycol, 2% gentisic acid ethanolamide, 1.6% polysorbate 80, 0.028% butylated hydroxytoluene, and 0.0005% butylated hydroxyanisole.

Vial 2: Contains 30% propylene glycol.

M.V.I. Adult Unit Vial: Contains 30% propylene glycol and 1% gentisic acid ethanolamide. Citric acid, sodium citrate, and NaOH are used to adjust pH. 0.8% polysorbate 80; 0.014% polysorbate 20, 0.001% butylated hydroxytoluene, and 0.0003% butylated hydroxyanisole.

Infuvite Adult

Vial 1: Contains 1.4% polysorbate 80.

Vial 2: Contains 30% propylene glycol.

Propylene glycol is added to parenteral drugs as a solubilizer. Rapid infusion of medications that contain propylene glycol has resulted in respiratory depression and cardiac dysrhythmias.[8] Its half-life is three times longer in neonates than in *adults*[9] and has caused hyperosmolality[10] and refractory seizures[11] in preterm neonates receiving 3 g/d.

Polysorbate 80 has been associated with hepatic and renal toxicity in low birth weight infants.[12,13]

Multivitamin products contain contaminant aluminum.[1,2] The M.V.I.-12 Unit vial 10-mL dose contains no greater than 0.78 mcg of contaminant aluminum; the M.V.I.-12 Dual vial 10-mL dose provides no more than 1.83 mcg; the MVI-12 multidose vial 10-mL dose provides no more than 0.43 mcg. For Infuvite Adult the amount of contaminant aluminum is ≤3.75 mcg in the 10-mL dose.[15]

Comments

Addition of these products to solutions containing bisulfites as antioxidants may result in thiamine inactivation.[14]

M.V.I. Adult and Infuvite Adult contain the recent FDA specifications of vitamin doses, including increased doses of vitamin C (200 mg), thiamine (6 mg), pyridoxine (6 mg), and folic acid (600 mcg). Of note, vitamin K in a dose of 150 mcg is also included.[1,2]

For patients receiving larger doses than usual or who are on parenteral vitamins for 4–6 months, serum concentration measurement of vitamins A, C, D, and folic acid should be performed to ensure that concentrations are within the normal range.[1,2]

Multivitamins (Pediatric)

Brand names	M.V.I. Pediatric, Infuvite Pediatric
Dosage	Dosages listed are in terms of the reconstituted single dose 5-mL vial. **Neonates <1 kg:** 1.5–3.25 mL/d[1-5] or 2 mL/kg/d.[6] (See Comments section.) **Neonates and infants 1–3 kg:** 3.25 mL/d[1-4] *or* 2 mL/kg/d up to 5 mL/d.[6] **Infants and children ≥ 2.5 kg and <11 years:** 5 mL/d.[1-4,6]
Dosage adjustment in organ dysfunction	Hypervitaminosis A and D are potential complications in patients with renal failure.[1,2]
Maximum dosage	Usually 5 mL. However, larger doses may be indicated during certain diseases.[1,2]
IV push	Contraindicated.[1,2]
Intermittent infusion	Infants <6 months of age have received PN solutions (including micronutrients) cycled over 18 h.[7]
Continuous infusion	Total daily dose is usually added to a PN solution.[1-4] The 5-mL dose of reconstituted M.V.I. Pediatric or Infuvite Pediatric should be added to at least 100 mL of compatible IV fluid.[1,2]
Other routes of administration	No information available to support administration by other routes.
Maximum concentration	5-mL dose added to at least 100 mL of infusate.[1,2] Do not give undiluted.[1,2]
Cautions related to IV administration	May cause dizziness, faintness, and tissue irritation if infused undiluted.[1,2]
Other additives	**M.V.I. Pediatric:** Contains 375 mg mannitol, 50 mg polysorbate 80, 0.8 mg polysorbate 20, 58 mcg butylated hydroxytoluene, and 14 mcg butylated hydroxyanisole. **Infuvite Pediatric** **Vial 1**: Contains 50 mg polysorbate 80. **Vial 2**: Contains 75 mg mannitol. Polysorbate 80 has been associated with hepatic and renal toxicity in low birth weight infants.[8,9] Multivitamin products contain contaminant aluminum.[1,2] For M.V.I. Pediatric the amount of contaminant aluminum is ≤42 mcg/L (0.21 mcg/5-mL dose) and for Infuvite Pediatric the amount of contaminant aluminum is ≤800 mcg/L in vial 1 (dose is 4 mL or 3.21 mcg) and 275 mcg/L in vial 2 (dose is 1 mL and 0.275 mcg) for a total 5-mL dose of 3.485 mcg.[13]

Multivitamins (Pediatric)

Comments

Does not result in optimal vitamin dosing in low birth weight infants.[5,6,10-12] Doses of 1.5 mL/d did not maintain vitamin E levels in therapeutic range (1–3 mg/dL) in 56% of infants <1 kg.[5,10] Doses of 2 mL/kg in premature infants will not provide adequate vitamin A.[6]

Muromonab-CD3

Brand names

Orthoclone OKT3

Dosage

The length of therapy depends on the type of transplant, the institution-specific protocol, and whether use is for induction of immunosuppression or rejection reversal.

Patients ≤30 kg: 2.5 mg/d for 10–14 days.[1-5] Alternatively, in one report those <12 years were given 0.1 mg/kg/d for 10–14 days (≤5 mg).[6] One study administered 1.25 mg/d to patients weighing <10 kg and 2.5 mg/d to those ≥10 kg up to 30 kg for 10 days.[7] One large retrospective study reported using 5 mg/d for 10–14 days in patients weighing >20 kg.[8]

Patients >30 kg: 5 mg/d for 10–14 days.[1-5] Alternatively, 1 mg/10 kg ≤5 mg/d for 10–14 days.[9]

Adjust dose to maintain CD3+ cell count at <25/mm^3[2] or OKT3 serum concentration >800 ng/mL.[1,2]

Acute viral myocarditis with left ventricular ejection fraction of 5% to 20%: As part of an institutional acute graft rejection protocol postcardiac transplant (therapy also included combinations of steroids, cyclosporine, azathioprine, and IVIG), five children from age 15 months to 16 years received 0.1 mg/kg/d for 10–14 days.[10] Four patients survived.[10]

Dosage adjustment in organ dysfunction

No information available to support the need for dosage adjustment.

Maximum dosage

15 mg.[1]

IV push

1 mg/mL over <1 min.[11]

Intermittent infusion

Not recommended.[1]

Continuous infusion

Not indicated.

Other routes of administration

No information available to support administration by other routes.

Maximum concentration

1 mg/mL.

Cautions related to IV administration

Anaphylactic and anaphylactoid reactions may occur following administration of any dose, usually within the first 10 min. Pretreatment with antihistamines and/or corticosteroids have not always been reliable in preventing this adverse reaction.[11]

A cytokine release syndrome may occur within 40–60 min and commonly includes fever, chills, generalized weakness, chest tightness, wheezing, nausea, and vomiting. Less common, patients could experience a spectrum of severe and life-threatening cardiorespiratory symptoms. It occurs less commonly and/or with less severity after the first three doses but may recur after a hiatus or a dosage increase. Pretreatment with corticosteroids, diphenhydramine, and acetaminophen before the first dose minimizes adverse effects.[3,6,9,13] Patients should be monitored for 48 h after the first dose is given.

Other additives	Each 5 mL (5 mg) contains 2.25 mg monobasic sodium phosphate, 9 mg dibasic sodium phosphate, 43 mg NaCl, and 1 mg polysorbate 80.[11]
Comments	Contraindicated in patients with volume overload or uncompensated heart failure or in patients who are predisposed to or have a history of seizures. Pediatric patients should be carefully evaluated for fluid retention and elevated blood pressure before initiating muromonab CD3 due to the risk of cerebral edema and herniation.[11] Immunologic monitoring during therapy should include drug serum concentration,[1,4] antidrug antibody formation,[2,3,10] and CD3+ cell count.[1,3-5,9,12,13] Do not shake solution.[11] Withdraw the solution from the ampul through a low protein-binding 0.2- or 0.22-micron filter. Discard this filter and attach a new needle prior to bolus injection.[11]

Nafcillin Sodium

Brand names	Nafcil, Nallpen, Unipen

Dosage

Serious anaphylactoid reactions may require immediate emergency treatment with epinephrine, oxygen, IV steroids, and airway management.

Neonates

PNA	<1200 g	≤2000 g	>2000 g
≤7 d	50 mg/kg/d divided q 12 h[1]*	50–100 mg/kg/d divided q 12 h[1-3]	75 mg/kg/d divided q 8 h[1-3]
>7 d	50–75 mg/kg/d divided q 12 h[1]*	50–75 mg/kg/d divided q 6–8 h[1-3]	100–140 mg/kg/d divided q 6 h[1-3]
≤4 weeks	50 mg/kg/d divided q 12 h[1]	75 mg/kg/d divided q 8 h[1-3]	100–200 mg/kg/d divided q 6 h[1-3]

*Until 4 weeks of age.

Infants and children

Mild to moderate infections: 50–100 mg/kg/d divided q 6 h.[1,4-6]

Severe infections: (e.g., osteomyelitis, pericarditis, endocarditis) 100–200 mg/kg/d divided q 4–6 h.[1,7-9]

Endocarditis (oxacillin-susceptible): 200 mg/kg/d divided q 4–6 h for 6 weeks with or without gentamicin.[7] If prosthetic valve related, add rifampin.[7]

Meningitis (staphlycoccus aerus methicillin susceptible)

≤7 days and >2000 g: 100–150 mg/kg/d divided q 8–12 h.[7-11]

>7 days and >2000 g: 150–200 mg/kg/d divided q 6–8 h.[7-11]

Dosage adjustment in organ dysfunction

Dosage adjustment is unnecessary in either renal[11,12] or hepatic failure alone[11]; however, the dosage should be adjusted in patients with combined renal and hepatic dysfunction.[11]

Maximum dosage

200 mg/kg/d, not to exceed 6[13] to 12 g/d.[13] 18 g/d has been given to *adults* with severe infections.[14]

IV push

Dilute dose in 15–30 mL ½NS, NS, or SW (paraben and benzyl alcohol free for neonates) and give over 5–10 min through running IV.[13,16]

Intermittent infusion

2–40 mg/mL in D5W, NS, or R and infuse over 30–60 min.[16]

Continuous infusion

Although no specific information is available to support infusion of nafcillin by this method, other beta-lactam antibiotics have been given by this method.[17]

Other routes of administration

250 mg/mL in SW, BW, or NS by deep IM injection.[11] No information available to support administration by other routes.

Maximum concentration

40 mg/mL for IV infusion.[15] Maximum concentration of 128 mg/mL in SW results in a recommended osmolality for peripheral infusion in fluid-restricted patients.[15,18]

Cautions related to IV administration

If a decision is made to give this medication to a patient with known penicillin hypersensitivity, the patient should be closely observed for allergenicity.[20-24] (See Comments section.)

Phlebitis was reported with a 15-min infusion in a child.[12]

Extravasation may cause tissue sloughing and necrosis.[17,18] A 15-unit dose of a 1:10 dilution of a 150-unit vial of hyaluronidase in NS should be prepared and injected in approximately five 0.2 mL aliquots around the extravasated are using a 25-gauge hypodermic needle with 12 h of the extravasation.[19]

For PN compatibility information, please see Appendix C.

Other additives

Contains 2.9 mEq sodium/g of nafcillin sodium.[13,15]

Comments

Patients with a history of type I reaction to penicillin should not receive beta-lactam antibiotics. From 5% to 15% of patients allergic to penicillin will also be allergic to cephalosporins. Certain infections (e.g., syphilis) require penicillin for cure. It is recommended that a desensitization protocol for penicillin-allergic individuals should be performed in a hospital setting. This can usually be completed in about 4 h, at which time the first dose of penicillin can be given.[1]

The beta-lactam ring of penicillins can link with an amino sugar of the aminoglycoside and inactivate the aminoglycoside.[21-23] To avoid this potential interaction, administer penicillins 1 h before or after an aminoglycoside, adequately flush the infusion line between each infusion, or infuse them through separate lines. *In vivo* inactivation that is dose dependent can also occur particularly in patients with renal failure.[23-25] In patients with end-stage renal failure, gentamicin half-life was decreased by 22–31 h after carbenicillin or ticarcillin was added to the drug regimen.[24]

Naloxone HCl

Brand names	Narcan

Dosage

When used for acute opiate overdose, other resuscitative measures (e.g., maintenance of an adequate airway, artificial respiration, cardiac massage, vasopressor agents) should be readily available.

Neonatal opioid depression/asphyxia

Naloxone may be used to treat asphyxia in a neonate whose mother was given opiates during labor and delivery. Although it has been given to the mother shortly before delivery, it is preferable to administer naloxone directly to the neonate after delivery.[1]

0.01 mg/kg (IV) administered into the umbilical vein and repeated q 2–3 min until clinical response; repeat q 1–2 h as needed.[1-3] Additional doses may be necessary at 1–2 h intervals depending on the response of the neonate and the dosage and duration of action of the opiate administered to the mother. When the IV route cannot be used, the drug may be administered by IM or SC injection.

Opiate intoxication/dependency (known or suspected)

Smaller doses may be used to reverse respiratory depression associated with therapeutic opioid use.[4]

Monitor for at least 24 h since relapse may occur as naloxone is metabolized.[1]

> **<5 years or ≤ 20 kg (including neonates):** 0.1 mg/kg q 2–3 min as needed until opiate effects are reversed.[1,4,5-10] Repeat q 1–2 h if inadequate response or symptoms recur.[1]
>
> **≥5 years or >20 kg:** 2 mg[1,6,8,11-13] with subsequent doses of 0.1 mg/kg q 1–2 min if no improvement occurs.[1,8,12,13] Repeat q 20–60 min if symptoms recur.[1]

When repeated doses are required, some suggest the use of continuous infusion (i.e., 2.5–160 mcg/kg/h).[12-14] After titrating clinical effectiveness, decrease by 25%.[13-16] Wean infusion in 50% increments over 6–12 h, depending on the half-life of the opiate.[16]

Postoperative opioid respiratory depression: Abrupt reversal of postoperative opioid depression may cause nausea, vomiting, sweating, trembling, tachycardia, hypertension, seizures, ventricular tachycardia and fibrillation, pulmonary edema, and cardiac arrest, which has resulted in death.[1]

Dose is one-tenth that used for opiate intoxication. 0.005–0.01 mg/kg q 2–3 min until clinical response is seen and then at 1–2 h intervals as necessary.[1,2,17]

Septic shock: Dose and dosage regimens have not been established. Although naloxone causes a sustained increase in the blood pressure of those with septic shock,[18-20] it does not appear to improve survival.[21] To date, there have not been any controlled trials in children. Three case reports have described success with 0.01–0.05 mg/kg/dose intermittently in infants and children with septic shock secondary to *Neisseria meningitides, Escherichia coli,* and group B streptococcus.[15,22,23] Intermittent doses have been followed by infusions of 0.13–0.45 mg/kg/h.[15]

Dosage adjustment in organ dysfunction	Although one reference notes no adjustment necessary in renal dysfunction,[24] the manufacturer recommends use with caution in patients with renal or hepatic dysfunction.[1]

Maximum dosage	Not established.[1] 0.4 mg/kg in neonate[25] or 2 mg/dose in those >5 years or weighing >20 kg.[1,4,10,13] If no response is seen after 10-mg total dose, diagnosis of opioid toxicity is questionable.[16] An 8-day-old received 0.45 mg/kg/h for 2 h without toxicity.[15] A total of 0.8 mg/kg was given in 27 h to a 1-month-old without adverse effects.[26] A 0.16-mg/kg/h continuous infusion was given to infants for 5 days without adverse effects.[14] A 4½-year-old received 11 doses of 0.2 mg (2.2 mg) and a 2½-year-old was accidentally given 20 mg without adverse effects.[1] A 13-year-old required a cumulative dose of 0.65 mg/kg over 65.6 h.[27] A 17-year-old received 0.8 mg/h for 15.5 h.[28]
IV push	0.2, 0.4, or 1 mg/mL undiluted over 30 sec.[29] The 0.02-mg/mL product is not recommended in neonates due to excessive fluid loads.[9]
Intermittent infusion	No information available to support administration by this method.
Continuous infusion	4 mcg/mL in D5W or NS for continuous infusion.[1,30] An 8-mcg/mL solution has been infused in an infant.[12] Diluted solutions should be used within 24 h.[30]
Other routes of administration	Naloxone can be given SC, IM, and ET.[2,4] The American Academy of Pediatrics does not recommend it be given IM or SC do to erratic absorption[10] but does suggest ET administration is acceptable.[10] Conversely, the American Heart Association notes that there is no evidence to support a specific ET dose.[4] When used, the ET doses is the same as that for opiate intoxication/dependency and should be followed by a 5-mL NS flush and five ventilations.[4] It can also be given intraosseously.[4]
Maximum concentration	1 mg/mL for IV push.[29]
Cautions related to IV administration	None.
Other additives	Some products contain methylparabens or propylparabens.[1] Paraben preservatives may cause hypersensitivity reactions that are more common with cutaneous exposure.[31] However, one case of pruritus and bronchospasm that occurred following infusion of hydrocortisone, which contained parabens, has been reported.[32]
Comments	Acute withdrawal may occur in patients who are dependent on opioids; therefore, individuals receiving naloxone should be monitored for at least 2 h after their last dose of naloxone.[5] A large dose may be required to antagonize buprenophine due to its prolonged duration, slow rate of binding, and slow dissociation from the opioid receptor.[1] Two adolescents developed acute pulmonary edema postoperatively after receiving 0.1 and 0.5 mg of naloxone, respectively.[33] Some clinicians advocate administration of half the initial bolus dose 15 min after the start of a continuous infusion to prevent a decrease in serum naloxone concentrations, but this practice has not been substantiated in children.[16]

Nesiritide

Brand names	Natrecor
Dosage	Safety and effectiveness in pediatric patients has not been established. **Congestive heart failure:** 1–2 mcg/kg IV bolus (see Comments section) followed by a continuous infusion of 0.01 mcg/kg/min.[1-10] Increases in continuous infusion rates by 0.005 mcg/kg/min are recommended at 2–3 h intervals to a maximum of 0.03 mg/kg/min.[1-10] Infusions of up to 0.09 mcg/kg/min have been reported in children on ECMO.[11] Higher dosing requirements in patients on ECMO may be related to drug's incompatibility with heparin. **Pulmonary hypertension:** Limited success reported in children with pulmonary hypertension following postcardiac repair. Intermittent infusion up to 0.2 mcg/kg/min has been given directly into the pulmonary artery.[12] **Septic shock/trauma:** Variable results reported in cases following infusions of 0.01–0.04 mcg/kg/min.[13-15]
Dosage adjustment in organ dysfunction	Although no dose modifications are recommended by the manufacturer, patients with cirrhosis and ascites have had reduced responses to nesiritide.[2] Increased dosing and/or avoidance of its use are suggested.[2] No dose adjustment is recommended for renal failure; however, increases in serum creatinine have been reported during therapy.[1,2]
Maximum dosage	The maximum recommended dose by the manufacturer is 0.03 mcg/kg/min.[1] Reports of up to 0.09 mcg/kg/min in a pediatric ECMO patient treated for hypertension[11]; however, larger dosing requirements may be due to drug's incompatibility with heparin in the ECMO circuit. Doses of 0.1 mcg/kg/min have been used in *adults* with congestive heart failure.[5] The manufacturer recommends the duration of infusion not exceed 72 h[1-3]; however, it has been given for up to 45 days in a patient awaiting heart transplantation.[7]
IV push	Loading doses of 1–2 mcg/kg should be administered over 60 sec.[1-3]
Intermittent infusion	Not recommended due to short half-life of agent.[1,16]
Continuous infusion	The contents of a vial (1.5 mg) should be reconstituted and 6 mcg/mL in D5W, NS, D5½NS, or D5¼NS.[1-3]
Other routes of administration	No information available to support administration by other routes.
Maximum concentration	The maximum concentration for administration recommended by the manufacturer is 6 mcg/mL.[1-3]

Cautions related to IV administration

Because hypotension is a dose-limiting adverse effect that may be prolonged, nesiritide should not be titrated at frequent intervals as done with other medications that have a short half-life.[1-3] (See Comments section.)

Nesiritide is an *E. coli* derived product; therefore, appropriate precautions should be taken during infusions in case of allergic reactions.[1]

Although information on infusion compatibility is limited, known incompatibilities include heparin, bumetanide, enalaprilat, ethacrynic acid, furosemide, hydralazine, insulin,[3] nitroglycerin,[11] and injectable drugs or solutions containing sodium metabisulfite.[2]

Due to its incompatibility with heparin, infusion through a heparin-coated catheter is not recommended.[1]

Other additives

None.

Comments

Hypotension is the dose-limiting adverse effect of nesiritide. Some pediatric intensivists recommend that the bolus dose be eliminated and that therapy begin with a continuous infusion at the recommended dose rate.[7,11] Others continue to recommend bolus dose.[6,9,10] When it occurs, hypotension may be prolonged (mean 2.2 h); therefore, observation for a prolonged period of time may be necessary.[1] Dose reductions, discontinuation of therapy, and/or supportive measures may be required.[3]

Premature ventricular contractions have been reported in children with congestive heart failure.[6] Ventricular arrhythmias and bradycardia have been reported in *adults.*[1-3]

Concerns regarding increasing serum creatinine in *adults* given the recommended infusion rates prompted an FDA MedWatch to alert practitioners of its potential effects on renal function.[16] It is unclear whether increases in serum creatinine reflect hemodynamic effects or renal effects.[3,5,16] A recent report indicated the successful management of heart failure in a term infant with polycystic kidney disease without worsening of renal function.[17] Additionally, concerns for increased mortality rates in *adults* receiving nesiritide have prompted further investigation into its impact on survival of patients with congestive heart failure.[16]

An overdose of 36 mcg/kg was reported in a child with decompensated heart failure resulting in no hemodynamic change, renal function, and/or changes in inotropic and/or vasopressor support.[17] The patient later underwent successful heart transplantation and developed no untoward long-term effects.

Nicardipine

Brand names	Cardene

Dosage

Hypertensive emergency/severe hypertension, hypertension on ECMO, during or postsurgery, and hypertension related to renal disease or postcoarctectomy

Neonates (preterm)[1,2]

Initial: 0.5 mcg/kg/d.

Maintenance: 0.5–2 mcg/kg/min; titrate q 15–30 min until target blood pressure achieved.

Has been given for up to 36–43 days.

Neonates (term) and infants

Initial: 0.5–1 mcg/kg/d[3,4]; one patient received 5 mcg/kg/min.[5]

Maintenance: 1.5–3 mcg/kg/min[3,6]; titrate q 15–30 min until target blood pressure achieved.

Children 1–17 years

Initial: 1–5 mcg/kg/min[3,5,7-11]; some patients have received an initial dose of 10 mcg/kg/min.[5,9,10]

Maintenance: Typically 2–3 (range 1–6) mcg/kg/min; titrate q 15–30 min until target blood pressure achieved.[4,5,7-17]

In hypertensive emergencies, blood pressure should be frequently monitored to ensure that it does not decrease too quickly.[18-20] One group recommended that the blood pressure decrease by one-third of the desired total blood pressure decrease within 6–12 h, a further one-third decrease within the next 24 h, with the final one-third decrease achieved over the next 2 days.[13] Alternatively, a blood pressure decrease of <25% within minutes to 1 h followed by further decreases over the next 2–6 h if the patient is stable has been suggested.[18]

Dosage adjustment in organ dysfunction

No dose adjustment is recommended for renal impairment; however, conservative doses are recommended since patients with renal insufficiency may respond to lower doses or accumulate drug.[15,21]

Since nicardipine is extensively metabolized by the liver, plasma concentrations will be elevated and half-life prolonged with hepatic failure; therefore, dose adjustment is warranted.[15,19]

While one reference suggests that nicardipine may be used in children with cardiac disease,[22] the manufacturer recommends caution when administering nicardipine to patients with heart failure or significant left ventricular dysfunction due to a potential negative inotropic effect.[19]

Maximum dosage

Initial: 10 mcg/kg/min.[5,9]

Maintenance: 6 mcg/kg/min.[17]

IV push

Not recommended.[19,23]

Intermittent infusion

Not recommended.[19,23]

Nicardipine

Continuous infusion	10 mL of nicardipine (25 mg) must be diluted before infusion by adding to 240 mL of D5W, D5½NS, D5NS, D5+40 mEq/L potassium, ½NS, or NS to achieve a final concentration of 0.1 mg/mL. Titrate to desired effect.[19,23] More concentrated solutions (0.5 mg/mL) have been used in volume-restricted patients,[4,8,11] but thrombophlebitis has occurred.[8,11] A concentration of 3.6 mg/mL has been infused safely via a central line.[11]
Other routes of administration	No information available to support administration by other routes.
Maximum concentration	0.1 mg/mL per manufacturer.[19] A 3.6-mg/mL concentration has been infused safely via a central line.[11]
Cautions related to IV administration	If administered via peripheral line, change sites q 12 h to avoid venous irritation/thrombophlebitis.[23] Nicardipine is not compatible with sodium bicarbonate or LR.[19]
Other additives	Each ampule contains 48 mg sorbitol/mL.[19,23]
Comments	May see reflex tachycardia[5,12,13,15]; propranolol has been used to treat tachycardia.[5] Avoid use in patients with space-occupying cerebral lesions due to increased intraocular pressure.[7] One report describes the sudden drop in blood pressure in two of four severely asphyxiated term neonates; use nicardipine in asphyxiated patients with caution and under careful blood pressure monitoring.[24] An accidental nicardipine overdose in a pregnant patient resulted in no serious maternal or neonatal consequence.[25] Nicardipine may have drug interactions with concomitant medications, including cyclosporine (increased cyclosporine concentrations), beta-blockers, cimetidine, and fentanyl.[19] Consult appropriate resources for dosing recommendations before combining any drug with a potential interaction.

Nitroglycerin

Brand names	Nitro-Bid I.V., Nitrostat I.V., Tridil
Dosage	When standard polyvinyl chloride (PVC) IV tubing is used, significant drug is absorbed to the tubing.[1,2] Thus, the apparent doses required to achieve a desired clinical response are increased.[1,2] **Neonates, infants, and children:** Begin infusion at 0.1–1 mcg/kg/min and increase by 0.5–1 mcg/kg/min q 3–5 min until desired clinical response,[3-5] usually ≤20 mcg/kg/min.[6] **Adolescents and adults:** Begin infusion at 5 mcg/min and increase by 5 mcg/min q 3–5 min. If the desired response is not achieved at 20 mcg/min, increase by 10 mcg/min and later by 20 mcg/min until desired clinical response.[1,2] Responses are usually noted with infusion rates from 5–100 mcg/min.[2] In hypersensitive emergencies, blood pressure should be frequently monitored to ensure that it does not decrease too quickly.[2] One group recommended that the blood pressure decrease by one-third of the desired total blood pressure decrease within 6–12 h, a further one-third decrease within the next 24 h, with the final one-third decrease achieved over the next 2 days.[7] A blood pressure decrease of <25% within min to 1 h followed by further decreases over the next 2–6 h if the patient is stable has been suggested.[2] (See Cautions related to IV administration section.)
Dosage adjustment in organ dysfunction	No dosage adjustment required.
Maximum dosage	60 mcg/kg/min was infused for ≤30 min to infants and children with congenital heart defects who had a low cardiac index postoperatively; however, the type of tubing used for the infusion was not stated.[4] In *adults* with hypertension, doses up to 100 mcg/min have been used.[1,2] In *adults* with acute MI, the risk of hypotension increases with doses approaching 200 mcg/min.[1,2]
IV push	Not indicated.
Intermittent infusion	Not indicated.
Continuous infusion	Initial concentrations of 50–100 mcg/mL in D5W or NS using an infusion control device are recommended; however, patient factors such as fluid requirements and duration of therapy may warrant use of more concentrated solutions.[1,2,8] Nitroglycerin readily absorbs to many plastics; therefore, glass infusion bottles and non-PVC administration sets are recommended. If PVC sets are used, larger doses are required.[1,2,8] Avoid filters, some of which absorb nitroglycerin.[1,2,8]
Other routes of administration	Not indicated.
Maximum concentration	400 mcg/mL.[1,7]

Cautions related to IV administration

Severe hypotension and shock can occur with small doses.[1] Monitor blood pressure and heart rate closely.[1]

For PN compatibility information, please see Appendix C.

Other additives

Nitroglycerin injection contains 30% ethanol and 30% propylene glycol in water.[1,2] Nitroglycerin in dextrose solution also contains ethanol and propylene glycol.[1,2]

Propylene glycol is added to parenteral drugs as a solubilizer. Rapid infusion of medications that contain propylene glycol has resulted in respiratory depression and cardiac dysrhythmias.[9] Its half-life is three times longer in neonates than in *adults*[10] and has caused hyperosmolality[11] and refractory seizures[12] in preterm neonates receiving 3 g/d.

Comments

In *adults*, tolerance to hemodynamic effects of nitroglycerin is observed within 12–48 h after beginning continuous infusion. If such tolerance occurs, intermittent therapy or a nitrate-free interval ≥8 h after 12–48 h of continuous infusion is recommended.[13]

Methemoglobinemia was associated with doses >7 mcg/kg/min in *adults*.[14,15] However, methemoglobinemia did not occur in 16 pediatric patients (3 days–23.7 months) who received concomitant IV nitroglycerin (0.5–4 mcg/kg/min) and sodium nitroprusside (0.3–8.4 mcg/kg/min) for 0.5–7.6 days.[16]

Norepinephrine Bitartrate

Brand names	Levophed
Dosage	**Infants and children:** Initially, 0.05–0.1 mcg/kg/min titrated to the desired blood pressure.[1-3] Usual maximum doses are 1–2 mcg/kg/min. **Adolescents and adults:** Initially, 4 mcg/min titrated to the desired blood pressure.[1,4] Usual maintenance doses are 2–4 mcg/min and usual maximum doses are 8–12 mcg/kg/min.[4] The intravascular volume should be corrected as fully as possible before starting norepinephrine.[1,4] Avoid abrupt withdrawal by gradually reducing the dose.[4] Abrupt discontinuation may cause acute, severe hypotension due to the short half-life and duration of effect (1–2 min after cessation of infusion).[1]
Dosage adjustment in organ dysfunction	No dosage adjustment required in renal dysfunction.
Maximum dosage	In *adults* with refractory shock an infusion of up to 30 mcg/min or 68 mg/d has been used.[1,4]
IV push	Not indicated.
Intermittent infusion	Not recommended.
Continuous infusion	4–16 mcg/mL in D5S or D5W infused into a large vein.[4-6] Dilution with dextrose-containing solutions protects against significant loss of potency from oxidation.[1,4] (See Comments section.)
Other routes of administration	Not indicated.
Maximum concentration	16 mcg/mL in D5W.[5]
Cautions related to IV administration	If possible, infuse via central,[7] antecubital, or femoral vein using a plastic catheter to decrease the risk of necrosis of overlying skin.[1] Extravasation may cause local ischemia and tissue necrosis.[1,4,8,9] Aliquots of phentolamine mesylate 5–10 mg in 10 mL of NS, infiltrated with a fine hypodermic needle into and around the extravasation area, should reverse blanching immediately. This should be done within the first 12 h of extravasation.[1,4] For PN compatibility information, please see Appendix C.
Other additives	Contains sodium metabisulfite. Sulfites may cause hypersensitivity reactions and these are more common in *adults* with asthma. Most reactions are mild but can include anaphylactic symptoms and life-threatening or less severe asthma episodes.[10-12] Epinephrine may be required in severe cases; and if the sulfite-free product is not available, the sulfite-preserved epinephrine should be used.[10]

Norepinephrine Bitartrate

Comments

Norepinephrine is easily destroyed by oxidants and in alkaline solutions; therefore, solutions should be protected from light.[4] Do not infuse if solution is pinkish or darker than slightly yellow or if it contains a precipitate.[4]

Several drugs (e.g., tricyclic antidepressants, MAO inhibitors, etc.) may potentiate the pressor effects of norepinephrine.[4] Atropine may block the reflex bradycardia and enhances the pressor response caused by norepinephrine.[1] Therefore, consult appropriate resources before combining any drug with norepinephrine.

Octreotide Acetate

Brand names	Sandostatin

Dosage

Chylothorax/chyloperitoneum: 0.3–2 mcg/kg/h via continuous IV infusion initially; gradually increase dose until effect seen.[1-6]

10 mcg/kg/d in three divided SQ doses; increase dose by 5–10 mcg/kg/d at 48- to 72-h intervals until effect seen (typically up to 20–40 mcg/kg/d).[1,5,7-10]

Diarrhea/increased gastrointestinal output: 13–200 mcg/d SC or IV in two divided doses.[11-16] Doses of 1.4–20 mcg/kg/d divided q 12 h have been used.[11,12,14-16] An alternative method is continuous infusion 1 mcg/kg/h.[17] Begin at low end of dosage range and increase by 0.3 mcg/kg/dose q 3 d.[11]

Excessive growth hormone (GH) secretion/tall stature (use not established): 100–500 mcg two to three times daily up to 1500 mcg/d has been used but has not fully suppressed GH levels.[16,18]

Children: 300–600 mcg/d in three divided doses.[16,18]

Adolescents: 500–1500 mcg/d in two to three divided doses.[16]

One study found 37.5 mcg (prepubertal) or 50 mcg (pubertal) given via SQ injection 1 h before bedtime to be effective in children.[19] Continuous SC infusion with the bulk of the total daily dose given overnight has been found to be superior to SC or depot injection therapy.[18]

Fistula closure

Neonates: 1.4 mcg/kg/d SC divided bid, gradually increased up to 5 mcg/kg/d SC divided bid.[20]

Children: 50–300 mcg/d SC divided in two to three doses. Start at lower end of dosage range and increase gradually.[21,22]

Gastrointestinal bleeding: 1–2 mcg/kg bolus, followed by either 1 mcg/kg/h IV infusion or 3 mcg/kg/d IV divided q 8 h. Older children have received an *adult* dose of 50 mcg bolus over 5 min followed by 50 mcg/h. Continuous infusion can be increased q 8 h if no decrease in bleeding. Dose is tapered by 50% q 12 h when no active bleeding for 24 h and can be stopped when dose is 25% of initial dose.[23-25] For chronic GI bleeding, 4–8 mcg/kg/d SC has been given with concurrent iron therapy.[26]

Hyperinsulinemia/hypoglycemia of infancy: Initial doses of 2–10 mcg/kg/d in two to six doses SC.[27-34] Doses are titrated up to 40 mcg/kg/d based on glucose concentrations. Total daily dose may be given SC in divided doses or continuous infusion via a SC or IV infusion pump.[16,27,30]

Pancreatitis/pancreatic tumors: A 10-year-old child received 1.5 mcg/kg/h IV for pancreatic pseudocyst.[35] A 15-month-old infant received 2 mcg/kg SC q 6 h increased up to 20 mcg/kg for recurrent acute pancreatitis and ascites.[36]

Sulfonylurea poisoning: In children, a single 25-mcg dose can be given IV. Dose and duration vary depending on amount of sulfonylurea ingested and its half-life.[37-41] SC, IV, and continuous infusion are appropriate routes, and 2 mcg/kg/d SC divided q 12 h has also been cited as appropriate.[37]

Dosage adjustment in organ dysfunction

In patients with renal failure requiring dialysis, the dose may need to be adjusted secondary to increased half-life.[42]

Maximum dosage

No data for maximum dosage in children. (See Comments section.) In *adults*, the maximum dose is 1500 mcg/d divided q 8 h.[42] An infant has received as much as 2000 mcg/d.[13]

IV push	In emergency situations, octreotide may be administered undiluted over 3 min.[43]
Intermittent infusion	Dilute with 50–200 mL of D5W or NS and infuse over 15–30 min.[43]
Continuous infusion	Dilute with NS or D5W and infuse over 24 h.[43] Manufacturer states that octreotide should not be added to PN because of the formation of glycosyl octreotide conjugate[42]; however, this is controversial.[43,44]
Other routes of administration	SC injection is the usual route of administration.[42] IM administration with depot form only (Sandostatin LAR® Depot). Reconstitute with provided diluent and administer immediately after reconstitution into gluteal area at 4-week intervals.[42]
Maximum concentration	No information available.
Cautions related to IV administration	None known. For PN compatibility information, please see Appendix C.
Other additives	None.
Comments	Do not confuse with Sandostatin LAR® Depot. SC injection sites should be rotated.[42,43] A 6-month-old infant died of fulminant colitis after receiving somatostatin analogue in a dose of 18 mcg/kg/d.[45] Prior to the infant's death, the dose had been decreased to 3.5 mcg/kg/d. A 16-month-old with enterocutaneous fistula developed sudden abdominal pain and increased nasogastric drainage and died 8 h after receiving a single 100 mcg SC dose of somatostatin analogue.[42] One report associated the use of octreotide for postoperative chylothorax to the development of necrotizing enterocolitis in an infant.[3] A neonate receiving 30 mcg/kg/d developed an increase in direct bilirubin and gamma glutamine transferase on day 7 of therapy. Ultrasound revealed ascites and biliary sludging. All symptoms resolved with termination of therapy.[7] Asymptomatic gallstones were found in an infant 1 year after being started on octreotide.[27] Fat malabsorption documented by fecal fat testing was observed in one infant on prolonged octreotide therapy.[34] Tachyphylaxis is a common occurrence, requiring larger doses to maintain similar effect, especially when used in patients with hyperinsulinism.[28,30,31]

Ondansetron HCl

Brand names Zofran

Dosage

Chemotherapy-induced nausea and vomiting: 0.15 mg/kg q 4 h for two or three doses. The first dose infusion should be started 30 min before emetogenic chemotherapy.[1-7] Alternatively, a single 0.6-mg/kg dose (≤32 mg/dose) was as effective as 0.15 mg/kg (≤8 mg) q 4 h for four doses in pediatric oncology patients.[6] Another group of investigators compared 5 or 10 mg/m^2 (≤16 mg) and found no difference in efficacy.[8] A third group noted a dose-dependent reduction in vomiting in children (n = 26; 18 months–15 years) given 0.15 mg/kg or 0.45 mg/kg 30 min prior to intrathecal chemotherapy.[9] (See Comments section.)

In *adults*, a single 32-mg dose is given before chemotherapy.[3] A loading dose of 8 mg followed by a continuous infusion of 1 mg/h for 24 h has also been used in *adults*.[3,10] (See Continuous infusion section.)

Prevention of postoperative nausea and vomiting: The manufacturer recommends a single dose of 0.1 mg/kg for those <1 month old and ≤40 kg or a single dose of 4 mg for those >40 kg and up to 12 years of age.[1] Other investigators report infusing 0.025–0.15 mg/kg immediately before induction of anesthesia or postoperatively in symptomatic patients.[11-18] One study noted that 0.075 mg/kg was as effective as 0.1–0.15 mg/kg.[17] Another study in infants (1–24 months; n = 670) undergoing general anesthesia and general surgery, established both safety and efficacy of a single dose of 0.1 mg/kg for the prevention of postoperative vomiting.[19] Administration of a second dose in patients who fail to respond will not improve control.[1] (See Comments section.)

Emergency department treatment of acute gastroenteritis: 0.15 mg/kg, infused over 2 min in children 1 month–22 years, reduced the need for hospital admission and decreased the number of vomiting episodes in the acute period of illness.[20]

Dosage adjustment in organ dysfunction

No dosage adjustment required in renal dysfunction.[1,21] In severe liver disease, a single dose of 8 mg in *adults* is recommended.[1]

Maximum dosage

0.45 mg/kg[8] up to 32 mg.[6] In *adults*, up to 150 mg/dose and total daily doses of 252 mg have been inadvertently given without adverse effects.[1]

IV push

Undiluted, over >30 sec. It is preferable to administer over 2–5 min.[1]

Intermittent infusion

Dilute in D5W or NS (if not premixed) and infuse over 15 min.[1,4,21]

Continuous infusion

Although continuous infusion has been used in *adults*,[3] its use has not been reported for pediatric patients. (See Dosage section.)

Other routes of administration

Can be given IM in *adults*.

Maximum concentration	2 mg/mL (undiluted).[1]
Cautions related to IV administration	An anaphylactoid reaction occurred in an 11-year-old girl.[22] Blood pressure changes and increased QTc interval have been reported in *adults*.[23] For PN compatibility information, please see Appendix C.
Other additives	Each mL of the 2-mL single-dose vial contains 9 mg NaCl, 0.5 mg of citric acid monohydrate, and 0.25 mg of sodium citrate dihydrate. Each mL of the 20-mL multidose vial contains 8.3 mg NaCl, 0.5 mg citric acid monohydrate, 0.25 mg of sodium citrate dihydrate, 1.2 mg of methylparaben, and 0.15 mg of propylparaben.[1] Paraben preservatives may cause hypersensitivity reactions that are more common with cutaneous exposure.[24] However, one case of pruritus and bronchospasm that occurred following infusion of hydrocortisone, which contained a paraben, has been reported.[25]
Comments	Compared to those 4–12 months old, infants 1–4 months have decreased clearance resulting in a prolonged half-life.[1] Those <4 months should be closely monitored.[1] Adolescents and children have a higher clearance and shorter half-life than *adults*.[1] 0.15 mg/kg prior to and again immediately following chemotherapy did not prevent nausea in children receiving cyclophosphamide.[4] The manufacturer reports a vasovagal episode with transient second-degree heart block was observed in a patient (age not specified) given 32 mg over 4 min, and sudden blindness lasting 2–3 min and severe constipation occurred in another patient (age not specified) given a single, 72-mg dose.[1] Because ondansetron is metabolized by the cytochrome P450 isozymes, it may serve as a substrate and can be inhibited or induced by other drugs. Consult appropriate resources for dosing recommendations before combining any drug with ondansetron.[26]

Oxacillin Sodium

Brand names	Bactocill, Prostaphlin

Dosage

Serious anaphylactoid reactions may require immediate emergency treatment with epinephrine, oxygen, IV steroids, and airway management.[10]

Neonates

PNA	≤1200 g	≤2000 g	>2000 g
≤7 d	50 mg/kg/d divided q 12 h.[1,2]*	50–100 mg/kg/d divided q 12 h[2-5]	75–150 mg/kg/d divided q 8 h[2-5]
>7 d		75–150 mg/kg/d divided q 8 h[2-4]	100–200 mg/kg/d divided q 6 h[2-5]

*Until 4 weeks of age.

Infants and children: 100–200 mg/kg/d divided q 4–6 h depending on disease severity.[2,3,5-8]

Dosage adjustment in organ dysfunction

Adjust dosage in patients with severe renal dysfunction by using the lower end of the dosage range if CrCl <10 mL/min.[9,10]

Maximum dosage

≤12 g/d was recommended for *adults* with endocarditis osteomyelitis.[11,12] Although doses of 400 mg/kg/d have been given, they have been associated with hepatotoxicity.[13]

IV push

100 mg/mL in SW, ½NS, and NS.[10,11,14] Should be infused over at least 10 min.[10,11,14] To minimize vein irritation, inject as slowly as possible.[10]

Intermittent infusion

0.5–40 mg/mL[10,11,14] in D5W, LR, NS, D5NS, or ½NS[10] administered over 15–30 min.[10,11] If given peripherally, consider infusing over 60 min at a maximum concentration of 20 mg/mL.[15] Slowing the infusion (e.g., 60 min) may minimize vein irritation.[10]

Continuous infusion

Although solution concentration and type were not specified, oxacillin has been given by this method.[11] Rate of infusion should be adjusted so total dose of oxacillin is administered before >10% of potency is lost.[10]

Other routes of administration

167 mg/mL in SW, NS, or ½NS may be given by deep IM injection in same doses as IV.[3,10,11]

Maximum concentration

100 mg/mL for IV push and ≤40 mg/mL for infusion.[14]

Cautions related to IV administration

If a decision is made to give this medication to a patient with known penicillin hypersensitivity, the patient should be closely observed for allergenicity.[13-19] (See Comments section.)

For PN compatibility information, please see Appendix C.

Other additives

Contains 2.5–3.1 mEq sodium/g of oxacillin sodium.[11]

Comments

Patients with a history of type I reaction to penicillin should not receive beta-lactam antibiotics. From 5% to 15% of patients allergic to penicillin will also be allergic to cephalosporins. Certain infections (e.g., syphilis) require penicillin for cure. It is recommended that a desensitization protocol for penicillin-allergic individuals should be performed in a hospital setting. This can usually be completed in about 4 h, at which time the first dose of penicillin can be given.[2]

The beta-lactam ring of penicillins can link with an amino sugar of the aminoglycoside and inactivate the aminoglycoside.[20-22] To avoid this potential interaction, administer penicillins 1 h before or after an aminoglycoside, adequately flush the infusion line between each infusion, or infuse them through separate lines. *In vivo* inactivation that is dose dependent can also occur particularly in patients with renal failure.[22-24] In patients with end-stage renal failure, gentamicin half-life was decreased by 22–31 h after carbenicillin or ticarcillin was added to the drug regimen.[23]

Palivizumab

Brand names	Synagis
Dosage	**Premature neonates born at ≤35 weeks gestation who are ≤1 year of age and infants <2 years of age with chronic lung disease (CLD) or bronchopulmonary dysplasia (BPD) or stable hemodynamically significant (cyanotic or acyanotic) congenital heart disease** **Outpatient prevention of RSV disease:** 15 mg/kg IM in the anterolateral aspect of the thigh repeated q 30 d during the RSV season for up to five doses (November through March).[1-5] Smaller doses (3–10 mg/kg) were associated with insufficient serum antibody concentrations.[6,7] **Inpatient prevention of RSV disease:** Two reports from different NICUs with RSV outbreaks stated that none of the infants who received 15 mg/kg IM q 4 weeks contracted RSV.[8,9] Another study in an NICU setting noted that only 23% of infants ≤30 weeks gestation had acceptable antibody concentrations prior to the second dose.[10] None of these infants experienced an adverse event other than injection site reactions nor did any treated infant develop RSV.[10]
Dosage adjustment in organ dysfunction	No specific information available.
Maximum dosage	15 mg/kg monthly.[5]
IV push	In pharmacokinetic studies, the drug was infused over 2–5 min or 1–2 mL/min (10 mg/mL).[7,11]
Intermittent infusion	Not indicated.
Continuous infusion	Not indicated.
Other routes of administration	100 mg/mL preferably administered in the anterolateral aspect of the thigh. Administration into the gluteal muscle may be associated with damage to the sciatic nerve and is, therefore, not recommended.[5]
Maximum concentration	10 mg/mL for IV use[7,11] and 100 mg/mL for IM use.[4,5]
Cautions related to IV administration	The manufacturer does not recommend IV administration.

Other additives	**Liquid solution formulation:** The 100-mg product contains 4.7 mg of histidine and 0.1 mg of glycine. The 50-mg product contains 2.7 mg of histidine and 0.08 mg of glycine.[5] **Lyophilized powder formulation:** The 100-mg product contains 67.5 mg of mannitol, 8.7 mg of histidine, and 0.3 mg of glycine. The 50-mg product contains 40.5 mg of mannitol, 5.2 mg of histidine, and 0.2 mg of glycine.[5] Since neither product contains a preservative, the vial should not be re-entered to draw additional doses.

Comments

Infants receiving monthly injections of 15 mg/kg of palivizumab may not have protective antibody levels (>40 mcg/mL) until after the second injection,[5] especially in premature infants with a gestational age ≤30 weeks when administered a month or more before anticipated discharge.[10]

Administration of palivizumab IV to patients in the acute phase of RSV illness will not improve clinical outcomes nor cause an exacerbation of the infection[11]; however, concentrations of virus in tracheal aspirates were reduced when administered at standard prophylactic doses.[12]

Studies with RSV Immunoglobulin Intravenous (Respigam) showed a higher risk of adverse events in patients with cyanotic congenital heart disease. This phenomenon was not observed in patients with cyanotic and acyanotic congenital heart disease who received palivizumab.[13]

It is available as a lyophilized powder and as a premixed solution. According to package labeling, once opened or reconstituted, vials of palivizumab must be used within 6 h.[5]

It is not recommended that either product be administered intravenously.[5] Palivizumab should be administered IM in divided doses if the dosage volume exceeds 1 mL. Additional doses should be given as indicated during the RSV season to complete five doses even if the patient develops RSV infection.

Serum concentrations decreased by a mean of 58% following cardiopulmonary bypass in pediatric patients receiving open heart surgery, thus additional dosing after surgery may be required.[5]

Rare cases of acute hypersensitivity reactions or anaphylaxis have been reported in patients receiving palivizumab.[5]

Pamidronate

Brand names	Aredia
Dosage	Little information is available on the use of pamidronate in children. **Hypercalcemia:** 0.5–1 mg/kg[1-5] or 35–50 mg/m^2[6] over 2–6 h as a single dose or repeated for 1[6] or 2 more days.[5] One group repeated the initial 0.5-mg/kg dose on days 1–3 and then decreased the dose to 0.25 mg/kg on day 4 and 0.125 mg/kg on day 5.[7] One report described three children with renal failure who became hypercalcemic; one developed fractures, one had symptomatic hypercalcemia, and the third developed avascular necrosis related to high-dose steroids.[8] Doses ranged from 0.4–0.5 mg/kg, and in the 11-year-old boy with fractures, were repeated at least three times.[8] Most who were treated for hypercalcemia had failed conventional therapy. (See Comments section.) **Osteogenesis imperfecta:** Regimens vary[9-12] but in general range from 1–1.5 mg/kg given every other month or q 3 mo (6 or 9 mg/kg/y).[13-15] Calcium and vitamin D supplements are usually provided. Treatment has continued for several years. Because of concerns over growth, one group discontinued treatment for 2 years and found that bone metabolism continues to be suppressed, improvements in bone mass continue, but children fail to achieve normal bone growth.[16] **McCune Albright syndrome:** 0.5 mg/kg over 4 h for 2–3 days each year[17] then 1 mg/kg daily for 3 days q 4–6 mo for up to 6 years.[17,18] **Osteoporosis/osteopenia:** 0.4–0.5 mg/kg over 2–4 h for 3 days q 3–6 mo for up to 13 months in children with cerebral palsy.[19,20] Seventeen children on steroids for endocrine or renal disease who developed fractures were given 1 mg/kg q 2 mo for 1 or 2 years.[21] Patients were also prescribed calcium and vitamin D supplements.[20,21]
Dosage adjustment in organ dysfunction	None recommended by manufacturer.[22] Excessive accumulation of pamidronate is not anticipated when the drug is administered monthly.[22] In cancer patients, renal clearance was found to correlate closely with creatinine clearance.
Maximum dosage	1.5 mg/kg has been used in osteogenesis imperfecta.[15] 90 mg in *adults*.[22]
IV push	Contraindicated.
Intermittent infusion	In *adults*, 30–90 mg to be infused over ≥2–4 h. Longer infusion times decrease the risk for renal toxicity.[22]
Continuous infusion	90 mg infused over 24 h in *adults*.
Other routes of administration	No information available to support administration by other routes.
Maximum concentration	90 mg diluted in 250 mL (0.36 mg/mL).[22]
Cautions related to IV administration	Infusion site reactions occur.[23]

Other additives	Each 30- and 90-mg vial contains 470 mg and 375 mg, respectively, of mannitol.

Comments

A transient, low-grade fever 24–48 h after the initial infusion is common and not usually present with subsequent infusions.[1,9,13,14,17,21]

Symptomatic and asymptomatic hypocalcemia has been reported.[4,9,23]

Pamidronate has been used in children with renal disease with no worsening of renal function.[8]

Osteonecrosis of the jaw has been reported in cancer patients on chemotherapy who also receive pamidronate. It is recommended that while on pamidronate extensive dental surgery should be avoided.[22]

Albumin-corrected serum calcium = serum calcium (mg/dL) + 0.8 (4.0 – serum albumin [mg/dL]).[22]

Pancuronium Bromide

Brand names	Pavulon
Dosage	Respiratory function must be supported during use of this agent. Concurrent administration of a sedative is also necessary. Monitoring of neuromuscular transmission with a peripheral nerve stimulator is recommended during continuous infusion or with repeated dosing.[1] **Endotracheal intubation and maintenance of neuromuscular blockade** **Neonates**: Because neonates are particularly sensitive to nondepolarizing agents, a test dose of 0.02 mg/kg should be given to assess responsiveness.[1] 0.03–0.1 mg/kg repeated as necessary q 1–2 h to maintain muscle relaxation or 0.02–0.04 mg/kg/h as continuous infusion.[2-8] **Infants and children:** 0.08–0.15 mg/kg initially and then 0.02–0.2 mg/kg repeated as required or 0.03-0.1 mg/kg/h as continuous infusion.[1,9-12]
Dosage adjustment in organ dysfunction	Adjust dosage in patients with renal dysfunction.[1,13,14] If CrCl is 10–50 mL/min, give 50% of a normal dose; if CrCl is <10 mL/min, do not use.[13,14] Although clearance is decreased, volume of distribution is significantly increased in patients with liver dysfunction; hence, these patients may require large doses.[1,15]
Maximum dosage	Cumulative dose of 0.3 mg/kg was given within several minutes to a newborn infant without adverse effects.[7] One study used up to 0.5 mg/kg as a single dose in neonates with hyaline membrane disease.[19] Although doses up to 0.16 mg/kg have been used, large doses may increase frequency and severity of tachycardia.[1,16]
IV push	1 or 2 mg/mL given rapidly over seconds.[1]
Intermittent infusion	No information available to support administration by this method.
Continuous infusion	0.01–0.8 mg/mL in D5NS, D5W, LR, or NS.[1]
Other routes of administration	IM administration is not recommended.[1]
Maximum concentration	2 mg/mL for IV push or 0.8 mg/mL for continuous infusion.[1]
Cautions related to IV administration	Cardiac dysrhythmias, tachycardia, and hypertension have been reported.[6,10,17] Joint contractures have occurred in neonates.[18] Anaphylaxis has occurred in *adults*.[19]

Other additives

Benzyl alcohol: Multidose vials contain benzyl alcohol 0.9% as a preservative.[1] Administration of flushes containing benzyl alcohol (bacteriostatic water for injection) was associated with a fatal gasping syndrome, intraventricular hemorrhage, metabolic acidosis, and increased mortality in preterm infants.[20] While benzyl alcohol in small doses as a preservative in drugs is considered safe in newborns,[21] a 3-week-old, very low birth weight (710 g) infant experienced a profound desaturation that required resuscitation after receiving clindamycin (third and fourth doses), which was subsequently related to the benzyl alcohol preservative.[22]

Hypersensitivity reactions to benzyl alcohol in parenteral products have been reported in *adults*.[23,24]

Comments

Prolonged paralysis (mean duration of 9 weeks) has been reported following pancuronium infusion.[25-27] Concomitant administration of corticosteroids with neuromuscular blockers has been shown to be a risk factor for this adverse effect.[28] Likewise, concomitant administration of pancuronium with certain antibiotics (e.g., aminoglycosides, clindamycin, and vancomycin) and other drugs such as ketamine, magnesium, and quinidine may also prolong neuromuscular blockade. Consult appropriate resources for additional information on drug interactions. Other factors that potentiate the duration of neuromuscular blockage include acidosis, hyponatremia, hypocalcemia, hypokalemia, and hypermagnesemia.[1,3]

Pantoprazole

Brand names	Protonix

Dosage

Experience with IV pantoprazole in children, particularly neonates and infants, is limited; currently there is no established IV dose range for pediatric patients.[1]

Initial pharmacokinetic studies of oral and IV pantoprazole in children 2–16 years of age have found similar pharmacokinetics to that observed in *adults*.[2-4] In *adults*, oral and IV dosage are similar in potency.

Doses used in pediatric IV pharmacokinetic studies[2,3]: 0.47–1.88 mg/kg/dose, maximum 80 mg (children 2–16 years).

General dosing ranges from pediatric oral dosing studies

Gastroesophageal reflux/reflux esophagitis[5]: 20 mg every day (0.5–1 mg/kg/d) for 28 days (children 6–13 years).

Adult dosing ranges (IV pantoprazole)

Gastroesophageal reflux/reflux esophagitis[1]: 40 mg every day for 7–10 days; oral formulation for maintenance.

Hypersecretory conditions[1]: 80 mg q 12 h for up to 6 days; may increase frequency to q 8 h as needed to suppress acid production.

Peptic ulcer (use not established)[6-8]: 80 mg bolus followed by continuous infusion of 8 mg/h for 3 days, followed by 40 mg q 12 h for 4–7 days.

Stress ulcer prophylaxis (use not established)[9]: 80 mg q 8–12 h.

Dosage adjustment in organ dysfunction

No dosage adjustment recommended for renal or hepatic dysfunction.[1] Doses >40 mg/d have not been used in patients with hepatic dysfunction.[1] Elimination half-life may be prolonged with hepatic dysfunction.[10]

Maximum dosage

80 mg/dose in children.[3] 240 mg/d in *adults*.[1]

IV push

May administer reconstituted 4 mg/mL solution over a minimum of 2 min.[1]

Intermittent infusion

Dilute reconstituted drug (4 mg/mL) to 0.4–0.8 mg/mL with NS, D5W, or LR and infuse over 15 min at a maximum rate of 7 mL/min.[1]

Continuous infusion

Not recommended in labeling.[1] In *adults*, a single 80-mg IV load followed by 8 mg/h has been used for 3 days.[6-8]

Other routes of administration

No information available to support administration by other routes.

Maximum concentration

4 mg/mL.[1]

Cautions related to IV administration

Injection site reactions (e.g., thrombophlebitis) have been reported with the use of IV pantoprazole.[1] Administer via a dedicated line or Y-site administration after flushing the line before and after with NS, D5W, or LR. Observe for any signs of precipitation when administering via Y-site.[1] Incompatible with midazolam, dobutamine, esmolol, norepinephrine, octreotide[10] and may be incompatible with zinc-containing solutions.[1]

Anaphylaxis has been reported.[1]

Other additives

Edetate disodium (1 mg/40-mg vial).[1]

Comments

An *adult* patient developed generalized edema following the initiation of intermittent IV pantoprazole for the treatment of pyloric stenosis.[11] Peripheral edema has been more commonly reported in patients receiving proton pump inhibitors via continuous infusion of large volumes.

Administration of proton pump inhibitors has been associated with increased risk of developing gastroenteritis and pneumonia in children.[12]

Adverse effects may include mild elevation of liver function tests.[1]

False positive urine THC has been reported in patients taking proton pump inhibitors, including pantoprazole.[1]

Pantoprazole is metabolized primarily by CYP2C19 and to a lesser extent by CYP3A4, CYP2D6, and CYP2C9. *In vivo* drug–drug interaction studies have found that pharmacokinetics are not significantly altered; therefore, there is no need for dosage reductions in general. Drug interaction potential is unknown in patients with hepatic dysfunction or in those receiving large doses.[1]

Papaverine HCl

Brand names	Generic
Dosage	**Prolongation life of arterial catheters in neonates and children**[1-3]**:** 30 mg/250 mL heparinized (1 unit/mL) NS or ½NS. (See Comments section.) **Flush of femoral artery catheter after cardiac catheterization:** A single intra-arterial flush of 1.5 mg/kg papaverine or 1 unit heparin/0.25 mL NS was mixed to a volume of 4 mL and infused over 2 min in children (3–69 months; n=56) after cardiac catheterization. Papaverine and heparin flush performed similar in terms of prevention of pulse loss.[4] **Acute vascular occlusion:** In children, 6 mg divided into four IM or IV doses.[5]
Dosage adjustment in organ dysfunction	No information available to support the need for dose adjustment.
Maximum dosage	Not established.
IV push	Not recommended. (See Cautions related to IV administration section.)[6]
Intermittent infusion	Diluted in NS and infused over at least 2 min.[6,7]
Continuous infusion	0.12 mg/mL in NS or ½NS. (See Comments section.)
Other routes of administration	Has been given IM.[5,6,8]
Maximum concentration	30 mg/mL for vasospasm in *adults* (commercially available).
Cautions related to IV administration	May cause arrhythmias, apnea, or death if administered by rapid IV push.[6]
Other additives	Available in single-dose (preservative-free) 2-mL amps or vials. 10-mL multiple-dose vials contain preservatives.[6]
Comments	Papaverine is a vasodilator that may add to the risk for intraventricular hemorrhage (IVH) in preterm neonates. A group of investigators compared papaverine (30 mg/250 mL) to standard heparin (1 unit/mL) for maintenance of arterial catheters in 141 neonates. The addition of papaverine significantly prolonged the functional duration of peripheral arterial catheters without increasing the risk of IVH.[1] Forms a precipitate in alkaline solutions. The data is conflicting on compatibility in LR.[5,8]

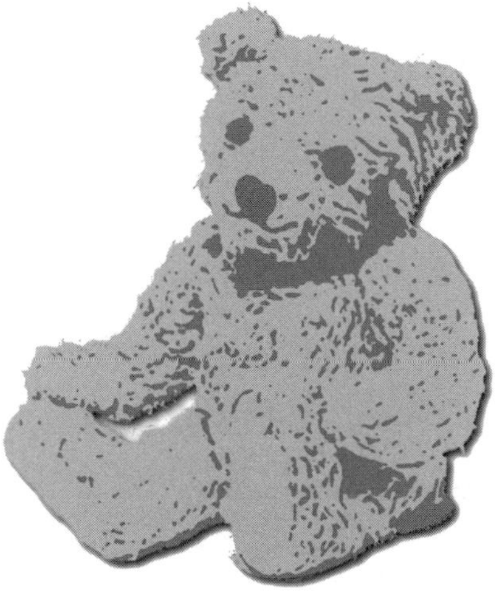

Peginterferon Alfa (alpha-2a, alpha-2b)

Brand names PEGASYS (alpha-2a), PEG-intron (alpha-2b)

Dosage

Prior to initiation, standard hematology and biochemistry evaluations should be done. Hematologic studies should be repeated at 2 and 4 weeks; biochemistry studies should be done at 4 weeks. Additional testing should be done periodically. If a virologic response has not occurred by 12 to 24 weeks of therapy, discontinuation should be considered.

Interferon-pegylated alpha-2a: 0.5 mcg/kg SC once a week (with ribavirin) has been used in children.[4] 180 mcg SC once a week is the usual *adult* dose.[5]

Interferon-pegylated alpha-2b: 1.5 mcg/kg SC once a week (with ribavirin) have been used in children 2–17 years of age.[1,2] In *adults* dosing (SC once a week) is based on weight and concentration of product as follows[3]:

Weight	Dose	Product Concentration	Amount to Be Given SC
<40 kg	50 mcg	50 mcg/0.5 mL	0.5 mL
40–50 kg	64 mcg	80 mcg/0.5 mL	0.4 mL
51–60 kg	80 mcg	80 mcg/0.5 mL	0.5 mL
61–75 kg	96 mcg	120 mcg/0.5 mL	0.4 mL
76–85 kg	120 mcg	120 mcg/0.5 mL	0.5 mL
>85 kg	150 mcg	150 mcg/0.5 mL	0.5 mL

Dosage adjustment in organ dysfunction

Peginterferon alpha-2a[5]: Use with caution and observe for toxicity in those with CrCl <50 mL/min. In *adults* with end-stage renal disease and on hemodialysis, clearance is reduced by 25% to 45%, and it is recommended that the dose be decreased to 135 mcg (a 25% decrease in usual dose). In addition, if there are progressive increases in ALT and bilirubin, the dose should be decreased or withheld. Therapy can be restarted when the ALT decreases to baseline.

Peginterferon alpha-2b[3]: Patients with CrCl 30–50 mL/min should have the dose reduced by 25%. For CrCl 10–29 mL/min (including during hemodialysis), the dose should be reduced by 50%. Discontinue if CrCl decreases during treatment. Dosing for patients with hematologic adverse effects is as follows:

Hemoglobin	<8.5 g/dL	Permanently discontinue
WBC	$<1.5 \times 10^9$/L	Reduce dose by 50%
	$<1.0 \times 10^9$/L	Permanently discontinue
Neutrophils	$<0.75 \times 10^9$/L	Reduce dose by 50%
	$<0.5 \times 10^9$/L	Permanently discontinue
Platelets	$<80 \times 10^9$/L	Reduce dose by 50%
	$<50 \times 10^9$/L	Permanently discontinue

Maximum dosage

Peginterferon alpha-2a: 3.45 mcg/kg/week over a period of 12 weeks; this overdosage did not result in serious adverse effects.[3]

Peginterferon alpha-2b: 180 mcg daily for 1 week; the associated toxicities included fatigue, increased liver enzymes, neutropenia, and decreased platelets.[5]

IV push Not indicated.

Intermittent infusion Not indicated.

Continuous infusion	Not indicated.
Other routes of administration	Given by SC injection. IM not indicated.
Maximum concentration	300 mcg/mL.[3]
Cautions related to IV administration	Not intended for intravenous use.

Other additives

Interferon-pegylated alpha-2a

Vial: Each vial contains 8.0 mg of sodium chloride, 0.05 mg of polysorbate 80, 10.0 mg of benzyl alcohol, 2.62 mg of sodium acetate trihydrate, and 0.05 mg of acetic acid.[5]

Prefilled syringe: Each syringe contains 4.0 mg of sodium chloride. 0.025 of polysorbate 80, 5.0 mg of benzyl alcohol, 1.3085 mg of sodium acetate trihydrate, and 0.0231 mg of acetic acid.[5]

Benzyl alcohol in small doses as a preservative in drugs is considered safe in newborns.[6] However, a 3-week-old, very low birth weight (710 g) infant who received clindamycin experienced a profound desaturation that required resuscitation after the third and fourth doses, which was subsequently related to the benzyl alcohol preservative.[7]

Administration of saline flushes containing benzyl alcohol (bacteriostatic water for injection) was associated with a fatal gasping syndrome, intraventricular hemorrhage, metabolic acidosis, and increased mortality in preterm infants.[8] This should not be used in neonates.

Hypersensitivity reactions to benzyl alcohol in parenteral products have been reported in *adults*.[9,10]

Interferon-pegylated alpha-2b: Each vial contains 1.11 mg of dibasic sodium phosphate anhydrous, 1.11 mg of monobasic sodium phosphate dehydrate, 59.2 mg of sucrose, and 0.074 mg of polysorbate 80. The PEG-Intron Redipen contains 1.013 mg of monobasic sodium phosphate dehydrate, 54 mg of sucrose, and 0.0675 mg of polysorbate 80.[3]

The Peg-Intron Redipen and Peg-Intron vials are single-use products, which do not contain preservatives. Once reconstituted, they should be used immediately or refrigerated and used within 24 h.[3]

Comments

Alpha interferons cause or aggravate fatal or life-threatening neuropsychiatric, autoimmune, ischemic, and infectious disorders. Patients should be monitored closely, and periodic clinical and laboratory evaluations should be performed. Patients with persistently severe or worsening signs or symptoms of these conditions should be withdrawn from therapy. In many cases, but not all, these disorders resolve after therapy is discontinued.[3,4]

Cutaneous eruptions and serious acute hypersensitivity reactions, including anaphylaxis, have been reported with the use of alpha interferon. If such a reaction should occur, treatment should be discontinued immediately and appropriate medical treatment should be initiated.[3]

Hemolytic anemia is a significant adverse effect with ribavirin. It is important that baseline and follow-up hematologic studies be performed as recommended.

Penicillin G Potassium/Sodium

Brand names	Pfizerpen (penicillin G potassium)

Dosage

Serious anaphylactoid reactions may require immediate emergency treatement with epinephrine, oxygen, IV steroids, and airway management.

Neonates

Congenital syphilis: If ≤7 days of age, give 100,000 units/kg/d divided q 12 h for 10 days.[1-4] If >7 days of age, give 100,000–150,000 units/kg/d divided q 8 h for 10 days.[1-4] If more than 1 day of therapy is missed, the entire therapy should be repeated.[1]

Mild-to-moderate infections

PNA	<1200 g	≤2000 g	>2000 g
≤7	25,000–50,000 units/kg/d divided q 12 h[5]	50,000–100,000 units/kg/d divided q 12 h[2,6,7]	75,000–150,000 units/kg/d divided q 8 h[2,6,7]
>7	25,000–50,000 units/kg/d divided q 12 h[5]*	75,000 units/kg/d divided q 8 h[2,6,7]	100,000–200,000 units/kg/d divided q 6 h[2,6,7]

*Until 4 weeks of age.

Meningitis: If ≤ 7 days of age, give 250,000–450,000 units/kg/d divided q 8 h.[2,6] Recent guidelines recommend 150,000 units/kg/d divided q 8–12 h.[8] Smaller doses and prolonged intervals may be needed in very low birth weight infants. If ≥7 days of age, give 450,000–500,000 units/kg/d divided q 4–6 h.[1,3,4] Recent guidelines recommend 200,000 units/kg/d divided q 6–8 h.[8]

Infants and children: Give 100,000–200,000 units/kg/d divided q 6 h for mild-to-moderate infections,[2] and 250,000–400,000 units/kg/d divided q 4–6 h for severe infections.[2]

Bacterial endocarditis

Enterococcal endocarditis: 300,000 units/kg/d divided q 4–6 h for 4–6 weeks (plus gentamicin for 2 weeks).[9]

Viridans group, streptococcal or S. bovis (penicillin sensitive): 200,000 units/kg/d divided q 4–6 h for 4 weeks if native valve and 6 weeks if prosthetic valve (plus ceftriaxone and gentamicin for 2 weeks).[9]

Viridans group, streptococcal or S. bovis (relatively resistant): 300,000 units/kg/d divided q 4–6 h for 4 weeks if native valve and 6 weeks if prosthetic valve (plus gentamicin and ceftriaxone for 2 weeks).[9]

Congenital syphilis: (>1 month after neonatal period) 200,000–300,000 units/kg/d divided q 4–6 h for 10 days.[1] If >1 day of therapy is missed, the entire course of therapy should be repeated.[1]

Meningitis: 250,000–400,000 units/kg/d divided q 4–6 h.[2,8]

Dosage adjustment in organ dysfunction

Adjust dosage in patients with renal dysfunction.[10,11] If CrCl is 10–50 mL/min, administer 75% of normal dose; if CrCl is <10 mL/min, give 20% to 50% of normal dose.[10] Additional reduction in dose may be necessary in combined renal and hepatic dysfunction.[11]

Maximum dosage

500,000 units/kg/d,[2] not to exceed 24 million units/d[2] in those with normal renal function and 10 million units/d in end stage renal failure.[10]

IV push

Not recommended. Rapid administration of large doses my cause electrolyte imbalances due to the potassium content. Cardiac arrest occurred in an infant who erroneously received 500,000 units/kg (containing 1 mEq/kg of potassium) over 2 min.[12]

Penicillin G Potassium/Sodium

Intermittent infusion	Reconstitute with D5W, NS, or SW according to manufacturers' recommendation[13] and infuse over 15–30 min.[11] The electrolyte (potassium) content should be considered when determining the infusion rate. (See Other additives section.)
Continuous infusion	Not generally administered by this method.[11] If given, the volume of IV fluid and rate of administration in 24 h should be determined and the appropriate daily dosage added to the fluid. Sensitization, due to degradation or transformation of penicillin G products, may be increased with continuous infusions over 6–24 h.[14,15]
Other routes of administration	≤100,000 units/mL cause little discomfort,[13] but higher concentrations may be used.[13]
Maximum concentration	1 million units/mL in D5W, NS, or SW.[16] 146,000 units/mL in SW results in a maximum recommended osmolality for peripheral infusion in fluid-restricted patients.[16,17]
Cautions related to IV administration	Large-dose penicillin therapy can induce electrolyte abnormalities.[13] The total dose of potassium or sodium content should influence rate of administration.[13] Because degradation or transformation penicillin G products form rapidly and may be responsible for sensitization, reconstituted solutions should be used immediately.[13] For PN compatibility information, please see Appendix C.
Other additives	Each million units of penicillin G potassium contain 1.7 mEq potassium and 0.3–1.02 mEq sodium, and each million units of penicillin G sodium contain 2 mEq sodium.[13]
Comments	Penicillin has been the drug of choice for *naturally* occurring anthrax; however, because of possible penicillin resistance or induction of resistance, the CDC does *not* recommend penicillin monotherapy to treat inhalational anthrax that occurs as the result of biologic warfare or bioterrorism.[18,19] Appropriate combination regimens include ciprofloxacin or doxycycline *and* one or two anti-infective agents that are predicted to be effective. Patients with a history of type I reaction to penicillin should not receive beta-lactam antibiotics. From 5% to 15% of patients allergic to penicillin will also be allergic to cephalosporins. Certain infections (i.e., syphilis) require penicillin. A desensitization protocol for penicillin-allergic patients should be performed in a hospital setting. This can usually be completed in 4 h and followed by the first dose of penicillin.[2] The beta-lactam ring of penicillins can link with an amino sugar of the aminoglycoside and inactivate the aminoglycoside.[13] This is dose-dependent and particularly problematic in patients with renal failure. To avoid this potential interaction, administer penicillins 1 h before or after an aminoglycoside, adequately flush the infusion line between each infusion, or infuse them through separate lines. Large doses (e.g., 12 million units/d)[20,21] have produced seizures in a 5-month-old.[21] Penicillin may cause false-positive urinary glucose results when cupric sulfate solution–based tests (Clinitest, Benedict's solutions, or Fehling's solution) are used.[22] Glucose oxidase methods (Clinistix) are not associated with false-positive test results.[22]

Pentamidine Isethionate

Brand names	Pentam 300
Dosage	**Infants and children** (see Comments section) **Parasitic infections (Leishmaniasis):** 2–4 mg/kg/d or q 2 d for up to 15 doses.[1,2] **Pneumocystis jiroveci (formerly carinii)** **Pneumonia:** 3–4 mg/kg/d as a single daily infusion over 1 to 2 h for 14–21 days[1,3] or 150 mg/m²/d for 5 days followed by 100 mg/m² for remainder of therapy, usually ≤21 days.[3,4] Current treatment guidelines recommend 4 mg/kg IV once daily for 7–10 days followed by oral atovaquone.[5] **Prophylaxis:** 4 mg/kg once q 2 or 4 weeks[6,7]; however, this use is controversial.[7]
Dosage adjustment in organ dysfunction	Adjust dosage in patients with renal dysfunction.[8] Some suggest if CrCl is 10–50 mL/min, give a normal dose q 24–36 h; if CrCl is <10 mL/min, give a normal dose q 48 h.[3] Renal toxicity is common following the use of parenteral pentamidine, and usually occurs after 2 weeks of therapy.[5] Maintaining adequate hydration and monitoring electrolytes and renal function can help minimize these effects.
Maximum dosage	4 mg/kg.[3]
IV push	Not indicated. Severe hypotension occurs with rapid infusion.[3]
Intermittent infusion	Over 60–120 min.[3,9]
Continuous infusion	Not indicated.
Other routes of administration	100 mg/mL is used for deep IM injection in *adults*.[3] To minimize local adverse effects, the Z-track injection technique should be used.[3] Pentamidine has also been given by inhalation for prophylaxis of pneumocystis.[3,5,7] This route is not used in children ≤5 years of age.[7]
Maximum concentration	~6 mg/mL. 300 mg is reconstituted with 3 mL of sterile water or D5W (100 mg/mL for IM use). This is further diluted in 50–250 mL D5W.[3] Do not use NS to reconstitute because precipitation will occur.[9]
Cautions related to IV administration	Severe hypotension, hypoglycemia, and cardiac arrhythmias have occurred following rapid administration.[3,10-12] Because of the risk of hypotension, the patient should be supine and have blood pressure monitored during infusion or injection.[3] After the dose is given, blood pressure should be monitored until stable.[3] The manufacturer recommends that emergency equipment for resuscitation be readily available because of the potential for sudden, severe hypotension during infusion. Some clinicians routinely administer a NS bolus (10 mL/kg; usually ≤500 mL) before and after pentamidine to minimize hypotension.

Other additives	None.
Comments	In neonates, primary but not secondary prophylaxis should be delayed because of the potential for adverse effects.[3] Nephrotoxicity is usually reversible with discontinuation of the drug.[3] Hypoglycemia and hyperglycemia can occur with parenteral or inhalational therapy and may persist for months after discontinuation. Monitor serum glucose concentrations before, during, and after treatment with pentamidine. Use with caution in patients predisposed to hypoglycemia or hyperglycemia.[3] Torsades de pointes occurred in a 7-month-old infant and in an 11-year-old child.[12,13] Although rare, acute pancreatitis has been reported.[14] Pentamidine should be discontinued if there are signs or symptoms of acute pancreatitis. Extravasation may lead to ulceration, tissue necrosis, and/or sloughing at the injection site.[3] Each 1.74 mg pentamidine isethionate is equivalent to 1 mg pentamidine.[3,9] Aerosolized pentamidine should be given via Respigard II nebulizer that is not used for bronchodilators.[7]

Pentobarbital Sodium

Brand names	Nembutal Sodium
Dosage	Respiratory depression and arrest requiring mechanical ventilation may occur. Monitor oxygen saturation. **Procedural sedation:** 1–6 mg/kg over 30 sec (≤50 mg/min).[1-8] If no response within 1 min, give 1–2 mg/kg to desired effect.[5] Repeat up to a total dose of 7.5 mg/kg.[3] Patients chronically receiving barbiturates may require doses of 9 mg/kg.[7,8] **Sedation with mechanical ventilation:** A loading dose of 1–2 mg/kg followed by a continuous infusion of 1–2 mg/kg/h.[8,9] Reload and titrate infusion to desired effect. **Therapeutic coma (for persistently elevated ICP or refractory status epilepticus:** A loading dose of 15–35 mg/kg over 60–120 min[11,13-16] followed by 1.5–3.5 mg/kg/h.[12-16] Reload and titrate infusion to desired effect. If hypotension occurs, decrease infusion rate or treat with IV fluids and vasopressors.
Dosage adjustment in organ dysfunction	No dosage adjustment required in renal failure.[17] Use cautiously and decrease dose in hepatic dysfunction.[17]
Maximum dosage	**Sedation:** Total cumulative doses have ranged from 1.3–9.5 mg/kg,[2,3,18] with a mean of 4.4 mg/kg,[2] up to 100 mg/dose.[5,17] **Therapeutic coma:** Individualize therapy by titrating dosage based on EEG, ICP, cerebral perfusion pressure, and blood pressure.[11,19,20] Serum pentobarbital concentrations of 20–40 mg/L should produce an isoelectric EEG.[19]
IV push	Not recommended. Rapid infusion may cause vasodilatation (hypotension) and decreased myocardial contractility.[5,17]
Intermittent infusion	50 mg/mL given over 10–30 min,[17] not to exceed 50 mg/min.[17] In order to decrease hypotension, a loading dose should be given over 60–120 min.[11,13-16]
Continuous infusion	50 mg/mL in D-LR, D-R, D-NS, D-W, LR, NS, ½NS, or R.[21]
Other routes of administration	2–6 mg/kg as a single injection given deep into a large muscle.[17] The volume of the injection at any one site should not exceed 5 mL.[17]
Maximum concentration	50 mg/mL for intermittent infusion.[21]
Cautions related to IV administration	Rapid administration may cause respiratory depression, apnea, and laryngospasm.[13,22] If hypotension occurs, the infusion rate should be decreased and the patient should be treated with IV fluids and/or vasopressors. Pentobarbital is an alkaline solution (pH = 9–10.5); therefore, extravasation may cause tissue necrosis.[17,21] Gangrene may occur following inadvertent intra-arterial injection. For PN compatibility information, please see Appendix C.

Other additives	**Propylene glycol:** Contains propylene glycol (40% v/v). Propylene glycol is added to parenteral drugs as a solubilizer. Rapid infusion of medications that contain propylene glycol has resulted in respiratory depression and cardiac dysrhythmias.[23] Its half-life is three times longer in neonates than in *adults*[24] and has caused hyperosmolality[25] and refractory seizures[26] in preterm neonates receiving 3 g/d.
Comments	Neonates may have an increased risk for complications from pentobarbital coma.[27] Administration of larger doses of pentobarbital for more than 4 days may be associated with pulmonary edema, pneumonia, and ileus.[28] For these reasons, some practitioners suggest that tapering of pentobarbital should be attempted 12 h after a burst-suppression pattern is obtained.[29] One case report described pentobarbital desensitization in a 3-month-old with refractory status epilepticus who had a known allergy to phenobarbital.[30]

Phenobarbital Sodium

Brand names Luminal Sodium

Dosage

Increased incidence of apnea when combined with other sedatives. Be prepared to provide respiratory support. Monitor oxygen saturation.

Hyperbilirubinemia: Studies evaluating the use of phenobarbital to prevent or treat neonatal hyperbilirubinemia and decrease the need for phototherapy and exchange transfusion are mixed.[1-4] 5 mg/kg/d within 6 h of life for 5 d reduced the duration of phototherapy[1]; however, 5 mg/kg/d for 3 days did not decrease the need for phototherapy or exchange transfusion.[2] 12 mg/kg as a single dose within hours of life significantly increased the rate of bilirubin disappearance, but the effect was not noted until day 7.[3] 20 mg/kg followed by 5 mg/kg/d for 1 week did not produce a clinically important difference when used with phototherapy.[4]

Neonatal abstinence syndrome: An opiate is the preferred initial therapy; however, addition of phenobarbital may decrease severity.[5,6] A loading dose of 20 mg/kg followed by 2–6 mg/kg/d.[7] If the severity score is <8, then a serum concentration of 20 mg/L is adequate.[7] If the score is >8, then 10 mg/kg q 12 h until the syndrome is better or serum concentrations reach 70 mg/L.[7] Once the infant is stable for 72 h, the dose should be decreased 15%/d.[7] When the severity score is <8 and serum concentration <15 mg/L, phenobarbital should be stopped.[7]

Prophylactic seizure therapy in severe perinatal asphyxia: There is little evidence from randomized controlled trials to support the use of any of the anticonvulsants.[8] 40 mg/kg over 60 min given as soon as possible is associated with a 27% reduction in seizures and significant improvement in neurological outcome at 3 years of age.[9] Term infants with asphyxia had higher trough serum concentration than those without asphyxia[10] and require about half the maintenance dose of nonasphyxiated neonates.[11]

Seizures—nonstatus epilepticus

Neonates: Loading dose (see status epilepticus section). Maintenance doses of 3.5–4.5 mg/kg/d if ≤35 weeks and 4 to 5 mg/kg/d if >35 weeks' gestational age.[11] Dose >5 mg/kg/d are generally associated with toxicity.[12] Serum phenobarbital concentrations should be ≥40 mg/L before an additional anticonvulsant is used.[13]

Infants and children: Loading dose (see status epilepticus section). Maintenance doses of ≤5 mg/kg/d.[14-16] If 1–5 years of age then 6–8 mg/kg/d, if 5–12 years of age then 4–6 mg/kg/d, and if 12 years of age give 1–3 mg/kg/d.[14] All doses may be given bid or once daily.[14-16]

Seizures—status epilepticus (persistent or recurrent)

Neonates: Some suggest that a benzodiazepine is the initial treatment of choice.[17] A loading dose of 8–10 mg/kg for 2 d,[18] 15–20 mg/kg,[12,19] or 30 mg/kg[20] has been suggested. Maintenance dose of ≤5 mg/kg/d given bid or qid.[12]

Infants and children: Some suggest that this should only be used when maximum doses of benzodiazepine and hydantoin have failed.[21] Loading dose of 20 mg/kg[21-23] up to 1000 mg.[22] Some have advocated an additional 20 mg/kg if no response within 15 min.[22]

Refractory status: May use a continuous infusion of a short-acting barbiturate (see Pentobarbital monograph). 10 mg/kg q 30 min (maximum 120 mg/kg in 24 h),[24] 5–10 mg/kg/dose to a total dose of 80 mg/kg/d.[25] (See Maximum dosage section.)

Maintenance dose: (see Seizures—nonstatus epilepticus above).

Dosage adjustment in organ dysfunction

Adjust dosage in patients with severe renal dysfunction.[26] Larger dosages are necessary in children undergoing continuous cycling peritoneal dialysis[27] and in neonates on ECMO.[28,29]

Phenobarbital Sodium

Maximum dosage

<30[20]– 40[17,22] mg/kg as a loading dose. Up to 300 mg/dose[30] or 1 g/dose[22] for status epilepticus. Total doses of 70–120 mg/kg were given over 24 h to children with refractory status epilepticus.[24,25] Because of interpatient variability in phenobarbital elimination, individualize dosage based on serum concentrations.

IV push

Not recommended.

Intermittent infusion

<30, 60, 65, or 130 mg/mL undiluted (available commercially) or dilute in an equal volume of D–LR, D–R, D–S, D5W, D10W, LR, NS, ½NS, or R[31] and infuse over 3–5 min, not to exceed 50–75 mg/min[21] or 2 mg/kg/min.[20,32]

Large loading doses (e.g., 40 mg/kg) may be infused over 60 min.[9]

Continuous infusion

No information available to support administration by this method.

Other routes of administration

May be given IM deep into muscle at a volume <5 mL.[33] No information available to support administration by other routes.

Maximum concentration

130 mg/mL.[31]

Cautions related to IV administration

May cause respiratory depression if administered too rapidly[33] or when combined with other sedatives.[22]

Extravasation may cause tissue necrosis.[33] Inadvertent intra-arterial injection can cause spasms, severe pain, and other symptoms (e.g., discolored skin or white hand with cyanosed skin) along the involved artery, which can result in local reactions varying from transient pain to gangrene.[33]

For PN compatibility information, please see Appendix C.

Other additives

Benzyl alcohol: May contain benzyl alcohol as a preservative.[33] Benzyl alcohol in small doses is considered safe in newborns.[34] However, a 3-week-old, very low birth weight (710 g) infant who received clindamycin experienced a profound desaturation that required resuscitation after the third and fourth doses, which was subsequently related to the benzyl alcohol preservative.[35]

Administration of saline flushes containing benzyl alcohol (bacteriostatic water for injection) was associated with a fatal gasping syndrome, intraventricular hemorrhage, metabolic acidosis, and increased mortality in preterm infants.[36] This should not be used in neonates.

Hypersensitivity reactions to benzyl alcohol in parenteral products have been reported in *adults*.[37,38]

Propylene glycol: Propylene glycol is added to parenteral drugs as a solubilizer. Rapid infusion of medications that contain propylene glycol has resulted in respiratory depression and cardiac dysrhythmias.[39] Its half-life is three times longer in neonates than in *adults*[34] and has caused hyperosmolality[40] and refractory seizures[41] in preterm neonates receiving 3 g/d.

Comments

Large variability exists in patient response to initial and maintenance doses, individualize dosage based on serum concentration and clinical response.

Because phenobarbital induces the CYP2C and CYP3A families and UGT, it is associated with numerous drug interactions[42]; consult appropriate resources for dosing recommendations before combining any drug with phenobarbital.

Phenytoin Sodium

Brand names	Dilantin, Phenytek

Dosage

In obese patients the loading doses should be calculated on adjusted body weight using the following equation[1]: (See Appendix B.)

Dosing weight (kg) = Ideal Body Weight (IBW) + 1.33 (measured weight − IBW)

Anticonvulsant

Post-traumatic epilepsy (see status epilepticus for dosing): Although prophylactic phenytoin for the prevention of epilepsy following head trauma is controversial, some have reported that it reduces early post-traumatic epilepsy.[2,3] It should not be used for the prevention of late epilepsy.[4] Children with severe, acute neurotrauma have markedly altered protein binding and phenytoin metabolism and may require larger doses and more frequent dosing.[5] Free serum phenytoin concentration should be monitored.[6]

Status epilepticus

Loading dose (assumes no previous phenytoin)

Neonates: 8–20 mg/kg[7-9] (may prefer to use phenobarbital or a benzodiazepine).

Infants and children: 10–20 mg/kg[10-12] not to exceed 1 g.[10]

Maintenance dose

Neonates: 4–8 mg/kg/d divided q 12–24 h.[7,8] Some suggest smaller doses of 3–5 mg/kg/d.[9] Extremely difficult to obtain serum concentrations following conversion to oral therapy; therefore, consider an alternative anticonvulsant for oral dosing.[6,9]

Infants and children: For 4 weeks to <1 years, 4–8 mg/kg/d.[9] For 1–12 years, 8–10 mg/kg/d divided q 8 h.[9,11-13] For ≥12 years, 4–8 mg/kg/d divided q 8–12 h.[9]

Arrhythmias (Class 1B) (digoxin-induced tachyarrhythmias): 1.25 mg over 5 min. May repeat q 5 min titrated up to a total of 15 mg/kg.[14]

Dosage adjustment in organ dysfunction

Dosage adjustment may be required in patients with hepatic[15] or renal dysfunction[16,17] and in obese patients.[1]

Maximum dosage

20 mg/kg as a single dose,[18] not to exceed 1 g.[19,20] Doses as high as 25 mg/kg/d divided q 6 h were used to achieve total serum phenytoin concentrations within the "therapeutic range" in a neonate.[21] These authors did not measure free phenytoin concentrations. If large doses are used, free phenytoin concentrations should be monitored. Because of age-dependent variation in phenytoin elimination, individualize dosage based on total or free serum concentrations.

IV push

Not recommended.[15,21]

Intermittent infusion

50 mg/mL (available commercially).[19] If necessary, dilute with NS[21] to a concentration <6 mg/mL[22] and infuse at a rate of 1–3 mg/kg/min in neonates, infants, and young children[18,20] or 50 mg/min in older children and *adults*.[15,18,23] Some advocate the use of a 0.22-micron filter.[21] Following administration, flush needle or catheter with NS.

Continuous infusion	Not recommended.[14]
Other routes of administration	Although the manufacturer suggests that IM administration is acceptable, most practitioners would not administer phenytoin IM because of severe pain at the injection site, erratic absorption, and possible precipitation of drug in tissue.[24] (See Comments section.) Has been given intraosseously.
Maximum concentration	50 mg/mL.[18]
Cautions related to IV administration	Rapid administration has resulted in hypotension, cardiovascular collapse, and CNS depression.[15,25] Heart rate should be monitored during administration and the infusion rate should be decreased if the heart rate decreases by more than 10 beats/min.[19] Phenytoin-induced, purple glove syndrome is the development of progressive distal limb edema, discoloration, and pain after peripheral administration of IV phenytoin. Although this condition is thought to occur from a reaction of the interstitial tissue to extravasation of the alkaline phenytoin solution, it can occur in the absence of infiltration.[15] It may result in extensive skin necrosis, limb ischemia, and compartmental syndrome that requires fasciotomies, skin grafting, or limb amputation. Because of the high risk of extravasation and local tissue irritation with peripheral administration of phenytoin, especially in neonates with peripheral scalp IV lines, fosphenytoin should be considered. (See Fosphenytoin monograph.) For PN compatibility information, please see Appendix C.
Other additives	**Benzyl alcohol:** 50 mg/mL contains 10% benzyl alcohol.[15] Benzyl alcohol in small doses as a preservative in drugs is considered safe in newborns.[26] However, a 3-week-old, very low birth weight (710 g) infant who received clindamycin experienced a profound desaturation that required resuscitation after the third and fourth doses, which was subsequently related to the benzyl alcohol preservative.[27] Administration of saline flushes containing benzyl alcohol (bacteriostatic water for injection) was associated with a fatal gasping syndrome, intraventricular hemorrhage, metabolic acidosis, and increased mortality in preterm infants.[28] This should not be used in neonates. Hypersensitivity reactions to benzyl alcohol in parenteral products have been reported in *adults*.[29,30] **Propylene glycol:** Contains 40% propylene glycol as a solubilizer. Rapid infusion of medications that contain propylene glycol has resulted in respiratory depression and cardiac dysrhythmias.[31] Its half-life is three times longer in neonates than in *adults*[26] and has caused hyperosmolality[32] and refractory seizures[33] in preterm neonates receiving 3 g/d. **Sodium:** Undiluted injection contains 0.2 mEq sodium/mL of phenytoin.[21]
Comments	Because large variability exists in patient response to initial and maintenance doses, individualize dosage based on serum concentration and clinical response. Free phenytoin serum concentrations should be measured in newborns, in patients with renal dysfunction, or in those who are hypoalbuminemic. Phenytoin is highly unstable in any IV solution; therefore, use only NS for dilution and do not mix with any other medication.[21] Because phenytoin induces the CYP2C19 and CYP3A families and UGT, it is associated with numerous drug interactions.[34] Phenytoin may also serve as a substrate and can be inhibited or induced by other drugs.[34] Consult appropriate resources for dosing recommendations before combining any drug with phenytoin.

Physostigmine Salicylate

Brand names	Antilirium
Dosage	Atropine sulfate injection should be available as an antagonist and antidote for physostigmine-associated, life-threatening symptoms.[1,2] The dose of atropine should be 50% of the administered dose of physostigmine.[2] **Anticholinergic toxicity** **Pediatric patients:** 0.02 mg/kg up to 0.5 mg/dose to reverse anticholinergic effects. If toxic effects persist, give 0.5 mg q 5–10 min up to 2 mg.[1-7] **Adolescents and adults:** 1–2 mg to reverse anticholinergic effects. If toxic effects persist, give 1 mg q 10–20 min up to 4 mg.[1-4,8] Doses should be repeated q 30–60 min if life-threatening signs or symptoms recur.[1,2,4]
Dosage adjustment in organ dysfunction	No information is available regarding dosage adjustment in organ dysfunction.
Maximum dosage	2 mg in pediatric patients[1-5] and 4 mg in adolescents or *adults*.[2] No maximum cumulative dose established. A total of 22 mg was administered IV over 48 h to a 22-year-old patient.[9]
IV push	Not recommended. Bradycardia, asystole, convulsions, and hypersalivation have occurred following rapid injection.[1,2,4]
Intermittent infusion	1 mg/mL or dilute with 10 mL D5W, NS, or SW[10] and infuse over 5–10 min, not to exceed 0.5 mg/min in children or 1 mg/min in *adults*.[1]
Continuous infusion	Although concentration was not specified, physostigmine has been diluted in NS or D5W.[11] It has been given by continuous infusion (0.02 mg/mL in D5W) to a 20-year-old patient.[12]
Other routes of administration	May be given IM at same doses as IV.[1]
Maximum concentration	1 mg/mL.[1]
Cautions related to IV administration	Bradycardia, asystole, convulsions, and hypersalivation have occurred following rapid injection.[1,2,4]

Other additives

Contains benzyl alcohol 2% as a preservative.[1]

Benzyl alcohol in small doses as a preservative in drugs is considered safe in newborns.[13] However, a 3-week-old, very low birth weight (710 g) infant who received clindamycin experienced a profound desaturation that required resuscitation after the third and fourth doses, which was subsequently related to the benzyl alcohol preservative.[14]

Administration of saline flushes containing benzyl alcohol (bacteriostatic water for injection) was associated with a fatal gasping syndrome, intraventricular hemorrhage, metabolic acidosis, and increased mortality in preterm infants.[15] This should not be used in neonates.

Hypersensitivity reactions to benzyl alcohol in parenteral products have been reported in *adults*.[16,17]

Contains sodium metabisulfite 0.1%.[1]

Sulfites may cause hypersensitivity reactions and these are more common in *adults* with asthma. Most reactions are mild but can include anaphylactic symptoms and life-threatening or less severe asthma episodes.[13,18,19] Epinephrine may be required in severe cases; and if the sulfite-free product is not available, the sulfite-preserved epinephrine should be used.[13]

Physostigmine should not be withheld from an individual with life-threatening anticholinergic toxicity who is sulfite sensitive.[4] Epinephrine should be available.

Comments

Contraindicated in those with asthma, gangrene, diabetes, cardiovascular disease, and mechanical obstruction of the gastrointestinal or urogenital tract.[1] It should also not be used in patients receiving choline esters or depolarizing neuromuscular blocking agents (e.g., decamethonium, succinylcholine).[1]

Although physostigmine has been used previously for tricyclic antidepressant toxicity in *adults* and children,[5,20] it now is recommended only for life-threatening symptoms unresponsive to other therapies.[11]

Two *adults* developed sinus bradycardia after receiving physostigmine for tricyclic overdose. Following 1 mg of atropine, both patients developed asystole.[21]

The use of physostigmine in the central anticholinergic syndrome has been described in an infant and a child.[22,23]

Piperacillin Sodium

Brand names	Pipracil
Dosage	Serious anaphylactoid reactions may require immediate emergency treatment with epinephrine, oxygen, IV steroids, and airway management. **Neonates:** 200 mg/kg/d divided q 12 h.[1] If <36 weeks gestational age, give 150 mg/kg/d divided q 12 h for 1 week and then 225 mg/kg/d divided q 8 h.[2] If >36 weeks gestational age, give 225 mg/kg/d divided q 8 h for 1 week and then 300 mg/kg/d divided q 6 h.[2] **Infants and children** **Mild-to-moderate infections:** 100–150 mg/kg/d divided q 6 h, up to 8 g/d.[3] **Severe infections:** 200–300 mg/kg/d divided q 4–6 h, up to 18 g/d.[3-5] **Appendectomy (perforated):** 200 mg/kg/d divided q 8 h.[6] **Cystic fibrosis:** 300–600 mg/kg/d divided q 4–6 h.[7,8] **Febrile neutropenia:** Administer 300 mg/kg/d divided q 8 h in conjunction with other antibiotics.[9,10] **Perioperative prophylaxis:** In adolescents, give 2 g 30 min before the procedure.[11]
Dosage adjustment in organ dysfunction	Adjust dosage in patients with renal dysfunction.[12,13] If CrCl is 10–50 mL/min, give normal dose q 6–12 h; if CrCl is <10 mL/min, give normal dose q 12 h.[12]
Maximum dosage	500 mg/kg/d,[7] 600 mg/kg/d in patients with cystic fibrosis[7,14] not to exceed 18 g/d.[3]
IV push	200 mg/mL in D5NS, D5W, NS, BW, or SW infused over 3–5 min.[15]
Intermittent infusion	45–70 mg/mL in D5NS, D5W, LR, or NS.[15] Concentration as high as 163 mg/mL may be given to fluid restricted patients.[16] Give over 20–60 min.[14]
Continuous infusion	Although no specific information is available to support administration of piperacillin by this method, piperacillin/tazobactam and other beta-lactam antibiotics have been given by this method.[17-20]
Other routes of administration	May be given by IM administration using 400 mg/mL in SW, NS, bacteriostatic SW or NS, D5W or D5NS, or lidocaine HCl 0.5% to 1% (without epinephrine).[15] Should be injected deep into the upper-outer quadrant of the buttock. Maximum dose injected into one site should not exceed 2 g.[15]
Maximum concentration	200 mg/mL for IV push,[15] 163 mg/mL for IV infusion,[16] and 400 mg/mL for IM administration.[15]
Cautions related to IV administration	If a decision is made to give this medication to a patient with known penicillin hypersensitivity, the patient should be closely observed for allergenicity.[21-25] For PN compatibility information, please see Appendix C.

Other additives	Contains 1.85 mEq sodium/g of piperacillin sodium.[15]

Comments

Patients with a history of type I reactions to penicillin should not receive beta-lactam antibiotics. From 5% to 15% of patients allergic to penicillin will also be allergic to cephalosporins. Certain infections (e.g., syphilis) require penicillin for eradication. It is recommended that a desensitization protocol for penicillin-allergic individuals should be performed in a hospital setting. This can usually be completed in about 4 h, at which time the first dose of penicillin can be given.[3]

Piperacillin is more allergenic (e.g., fever, rash) in patients with cystic fibrosis.[26]

Serum-like sickness and coagulopathy associated with fever, rash, and abnormal liver function tests occurred in two patients with cystic fibrosis.[27]

Thrombophlebitis was reported in 4% to 13% of patients.[28] Abnormal coagulation tests (e.g., clotting time, platelet aggregation, and prothrombin time) may occur, especially in patients with renal failure. Piperacillin should be discontinued if bleeding occurs.[14]

Tonic-clonic seizures have been reported in an 11-year-old child receiving IV piperacillin (3 g q 4 h) over 30 min.[29]

The beta-lactam ring of penicillins can link with an amino sugar of the aminoglycoside and inactivate the aminoglycoside.[30-32] To avoid this potential interaction, administer penicillins 1 h before or after an aminoglycoside, adequately flush the infusion line between each infusion, or infuse them through separate lines. *In vivo* inactivation that is dose dependent can also occur particularly in patients with renal failure.[32-34] In patients with end-stage renal failure, gentamicin half-life was decreased by 22–31 h after carbenicillin or ticarcillin was added to the drug regimen.[33]

Piperacillin Sodium–Tazobactam Sodium

Brand names	Zosyn
Dosage	Serious anaphylactoid reactions may require immediate emergency treatment with epinephrine, oxygen, IV steroids, and airway management.[1] Piperacillin/tazobactam is available in a ratio of 8:1 (piperacillin:tazobactam).[1] Tazobactam is a beta-lactamase inhibitor that extends the spectrum of piperacillin but has little antibacterial activity. Doses are based on piperacillin component.[1] **Neonates:** 100–300 mg/kg/d divided q 8–12 h.[2-4] **Infants and children:** Use is inappropriate in mild-to-moderate infections.[5] For severe infections, give 240 mg/kg/d divided q 8 h up to 18 g/d.[5] Based on a single-dose pharmacokinetic study, doses of 100 mg/kg q 8 h for bacteria whose MIC is 2 mg/L and q 6 h if the MIC is between 4 and 8 mg/L should be effective.[6] **Cystic fibrosis:** 350–450 mg/kg/d divided q 6 h.[7,8]
Dosage adjustment in organ dysfunction	Adjust dosage in patients with renal dysfunction.[1] If CrCl is 10–50 mL/min, give normal dose q 6–8 h; if CrCl <10 mL/min, give normal dose q 8 h.[9] No adjustment necessary in liver impairment.[10]
Maximum dosage	450 mg/kg/d[7,8] up to 16 g of piperacillin component daily.[1,5]
IV push	No information available to support administration by this method.
Intermittent infusion	Infuse over at least 30 min.[1] Reconstitute vials with 5 mL of NS, SW, D5W, bacteriostatic saline, or BW. Reconstituted drug should be further diluted with 50–150 mL of NS, SW, D5W, or Dextran 6% in saline.[1,11]
Continuous infusion	Continuous infusions of 8–12 mg piperacillin/24 h have been studied in *adults*.[12-14]
Other routes of administration	No information available to support administration by other routes.
Maximum concentration	200 mg/mL (piperacillin component); however, 20 mg/mL preferred.[11]
Cautions related to IV administration	Piperacillin is more allergenic in patients with cystic fibrosis.[1,15] If a decision is made to give this medication to a patient with known penicillin hypersensitivity, the patient should be closely observed for allergenicity. (See Comments section.) For PN compatibility information, please see Appendix C.

Other additives 2.35 mEq of sodium/g of piperacillin.[1,11]

Comments

Patients with a history of type I reaction to penicillin should not receive beta-lactam antibiotics. From 5% to 15% of patients allergic to penicillin will also be allergic to cephalosporins. Certain infections (e.g., syphilis) require penicillin for cure. It is recommended that a desensitization protocol for penicillin-allergic individuals should be performed in a hospital setting. This can usually be completed in about 4 h, at which time the first dose of penicillin can be given.[5]

Serum-like sickness and coagulopathy associated with fever, rash, and abnormal liver function tests occurred in two patients with cystic fibrosis.[16]

Thrombophlebitis was reported in 4% to 13% of patients.[17,18]

Tonic clonic seizures have been reported in an 11-year-old patient receiving IV piperacillin (3 g q 4 h) over 30 min.[19]

The beta-lactam ring of penicillins can link with an amino sugar of the aminoglycoside and inactivate the aminoglycoside.[20-24] To avoid this potential interaction, administer penicillins 1 h before or after an aminoglycoside, adequately flush the infusion line between each infusion, or infuse them through separate lines. *In vivo* inactivation that is dose dependent can also occur particularly in patients with renal failure.[19-21] In patients with end-stage renal failure, gentamicin half-life was decreased by 22–31 h after carbenicillin or ticarcillin was added to the drug regimen.[24]

Piperacillin may cause false-positive urinary glucose results when cupric sulfate solution-based tests (Clinitest, Benedict's solution, or Fehling's solution) are used.[1] Glucose oxidase methods (Clinistix) are not associated with false-positive test results.[1]

Potassium Chloride

Brand names	Various manufacturers
Dosage	The rate of potassium infusion should not exceed 0.5–1 mEq/kg/h and all sources should be considered.[1-5] Intermittent doses range from 0.5–1 mEq/kg.[2] During loop and thiazide diuretic therapy up to 4 mEq/kg/d may be required.[3] Intermittent infusions of 1 mEq/kg over 2 h are usual.[4] Dosing is based on serum potassium concentrations.
Dosage adjustment in organ dysfunction	Potassium is renally eliminated; therefore, extreme caution is required when dosing patients with renal insufficiency.[6] (See Comments section about sickle cell disease.)
Maximum dosage	Maximum recommended total daily dose in *adults* is 200 mEq.[8] 40 mEq/h in *adults* with electrocardiographic changes or muscle paralysis and serum potassium <2 mEq/L.[7] Close monitoring of ECG and serum concentrations is required.
IV push	Contraindicated.[1,8]
Intermittent infusion	≤0.5–1 mEq/kg/h.[1,3,5] (See Cautions related to IV administration section.) ECG monitoring should accompany infusion of individual doses >0.5 mEq/kg/h.[6] Usually <80 mEq/L.[6] The rate of delivery should not exceed 0.5–1 mEq/kg/h.[1,3-5]
Continuous infusion	≤40 mEq/L in D-LR, D-R, D-S, D5LR, D5NS, D5W, D10W, D20W, LR, NS, ½NS, or R for continuous administration via peripheral vein.[7] ≤60 mEq/L have been used for peripheral infusion in *adults*.[1] Usually ≤80 mEq/L.[1,4,7] Greater concentrations may be used when the potassium concentration is ≤2 mEq/L and cardiac arrhythmias are present. The rate of delivery should not exceed 0.5–1 mEq/kg/h.[1,3,7] (See Cautions related to IV administration section.)
Other routes of administration	Contraindicated.[8]
Maximum concentration	40[3]–60 mEq/L[1] for peripheral IV and ≤200 mEq/L for central lines.[3,10]
Cautions related to IV administration	Inadequate mixing of concentrated potassium chloride with a diluent, including the addition of potassium to a flexible container such as a Buretrol or Soluset, may result in inconsistent potassium concentrations.[6,7] Infusion of such a solution could deliver potassium at variable rates that may exceed recommendations.[6,7] Phlebitis occurs frequently with concentrations >40 mEq/L.[1,8] Extravasation may cause tissue sloughing and necrosis.[11] Administration of potassium chloride at excessive rates may result in fatal dysrhythmias.[9] For PN compatibility information, please see Appendix C.

Other additives	The 60-mEq/30 mL multidose vial contains methylparaben 0.05% and propylparaben 0.005%.[6-8] Paraben preservatives may cause hypersensitivity reactions that are more common with cutaneous exposure.[12] However, one case of pruritus and bronchospasm that occured following infusion of hydrocortisone, which contained a paraben, has been reported.[13] Contains contaminant aluminum.[1]
Comments	In six patients from 19–37 years old with sickle cell disease and normal glomerular filtration, urinary potassium excretion was significantly less than normal individuals during a 0.75 mEq/kg infusion over 2 h.[14] In *adults*, the addition of lidocaine (50 mg/65 mL of infusate) decreased the pain associated with infusion.[15]

Potassium Phosphates

Brand names	Various manufacturers
Dosage	Potassium phosphates are used to replace phosphate and not to replace potassium. The rate of potassium infusion should not exceed 0.5–1 mEq/kg/h and all sources should be considered.[1,2] (See Comments for conversion of mEq to mmol.) **Diabetic ketoacidosis**: If the phosphate concentration is low, consider providing one-third to one-half the potassium replacement as phosphates.[4] Alternatively, 1.5–2 mmol/kg (estimated deficit) can be infused over 24 h.[5] These patients should be monitored for hypocalcemia and hypomagnesemia.[4,5] **Hypophosphatemia** **Children:** 0.16–0.32 mmol/kg over 6 h (≤0.1 mmol/kg/h)[2] **Adults receiving 15 mmol potassium phosphate/L in PN solutions:** Additional phosphate via intermittent infusions according to the degree of hypophosphatemia.[3] **Mild (serum concentration of 2.3–3 mg/dL):** 0.16 mmol/kg infused over 4–6 h. **Moderate (1.6–2.2 mg/dL):** 0.32 mmol/kg infused over 4–6 h. **Severe (<1.5 mg/dL):** 0.64 mmol/kg infused over 8–12 h.
Dosage adjustment in organ dysfunction	Potassium and phosphate ions are renally eliminated; therefore, extreme caution is required when dosing patients with renal insufficiency.[6]
Maximum dosage	1.5 mmol/kg over 24 h.[2] Of note, infants and children receiving PN may require daily doses of up to 2 mmol/kg (depending on the dose of calcium in PN) for optimal bone growth.[7,8]
IV push	Contraindicated.[8]
Intermittent infusion	The required dose for *adults* has been diluted in 100 or 150 mL of NS or D5W and infused over 4–6 h (mild/moderate hypophosphatemia) and over 8–12 h (severe hypophosphatemia).[3] The final potassium concentration of the solution should be considered. (See Dosage and Cautions related to IV administration sections.)
Continuous infusion	10–20 mmol/L in PN solutions.[3]
Other routes of administration	Contraindicated.[8]
Maximum concentration	Add dose to 100 mL of NS or D5W for intermittent infusion[3] or 10–20 mmol/L in PN solutions for continuous infusion.[3]

Potassium Phosphates

Cautions related to IV administration	Inadequate mixing of concentrated potassium chloride with a diluent, including the addition of potassium to a flexible container such as a Buretrol or Soluset, may result in inconsistent potassium concentrations.(4,9) Infusion of such a solution could deliver potassium at variable rates that may exceed recommendations.(5,9) Extravasation may cause tissue sloughing and necrosis.(10) Administration of potassium phosphate at excessive rates may result in fatal dysrhythmias.(11) ECG monitoring should accompany infusion of individual doses >0.5 mEq/kg/h. Compatibility with calcium is limited and depends on the pH of the final solution. Potassium phosphate should not be administered through a Y-site with a calcium-containing solution. For PN compatibility information, please see Appendix C.
Other additives	Contains contaminant aluminum.(8)
Comments	Administration of large amounts of phosphate may cause hypocalcemia.(5,8,9) 4.4 mEq of potassium and 3 mmol of phosphate/mL.(5,8,9) 1 mmol phosphorus = 31 mg phosphorus.(9) The valence of phosphate changes with pH; therefore, the preferred units in which to express the amount of phosphate are mmol.(9)

Pralidoxime Chloride (2-PAM Chloride)

Brand names	Protopam Chloride
Dosage	**Chemical warfare:** Dose and route are based on severity of symptoms. **Outpatient setting, usually given IM as follows**[1] **Mild-to-moderate symptoms:** 15 mg/kg. **Severe symptoms:** 25 mg/kg. **Emergency department, usually given as slow IV injection**[1] **Mild-to-moderate symptoms:** 15 mg/kg. **Severe symptoms:** 15 mg/kg. **Organophosphate poisoning:** For nicotinic (e.g., fasciculation, muscle weakness, paralysis, and decreased respiratory effort) and CNS symptoms. **Intermittent dosing:** 25–50 mg/kg, up to 2 g/dose, over 5–30 min; repeat dose after 1–2 h and then q 6–12 h if cholinergic signs recur.[2-7] **Continuous infusion:** 25-50-mg/kg loading dose infused over 15–30 min followed by continuous infusion of 10–20 mg/kg/h for ≤60 h while symptoms persist.[8,9] A loading dose of 50 mg/kg may be more appropriate in patients with severe organophosphate poisoning.[9]
Dosage adjustment in organ dysfunction	Should be used with caution and in reduced dosage in patients with renal dysfunction.[1,6]
Maximum dosage	As much as 2 g/dose,[3] 12 g in 24 h,[6] and 0.5 g/h by continuous infusion[1,10] have been used in *adults*, with the total dosage titrated according to cholinergic signs and clinical symptoms.
IV push	20 mg/mL in NS or SW over at least 5 min in children.[1,4] In fluid-restricted patients, 50 mg/mL may be used.[1] Not to exceed 200 mg/min in *adults*.[6] (See Cautions related to IV administration section.)
Intermittent infusion	20 mg/mL in NS or SW over 15–30 min.[8]
Continuous infusion	Although concentration and solution type were not provided, pralidoxime has been given by this method.[8,9]
Other routes of administration	300 mg/mL in NS or SW may be given IM.[1] May produce mild pain at the injection site.[1]
Maximum concentration	50 mg/mL.[1]

Pralidoxime Chloride (2-PAM Chloride)

Cautions related to IV administration

Side effects (e.g., tachycardia, laryngospasm, and muscle rigidity) may be more common after rapid IV infusion of >30-mg/kg doses.[7,8] Weakness, blurred vision, dizziness, headache, nausea, and tachycardia have been noted when infusion rates exceed 0.5 g/min in *adults*.[2] Asystole has been reported following infusion of 2 g over 10 min.[2]

Transient dose-dependent increases in blood pressure have been reported in *adults*.[2] If hypertension occurs, the drug should be discontinued or the rate reduced.[1] IV administration of 5 mg of phentolamine has been reported to reverse the hypertension.[1]

Other additives

None. Diluents should be preservative-free due to larger volume required.[1]

Comments

Use with caution in patients with myasthenia gravis because drug may precipitate a crisis.[1]

Most effective if administered within 24–48 h of exposure; however, patients presenting late (i.e., 2–6 days) may still benefit.[3,6]

Concomitant administration of pralidoxime may increase side effects of atropine.[6,7]

Morphine, theophylline, aminophylline, and succinylcholine are contraindicated.[1,4,7] Pralidoxime has been given for up to 22 days following poisoning with highly lipophilic organophosphates.[6]

Procainamide HCl

Brand names	Pronestyl
Dosage	Monitor EKG. If QRS widens >50% or if the patient develops hypotension during the loading dose, the infusion should be discontinued and the maintenance dose held until signs of toxicity resolve.[1,2] **Tachycardia** **Loading dose:** Two alternative regimens for IV loading are recommended. 2–5 mg/kg (max 100 mg) repeated q 5–10 min until the arrhythmia is controlled to a maximum of 15 mg/kg (500 mg) over 30 min.[1,3-6] or 10–15 mg/kg over 30–60 min followed by maintenance infusion. **Maintenance dose:** 20–120 mcg/kg/min[1-6] or 50–100 mg/kg/d divided q 4 h.[4]
Dosage adjustment in organ dysfunction	Change dosing intervals in moderate to severe renal dysfunction. If CrCl is 10–50 mL/min, give normal dose q 6–12 h. If CrCl is <10 mL/min, administer normal dose q 8–24 h.[4]
Maximum dosage	Maximum IV daily dose is 2 g.[3,4] Maximum IM dose is 4 g/d.[3,4] In *adults* 20 mg/min up to 17 mg/kg.[2]
IV push	20–30 mg/mL in D5W, NS, or SW given over 5–10 min at a maximum infusion rate of 20–30 mg/min (50 mg/min in *adults*).[3,4] Severe hypotension may occur with rapid administration.[2]
Intermittent infusion	Infuse the loading doses at a concentration of 20–30 mg/mL over 25–30 min.[7] For intermittent maintenance infusions, use 2–4 mg/mL concentration solution.[6,7]
Continuous infusion	2 or 4 mg/mL for continuous infusion preferably in NS or SW.[6] Variable stability has been reported in dextrose containing solutions with significant drug loss in as little as 4 h, depending upon the pH adjustment of dextrose solution.[6]
Other routes of administration	Has been given IM in doses of 20–30 mg/kg/d divided q 4–6 h, not to exceed 4 g/d.[3] Has been given IO.[2]
Maximum concentration	20–30 mg/mL for loading doses[3] or 4 mg/mL for intermittent infusions.[6]
Cautions related to IV administration	To avoid the development of significant hypotension, limit the infusion rate to 20–30 mg/min.[3] Hypotension, atrioventricular block, cardiac dysrhythmias, and cardiac arrest may occur.[3,4]

Other additives

Sulfites: Some products contain sodium bisulfite.[3] Sulfites may cause hypersensitivity reactions and these are more common in *adults* with asthma. Most reactions are mild but can include anaphylactic symptoms and life-threatening or less severe asthma episodes.[8-10] Epinephrine may be required in severe cases; and if the sulfite-free product is not available, the sulfite-preserved epinephrine should be used.[8]

Benzyl alcohol: Some 100- and 500-mg/mL vials contain benzyl alcohol 0.9% as a preservative.[3] Benzyl alcohol in small doses as a preservative in drugs is considered safe in newborns.[11] However, a 3-week-old, very low birth weight (710 g) infant who received clindamycin experienced a profound desaturation that required resuscitation after the third and fourth doses, which was subsequently related to the benzyl alcohol preservative.[12]

Administration of saline flushes containing benzyl alcohol (bacteriostatic water for injection) was associated with a fatal gasping syndrome, intraventricular hemorrhage, metabolic acidosis, and increased mortality in preterm infants.[13] This should not be used in neonates.

Hypersensitivity reactions to benzyl alcohol in parenteral products have been reported in *adults*.[14,15]

Comments

Because large variability exists in patient response to initial and maintenance doses, individualize dosage based on serum concentration and clinical response.

Reference range[3,16,17]: For procainamide, 4–10 mg/L. For combination of procainamide plus n-acetyl procainamide, 5–30 mg/L.

Because procainamide is associated with numerous pharmacokinetic and pharmacodynamic drug-drug interactions,[3] consult appropriate resources for dosing recommendations before combining any drug with procainamide.[17]

Promethazine HCl

Brand names	Anergan, Pentazine, Phenazine, Phencen-50, Phenergan, Phenoject, Pro-50, Promet, Prorex, Prothazine, V-Gan, and others

Dosage

A black box warning was added to prescribing information in 2004 as follows[1]:

Promethazine contraindicated in pediatric patients <2 years of age because of the potential for fatal respiratory depression. Postmarketing cases of respiratory depression, including fatalities, have been reported with promethazine use in patients <2 years of age. A wide range of weight-based doses have resulted in respiratory depression in these patients.

Caution should be exercised when administering promethazine to pediatric patients >2 years of age. Use the lowest effective dose and avoid the use of concomitant therapy with respiratory depressant effects.

Antiemetic/sedation

Children >2 years of age: 0.25–1 mg/kg (not to exceed 25 mg) q 4–6 h as needed.[2-4]

Dosage adjustment in organ dysfunction

No dosage adjustment required in patients with renal dysfunction. May cause excessive sedation in end stage renal disease.[5]

Maximum dosage

The dose should not exceed half of the suggested *adult* dose or up to 25 mg/dose in children or 50 mg/dose in adolescents.[1]

IV push

≤ 25 mg/mL; administer into tubing of a compatible infusion fluid (D–LR, D–R, D–S, D5W, D10W, LR, R, NS, ½NS) at a rate <25 mg/min.[1,6]

Intermittent infusion

No information available to support administration by this method.

Continuous infusion

No information available to support administration by this method.

Other routes of administration

≤25 mg/mL via deep IM injection is the preferred route of administration.[1]

Maximum concentration

25 mg/mL.[1]

Cautions related to IV administration

Tissue irritation and damage can occur from promethazine injection regardless of the route of administration.[1] Extravasation may cause tissue necrosis.[1,7]

In an effort to increase awareness of the risk of severe tissue injury with IV promethazine administration, the Institute for Safe Medication Practices has recommended that institutions only stock the 25-mg/mL concentration, limit doses used, further dilute the 25-mg/mL concentration prior to administration, use large veins for administration, administer via a running IV at the furthest port from the patient, and administer slowly.[8]

Intra-arterial injection may result in gangrene of the affected extremity.[1,7]

For PN compatibility information, please see Appendix C.

Other additives

Each mL of solution (25 mg/mL and 50 mg/mL) contains 0.1 mg edetate disodium, 0.04 mg calcium chloride, 0.25 mg sodium metabisulfite, and 5 mg phenol.

Sulfites may cause hypersensitivity reactions and these are more common in *adults* with asthma. Most reactions are mild but can include anaphylactic symptoms and life threatening or less severe asthma episodes.[9-11] Epinephrine may be required in severe cases; and if the sulfite-free product is not available, the sulfite-preserved epinephrine should be used.[9]

Comments

All FDA-reported cases of serious adverse events (respiratory depression, apnea, cardiac arrest, dystonias, CNS effects, seizures, neuroleptic malignant syndrome) in children (0 to 16 years of age) were evaluated.[12] Respiratory depression occurred in 22 patients (1.5 months–2 years of age) and seven of these patients died. A wide range of doses was represented (0.45–6.4 mg/kg). Nine patients received ≤1 mg/kg in addition to another drug with respiratory depressant effects.[12]

Excessively large doses of antihistamines may cause hallucinations, convulsions, and sudden death in infants and children. Acutely ill children who are dehydrated may be more susceptible to dystonias. For these reasons, antiemetics are not recommended for the treatment of uncomplicated vomiting in children; their use should be limited to prolonged vomiting of unknown etiology.[1]

Meperidine, promethazine, and chlorpromazine have been used in combination (Demerol, Phenergan, Thorazine [DPT] cocktail) to sedate pediatric patients.[2,3,13-16] However, with the availability of safer and more effective agents,[14,17,18] this combination is no longer recommended.[16]

An increase in blood glucose and false positive or false negative pregnancy tests (diagnostic tests utilizing HCG and anti-HCG) may occur with promethazine therapy.[1]

Steroid-induced psychosis in a 32-month-old child with acute lymphocytic leukemia resolved with promethazine (0.5 mg/kg) therapy.[19]

Propofol

Brand names	Diprivan 1% and 2%, Propofol Injectable Emulsion 1% (generic)

Dosage

Anesthesia

Induction doses (>3 years of age): Mean dose 2.5 mg/kg (range of 1–4 mg/kg) given over 20–30 sec until onset of induction.[1-10] Noncommunicative and nonverbal children (ASA III and IV) with cerebral palsy require less propofol for induction than healthy children.[11]

Those older than 16 years should be given 40 mg (2–2.5 mg/kg) q 10 sec until onset of induction.[1] *Adults* >16 years who have neurosurgical diagnosis should receive smaller doses 20 mg (1–2 mg/kg) q 10 sec.[1]

Maintenance (>2 months of age): If clinical signs of light anesthesia are not present following the first 30 min, the infusion rate should be decreased.[1]

133–400 mcg/kg/min.[8,10,12] Younger children may require larger doses. During clinical trials mean doses were 125–300 mcg/kg/min (7.5–18 mg/kg/h).[1] Those >16 years received doses of 100–200 mcg/kg/min (6–12 mg/kg/h) or 40 mg (2–2.5 mg/kg) q 10 sec.[1]

Although rare, the propofol infusion syndrome has been reported following anesthesia. (See Comments section.)

Epilepsy (refractory status epilepticus): Use in refractory status is based on nonrandomized studies and case reports; hence, it should be used cautiously. Initial loading doses of 3 mg/kg followed by continuous infusion of 40–300 mcg/kg/min (2.4–18 mg/kg/h) for up to 48 h have been used in patients from 9 months to 19 years.[13-17] (See Comments section.)

Procedural sedation: 0.5–3 mg/kg initially followed by 50–200 mcg/kg/min (3–12 mg/kg/h)[18-20] with additional 1 mg/kg boluses as needed.[18,19] For the initial bolus, one group used 2.5 mg/kg in children and 3 mg/kg in infants.[19] As an alternative to continuous infusion, 0.2 to ≤1 mg/kg boluses as needed for patient comfort have been used.[18,21] (See Comments section.)

Sedation: The manufacturer stresses that propofol lacks approved labeling for sedation in critically ill, mechanically-ventilated pediatric patients.[1]

Given the current controversy regarding the Propofol Related Infusion Syndrome (PRIS), the lowest effective dose should be used and the dose should not exceed 4 mg/kg/h.[22] The infusion rate should be increased by 5–10 mcg/kg/min (0.3–0.6 mg/kg/h) until the desired effect is achieved.[1] A minimum period of 5 min should be allowed for peak effect between titration events.[1] The patient should be switched to a benzodiazepine (i.e., midazolam or lorazepam) if adequate sedation can not be achieved with dose of 4 mg/kg/h or if prolonged therapy (≥48 h) is required.[22] While on propofol the patient should be monitored for clinical features and laboratory findings that have been attributed to the syndrome. (See Comments section.) Should symptoms occur propofol should be discontinued.

Dosage adjustment in organ dysfunction	No dosage adjustment required in hepatic or renal dysfunction.[1,23] Although rare, at large doses (2–3 g/d), EDTA (antimicrobial agent in Diprivan) may be toxic to the renal tubules.[1] In those predisposed to renal impairment, urinalysis and urine sediment should be assessed prior to initiation and on alternate days during therapy.[1]
Maximum dosage	Not established. (See Comments section.)
IV push	10 mg/mL[1] given over 20–30 sec.[1,2-6] Has been given safely over 10 sec.[2] (See Cautions related to IV administration section.)

Intermittent infusion	Not routinely recommended.
Continuous infusion	2–10 mg/mL in D5W.[1] Do not dilute <2 mg/mL due to emulsion instability.[1]
Other routes of administration	IM administration is not recommended.[1] No information available to support administration by other routes.
Maximum concentration	10 mg/mL.[1] Should not be diluted to <2 mg/mL.[1]
Cautions related to IV administration	Should not be given to patients allergic to eggs and/or soybean products.[1] Cardiorespiratory depression may result from bolus dosing or rapid increase in infusion rate. Therefore, wait 3–5 min between dosage adjustments to assess patient response.[1] Abrupt discontinuance of propofol may cause flushing of the hands and feet, agitation, tremors, hyperirritability, bradycardia, agitation, or jitteriness.[24] For PN compatibility information, please see Appendix C.
Other additives	**Eggs and soybean:** Each mL of Diprivan contains 100 mg soybean oil, 22.5 mg glycerol, 12 mg egg lecithin, and disodium edetate 0.005%. NaOH is used to adjust pH.[1,25] The generic contains 100 mg soybean oil, 22.5 mg glycerol, 12 mg egg yolk phospholipid, and 0.25 mg sodium metabisulfite. NaOH is used to adjust pH.[25] Patients who are allergic to eggs and/or soybean products should not be given propofol.[1] A 14-month-old patient with a history of egg and peanut allergies developed anaphylaxis after receiving propofol.[26] **Sulfites:** The generic formulation contains sodium metabisulfite. Sulfites may cause hypersensitivity reactions and these are more common in *adults* with asthma. Most reactions are mild but can include anaphylactic symptoms and life-threatening or less severe asthma episodes.[27-29] Epinephrine may be required in severe cases; and if the sulfite-free product is not available, the sulfite-preserved epinephrine should be used.[27] **EDTA:** Diprivan contains EDTA. Although this formulation has not been associated with decreased zinc levels or zinc deficiency-related adverse events, it should not be infused for longer than 5 days without providing a drug-free period.[1]
Comments	The Propofol Related Infusion Syndrome (PRIS) is associated with a variety of symptoms, including progressive metabolic acidosis, lipemia, hypotension, MSOF, and rhabdomyolysis, which may culminate in cardiovascular collapse.[22] Several practitioners have successfully managed PRIS with venovenous hemodiafiltration and charcoal hemofiltrationor ECMO.[22] Plasmapheresis was not beneficial.[22] Although the propofol emulsion contains an antimicrobial agent, it is not to USP standards; hence, it can support growth of microorganisms.[1] Accordingly, strict aseptic technique must still be used. Several incidences of bacterial contamination have been reported following repackaging[30] or improper storage of propofol[31] and Intralipid.[32] Administration should commence promptly and be completed within 12 h after the vial has been spiked.[1] The tubing and any unused portions of propofol emulsion must be discarded after 12 h. If propofol is transferred to a syringe or other container, the transfer should be done as soon as the vial is opened and the product should be discarded and administration lines changed after 6 h.[1] Acute dystonia and seizures have also been reported in those with and without a history of epilepsy.[33-38] Subtherapeutic doses or withdrawal may contribute to this effect since increasing the dose can result in termination of the seizure activity. To ensure proper delivery of propofol, in-line IV filters should be >5 microns.[1]

Propranolol HCl

Brand names	Inderal
Dosage	**Arrhythmias:** 0.01–0.25 mg/kg over 10 min[1-7] not to exceed 1 mg/min.[1] Repeat dose q 2 min.[2,3] (See Maximum dosage section.) **Burn patients:** (not established use) 0.5–1 mg/kg q 8 h for 5–10 days.[7,8] Used to decrease heart rate, cardiac work, and metabolic stress associated with severe burn. **Hypertensive emergency:** The 4th report on the diagnosis, evaluation and treatment of high blood pressure in children and adolescents does not include propranolol in its discussion of hypertensive emergencies in children.[9] Intravenous labetalol appears to be the preferred beta-blocker.[9,10] When propranolol is used, give 0.01–0.05 mg/kg over 1 h.[11] **Infundibular spasm ("Tet" spell):** Oxygen should be given before propranolol. 0.01–0.02 mg/kg over 10 min.[12-14] May repeat dose in 15 min.[13,14] Maximum initial dose 1 mg.[12]
Dosage adjustment in organ dysfunction	No dosage adjustment required in renal dysfunction.[15]
Maximum dosage	0.2 mg/kg,[2,13] not to exceed 1 mg as initial dose for infants.[2,6,12] Although the AAP recommends that the maximum initial dose in children is 10 mg,[2] the usual dose for *adults* is 1–3 mg.[16]
IV push	Not recommended. Although rapid administration may cause hypotension and cardiac standstill,[16] doses have been given over 2 min.[17]
Intermittent infusion	1 mg/mL dilute dose in D5W or NS.[18] Generally, administered over 10 min.[2] Not to exceed 1 mg/min in *adults*.[16]
Continuous infusion	No information available to support administration by this route.
Other routes of administration	No information available to support administration by other routes.
Maximum concentration	1 mg/mL.[18]
Cautions related to IV administration	Use with caution in patients with asthma.[16]
Other additives	None.
Comments	EKG and central venous pressure should be monitored during IV administration. Propranolol-induced bradycardia should be treated with atropine.[16] If there is no response to atropine, then isoproterenol should be tried.[1]

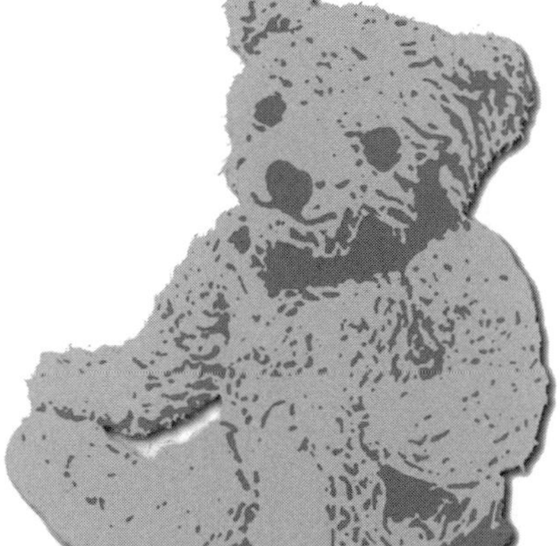

Protamine Sulfate

Brand names	Generic

Dosage

Heparin: 1 mg of protamine sulfate will neutralize about 100 USP heparin units.[1,2] Because heparin's half-life is short, over time less protamine is required. Only one-half the dose of protamine should be used if IV heparin has been discontinued for 30 min.[1] If the heparin was administered SC, *adults* should receive 25–50 mg followed by an infusion of the remaining calculated dose over 8–16 h.[2]

The following doses have been recommended for pediatric patients following IV injection of heparin[2]:

Time since Last Heparin Dose Received	Protamine Dose (mg of protamine/100 units of heparin received)
<30 min	1 mg
30–60 min	0.5–0.75 mg
60–120 min	0.375–0.5 mg
>120 min	0.25–0.375 mg

Low molecular weight heparin (LMWH): 1 mg protamine will neutralize about 1 mg enoxaparin or dalteparin. If the LMWH was given >8 h prior, 0.5 mg protamine should be given for each mg LMWH.[2] Repeat doses may be required after SC LMWH.[3]

Dosage adjustment in organ dysfunction

No information available to support the need for dosage adjustment.

Maximum dosage

50 mg.[1,2]

IV push

Not recommended. Rapid administration may result in hypotension, bradycardia, pulmonary hypertension, etc.[1,2]

Intermittent infusion

50 mg over 10 min,[1,2] and ≤5 mg/min.[3] (See Cautions related to IV administration section.)

May be diluted with D5W or NS.[1,2,4]

Continuous infusion

No information available to support administration by this method.

Other routes of administration

No information available to support administration by other routes.

Maximum concentration

10 mg/mL.[1,2]

Cautions related to IV administration

Anaphylaxis may occur.[1,2] Patients with known hypersensitivity reactions to fish and those who have received protamine containing insulin or previous protamine therapy are at greatest risk for hypersensitivity reactions.[1,2,5] However, fatal anaphylaxis occurred in one patient with no previous history of allergies.[1] In two case reports, doses of 3 and 4.5 mg/kg after cardiopulmonary bypass resulted in an anaphylactoid response in a 6- and a 2.5-year-old child, respectively.[6,7]

Hypotension, bradycardia, and flushing are caused by rapid IV injection.[1] In *adults* after cardiopulmonary bypass, those who received 5 mg/kg protamine over 5 min had significant changes in cardiovascular parameters while those who received protamine with a calcium chloride infusion did not.[8] In another study, hemodynamic changes were noted with protamine infusion in patients who had poor left ventricular (LV) function but not in those who had good LV function.[9]

Other additives

Contains 9 mg NaCl/10 mg.[2]

Comments

When administered before protamine, IV famotidine (0.4 mg/kg), but not diphenhydramine prevented hypotension associated with protamine in *adults*.[10]

A neonate experienced pulmonary hypertension and impending respiratory failure immediately after receiving protamine for heparin reversal after cardiopulmonary bypass.[11] This episode was attributed to a presumed pulmonary embolism. The infant underwent a second procedure and was again given protamine. Similar respiratory decompensation occurred and was attributed to protamine. The child was treated with high-frequency oscillation ventilation, nitric oxide, and prostacycline, and recovered.

Ranitidine

Brand names	Zantac
Dosage	**Active GI bleeding, peptic ulcer disease, or hypersecretory conditions**: 0.5–5 mg/kg/d given in divided doses or via continuous infusion.[1-4] **Prophylaxis against dexamethasone-associated ulceration in premature infants with bronchopulmonary dysplasia:** 0.031–1.25 mg/kg/h during dexamethasone therapy.[5] An infusion of 0.0625 mg/kg/h was sufficient to increase and maintain gastric pH >4.[5] **Prophylaxis against stress ulceration** **Premature neonates:** 0.5 mg/kg q 12 h.[6] **Term neonates:** Although one study recommended 1.5 mg/kg q 8 h,[6] another study reported that term neonates receiving 2 mg/kg/dose did not require dosing more frequently than q 12 h.[7] Ranitidine has also been given as a 2-mg/kg loading dose over 10 min followed by 0.083 mg/kg/h.[7] **Infants and children:** Although doses of 1–6 mg/kg/d divided q 6–8 h have been used,[8-12] it has been suggested that critically ill infants and children require larger doses (i.e., >3 mg/kg/d) and more frequent dosing.[8,12-14] Alternatively, a loading dose of 0.15–0.6 mg/kg[1,2,12,15] over 15 min followed by a continuous infusion of 0.031–0.25 mg/kg/h has been used.[1,3,5,10-12,16-18]
Dosage adjustment in organ dysfunction	Adjust dosage in patients with severe renal dysfunction.[4,19] If CrCl >50 mL/min, give 75% of normal dose; if CrCl is 10–50 mL/min, give 50% of a normal dose; if CrCl <10 mL/min, give 25% of normal dose.[4,19]
Maximum dosage	200 mg/d in infants and children and 400 mg/d in *adults*.[4] 2.5 mg/kg/h and infusion rates of 220 mg/h have been used in *adults* with hypersecretory conditions.[4]
IV push	Not generally recommended because of risk of bradycardia and hypotension.[20] Dilute to ≤2.5 mg/mL in D5W, D10W, LR, or NS and inject over at least 5 min,[4,21] not to exceed 4 mL/min (10 mg/min).[4,21]
Intermittent infusion	Dilute to ≤0.5 mg/mL in D5W, D10W, LR, or NS and infuse at 5–7 mL/min (15–20 min).[4,21]
Continuous infusion	<0.5 mg/mL in D5W, D10W, LR, NS, or sodium bicarbonate 5%.[4,21] Visually compatible with PN[21] and stable in PN and TNA solutions for 24 h at room temperature.[22-24]
Other routes of administration	May be given IM (25 mg/mL).[4]
Maximum concentration	2.5 mg/mL for IV and 25 mg/mL for IM administration.[4,21]
Cautions related to IV administration	Infusion of 50 mg over <5 min has resulted in transient hypotension in critically ill *adults*.[20] For PN compatibility information, please see Appendix C.

Other additives	Each mL of the premixed solution (50 mg/50 mL) contains 4.5 mg NaCl, 0.3 mg citric acid, and 1.8 mg dibasic sodium phosphate.[4] Each mL of the sterile injection (25 mg/mL) contains 5 mg phenol, 2.4 mg dibasic sodium phosphate, and 0.96 mg monobasic potassium phosphate.[4]

Comments

Several critically ill children have failed to respond to 6 mg/kg/d.[10,14] Tolerance developed in five of six infants who received continuous infusion ranitidine in PN solutions for 2–6 weeks.[16]

Bradycardia began 2 h after ranitidine was infused in a neonate and gradually resolved within 24 h of discontinuation.[25] No other cause of bradycardia could be determined.

Ranitidine has produced a negative chronotropic effect in children receiving concomitant tolazoline.[26]

The use of H2-blocker therapy has been associated with the incidence of necrotizing enterocolitis in very low birth weight infants.[27]

Because ranitidine inhibits a variety of isoenzymes and is associated with numerous drug interactions,[4] consult appropriate resources for dosing recommendations before combining any drug with ranitidine.

Rasburicase

Brand names	ELITEK
Dosage	Indicated for the initial management of plasma uric acid levels in pediatric patients who are expected to develop tumor lysis syndrome and subsequent elevations in uric acid as a result of their disease (lymphoma, leukemia, and solid tumor malignancies) and/or treatment regimen.[1] Rasburicase may elicit an antibody response that may increase hypersensitivity reactions and decrease efficacy.[2] For this reason, the manufacturer recommends that it should be used for a single course of therapy only.[1] Rasburicase has been administered safely and effectively to pediatric and *adult* patients who had received prior therapy.[2,3] **Hyperuricemia:** 0.15–0.2 mg/kg/d for up to 5–7 days.[1-8] Chemotherapy should begin 4–24 h after administration of rasburicase.[1] Some trials have given 0.15–0.2 mg/kg q 12 h for the first 48–72 h in patients at greatest risk of developing hyperuricemia.[2,3,5-8] A single dose of 0.15 mg/kg was effective at decreasing uric acid levels in patients (18 months–72 years) with bulky tumor.[9] A single 6-mg dose has been found to be effective in *adults*.[10]
Dosage adjustment in organ dysfunction	Not established.
Maximum dosage	0.2 mg/kg/dose or 0.4 mg/kg/d.[1]
IV push	Not recommended.[1]
Intermittent infusion	Dilute rasburicase vials with 1 mL of provided diluent and add desired rasburicase dose to an infusion bag of NS for a final volume of 50 mL to be infused over 30 min.[1] Total dosing volumes of 10–50 mL have been given in infants.[6]
Continuous infusion	No information available to support administration by this method.
Other routes of administration	No information available to support administration by other routes.
Maximum concentration	Not established. Desired dose of reconstituted rasburicase should be added to NS for a final total volume of 50 mL.[1]
Cautions related to IV administration	Hypersensitivity reactions have been reported.[2] Do not filter infusion. A separate line is preferred. Flushing the line with 15 mL of NS before and after administration is also acceptable.[1] Give concomitant IV hydration.

Other additives	None.

Comments

Rasburicase has the following black box warnings: anaphylaxis (incidence <1%), hemolysis (incidence <1%), methemoglobinemia (incidence <1%), and interference with uric acid measurements.[1]

Anaphylaxis may occur at any point during infusion. Immediately and permanently discontinue rasburicase should anaphylaxis occur.[1]

Patients with glucose-6-phosphate dehydrogenase deficiency (G6PD) are at increased risk of developing severe hemolysis. Rasburicase is contraindicated in G6PD since hydrogen peroxide is a major by-product in the conversion of uric acid to allantoin. High-risk G6PD populations should be screened prior to administration.[1]

Methemoglobinemia and severe hypoxemia have occurred in two clinical trial patients. Immediately and permanently discontinue rasburicase and initiate supportive care.[1]

Rasburicase interferes with uric acid analysis. Collect blood in heparin-containing, prechilled tubes, which are immediately immersed in an ice bath. Analyze within 4 h of collection.[1]

Renal tubular damage was reported in a 7-year-old receiving rasburicase and alkalinization.[11] Renal damage has been related to alkalinization resulting in calcium phosphate precipitation.[2,11] Alkalinization should be avoided during rasburicase administration.[11]

Respiratory Syncytial Virus Immune Globulin Intravenous

Brand names	RespiGam

Dosage

RSV prophylaxis[1]

(1) Infants <24 months of age who have bronchopulmonary dysplasia (BPD) that have required medical therapy within 6 months of the expected RSV season.
(2) Infants <12 months of age who were born at ≤32 weeks gestation without chronic lung disease during the first RSV season of their life.
(3) Infants with congenital heart disease who meet criteria (1) or (2) may benefit. (Infants with cyanotic congenital heart disease should not receive RSV IG.)[2]
(4) Immunocompromised children who receive IGIV monthly may benefit from substituting RSV IG for IGIV.

Infants are dosed monthly during RSV season that varies regionally. Maximum monthly dose is 750 mg/kg.[3–5] It is recommended that a loop diuretic be available in case fluid overload occurs.[3]

Usual infusion rate

0 to 15 min	1.5 mL/kg/h
15 min to end (4 h)	3.6 mL/kg/h (see Comments section)

RSV treatment (highly controversial)

Bone marrow transplant patients (within 1–37 d of onset of RSV symptoms): 1500 mg/kg over 12 h.[6]

Treatment with 1500 mg did not benefit healthy children or infants and children <24 months with BPD, congenital heart disease, or prematurity.[7,8]

Dosage adjustment in organ dysfunction	None required.
Maximum dosage	1500 mg/kg.[6–8]
IV push	Contraindicated.
Intermittent infusion	750 mg/kg infused over about 4.5 h.[3]
Continuous infusion	Not indicated.
Other routes of administration	Contraindicated.
Maximum concentration	Undiluted, 50 mg/mL.[3]
Cautions related to IV administration	In certain cases (severe BPD), a slower infusion rate may be required to avoid complications related to fluid overload.[3]

Respiratory Syncytial Virus Immune Globulin Intravenous

Other additives	The product has 5% sucrose as a stabilizer and 1% albumin. Immune globulin products that contain sucrose as a stabilizer have a disproportionate number of patients who develop renal insufficiency. Use cautiously in patients with underlying renal disease.[3] May contain trace amounts of IgA and IgM. Sodium content varies from 20–30 mEq/L. Contains no preservatives.[3]
Comments	Adverse effects are similar to those seen with other immune globulin products and include fever, respiratory distress, vomiting, and wheezing and may be related to the infusion rate.[3] The infusion should begin within 6 h of opening the vial and be completed within 12 h.[3] Infants who receive RSV IG should not receive the measles-mumps-rubella, monovalent measles, or varicella vaccines until at least 9 months after the dose.[9]

Rifampin

Brand names	Rifadin I.V.
Dosage	**Neonates:** 10–20 mg/kg/d divided q 12 h.[1,2] **Infants and children:** 10–20 mg/kg/d divided q 12 h or given as a single dose q 24 h.[3,4] One study concluded that it may be more appropriate to shorten the dosing interval from 12 h to 8 h after 2 days of therapy to avoid prolonged periods of low plasma concentrations.[5] Rifampin IV has been used synergistically in patients with persistent staphylococcal bacteremia unresponsive to vancomycin therapy and in patients with methicillin-resistant *Staphylococcus aureus* and methicillin-resistant coagulase-negative staphylococci.[6,7] **Biologic warfare or bioterrorism:** The CDC and other experts recommend that treatment of inhalational anthrax spores due to biologic warfare or bioterrorism should be started on a multiple-drug parenteral regimen that includes ciprofloxacin or doxycycline and one or two additional anti-infective agents (e.g., chloramphenicol, clindamycin, rifampin, vancomycin, clarithromycin, imipenem, penicillin, or ampicillin).[8,9] **Prophylaxis following intraventricular shunt revision:** 20 mg/kg as a single dose 1 h prior to surgery.[10]
Dosage adjustment in organ dysfunction	No dosage adjustment required in patients with renal or hepatic dysfunction. However, if CrCl is <10 mL/min, a 50% decrease in dose has been recommended.[11]
Maximum dosage	20 mg/kg/d[10,12] not to exceed 600–1200 mg/d in *adults*.[2,13]
IV push	Not recommended.[11]
Intermittent infusion	Dilute with D5W or NS (slightly less stable in NS) to a final concentration ≤6 mg/mL.[11,14] Infuse over 30 min to 3 h.[1,10,11] Infusion solution should be administered within 4 h of preparation because rifampin may precipitate.[11]
Continuous infusion	Has been infused over 3 h.[11,14]
Other routes of administration	IM and SQ administration is not recommended.[11] Intraventricular administration (5 mg/d) has been used in cases of central nervous system tuberculosis.[15]
Maximum concentration	6 mg/mL.[11]
Cautions related to IV administration	Extravasation may cause local irritation and inflammation.[11]
Other additives	None.
Comments	May discolor body secretions (e.g., sweat, urine, and tears).[11] Rifampin induces the CYP2C19 isozymes to cause numerous drug interactions. Consult appropriate resources before combining any drug with rifampin. Rifampin may interfere with assays for serum folate and vitamin B_{12}.[11]

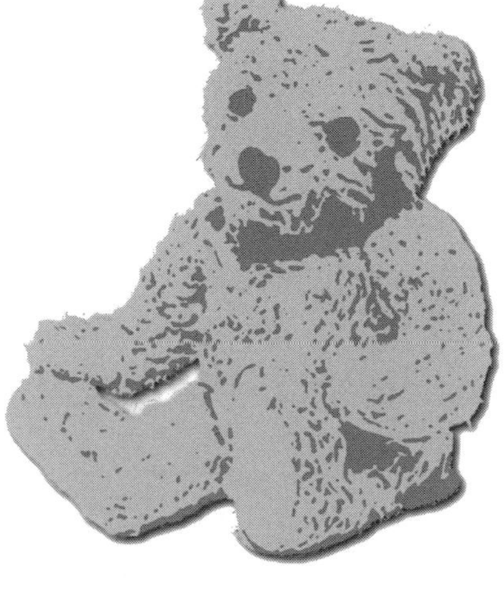

Rituximab

Brand names	Rituxan
Dosage	Consult institutional protocols for complete dosing information. Rituximab is part of combination therapy to treat newly diagnosed, relapsed, or refractory CD20 positive B-cell, non-Hodgkin's lymphoma or B-cell ALL, as well as other hematologic disorders. **CD20 positive B-cell, non-Hodgkin's lymphoma** **Initial:** 375 mg/m^2 once weekly for four to eight doses as monotherapy or in combination with CHOP (i.e., cyclophosphamide, doxorubicin, vincristine, and prednisone).[1-3] **Retreatment:** 375 mg/m^2 once weekly for four doses or once weekly for four doses given q 6 mo for up to 2 years.[1,4] **Refractory:** 375 mg/m^2 on days 1 and 3 in combination with ifosfamide, mesna, carboplatin, and etoposide.[5] **B-cell ALL:** 375 mg/m^2 to conventional salvage therapy.[6] **Relapsed or refractory low-grade, follicular, or transformed B-cell non-Hodgkin's lymphoma:** 250 mg/m^2 administered 4 h prior to Indium-111 ibritumomab; 7–9 days later, 250 mg/m^2 administered within 4 h of Yttrium-90 ibritumomab.[1,7] **Post-transplant lymphoproliferative disorder:** 375 mg/m^2 once weekly for three to four doses.[8,9] **Autoimmune hemolytic anemia:** 375 mg/m^2 once weekly for three to six doses.[10,11]
Dosage adjustment in organ dysfunction	Not established.
Maximum dosage	Clinical trials have reported single dosages up to 500 mg/m^2.[1]
IV push	Not recommended.[1]
Intermittent infusion	Dilute with NS or D5W to a final concentration of 1–4 mg/mL and infuse at a beginning rate of 50 mg/h. If no hypersensitivity reactions occur, the rate may be escalated by 50 mg/h q 30 min to a maximum rate of 400 mg/h. In patients tolerating the first infusion, subsequent cycles may begin at a rate of 100 mg/h, escalating up to a maximum rate of 400 mg/h.[1]
Continuous infusion	No information available to support administration by this method.
Other routes of administration	No information available to support administration by other routes.

Maximum concentration	4 mg/mL.[1]

Cautions related to IV administration

Premedication with acetaminophen and diphenhydramine is recommended to reduce the incidence of hypersensitivity reactions (e.g., fevers, chills, rigors).[1]

Severe infusion reactions (hypotension, hypoxia, bronchospasm, or angioedema) are most common with the first dose and generally occur within 30–120 min after beginning the infusion. Treatment should include interruption of the infusion and the use of supportive care measures, including oxygen, bronchodilators, and IV fluids. Often the infusion can be resumed with a 50% reduction in the infusion rate. Close monitoring in subsequent courses should occur.[1]

Rituximab carries a black box warning regarding the development of a fatal infusion reaction complex (hypoxia, pulmonary infiltrates, respiratory distress, myocardial infarction, ventricular fibrillation or cardiogenic shock). This complex most commonly occurs with the first dose.[1]

Other less serious hypersensitivity reactions are common and can be treated with a 50% reduction in infusion rate and acetaminophen and diphenhydramine. Bronchodilators and IV saline may be used as needed.[1]

Other additives

Contains 9 mg/mL sodium chloride.[1]

Comments

Rituximab carries black box warnings for fatal infusion reactions (see Cautions related to IV administration section), tumor lysis syndrome, and severe mucocutaneous reactions. Tumor lysis syndrome (hyperkalemia, hypocalcemia, hyperuricemia, hyperphosphatemia, and acute renal failure) necessitating dialysis to prevent renal failure has been reported within 12–24 h after the first rituximab infusion. Treatment should include supportive care with electrolyte correction and dialysis, as needed. Prophylaxis may be warranted in patients with a high tumor burden. Severe mucocutaneous reactions with fatal outcomes have been reported 1–13 weeks after the initial rituximab dosage.[1]

Rituximab is associated with a minimal (<10%) risk of emesis.[12,13] Generally, prophylaxis for acute and delayed emesis is not needed. Patients may receive one time prophylaxis with a phenothiazine (e.g., prochlorperazine) or a butyrophenone (e.g., droperidol). Breakthrough medications should be offered, such as a phenothiazine (e.g., prochlorperazine), a butyrophenone (e.g., droperidol), a substituted benzamide (e.g., metoclopramide), or a benzodiazepine (e.g., lorazepam). Selection should be based on what the patient is currently receiving for acute antiemesis prophylaxis.[12,13]

Rocuronium Bromide

Brand names	Zemuron
Dosage	Respiratory function must be supported during use of this agent. Concurrent administration of a sedative is also necessary. Monitoring of neuromuscular transmission with a peripheral nerve stimulator is recommended during continuous infusion or with repeated dosing.[1] Dosing for rapid sequence intubation should be based on actual body weight, not ideal or lean body mass.[2,3] When administered with inhalational anesthetics, such as halothane, isoflurane, or sevoflurane, the dose of rocuronium should be reduced by 20% to 50%.[4,5] **Infants:** 0.5 mg/kg repeated q 20–30 min as needed to maintain pharmacological paralysis.[2,6] **Children:** 0.6–0.8 mg/kg initially, followed by repeated doses of 0.075–0.125 mg/kg q 20–30 min as needed to maintain pharmacological paralysis.[2,3,6-9] May also give 10–12 mcg/kg/min as continuous infusion.[2-5,8]
Dosage adjustment in organ dysfunction	An increased initial dosage may be required for complete neuromuscular blockade in patients with hepatic impairment.[2,3] Duration of neuromuscular blockade in these patients may also be prolonged.[2,3] No dosage adjustment required in those with renal impairment.[2,3] In children with renal failure who were older than 1 year of age, a single bolus dose did not cause prolonged neuromuscular blockade but was associated with a slower onset of action than that noted in healthy children.[11]
Maximum dosage	Not established.
IV push	10 mg/mL over 5–10 sec.[2]
Intermittent infusion	Not administered by this method.
Continuous infusion	0.5–1 mg/mL in D5W, D5NS, LR, or NS.[12]
Other routes of administration	Although a single IM dose of 1 mg/kg in infants and 1.8 mg/kg in children has been used,[11] rocuronium should not be used as an alternative to IM succinylcholine when rapid intubation is necessary. The use of IM administration is not recommended since it does not consistently provide satisfactory tracheal intubating conditions.[13] When given in the deltoid muscle of infants and children, serum concentrations peak at 13 min, with about 80% of the dose absorbed systemically.[14]
Maximum concentration	10 mg/mL for IV push; 1 mg/mL for infusion.[2]
Cautions related to IV administration	Hypersensitivity reactions, hypotension, arrhythmias, and bronchospasm have been reported but appear to be rare.[2,3]

Other additives	None.
Comments	Concomitant administration of other drugs (e.g., aminoglycosides, clindamycin, inhalational anesthetics, ketamine, magnesium, succinylcholine, or vancomycin) may prolong neuromuscular blockade. Consult appropriate resources for additional information on drug interactions. Other factors that potentiate the duration of neuromuscular blockade include acidosis, hypokalemia, hypermagnesemia, neuromuscular disease, and hepatic disease.[2,3,6] Patients with neurological diseases, such as myasthenia gravis, may exhibit increased sensitivity.[2] Decreased sensitivity to rocuronium may occur in patients with severe burns, muscle trauma, demyelinating lesions, neuropathy, or infection.[2,3]

Ropivacaine HCl

Brand names	Naropin
Dosage	**Not for IV infusion. Administered by epidural or caudal route.**[1] Dose varies with the anesthetic procedure, the area to be anesthetized, the vascularity of the tissues, the number of neuronal segments to be blocked, the depth and duration of anesthesia required, as well as individual response. Once the catheter is placed, negative aspiration of blood or cerebrospinal fluid[1,6-9] and the absence of cardiovascular changes following a test dose indicates correct position of the catheter.[1,3,6] (See Comments section.) **Caudal/epidural block**: Children 1.25–6.5 mg/kg.[1-8] or 1 mL/kg of 0.2% solution.[10] **Epidural continuous infusion** **Children 4 months to 7 years:** A loading dose of 1 mg/kg followed by 0.2–0.4 mg/kg/h for 48 h.[1,2,9-11] One group of investigators reported continuous infusion up to 96 h without adverse events.[9] **Children from 7 to 12 years:** 24 children assigned to a patient-controlled infusion of a loading dose of 3.6 mg followed by a continuous infusion of 3.2 mg/h with dose titration up to 27.2 mg/h if needed required less drug than 24 children assigned to a standard treatment of a continuous infusion of 0.4 mg/kg/h (239 mg/48 h compared to 576 mg/48 h, respectively).[12] **Adults:** A loading dose of 10–14 mg (5–7 mL of 0.2% solution) followed by 12–28 mg/h (6–14 mL/h of 0.2% solution) for up to 72 h.[1,2]
Dosage adjustment in organ dysfunction	Use with caution in patients with hepatic or cardiovascular disease.[1,2,10]
Maximum dosage	Not established.
IV push	Do not administer IV. Accidental IV injection may result in seizures, coma, or cardiac or respiratory arrest.[1,2.10]
Intermittent infusion	Do not administer IV.[1,2,10,13] 1 mg/kg over 10 min has been administered via epidural catheter.[10]
Continuous infusion	Do not administer IV. For epidural infusion only.[1,2,9-12] (See Dosage section.)[1,2,10,13]
Other routes of administration	Do not administer IM.[1,2,13]
Maximum concentration	1% (10 mg/mL).[1,2,13]
Cautions related to IV administration	Do not administer IV. Accidental IV injection may result in seizures, coma, or cardiac and respiratory arrest.[1,2,10]

Other additives	Sodium hydroxide and/or hydrochloric acid may be used for pH adjustment.[1,13]
Comments	The manufacturer does not recommend the use of ropivacaine with or without epinephrine in children <12 years.[1] A test dose of epinephrine with or without lidocaine has been used to verify that the needle is not in the vascular space.[5,12] Systemic absorption of local anesthetics may result in toxic plasma concentrations, resulting in cardiovascular adverse effects, including decreased cardiac output, heart block, hypotension, bradycardia, ventricular arrhythmias, and cardiac arrest. Patients should be carefully monitored during injection. Use with caution in patients with underlying cardiovascular disease.[1,2,10] Patients receiving class III antiarrhythmics (e.g., amiodarone) may be at increased risk for cardiac adverse effects.[1,2]

Sargramostim

Brand names

Leukine; yeast derived (*Saccharomyces cerevisiae*) recombinant human granulocyte-macrophage colony-stimulating factor (rhGM-CSF)

Dosage

The products derived from *Escherichia coli* and Chinese hamster ovaries are not available in the U.S. Some of the studies cited evaluated these products, which may have different potencies, specific activities, and adverse effects.[1]

Chemotherapy-induced neutropenia: 250–1000 mcg/m² IV over 2 h for up to 14 days[2-4] or 5–30 mcg/kg/d IV (bacteria [*Escherichia coli*] derived) over 4 h for up to 21 days.[5] Alternatively, 5 mcg/kg SC for up to 21 days following chemotherapy or irradiation.[6,7]

Bone marrow transplantation: 250 mcg/m² IV over 2 h beginning 2–4 h after transplant and not <24 h after chemotherapy or after radiation until absolute neutrophil count (ANC) >1500 cells/mm³ for 3 consecutive days[2] or 250 mcg/m² IV over 4 h beginning after transplant for 21 days.[8]

Neutropenia

Congenital neutropenia: Five children (age 1, 2, 3, 9, and 19 years) were started on 3 mcg/kg/d IV over 30–60 min for 14 days that was increased to 10 mcg/kg/d if the ANC failed to increase and finally to 30 mcg/kg/d. Only one had an increase in ANC.[8] One patient received 10 mcg/kg/d as a continuous infusion for 4 weeks followed by SC dosing for another week without response.[9]

Neutropenia associated with HIV or antiretroviral therapy: 250 mcg/m²/d IV or SC for 2–4 weeks.[1]

Neutropenic and septic premature and term neonates ≥28 weeks gestation: 5 mcg/kg over 2 h once daily for 5 days[10] or 4 mcg/kg over 2 h q 12 h for up to 6 days or until neutropenia resolved.[11]

Aplastic anemia: In nine children (0.7–19 years of age), induction phase continuous infusion doses of either 8 mcg/kg increased after 14 days to 16 mcg/kg for up to 14 more days if the hematologic response was inadequate or doses of 16 mcg/kg increased to 32 mcg/kg (Chinese hamster ovary cell derived).[12] After the induction phase, administration was changed to SC dosing.[12] Eighteen children received a standard immunosuppressive regimen for 5 days and then GM-CSF at 250 mcg/m² SC was started.[13]

Incomplete remission after treatment for neuroblastoma: phase II study in 45 children who also received a murine monoclonal antibody against neuroblastoma[14]

Days	1–5	6, 7	8–10	11, 12	13–17
Dose (mcg/m²)	250	250	500	500	
Route	SC	IV over 2 h	IV over 2 h	SC	IV over 2 h

Dosage adjustment in organ dysfunction

None. Patients with renal or hepatic impairment should have renal function or liver function monitored weekly.[1]

Maximum dosage

32 mcg/kg[12] or 1500 mcg/m².[3]

IV push

Not indicated.[1,2]

Intermittent infusion

Usually infused over 2 to 4 h[1-4] but has been given over 30 min.[9] (See Comments section.)

Continuous infusion

≥10 mcg/mL in NS.[1]

Other routes of administration	Not administered IM. The liquid product (500 mcg/mL) can be given SC undiluted.[1] The lyophilized product is reconstituted to 250 mcg/mL and given SC without further dilution.[1] (See Comments section.)
Maximum concentration	Reconstitute vials to 250 or 500 mcg/mL in SW and then dilute in NS.[1] (See Comments section.)
Cautions related to IV administration	With either IV or SC dosing, a first-dose response that includes respiratory distress, hypotension, tachycardia, and flushing is common with infusion of the first dose in *adults*.[1] Symptomatic treatment should include administration of oxygen, fluids and acetaminophen, or nonsteroidal anti-inflammatory agents.[1] For PN compatibility information, please see Appendix C.
Other additives	The liquid product contains 1.1% benzyl alcohol, 1.9 mg of edetate disodium, 40 mg mannitol, 10 mg sucrose, and 1.2 mg/mL tromethamine. After reconstitution, each mL of the lyophilized product contains 40 mg mannitol, 10 mg sucrose, and 1.2 mg/mL tromethamine. This should be used within 6 h of reconstitution because it contains no preservative.[1,2] Bacteriostatic water for injection can be used to reconstitute the lyophilized product; it contains benzyl alcohol. Benzyl alcohol in small doses as a preservative in drugs is considered safe in newborns.[15] However, a 3-week-old, very low birth weight (710 g) infant who received clindamycin experienced a profound desaturation that required resuscitation after the third and fourth doses, which was subsequently related to the benzyl alcohol preservative.[16] Administration of saline flushes containing benzyl alcohol (bacteriostatic water for injection) was associated with a fatal gasping syndrome, intraventricular hemorrhage, metabolic acidosis, and increased mortality in preterm infants.[17] This should not be used in neonates. Hypersensitivity reactions to benzyl alcohol in parenteral products have been reported in *adults*.[18,19]
Comments	The lyophilized product reconstituted with SW must be used within 6 h of reconstitution because it contains no preservatives.[1,2] A CBC with differential is recommended twice a week during therapy to evaluate for leukocytosis. If the ANC >20,000 cells/mm^3, or the platelet count >500,000 cells/mm^3, the dose should be decreased by 50% or held.[1,2] Children receiving multiple courses of SC GM-CSF have experienced acute toxicities at various times during their dosing including fever, tachycardia, hypotension and rash requiring discontinuation.[6] The severity of adverse reactions appears to be less with the yeast-derived product than those derived in Chinese hamster ovary cells or bacteria.[1] If significant adverse effects occur, discontinue the drug until the toxicity resolves, then restart at 50% of the initial dose.[2] Pericardial and pleural effusions, myalgias, and volume overload are dose-limiting side effects in *adults*.[1,2] Although adverse effects have been reported in children, they are usually mild[4,5] and unrelated to dose.[3] However, cardiopulmonary symptoms occurred in a child receiving continuous infusion of 24 mcg/kg/d[12] and a deep vein thrombosis occurred in a child being treated for myelosuppressive chemotherapy, who inadvertently received 1500 mcg/m^2/d for 7 days.[3] For more dilute solutions, albumin should be added to the NS diluent to achieve a final albumin concentration of 0.1% prior to the addition of sargramostim to prevent adsorption to the drug delivery system.[1,2,20] An in-line membrane filter should not be used when sargramostim is given IV.[1,2] One study presented evidence that GM-CSF has the potential to activate the coagulation system in pediatric patients receiving bone marrow or stem cell transplant.[21]

Sodium Bicarbonate

Brand names	Various manufacturers

Dosage

Cardiopulmonary resuscitation: Sodium bicarbonate should only be used after establishment of airway and adequate ventilation, administration of oxygen and medications (e.g., epinephrine and lidocaine), and restoration of effective circulation.[1,2,3]

Routine use of sodium bicarbonate does not improve the outcome of cardiac arrest in children; however, there are certain times when its use can be considered.[1] Doses range from 1–2 mEq/kg.[1,2] The 4.2% solution (0.5 mEq/mL) should be used in neonates and infants ≤2 years to decrease the osmotic load and the infusion rate should be slow.[1,4]

Cocaine-induced ventricular arrhythmia: 1–2 mEq/kg.[1,2]

Prolonged cardiac arrest: 1 mEq/kg.[1,2]

Tricyclic antidepressant, sodium channel blocker toxicity: 1–2 mEq/kg until arterial pH is >7.45; then use continuous infusion to maintain alkalosis.[1]

Metabolic acidosis: 1–2 mEq/kg.[2] Alternatively, the dose for correction can be calculated using the following equation[5]:

HCO_3 (mEq) = 0.3 (L/kg) × weight (kg) × base deficit (mEq/L)

Subsequent dosing should be based on current acid-base status.[1] Complete correction of the base deficit should occur over >24 h because the compensatory changes may be delayed.[5] (See Comments section.)

Urinary alkalinization

Rhabdomyolysis: Salicylate poisoning in a child[6]: 25 mEq infused over 1 h. Additional doses should be given to maintain urine pH 7.5–8.5. Keep arterial pH ≤7.5.

Tumor lysis syndrome (prevention): D5¼NS + 50 – 100 mEq/L $NaHCO_3$ (no potassium) infused at 3–6 L/m²/d and titrated to a urinary pH of 7–7.5. Serum bicarbonate concentration should be kept ≤30 mEq/L.[7] (See Comments section.)

Dosage adjustment in organ dysfunction

No information available to support the need for dosage adjustment.

Use caution in patients with renal insufficiency as administration may lead to metabolic alkalosis.[5]

Maximum dosage

2 mEq/kg/dose[2] or 8 mEq/kg/d.[4,5,8]

IV push

This method of administration is reserved for cardiac arrest.

Intermittent infusion

2–5 mEq/kg over 4–8 h in older children.[4,5]

Continuous infusion

Not the usual route of administration.

Other routes of administration

Generally not recommended.[5] Can be given SC if diluted to 1.5% (isotonicity).[5,9] May be administered IO if unable to establish adequate IV access during cardiac arrest.[5]

Cautions related to IV administration

Rapid infusion (>10 mL/min) of hypertonic sodium bicarbonate in neonates and children ≤2 years of age may produce hypernatremia, decreased CSF pressure, and possible intracranial hemorrhage.[5] Extravasation may cause local ischemia and tissue necrosis.[10]

For PN compatibility information, please see Appendix C.

Maximum concentration

4.2% (0.5 mEg/mL) in neonates and infants <2-years-old; 8.4% (1 mEq/mL) in those ≥2-years-old.[4,5]

Other additives

Each gram of sodium bicarbonate contains 12 mEq sodium.[4,5]

The 5% solution in 500-mL bottles also contains 0.9 mg/mL of edetate disodium.[5,9]

Comments

In neonates and infants, hypernatremia and hyperosmolality may occur and result in fluid overload or intracranial hemorrhage.[4,11,12]

Adjunctive IV bicarbonate therapy is commonly used in children with severe DKA and a pH <6.9.[13] However, a retrospective study reported no difference in rate of metabolic recovery and complications between patients treated with or without bicarbonate, and hospitalization was prolonged in the bicarbonate group.[14]

Arterial blood gas analysis may not accurately reflect tissue and venous pH during cardiac arrest or severe shock.[1]

Calcium precipitates with bicarbonate and bicarbonate inactivates catecholamines. It is important to adequately flush the IV lines between administration of resuscitation drugs and sodium bicarbonate.[1,5]

Metabolic alkalosis is a complication that may result in hypokalemia, hypocalcemia, and impaired delivery of oxygen to the tissue.[4,5,8]

In a retrospective review of 1771 *adults* with rhabdomyolysis due to trauma, bicarbonate and mannitol forced diuresis did not decrease renal failure when compared to a group that did not receive this treatment.[15]

Sodium Chloride

Brand names	Various manufacturers 0.45% saline (1/2 NS) = 77 mEq/L 0.9% saline (NS) = 154 mEq/L 3% saline = 513 mEq/L 5% saline = 855 mEq/L

Dosage

Hypotension/shock: 20 mL/kg of NS that may be repeated. Up to 80 mL/kg may be required during the first h; however, the child should continuously be assessed for fluid overload.[2]

Moderate-to-severe dehydration: 20 mL/kg of NS that may be repeated in severe dehydration.[1] This is followed by replacement of the fluid deficit (% dehydration × wt [kg]) over 24 h.[1]

Severe traumatic brain injury: 1.5% saline (268 mEq/L) infused to obtain a desired serum sodium concentration of 145–150 mEq/L[6] or 0.1–1 mL/kg/h 3% saline titrated to an intracranial pressure (ICP) of <20 mm Hg.[7-9]

Symptomatic hyponatremia (see Comments section): The sodium deficit can be estimated using the following equation[3]:

Sodium deficit (mEq) = 0.6 × weight (kg) × (desired serum sodium [usually 135 mEq/L] – measured serum sodium).[1]

Initially, the rate of infusion of 3% saline should increase the sodium concentration by 1 mEq/L/h until symptoms resolve.[4] As an estimate, 1 mL/kg of 3% sodium chloride will raise the serum sodium by 1 mEq/L.[4] More aggressive replacement may be required in patients with severe symptoms such as seizures.[5] Following resolution of symptoms, the infusion should be adjusted to increase serum sodium concentration by no more than 10–12 mEq/L/d.[1,3] (See Comments section.) Frequent monitoring of serum sodium concentrations is essential.

Dosage adjustment in organ dysfunction

None required.

Maximum dosage

None established.

IV push

20 mL/kg given rapidly may be indicated in severe hypotension/shock.[2]

Intermittent infusion

20 mL/kg over 20 min to 1 h in moderate dehydration.[1,3]

Continuous infusion

Usual method of administration.[10,11] 3% saline and greater concentrations should be infused via a central line.[10]

Other routes of administration

Not indicated.

Maximum concentration

154 mEq/L via a peripheral line.[10] 5% saline administered via a central line.[10]

Cautions related to IV administration

See Comments section regarding rapid correction of serum sodium concentration.

Other additives

May contain benzyl alcohol or parabens as a preservative.[10] Benzyl alcohol in small doses as a preservative in drugs is considered safe in newborns.[12] However, a 3-week-old, very low birth weight (710 g) infant who received clindamycin experienced a profound desaturation that required resuscitation after the third and fourth doses, which was subsequently related to the benzyl alcohol preservative.[13]

Administration of saline flushes containing benzyl alcohol (bacteriostatic water for injection) was associated with a fatal gasping syndrome, intraventricular hemorrhage, metabolic acidosis, and increased mortality in preterm infants.[14] This should not be used in neonates.

Hypersensitivity reactions to benzyl alcohol in parenteral products have been reported in *adults*.[15,16]

Paraben preservatives may cause hypersensitivity reactions that are more common with cutaneous exposure.[17] However, one case of pruritus and bronchospasm that occurred following infusion of hydrocortisone, which contained a paraben, has been reported.[18]

Comments

Because of the larger brain to intracranial volume, children are more likely to develop encephalopathy during hyponatremia. Symptoms associated with hyponatremia are primarily related to central nervous system effects. In general, a serum sodium concentration of 130 mEq/L results in symptoms including nausea, headache, and muscle aches. With concentrations below 125 mEq/L, symptoms progress to lethargy, confusion, agitation, and seizures. Those who slowly develop hyponatremia may be relatively asymptomatic; however, those with a more rapid rate of decline of the sodium concentration are likely to be symptomatic with mild hyponatremia.[5] And in those who develop hyponatremia rapidly, cerebral edema can occur.[5]

During hyponatremia, shifts of water and sodium occur to maintain normal cellular volume. After 48–72 h in an adaptive response, organic osmolytes are mobilized to maintain the cellular volume. Too rapid correction of hyponatremia can result in central pontine or extrapontine myelinolysis.[19-21]

Sodium Nitroprusside

Brand names	Nipride, Nitropress
Dosage	0.25–0.3 mcg/kg/min initially titrated by 0.25 mcg/kg/min q 5–10 min up to a maximum of 10 mcg/kg/min.[1-18] Infusion rates of up to 6 mcg/kg/min in neonates and 8 mcg/kg/min in children have been reported.[7,14] The manufacturer recommends that if blood pressure is not controlled after 10 min at 10 mcg/kg/min, the infusion should be discontinued.[1,2] The infusion may be tapered off to avoid potential rebound hypertension.[7,19,20] (See Comments section.) Usual maintenance dose requirement is <2 mcg/kg/min in neonates[17] and ≤3 mcg/kg/min in children and *adults*.[2] In hypertensive emergencies, blood pressure should be frequently monitored to ensure that it does not decrease too quickly.[1,4] One group recommended that the blood pressure decrease by one-third of the desired total blood pressure decrease within 6–12 h, a further one-third decrease within the next 24 h, with the final one-third decrease achieved over the next 2 days.[21] Alternatively, a blood pressure decrease of <25% within min to 1 h followed by further decreases over the next 2–6 h if the patient is stable has been suggested.[1] (See Cautions related to IV administration section.)
Dosage adjustment in organ dysfunction	Use cautiously in severe renal or hepatic disease.[2] The dose in anuric patients receiving a prolonged infusion should be ≤1 mcg/kg/min to ensure thiocyanate concentrations are <60 mcg/mL. [2] (See Comments section.)
Maximum dosage	10 mcg/kg/min for a maximum of 10 min.[1,2] In *adults*, 400 mcg/kg/min was infused for short periods.[22] A cumulative dose of 3–3.5 mg/kg has been associated with toxicity in *adults*.[23,24] A cumulative dose of 4.3–9.1 mg/kg was infused over 23–73 h in five children 2–169 months of age with normal renal and hepatic function without apparent toxicity.[13]
IV push	Not indicated.
Intermittent infusion	Not indicated.
Continuous infusion	50–200 mcg/mL in D5W, LR, or NS.[1,2,22,23] Although it is not necessary to protect IV tubing, the bottle, burette, and/or syringe pump should be covered with an opaque protective covering.[1,2] Amber plastic coverings are ineffective.[23] The PALS guidelines and AAP recommend the following formula for preparation of the infusion: 6 × weight (kg) = mg of drug to be added to IV solution for a total volume of 100 mL. An infusion rate of 1 mL/h provides 1 mcg/kg/min. This formula estimates an initial concentration. Ultimately, the concentration of the drug should consider the patient's fluid requirements or fluid limitations. Despite widespread use of the above formula, recent JCAHO® guidelines recommend the implementation of "standardized concentrations" of vasoactive medications.[24]
Other routes of administration	Not indicated.
Maximum concentration	200 mcg/mL[1] but 100 mcg/mL is usually used for pediatric patients.[8] In *adults*, a concentration of 800 mcg/mL has been used.[25]

Cautions related to IV administration

Too rapid decrease in blood pressure can result in serious unwanted side effects.[1,2] Because profound hypotension may occur, blood pressure should be continuously monitored with an arterial line.[1,2,4]

Use with caution in those with increased intracranial pressure and those with compensatory hypertension, such as infants with arteriovenous shunt or coarctation of the aorta.[1,2]

For PN compatibility information, please see Appendix C.

Other additives

Contains 0.335 mEq sodium/50 mg of sodium nitroprusside.[23,26]

Comments

A retrospective study reported rebound hypertension in *adults* with nitroprusside induced hypotension during a surgical procedure.[19]

Neonatal lambs experienced rebound hypertension after a nitroprusside infusion was abruptly discontinued and investigators postulated that immaturity of feedback mechanisms or metabolism of vasoactive mediators stimulated during the infusion may be responsible.[20]

Cyanide toxicity (and the development of metabolic acidosis) usually occurs with prolonged use; however, it has been reported after as short a time as a few hours.[1,2,22,27,28] No association between cumulative dose or duration of therapy and increased cyanide levels has been noted.[29] Those with decreased renal function may be at increased risk.[4]

Thiocyanate is a product of cyanide metabolism and a route for cyanide elimination. To minimize steady state thiocyanate concentrations, the infusion should be <3 mcg/kg/min in patients with normal renal function and ≤1 mcg/kg/min in those who are anuric.[1,2] Some recommend monitoring thiocyanate concentrations in patients receiving >3 mcg/kg/min, who receive an infusion for 24–48 h, and in patients with renal or hepatic dysfunction.[18] Sodium thiosulfate has been administered with sodium nitroprusside at infusion rates of five to 10 times that of nitroprusside to accelerate the metabolism of cyanide; however, further study is needed before this can be recommended.[1,2]

Methemoglobinemia can occur in those who have received >10 mg/kg. Patients with methemoglobinemia (>10% of hemoglobin) exhibit signs of impaired oxygen delivery despite adequate cardiac output and arterial PaO_2.[2] Methylene blue is an antidote but should be used cautiously.[2]

Succinylcholine Chloride

Brand names	Anectine, Quelicin
Dosage	Respiratory function must be supported during use and concurrent administration of a sedative is necessary.[1] Monitoring of neuromuscular transmission with a peripheral nerve stimulator is recommended with repeated dosing.[1,2] Dosing for rapid sequence intubation should be based on actual body weight, not ideal or lean body mass.[3] Because of potential vagal stimulation with succinylcholine, prophylactic atropine doses (0.01–0.02 mg/kg with minimum of 0.15 mg) should always be administered with or, preferably, before succinylcholine.[2] **Loading dose (for intubation or short surgical procedures):** 1–2 mg/kg[4-9]; 1 mg/kg is recommended for older children and adolescents.[5-9] **Maintenance dose:** 0.3–1 mg/kg q 5–10 min as needed.[4-9] Normal *adult* dosing is 0.04–0.07 mg/kg q 5–10 min as needed.[1]
Dosage adjustment in organ dysfunction	No adjustment necessary in renal failure.[1] However, use with caution because succinylcholine can cause hyperkalemia.[1] Dose should be decreased in hepatic failure.[1]
Maximum dosage	2 mg/kg IV or 4 mg/kg IM.[1] Not to exceed 150 mg when given IM.[2]
IV push	100 mg/mL (available commercially) given over 10–30 sec.[1] Flush needle or catheter with D5W or NS after administration.[1]
Intermittent infusion	No information available to support administration by this method.
Continuous infusion	1–2 mg/mL in D5W, NS, or D5NS.[1] Not routinely recommended. Although continuous infusion is generally preferred for long surgical procedures in *adults*[1] and has been used successfully for neuromuscular relaxation in infants, tachyphylaxis and phase II nerve block have occurred during continuous infusion in infants and children.[10] The risk of malignant hyperthermia also precludes continuous infusions in infants and children.[1]
Other routes of administration	2.5–4 mg/kg, not to exceed a 150-mg total dose, by deep IM injection.[1] No information available to support administration by other routes.
Maximum concentration	100 mg/mL for IV push and 2 mg/mL for continuous infusion.[1]
Cautions related to IV administration	If given by rapid administration may cause bradyarrhythmias secondary to vagal stimulation.[1,8,9,11] As mentioned above, pretreatment with atropine may reduce this risk.[1,8,9]

Other additives

Benzyl alcohol: Multidose vials contain benzyl alcohol 0.9% as a preservative.[1] Administration of flushes containing benzyl alcohol (bacteriostatic water for injection) was associated with a fatal gasping syndrome, intraventricular hemorrhage, metabolic acidosis, and increased mortality in preterm infants.[12] While benzyl alcohol in small doses as a preservative in drugs is considered safe in newborns,[13] a 3-week-old, very low birth weight (710 g) infant experienced a profound desaturation that required resuscitation after receiving clindamycin (third and fourth doses), which was subsequently related to the benzyl alcohol preservative.[14]

Hypersensitivity reactions to benzyl alcohol in parenteral products have been reported in *adults*.[15,16]

Comments

Infants and children are more resistant than *adults* to the neuromuscular blockade produced by succinylcholine.[1,8,9] Succinylcholine-induced prolonged apnea secondary to neuromuscular blockade has occurred in neonates.[17]

Hyperkalemia may occur, especially in patients who have trauma, severe burns, or neuromuscular disease.[1,8,9,18,19] If serum potassium is 5.5 mEq/L, succinylcholine should not be used.[1]

Acute rhabdomyolysis with hyperkalemia, followed by ventricular dysrhythmias, cardiac arrest, and death, occurred soon after administration of succinylcholine to apparently healthy children.[1,8,9,20,21] These children were found subsequently to have Duchenne's muscular dystrophy. This syndrome may present with peaked T-waves and sudden cardiac arrest within minutes of administration. It appears to be most common in males ≤8 years old.[1] If a healthy infant or child develops sudden cardiac arrest soon after administration of succinylcholine, and the arrest is not due to inadequate ventilation, oxygenation, or anesthetic overdose, immediate treatment for hyperkalemia should be instituted with calcium bicarbonate, glucose with insulin, and hyperventilation.[1]

Because succinylcholine is associated with numerous drug interactions, consult appropriate resources for dosing recommendations before combining any drug with succinylcholine.[1]

Sufentanil Citrate

Brand names	Sufenta

Dosage

Dosages vary depending on the desired degree of analgesia/anesthesia and adjunctive therapies (e.g., halothane, propofol).

Use lean body weight when dosing patients whose weight is >20% of their ideal body weight.[1] (See Appendix B.)

Analgesia (children >12 years): 10–25 mcg administered as needed or continuous or intermittent infusion of ≤1 mcg/kg/h.[4]

Anesthesia: The elimination half-life is shorter in infants and children and longer in neonates compared to that of adolescents and *adults*.[2,3] Clearance can be further reduced by up to a third in neonates with cardiovascular disease.[3]

Neonates: 5–10 mcg/kg initial dose followed by a continuous infusion or 1–2 mcg/kg/h.[4]

Infants and children (<2 years): 5–20 mcg/kg (0.5 mcg/kg dose when combined with halothane and nitric oxide)[6,7] followed by a continuous infusion of 1–1.5 mcg/kg/h.[6,7]

Children (2–12 years): An initial dose of 10–25 mcg/kg administered over 2–5 min with supplemental doses of up to 0.5–0.75 mcg/kg as needed.[6,7] The clearance of sufentanil in healthy children is about twice that reported for adolescents and *adults*.[3] Should be administered with 100% oxygen and a skeletal muscle relaxant.[7]

Adolescents and adults: 8–30 mcg/kg as an initial dose with doses of 0.5–10 mcg/kg given at the first incision and repeated as needed.[4] Repeat doses should be increased or decreased based on response to initial dose. Alternatively, doses up to 25 mcg and 50 mcg may be given as an intermittent or continuous infusion for minor and major surgical procedures, respectively.[8] For procedures lasting longer than 1 h, the total sufentanil dose should not exceed 30 mcg/kg.[8] For all procedures the total infusion dose should not exceed 1 mcg/kg/h of anticipated procedure time.[8]

Dosage adjustment in organ dysfunction

No dosage adjustment required in patients with renal dysfunction.[8,9] Sufentanil should be administered with caution in patients with hepatic or renal impairment, since the drug undergoes metabolism mainly in the liver.[9]

Maximum dosage

Doses should be titrated to an appropriate level of anesthesia or pain control with manageable adverse effects.[4] In *adults* a maximum dose of 30 mcg/kg has been recommended for anesthesia and 50 mcg/kg for analgesia.[4] For procedures lasting only 1–2 h, doses should not exceed 1 mcg/kg/h of anticipated surgical time.[9]

IV push

50 mcg/mL given over 2–5 min.[4,6,10,11]

Intermittent infusion

Not given by this method.

Continuous infusion

12 mcg/mL in D5W or NS.[4,5,7,11]

Other routes of administration

Although sufentanil has been given by IM administration,[9] it is generally not administered via this route. It can be given by epidural injection.[4]

Maximum concentration	50 mcg/mL.[11]
Cautions related to IV administration	Significant bradycardia, muscle or chest wall rigidity, and apnea may occur early in administration of sufentanil. Pretreatment with atropine and a nondepolarizing neuromuscular blocking agent may aid in minimizing these adverse effects. Ventilation support is indicated.[4]
Other additives	None.
Comments	Caution should be used when administering sufentanil to patients with head trauma. It has been associated with increases in intracranial pressure in this population.[12]

Tacrolimus

Brand names	Prograf
Dosage	In the absence of pre-existing renal or hepatic impairment, pediatric patients require larger doses per body weight compared to *adults*; and the risk of lymphoproliferative disorders is greater in pediatric patients.[1,2] **Cardiac transplantation:** 0.05–0.15 mg/kg/d starting ≥6 h after transplantation if urine output is >1 mL/kg/h. Initial monitoring of blood concentrations at 12 h.[14] **Graft-versus-host disease (GVHD) after bone marrow transplantation:** Limited research supports the administration of 0.03 mg/kg of tacrolimus plus mycophenolate mofetil or methotrexate as a 24-h continuous infusion beginning the day before transplantation for GVHD prophylaxis.[11,12] Another group treated an 18-year-old and a 9-year-old with steroid-resistant, severe, acute GVHD with 0.1 mg/kg as a 24-h continuous infusion, maintaining serum concentration at 25–35 ng/mL. (The specifics of the assay were not reported.)[13] (See Comments section.) **Liver or renal transplantation:** 0.03–0.15 mg/kg/d by continuous infusion.[3-9] The first dose should be given >6 h after liver transplant and within 24 h of kidney transplant if renal function has recovered (SCr <4 mg/dL).[2] Therapy should be postponed >48 h in renal transplant patients with postoperative oliguria.[2] Initial dose should be administered over ≥12 h.[2] Use lowest dose that attains the desired response or serum concentration and change to oral therapy as soon as possible.[1-6] Children who received an intact child's liver had a greater than expected clearance of tacrolimus, while those who received a cut-down liver from an *adult* had lower clearance than expected.[10]
Dosage adjustment in organ dysfunction	In renal and hepatic insufficiency (Pugh ≤10), initial doses should be the lowest in the recommended range.[2] Monitor trough serum concentration and change to oral therapy as soon as possible.[2]
Maximum dosage	Not established. 0.44 mg/kg/d has been given to *adults*.[9]
IV push	Not indicated.
Intermittent infusion	Not indicated.
Continuous infusion	0.004–0.02 mg/mL in D5W or NS[2,15] given over 4–24 h.[2-4,6,7,15]
Other routes of administration	No information available to support administration by other routes.
Maximum concentration	0.02 mg/mL.[2]
Cautions related to IV administration	Anaphylaxis to the polyoxyl 60 hydrogenated castor oil vehicle has occurred.[1,2] Observe patient continuously for ≥30 min after start of infusion and frequently thereafter.[1,2] Oxygen and an aqueous solution of epinephrine 1:1000 should be at the bedside during the infusion.[1,2] For PN compatibility information, please see Appendix C.

Other additives	Each mL contains 200 mg polyoxyl 60 hydrogenated castor oil (HCO-60) and dehydrated alcohol 80% w/v.[1,2]

Comments

Contraindicated in patients allergic to polyoxyl 60 hydrogenated castor oil.[1,2]

To minimize toxicity, monitor whole blood, serum, or plasma concentrations.[2,4] Use the same matrix and assay type consistently for a given patient.[2] Whole blood is the preferred matrix and samples should be collected in EDTA tubes.[2] Trough concentrations should range from 5–20 ng/mL for whole blood.[2] Accuracy of whole blood measurements is diminished when microparticle enzyme immunoassay methods are used and concentrations are <9 ng/mL. Liquid chromatography—tandem mass spectrometry assays are associated with greater sensitivity and precision.[16]

Absorbs to PVC; therefore, store in polyolefin containers or glass IV bottles. Infusion through PVC anesthesia extension tubing, PVC IV administration set tubing, or fat emulsion tubing does not result in decreased blood concentrations.[17,18] Surfactants in injectable products have been associated with leeching of the plasticizer DEHP when stored or administered in PVC containers. Only glass, polyethylene or non-DEHP plasticized administration sets should be used for tacrolimus infusions.[15]

Reversible left ventricular wall thickening was noted in pediatric and *adult* patients who had trough concentrations >15 ng/mL.[19]

Tacrolimus is a substrate of CYP3A4 and can be inhibited or induced by other drugs. Consult appropriate resources for dosing recommendations before combining any drug with tacrolimus.

Hypertension occurs frequently. Serum potassium should be monitored to be sure hyperkalemia has not developed.[2]

When converting from IV to oral dosing, the first oral dose should be given 8–12 h after the infusion is stopped.[2]

Terbutaline Sulfate

Brand names	Brethine, generic
Dosage	The National Asthma Education and Prevention Program (NAEPP) Expert Panel Report 2: Update on Selected Topics 2002 states that there is no proven advantage of systemic terbutaline therapy over aerosol.[1] However, the following doses have been reported in the literature. **Acute asthma:** 0.01 mg/kg SC q 20 min for three doses then q 2–6 h as needed (in *adults* 0.25 mg q 20 min for three doses).[1] SC administration of 10 mg/24 h, 3.6 mg divided q 12–15 min for 3 h, 0.2 mg q 4 h has been reported in adolescents.[2] In children 7–33 months old, SC infusion of 0.2–0.3 mcg/kg/min for 20 min followed by 0.1 mcg/kg/min for an average of 6 days.[3] IV loading dose of 2 mcg/kg over 5 min up to 10 mcg/kg over 30 min followed by 0.08–0.4 mcg/kg/min with increases of 0.1–0.2 mcg/kg/min q 30 min to desired response or toxicity.[4-6] Alternatively, an initial infusion of 0.5–1 mcg/kg/min increased by 0.1–0.2 mcg/kg/min q 2 h or according to respiratory symptoms up to 5–10 mcg/kg/min.[7,8] Usual doses are ≤5 mcg/kg/min.[5,6,8] (See Comments section.) **Chronic asthma:** In eight children (8–14 years old) with chronic severe asthma, SC infusion of 2.5–5 mg/24 h increased to 10 mg/24 h as indicated (improvement in symptoms) and tolerated was used for ≥2 months.[9]
Dosage adjustment in organ dysfunction	If CrCl is ≤ 50 mL/min, reduce usual dose 50%.[10]
Maximum dosage	10 mcg/kg as loading dose.[5,6] 10 mcg/kg/min for 6 h has been reported in an adolescent.[7]
IV push	Not indicated.[11]
Intermittent infusion	0.05 mg/mL in NS has been infused over 5 min in a pharmacokinetic study in seven children 8–11.7 years old.[12]
Continuous infusion	Diluted in D5W, ¼NS, or NS.[13]
Other routes of administration	Usually SC. IM administration is not indicated.
Maximum concentration	1 mg/mL (undiluted) for SC bolus administration.[13,14] 0.05 mg/mL for SC infusion.[9]
Cautions related to IV administration	The manufacturer does not recommend IV administration.[11] (See Comments section.)

Other additives Sodium chloride added for isotonicity.[11]

Comments

Current parenteral terbutaline products are marketed only for SC administration.[13]

Although larger doses are used in children than in *adults*, there is no pharmacokinetic basis to support the need for larger doses.[12]

In children, increased heart rate,[3,4,7,8] increased systolic and decreased diastolic blood pressure,[4,7] tremor,[4,9] headache,[4] and decreased serum potassium[8] have been reported. An 11-year-old who received 10 mcg/kg/min for 6 h had no evidence of arrhythmias, and creatine phosphokinase-MB (CPK-MB) cardiac isoenzymes were normal.[7] However, in that same study three children receiving a lower terbutaline dose (two of these three were also receiving aminophylline) did have an elevated CPK-MB concentration. Two of 18 children developed ST segment depression following terbutaline and epinephrine. There was no correlation between CPK values and arrhythmias or ST changes.[7]

The incidence of tremor and tachycardia may be increased in those receiving theophylline concomitantly.[4]

Bruising, tenderness, and site infection have been reported with continuous SC infusion.[9]

Terbutaline may increase theophylline clearance.[15]

Thiopental Sodium

Brand names	Pentothal

Dosage

Be prepared to provide respiratory support. Monitor oxygen saturation because large doses may cause hypotension and apnea. Use cautiously in patients with cardiac compromise or hypovolemia.

Anesthesia induction and maintenance: 4–8.6 mg/kg over 10–60 min.[1-6] Although rapid injection can cause hypotension and decreased cardiac output, 5 mg/kg have been given over 10 sec when rapid induction was needed.[3] If clinically indicated, 0.1 mg/kg/sec may be given until the face mask is tolerated.[7] If necessary, a second dose of 1 mg/kg may be infused. Although some have suggested that the induction doses of thiopental should be higher (relative to weight) in children[8] and lower in neonates,[9] others have found no difference in dosing based on age.[10,11]

Elevated intracranial pressure

Acute increases: 1.5–3.5 mg/kg, repeat as needed.[1,2]

Sustained elevations (medically induced coma)

Neonates: A loading dose of 10–30 mg/kg[12-14] followed by 2–4 mg/kg/h as a continuous infusion.[12,14] Two studies evaluated the effects of short-term[13] and prolonged coma with thiopental on outcome in neonates with asphyxia and reported no improvement; however, a greater complication rate (i.e., hypotension) was noted.[13,14]

Infants and children: A loading dose of 10–30 mg/kg.[12,15-18] Some investigators recommend administration of two loading doses: 20 mg/kg over 1 h followed by 10 mg/kg over 6 h.[13] The loading dose should be followed by a 1–2 mg/kg/h continuous infusion and should be titrated based on clinical response and/or serum thiopental concentration (20–40 mg/L).[12,15,18]

Procedural sedation (for procedures <15 min): Has been given rectally for this purpose[19]; however, other barbiturates are more frequently used. (See Pentobarbital monograph.)[19]

Status epilepticus

Loading: 10–30 mg/kg.[20,21]

Maintenance: 5–55 mg/kg/h.[20] Total doses of thiopental used to obtain and maintain burst suppression were 15–50 g over 48–120 h and correlated with plasma thiopental levels of 25–40 mg/dL.[20] Some clinicians begin at 5 mg/kg/h and gradually increase by 1–2 mg/kg/h for 6–8 h until all electrical brain activity is suppressed.[22,23]

Dosage adjustment in organ dysfunction

Because the hypnotic effect may be prolonged in renal or hepatic disease, thiopental should be used cautiously in these patients.[1,24] Adjust dose in patients with renal dysfunction.[24,25] If CrCl is <10 mL/min, give 75% of normal dose.[24] May need to reduce dosage in hepatic failure/cirrhosis, but specific recommendations have not been made.[25]

Maximum dosage

Not established.

IV push

When given via this method, thiopental should be administered over 20–30 sec; however, hypotension may occur.[26] Twenty infants, age 12 months, received 5 mg/kg over 10 sec for rapid anesthesia induction[7] and 10 mg was given over 2 min to neonates with resistant seizures without adverse effects.[21] (See Cautions related to IV administration section.)

Thiopental Sodium

Intermittent infusion	20–50 mg/mL in D5W, NS, or SW[1] given over 10–60 min with rate titrated according to blood pressure.[12,14,17,26]
Continuous infusion	2–4 mg/mL in D5W or NS for continuous infusion.[1,27] Sterile water for injection should *not* be used for preparing solutions <2% thiopental since use of the resulting hypotonic solutions will cause hemolysis.[27]
Other routes of administration	IM administration not recommended because of tissue necrosis.[1,2,26] No information available to support administration by other routes.
Maximum concentration	50 mg/mL is the highest concentration listed by the manufacturer.[1]
Cautions related to IV administration	Respiratory depression, apnea, laryngospasm, and hypotension may occur if administration is too rapid.[1] High alkaline pH may cause tissue necrosis upon extravasation.[1]
Other additives	Contains 4.9 mEq sodium/g of thiopental sodium.[27]
Comments	Use cautiously in patients who are receiving concomitant vasodilators (e.g., low-dose dopamine).[13,14,28] High-dose thiopental leads to a pronounced fall in serum potassium; therefore, measure diurnal urinary loss of potassium.[28] Renal failure may occur as a complication of barbiturate treatment. Monitor BUN and serum creatinine.[28] Recovery time after large or repeated doses may be more rapid for infants and children compared to *adults* because of a higher clearance.[29]

Ticarcillin

Brand names Ticar

Dosage

Serious anaphylactoid reactions may require immediate emergency treatment with epinephrine, oxygen, IV steroids, and airway management.

Neonates

PNA	<1200 g	≤2000 g	>2000 g
<7d	150 mg/kg/d divided q 12 h[1]*	150 mg/kg/d divided q 12 h[2-5]	225 mg/kg/d divided q 8 h[2-5]
≥7d		225 mg/kg/d divided q 8 h[2-5]	300 mg/kg/d divided q 6 h[2-5]

*Until 4 weeks of age.

Infants and children

Mild to moderate infections: 100–200 mg/k/d divided q 6 h up to 6 g/d.[2,6,7]

Severe infections: 200–300 mg/kg/d divided q 6 h up to 24 g/d.[2,6,7]

Cystic fibrosis: 400 mg/kg/d divided q 4–6 h not to exceed 24 g/d.[8-12]

Febrile neutropenia: 9 g/m^2/d divided q 6 h given in conjunction with other antibiotics.[13,14]

Dosage adjustment in organ dysfunction

Adjust dosage in patients with renal dysfunction.[16,17] If CrCl is 10–50 mL/min, give normal dose q 8 h; if CrCl is <10 mL/min, give normal dose q 12 h.[16] Ticarcillin-associated neurotoxicity has been reported in a patient with renal failure.[18]

Maximum dosage

300 mg/kg/d, not to exceed 18 g/d, in normal children.[3,6] 400 mg/kg/d, not to exceed 24 g/d, in patients with cystic fibrosis.[9]

IV push

Not given by this method.

Intermittent infusion

≤50 mg/mL is preferred for peripheral infusion to avoid vein irritation.[19] However, 90 mg/mL in SW results in a recommended osmolality for peripheral infusion in fluid-restricted patients.[20] Infuse over 30[4,11]–120 min.[8,11] The manufacturer recommends infusion over 10–20 min in neonates.[8] There is one report of infusion over 5–10 min in *adults*.[17]

Continuous infusion

10–100 mg/mL in D5W, LR, or NS.[19] Although 100 mg/mL has been used for intermittent or continuous infusion, a concentration of 50 mg/mL is recommended to minimize peripheral vein irritation.[19]

Other routes of administration

Has been given IM in concentrations of 385 mg/mL in SW, NS, or 1% lidocaine HCl (without epinephrine), not to exceed 1 g per injection.[8,19,21] Should only be used for uncomplicated UTI.[21] No information available to support administration by other routes.

Cautions related to IV administration	If a decision is made to give ticarcillin to a patient with known penicillin hypersensitivity, the patient should be closely observed for allergenicity.[22-26] (See Comments section.) For PN compatibility information, please see Appendix C.
Other additives	Contains 5.2–6.5 mEq sodium/g of ticarcillin sodium.[19]
Comments	Patients with a history of type I reactions to penicillin should not receive beta-lactam antibiotics. From 5% to 15% of patients allergic to penicillin will also be allergic to cephalosporins. Certain infections (i.e., syphilis) require penicillin for eradication. It is recommended that a desensitization protocol for penicillin-allergic individuals should be performed in a hospital setting. This can usually be completed in about 4 h, at which time the first dose of penicillin can be given.[2] With chronic administration, patients should be monitored for hypokalemia[9,27] and platelet dysfunction.[8] Thrombophlebitis has been reported.[8] The beta-lactam ring of penicillins can link with an amino sugar of the aminoglycoside and inactivate the aminoglycoside.[28-30] To avoid this potential interaction, administer penicillins 1 h before or after an aminoglycoside, adequately flush the infusion line between each infusion, or infuse them through separate lines. *In vivo* inactivation that is dose dependent can also occur particularly in patients with renal failure.[30-32] In patients with end-stage renal failure, gentamicin half-life was decreased by 22–31 h after carbenicillin or ticarcillin was added to the drug regimen.[31]

Ticarcillin Disodium–Clavulanate Potassium

Brand names Timentin

Dosage

Serious anaphylactoid reactions may require immediate emergency treatment with epinephrine, oxygen, IV steroids, and airway management.

Dosage is based on ticarcillin component. Although clavulanate is a beta-lactamase inhibitor that extends the spectrum of ticarcillin, it has little antibacterial activity.[1]

Neonates

PNA	1200–2000 g	≥2000 g
<7 d	150 mg/kg/d divided q 12 h[2-4]	225 mg/kg/d divided q 8 h[2,5]
≥7 d	225 mg/kg/d divided q 8 h[2,5]*	300 mg/kg/d divided q 6 h[2,5]

*Until 4 weeks of age.

Infants and children

Mild-to-moderate infections: Although several references recommend 200–300 mg/kg/d divided q 6–8 h,[6-16] the *2006 Red Book: Report of the Committee on Infectious Disease* recommends 100–200 mg/kg/d divided q 6 h.[2]

Severe infections: 200–300 mg/kg/d divided q 4–6 h[2,14-18] or 9 g/m^2/d divided q 6 h.[2,17-25]

Dosage adjustment in organ dysfunction

Adjust dosage in patients with renal dysfunction.[1,26-28] If CrCl is between 10 and 50 mL/min, give a normal dose q 8 h; if CrCl is <10 mL/min, give a normal dose q 12 h.[26,28] Alternatively, the manufacturer recommends if CrCl 30–60, give two-thirds normal dose q 4 h; if CrCl 10–30, give two-thirds dose q 8 h; if CrCl <10, give two-thirds dose q 12 h; and if CrCl <10 with hepatic insufficiency, give two-thirds dose q 24 h.[1]

Maximum dosage

400 mg/kg/d of ticarcillin,[1,2,29] not to exceed 3 g/dose or 24 g/d, in adolescents >12 years of age and *adults*.[1,2]

IV push

No information available to support administration by this method.

Intermittent infusion

10–100 mg/mL (ticarcillin) in D5W, LR, SW, or NS[1,30] given over 30[1,30,31]–60[23,24] min. Has been infused over 10–20 min in neonates.[5]

Continuous infusion

No information available to support administration by this method. One study has been conducted in *adults*, but it contained no concentration information.[32]

Other routes of administration

No information available to support administration by other routes.

Maximum concentration

100 mg/mL (ticarcillin).[1]

Cautions related to IV administration

If a decision is made to give this medication to a patient with known penicillin hypersensitivity, the patient should be closely observed for allergenicity. (See Comments section.) Epinephrine should be available.

For PN compatibility information, please see Appendix C.

Ticarcillin Disodium–Clavulanate Potassium

Other additives

Contains ~4.51 mEq of sodium and 0.15 mEq of potassium per g of ticarcillin.[1]

Comments

Patients with a history of type I reactions to penicillin should not receive beta-lactam antibiotics. From 5% to 15% of patients allergic to penicillin will also be allergic to cephalosporins. Certain infections (e.g., syphilis) require penicillin for eradication. It is recommended that a desensitization protocol for penicillin-allergic individuals should be performed in a hospital setting. This can usually be completed in about 4 h, at which time the first dose of penicillin can be given.[2]

The beta-lactam ring of penicillins can link with an amino sugar of the aminoglycoside and inactivate the aminoglycoside.[33-35] To avoid this potential interaction, administer penicillins 1 h before or after an aminoglycoside, adequately flush the infusion line between each infusion, or infuse them through separate lines. *In vivo* inactivation that is dose dependent can also occur particularly in patients with renal failure.[35-37] In patients with end-stage renal failure, gentamicin half-life was decreased by 22–31 h after carbenicillin or ticarcillin was added to the drug regimen.[37]

Thrombophlebitis may occur.[1]

Hypokalemia may occur.[1]

Tissue Plasminogen Activator (TPA)-Alteplase

Brand names	Activase, CathFlo Activase

Dosage

The current recommendations for use of thrombolytics in children are[1]

- in neonates with a major vessel occluded and perfusion of limbs or vital organs is being compromised. If thrombolytics are needed, plasminogen (FFP) should be given prior to infusion.
- in neonates with or without an umbilical artery catheter who develop an aortic thrombosis and have evidence of renal failure.
- in those with bilateral renal vein thrombosis that extends into the inferior vena cava (concomitant with unfractionated heparin).
- after femoral artery catherization when limb- or organ-threatening thrombosis does not respond to heparin and where no contraindication to thrombolytics is known.
- after catheter removal in children with peripheral artery catheter related thrombus, anticoagulation with or without thrombolytic therapy.

Thrombolytic therapy: 0.1–0.5 mg/kg over 10–20 min[2-4] followed by infusion of 0.04–0.6 mg/kg/h[1,2,5-9] for ≤58 h.[2] 0.47 mg/kg/h was infused for 3 h in an 820-g premature neonate with aortic thrombosis.[10] Several studies report continuous infusion of 0.27–0.5 mg/kg/h over 3 h, which can be repeated if clot resolution does not occur.[4,7,11,12] Because of bleeding tendencies in 50% of patients, some investigators suggest that initial doses of 0.1 mg/kg/h be increased gradually up to 0.5 mg/kg/h if clot dissolution does not occur at lower doses.[5] Another suggests 0.5 mg/kg/h for 1 h followed by 0.25 mg/kg/h for 4–11 h until clot lysis occurs, but the incidence of bleeding was still approximately 50% with the lower infusion rate.[13]

In a 19-month-old child with pulmonary embolism, 0.1 mg/kg/h was infused for 11 h via pulmonary artery.[14] One case report described the successful use of 2.5 mg TPA given in repeated small boluses intra-arterially for thrombolysis of middle cerebral artery occlusion.[15]

Central venous line occlusions have been successfully treated with TPA.[16-23] Depending on catheter volume, 0.5–2 mg (1 mg/mL) for a dwell time of 20 min–4 h.[16-23] Some catheters may require more than one instillation.[16,17,19,22]

Infusions of 0.1–0.2 mg/kg/h have been given for up to 8–11 days.[3,12]

Glaucoma or cataract surgery complicated by hyphema and/or fibrin: Intracameral injection of 5–25 mg postoperatively.[23-25] An additional dose may be required.[23]

Myocardial infarction: TPA was given postinfarction in a 7-year-old child with a thrombosed coronary aneurysm. 5 mg IV push was given <1.5 h after arrival, followed by 0.75 mg/kg over 0.5 h, then 0.5 mg/kg over 1 h and symptoms resolved.[26]

Occlusion of catheter used for thoracentesis: In a 16-month-old girl with parapneumonic effusion, 2 mg (2 mL) was infused via the catheter into the pleural space and the tube clamped for 4 h. Drainage was re-established after one dose.[27]

Infective endocarditis (IE): Seven high-risk infants with IE and overwhelming sepsis were treated with 0.2–0.3 mg/kg/h of TPA for 6 h, and the dose was then titrated to 0.5 mg/kg/h and continued until vegetations were no longer visible by ECHO.[28]

Dosage adjustment in organ dysfunction	No information available to support the need for dosage adjustment. Benefits should outweigh risks when using in patients with significant hepatic dysfunction.[29]

Maximum dosage

100 mg for pulmonary embolism, coronary artery thrombi, or MI, or 90 mg for acute ischemic stroke in *adults*.[29]

Doses ≥150 mg are associated with intracranial bleeding in *adults*.[29]

Tissue Plasminogen Activator (TPA)-Alteplase

IV push	No information is available.
Intermittent infusion	1 mg/mL, up to 2 mg/dose × two doses for catheter clearance.[16] ≥0.5 mg/mL in D5W or NS for IV infusion. Dilutions <0.5 mg/mL may result in precipitation.[30]
Continuous infusion	Usual method of administration. Length of infusion varies according to response.
Other routes of administration	No information available to support administration by other routes.
Maximum concentration	1 mg/mL.[29,31] Dilutions <0.5 mg/mL may result in precipitation.[30] For dwell therapy in catheter occlusion, 1 mg/mL.[29]
Cautions related to IV administration	Bleeding is the most common adverse effect.[29] In children bleeding from venipuncture sites, extension of intraventricular hemorrhage, bruising, and other internal bleeding have been reported.[4,5,13]
Other additives	Products contain arginine and polysorbate 80.[29,31]

Comments

50 mg = 29 million international units.[5]

One investigator commented that higher bleeding rates may be associated with concomitant heparin infusions, higher TPA doses, or use in patients with contraindications to antithrombolytic therapy, such as severe thrombocytopenia.[4]

Using appropriate aseptic technique, 50- and 100-mg vials have been reconstituted and frozen in aliquots of 0.5, 1, 2, and 2.5 mL at −20° to −70°C for 2 weeks to 6 months and retained activity.[17,21,32] This allows for multiple doses to be prepared to treat catheter occlusions and minimizes drug wastage.

A 2-year-old with a superior vena cava thrombus was treated successfully with 0.03 mg/kg/h for 48 h in combination with low molecular weight heparin.[33] A 22-month-old with SVC thrombosis received 1.5 mg/kg TPA over 2 h once daily for 2 days, after failing initial therapy with heparin.[34]

TPA (2 mg in 8 mL NS) was infused via intraperitoneal catheters to aid in drainage of abdominal abscesses in a 4-week-old infant, and the patient's course improved.[3]

A study comparing standard dose to low-dose TPA (0.01–0.06 mg/kg/h) for clot lysis showed promising benefits for the lower dose. The authors suggested a starting dose of 0.06 mg/kg/h in neonates and 0.03 mg/kg/h in older infants for thrombolysis.[36]

Two infants with fulminant meningogoccemia and purpura fulminans were given 0.5 mg/kg/h for 1–1.5 h followed by 0.25 mg/kg/h for 1.5–4 h and made a full recovery.[37] However, a retrospective review of 62 infants with meningococcal purpura fulminans treated with a median dose of 0.3 mg/kg/h (range: 0.008–1.13 mg/kg/h) for a median duration of 9 h (range of 1.2–83 h) reported that 29 (47%) patients died, 17 (51%) of the 33 survivors had amputations, and five (8%) experienced intracranial hemorrhage.[38] They questioned the use of TPA in patients with this disease.[38]

Tobramycin Sulfate

Brand names Nebcin

Dosage

Except in neonates, dosage should be based on the following equation[1]: Dosing weight = IBW + 0.4 (TBW − IBW). (See Appendix B.)

Neonates

Loading dose: Although limited data are available, some practitioners advocate an initial 4-mg/kg dose in neonates.[2,3]

Maintenance dose: Estimated using age and weight,[4,5] gestational age,[6-8] or postmenstrual and postnatal age.[1,4]

Based on age and weight

PNA	<1200 g	1200–2000 g	≥2000 g
<7 d	2.5 mg/kg q 18–24 h[4,5]	2.5 mg/kg q 12 h[4]	2.5 mg/kg q 12 h[4]
≥7 d	2.5 mg/kg q 18–24 h[4,5]*	2.5 mg/kg q 8–12 h[4]	2.5 mg/kg q 8 h[4]

*Until 4 weeks of age.

Based on gestational age[6-8]

Gestational Age	Weight	Dose
≤26 weeks		2.5 mg/kg q 24 h[6]
27–34 weeks		2.5 mg/kg q 18 h[6]
	<34 weeks and <1.25 kg	3 mg/kg q 24 h[7,8]
	<34 weeks gestation and ≥1.25 kg	2.5 mg/kg q 18 h[7,8]
35–42 weeks		2.5 mg/kg q 12 h[6-8]

Based on postmenstrual and postnatal age[9]

Postmenstrual Age	Postnatal Age	Dose
≤29 weeks or significant asphyxia, PDA, or treatment with indomethacin	≤7 d	5 mg/kg q 48 h
	8–28 d	4 mg/kg q 36 h
	≥29 d	4 mg/kg q 24 h
30–34 weeks	≤7 d	4.5 mg/kg q 36 h
	≥8 d	4 mg/kg q 24 h
≥35 weeks	ALL	4 mg/kg q 24 h

Infants and children: 2.5 mg/kg q 8 h.[4,6,10] Several investigators reported that once-daily dosing has comparable efficacy and perhaps less toxicity than classical 8–12 h dosing.[11-13] A single dose of aminoglycoside has been given once daily (over 20–30 min) in infants and children with severe gram-negative infections,[14-16] bone marrow transplantation,[17] or in febrile neutropenic patients with cancer.[18-22] At this time, the use of once-daily dosing in infants and children is controversial.[23] Once-daily dosing should only be done in combination with appropriate beta-lactam antibiotics in neutropenic patients and in those with *Pseudomonas aeruginosa* or *Serratia marcescens*.[11]

Cystic fibrosis: Patients require larger doses due to increased clearance and volume of distribution. Average dose is 10 mg/kg/d divided q 8 h[24,25]; however, doses have ranged from 7.5–20 mg/kg/d divided q 8 h.[24] Although several groups have investigated once-daily dosing in *adults*[26,27] and children,[25,27-29] this is not standard practice. Doses ranging from 7–15 mg/kg/d have been used.[26-28] No nephrotoxicity has been reported,[26,28] but one child given 15 mg/kg over 5 min developed transient ototoxicity.[28]

Dosage adjustment in organ dysfunction	If CrCl is >50 mL/min, give a normal dose q 8–24 h; if CrCl is between 10–50 mL/min, give a normal dose q 24–48 h; if CrCl is <10 mL/min, give a normal dose q 48–72 h.[30]
Maximum dosage	15 mg/kg/dose[24] up to 120 mg initially.[21] Because large variability exists in response to therapy, individualize dosage based on serum concentration and clinical response. Larger doses or shorter dosing intervals may be required in CF, major thermal burns or dermal loss, ascites, febrile granulocytopenia[31-33] and in patients undergoing veno-venous hemofiltration.[34] Based on similarities between aminoglycosides, prolonged dosing interval may be required in those on ECMO.[35]
IV push	Although aminoglycosides have been safely administered over 15 sec,[36] 1 min,[37] and 3–5 min,[38] rapid infusion is not recommended.
Intermittent infusion	10 or 40 mg/mL or dilute in appropriate volume of D5W or NS to allow more accurate dosage measurement and infusion over 30–60 min.[39]
Continuous infusion	Although aminoglycosides have been given by continuous infusion,[40-42] this is not recommended. Administration of a normal daily dose over 24 h results in low serum concentrations[41] and nephrotoxicity may occur more frequently.[42]
Other routes of administration	40 mg/mL may be given IM.[39] Solutions prepared from or commercially available in bulk packages, ADD-Vantage vials, and premixed solutions in 0.9% sodium chloride should *not* be given IM.[43]
Maximum concentration	40 mg/mL.[39] The volume must allow accurate measurement and delivery over 30 min.
Cautions related to IV administration	None. For PN compatibility information, please see Appendix C.
Other additives	**Bisulfites:** Contains sodium bisulfite.[39] Sulfites may cause hypersensitivity reactions, which are more common in *adults* with asthma. Most reactions are mild but can include anaphylactic symptoms and life-threatening or less severe asthma episodes.[44,45] Epinephrine may be required in severe cases; and if the sulfite-free product is not available, the sulfite-preserved epinephrine should be used.[45] **Sodium:** The premixed product contains 15.4 mEq/L of sodium/100 mL.[39]
Comments	Because large variability exists in response, individualize dosage based on serum concentrations, response, and renal function. Recommended peak and trough concentrations are 4–12 mg/L and <2 mg/L, respectively.[43] Desired peak concentrations are dependent on the site of infection. Serum concentrations may be falsely elevated when samples are collected through central venous Silastic catheters[46] or in patients with CF who are receiving inhaled tobramycin and have serum concentrations collected via finger stick.[47,48]

Comments *(cont.)*

Serum concentration monitoring is routine practice in many institutions, but not all patients require monitoring.[49,50] It is indicated if a patient is not clinically responding, is ≤3 months of age, requires large doses or high concentrations (CNS infections, endocarditis, pneumonia, ascites, burns), has decreased or unstable renal function, or will be treated >10 days.

The beta-lactam ring of penicillins can link with an amino sugar of the aminoglycoside and inactivate the aminoglycoside.[39] This is dose-dependent and particularly problematic in patients with renal failure. To avoid this potential interaction, administer penicillins 1 h before or after an aminoglycoside, adequately flush the infusion line between each infusion, or infuse them through separate lines.

Cochlear and/or vestibular ototoxicity are associated with all aminoglycosides.[11] Total AUC is a better indicator of risk than peak or trough concentrations.[51,52] Use with caution if other ototoxic drugs (e.g., macrolide antibiotics, loop diuretics, platinum-based chemotherapeutic agents) are given.

Aminoglycosides accumulate in renal cortical tissue and may damage proximal tubule cells. This has been associated with elevated trough concentrations or concurrent use with other nephrotoxic drugs.[11]

Aminoglycosides may cause neuromuscular blockade that is pronounced in patients with renal insufficiency, neuromuscular disease, and hypocalcemia.[53,54] The effects of nondepolarizing neuromuscular blockers may be prolonged during aminoglycoside use.[53]

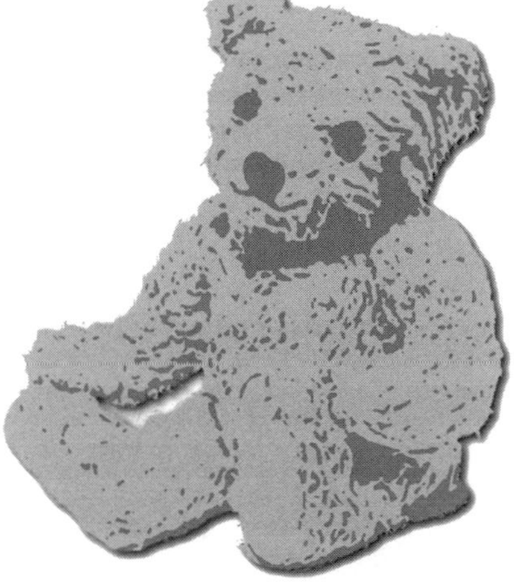

Topotecan HCl

Brand names	Hycamtin
Dosage	Consult institutional protocol for complete dosing information. Topotecan is a component of combination therapy or as single agent therapy to treat multiple pediatric solid tumors, including osteosarcoma, neuroblastoma, rhabdomyosarcoma, Ewing's sarcoma, retinoblastoma, ependymoma, as well as pediatric leukemia. **Combination therapy for solid tumors:** 0.75 mg/m^2/d over 30 min for 5 days; repeat q 21 d.[1] **Single agent therapy for refractory solid tumors:** 1.4–2.4 mg/m^2/d over 30 min for 5 days; repeat q 21 d.[2,3] **Pediatric solid tumors:** 1 mg/m^2/d (range: 0.6–1.9 mg/m^2/d) for 3 days as a continuous infusion; repeat q 21 d,[4,5] or over 30 min 5 days a week for 2 consecutive weeks; repeat q 24–28 d.[6] **Pediatric refractory acute leukemias:** 2.4 mg/m^2/d over 30 min for 9 days; repeat q 21 d.[7]
Dosage adjustment in organ dysfunction	No dosage adjustment necessary in patients with hepatic dysfunction or mild renal impairment (CrCl 40–60 mL/min).[8] The manufacturer recommends that patients with moderate renal failure (CrCl ≤ 20–39 mL/min) receive 50% of the standard dose.[8] Another reference recommends a 25% dose reduction for patients with CrCl >50 mL/min, a 50% reduction for CrCl of 10–50 mL/min, and a 75% reduction with CrCl <10 mL/min.[9]
Maximum dosage	Not established. One *adult* patient received a single dose of 35 mg/m^2 and developed reversible severe neutropenia.[8]
IV push	Not recommended.
Intermittent infusion	Dilute the 4-mg topotecan vial with 4 mL SW.[8] Dilute further in 50–250 mL NS or D5W and infuse over 30 min.[8,10]
Continuous infusion	Has been administered via continuous infusion for up to 72 h.[5]
Other routes of administration	No information available to support administration by other routes.
Maximum concentration	0.5 mg/mL.[11]
Cautions related to IV administration	Extravasation has been reported.[8,10]

Other additives	None.
Comments	Patients should have a baseline absolute neutrophil count >1500 cells/mm^3 and a platelet count >100,000 cells/mm^3 before drug administration.[8] The manufacturer recommends dose adjustments with severe neutropenia or thrombocytopenia.[8] Topotecan is associated with a low (10% to 30%) risk of emesis.[12] Patients should receive antiemetic therapy to prevent acute and delayed nausea and vomiting. The recommended therapy is a corticosteroid on every day chemotherapy is administered; alternatives are a phenothiazine (e.g., prochlorperazine) or a butyrophenone (e.g., droperidol).[12,13] Therapy for delayed nausea and vomiting is generally not needed. Breakthrough medications should also be offered, such as a phenothiazine (e.g., prochlorperazine), a butyrophenone (e.g., droperidol), a substituted benzamide (e.g., metoclopramide), or a benzodiazepine (e.g., lorazepam). Selection should be based on what the patient is currently receiving for acute emesis prophylaxis.

Tromethamine

Brand names	THAM
Dosage	Doses (mL) are based on 0.3 M solution; 100 mL = 3.6 g, 30 mEq, and 30 mmol.[1] **Metabolic acidosis:** In neonates, 1 mL/kg for each pH unit <7.4.[1-3] One study reported doses of 1.8–4.7 mmol/kg in six neonates (26–37 weeks gestation) with respiratory distress syndrome.[4] Alternatively, the dose to correct the base deficit can be calculated using the following equation[1,2]: dose (mL) = base deficit (mEq/L) × body weight (kg) × 1.1 THAM is contraindicated in neonates with chronic respiratory acidosis and salicylate intoxication.[1]
Dosage adjustment in organ dysfunction	THAM should not be used in patients who are anuric or uremic.[1] (See Comments section.)
Maximum dosage	In neonates, the maximum daily dose is 5–7 mmol/kg.[5] The manufacturer states that 1000 mL (300 mmol) may be needed in *adults* with severe acidosis.[1] Others report that the maximum dose in an *adult* in 24 h is 15 mmol/kg.[5,7]
IV push	Too rapid administration may decrease the respiratory drive.[8]
Intermittent infusion	The manufacturer recommends infusion over >1 h.[1] In acute acidosis, 25% to 50% of the calculated deficit can be given over 5–10 min with the remainder infused over >1 h.[5,6]
Continuous infusion	Not the usual method of administration.
Other routes of administration	No information available to support administration by other routes.
Maximum concentration	Undiluted.[1,2]
Cautions related to IV administration	Extravasations may result in tissue necrosis, severe inflammation, and sloughing.[1,2,5,6] Extravasations may be treated with procaine 1% with hyaluronidase or phentolamine.[2] Irreversible ischemia of the hand was reported in an *adult* receiving THAM 3.6% (pH 10.5) peripherally.[9] This product is not available in the U.S.
Other additives	Glacial acetic acid is added to decrease the pH to 8.6 and may be referred to as *THAM acetate*.[5]
Comments	THAM is renally eliminated and may accumulate in renal insufficiency.[6] Overdose or excessively rapid administration may cause prolonged hypoglycemia.[6,10] Respiratory depression and apnea may occur.[8] Hemorrhagic liver necrosis has occurred after infusion through umbilical vein catheters but not umbilical artery catheters.[1,11]

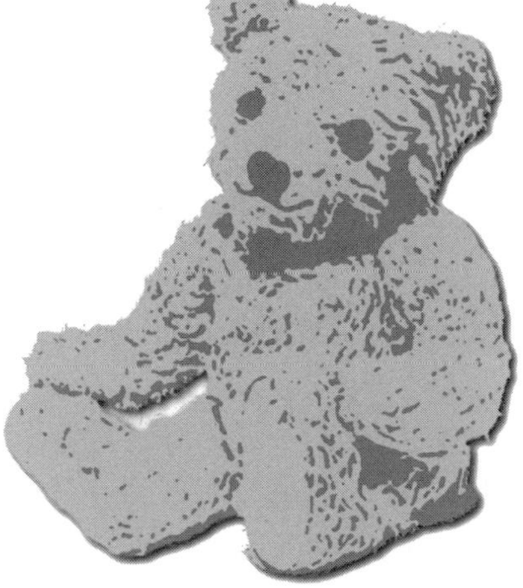

Tubocurarine Chloride

Brand names	Various manufacturers
Dosage	Respiratory function must be supported during use of this agent. Concurrent administration of a sedative is also necessary. Monitoring of neuromuscular transmission with a peripheral nerve stimulator is recommended during continuous infusion or with repeated dosing.[1,2] It is best to calculate the dosage based on actual body weight, not BSA. If BSA is used, the dose can lead to toxicity.[2] **Neonates:** 0.1–0.4 mg/kg/dose[1-4] repeated as needed to maintain desired level of muscle paralysis.[1-4] Premature infants and neonates may be more sensitive to nondepolarizing neuromuscular blocking agents.[1,2] **Infants and children:** 0.1–0.8 mg/kg/dose[1,2,5-7] repeated as needed to maintain desired level of muscle paralysis.[1,2,5-7]
Dosage adjustment in organ dysfunction	Use with caution in patients with renal dysfunction because prolonged neuromuscular blockade may occur. If CrCl is 10–50 mL/min, decrease dose by 50%.[8] If CrCl is <10 mL/min, do not use.[8] Patients with hepatic impairment may require larger doses.[1]
Maximum dosage	Not established.
IV push	3 mg/mL given over 60–90 sec.[1,9]
Intermittent infusion	No information available to support administration by this method.
Continuous infusion	Dilute to desired concentration in D5W, NS, D5NS, or LR.[1,9] A neonate received 16 mcg/kg/min until 70% to 90% depression of electromyelogram twitch height was achieved.[7]
Other routes of administration	May be given IM at same doses as IV.[1,9]
Maximum concentration	3 mg/mL.[1,9] Osmolality of 3-mg/mL solution is 296 mOsm/kg.[1,9]
Cautions related to IV administration	Histamine release resulting in hypotension and bronchospasm has occurred; thus, use cautiously in patients with cardiovascular disease or asthma.[2,10,11]
Other additives	**Sulfites:** May contain sodium bisulfite.[1,2] Sulfites may cause hypersensitivity reactions, and these are more common in *adults* with asthma. Most reactions are mild but can include anaphylactic symptoms and life-threatening or less severe asthma episodes.[12-14] Epinephrine may be required in severe cases; and if the sulfite-free product is not available, the sulfite-preserved epinephrine should be used.[12] **Benzyl alcohol:** Benzyl alcohol in small doses as a preservative in drugs is considered safe in newborns.[12] However, a 3-week-old, very low birth weight (710 g) infant who received clindamycin experienced a profound desaturation that required resuscitation after the third and fourth doses, which was subsequently related to the benzyl alcohol preservative.[15]

Other additives (cont.)

Administration of saline flushes containing benzyl alcohol (bacteriostatic water for injection) was associated with a fatal gasping syndrome, intraventricular hemorrhage, metabolic acidosis, and increased mortality in preterm infants.[16] This should not be used in neonates.

Hypersensitivity reactions to benzyl alcohol in parenteral products have been reported in *adults*.[17,18]

Comments

Young infants (<10 days) tend to require larger doses to achieve the same amount of twitch inhibition as older children.[1]

Concomitant administration of tubocurarine with certain antibiotics (e.g., aminoglycosides, clindamycin, tetracycline, and vancomycin) and other agents (e.g., magnesium sulfate, quinidine) may prolong neuromuscular blockade.[1,2,19,20] Azathioprine and theophylline may decrease neuromuscular blockade.[1,2] Consult appropriate resources for additional information on drug interactions.

Valproate Sodium

Brand names Depacon

Dosage

Because of the increased risk for hepatotoxicity, valproate should be used cautiously in children <2 years of age, especially if they are receiving multiple anticonvulsants, have congenital metabolic disorders, severe seizures accompanied by mental retardation, or organic brain disease.[1-4] (See Comments section.)

Headache: IV valproate has been safely and effectively used in *adults*[5-7] and adolescents.[8] Initial doses of 1000 mg were infused at 50 mg/min in 31 adolescents.[8] When response was not sufficient, a second 500 mg/dose was given.[8]

Seizures (acute, nonstatus epilepticus)

Replacement therapy: Individuals chronically receiving oral valproate may be converted to IV valproate using the same total daily dose (1:1 conversion); however, it should be administered q 6 h or by continuous infusion.[9]

Children (≥2 years) and adolescents: 10–15 mg/kg administered q 6 h; increase weekly by 5–10 mg/kg/d until seizures are controlled, therapeutic concentrations are reached, or the patient exhibits unacceptable toxicities.[9-16] Maintenance dose in children ≥2 years/adolescents: 30–60 mg/kg/d divided q 6 h.[10-16]

Seizures—generalize convulsive status epilepticus

Neonates and infants: Although IV valproate has been used safely in neonates to treat acute seizures and status epilepticus,[16,17] it should not be used unless all other options have failed. If used, it should be given with carnitine (see Comments section). A single dose of 10–25 mg/kg was given and an apparent Vd of 0.245 L/kg and clearance of 25 mL/h/kg were estimated.[17] The elimination of valproate is significantly reduced in neonates and infants; therefore, doses may need to be administered less frequently than in older children.

Children and adolescents: 13.4–40 mg/kg[18-21] loading dose or 500 mg.[22] The need for further loading doses should be guided by clinical response and serum concentrations. If the patient is on valproate monotherapy or other antiepileptics that do not induce the cytochrome P450 system, begin with 1 mg/kg/h; if the patient is on one or more inducers (e.g., phenobarbital, phenytoin, rifampin), begin with 2 mg/kg/h; if the patient is receiving inducers and is in pentobarbital coma, begin with 4–6 mg/kg/h.[18] Continue to increase the dose until seizures are controlled, desired serum concentrations are reached, or the patient develops unacceptable toxicity.

Seizures—nonconvulsive status epilepticus

Children and adolescents: A loading dose of 13.4–25 mg/kg[18,23] followed by 4 mg/kg q 6 h.[19]

Dosage adjustment in organ dysfunction

No dosage adjustment necessary in renal dysfunction.[24] However, renal failure may cause a disproportionate increase in free-to-total valproate ratios.[25,26] Use with caution in patients with pre-existing liver dysfunction.[9]

Maximum dosage

Maximum dose has not been established. A loading dose of 40 mg/kg[21] and a continuous infusion of 6 mg/kg/h have been used in children.[18] A loading dose of 1000 mg has been given to adolescents[8] and 240 mg/h has been given to *adults*.[27] Children receiving one or more medications known to increase the metabolism of valproate may require doses up to 100 mg/kg/d, while children in pentobarbital coma may require larger doses (150 mg/kg/d).[18,28] Because large variability exists in patient response to initial and maintenance doses, individualize dosage based on response and serum concentrations.

IV push	Not given by this method.
Intermittent infusion	The parenteral injection has been used undiluted; however, this results in severe vein irritation. Administer in a 1:1 or 2:1 dilution in D5W, NS, or LR.[9,30] Although the manufacturer recommends that infusion occur over 20 min, a loading dose of 20–40 mg/kg has been safely given over 1–5 min[21] or 1–6 mg/kg/min.[19,20] Others have given as fast as 82 mg/min (1000 mg)[8] or ≤15 min (8.2–15.4 mg/kg).[31] An 11-year-old girl received 30 mg/kg (480 mg) over 20 min (0.5 mg/kg/h) and developed significant, but reversible, hypotension 12 min into the infusion.[29]
Continuous infusion	2–4 mg/mL in D5W or NS at a rate of 1–6 mg/kg/h.[9,18]
Other routes of administration	No information available to support administration by other routes.
Maximum concentration	25–50 mg/mL in D5W.[22]
Cautions related to IV administration	Highly concentrated solutions may lead to pain and irritation at the infusion site.[9] (See Maximum dosage section.)
Other additives	None.
Comments	Dosing should be guided by clinical response and total serum valproate concentrations (50–150 mg/L). Life-threatening hemorrhagic pancreatitis has been reported in children and *adults* receiving valproate.[32-34] If valproate is used in children ≤2 years, those with neurological handicap, and those receiving multiple antiepileptic medications may be at risk for valproate-induced hepatotoxicity and routine monitoring of liver function tests is indicated.[9] In addition, prophylactic carnitine therapy (50–100 mg/kg/d) is recommended.[35-37] Because a clinical study in *adults* with head trauma showed a higher mortality rate than that observed for phenytoin, IV valproate is not recommended for seizure prophylaxis following head trauma.[38] Because valproate inhibits CYP2C9, epoxide hydroxylase, and beta-oxidation, it is associated with numerous drug interactions.[39] Valproate can also serve as a substrate and can be inhibited or induced by other drugs. Consult appropriate resources for dosing recommendations before combining any drug with valproate.

Vancomycin HCl

Brand names Lyphocin, Vancocin, Vancoled

Dosage

Obese individuals should be dosed using actual or total body weight.[1] Shorter dosing intervals may be needed in these patients to maintain trough serum vancomycin concentration above 5 mg/L.[1]

Neonates

Some advocate a 15–20-mg/kg loading dose.[2]

Although a variety of neonatal dosing recommendations have been published,[3-5] the following continue to be the most commonly used and are based on gestational age and weight or postconceptional age.

Based on weight and gestational age[6-11]:

PNA	<1200 g	1200–2000 g	≥2000 g
<7 d	15 mg/kg q 24 h*	20–30 mg/kg/d divided q 12–18 h	30–45 mg/kg/d divided q 8–12 h
≥7 d		30–45 mg/kg divided q 8–12 h*	40–60 mg/kg/d divided q 6–8 h

*Until 4 weeks of age.

Based on postconceptional age[12]:

Postconceptional Age	Dose
≤26 weeks	15 mg/kg q 24 h
27–34 weeks	15 mg/kg q 18 h
35–42 weeks	30 mg/kg/d divided q 12 h
≥43 weeks	45 mg/kg/d divided q 8 h

Infants and children

Mild-to-moderate infections: 40 mg/kg/d divided q 6–8 h up to 2 g/d.[6,12,13]

Severe infections (including meningitis): 60 mg/kg/d divided q 6 h up to 4 g/d.[6,14]

Bacterial endocarditis (prophylaxis): Genitourinary and gastrointestinal procedures in patients allergic to ampicillin. High-risk patients should be given a single 20-mg/kg dose (up to 1 g) and within 30 min of starting a procedure. Administered in conjunction with gentamicin (1.5 mg/kg, not to exceed 120 mg).[6] May omit gentamicin in those with only moderate risk.[6]

Bacterial endocarditis (treatment)

Culture negative (including Bartonella): Should not be used in native value diseases unless the patient can not tolerate penicillin.[14,15] If ≤1 year since prosthetic valve placement give 40 mg/kg/d divided q 8–12 h plus gentamicin (3 mg/kg/d divided q 8 h) plus cefepime (150 mg/kg/d divided q 8 h) plus rifampin (20 mg/kg/d divided q 8 h) for 6 weeks.[14,15]

Oxacillin-resistant staphylococci: Those without prosthetic material should receive 40 mg/kg/d divided q 8–12 h for 6 weeks.[14,15] Patients *with* prosthetic material should be given 40 mg/kg/d divided q 8–12 h for 6 weeks plus rifampin (20 mg/kg/d divided q 8 h for 6 weeks) and gentamicin (3 mg/kg/d divided q 8 h for 2 weeks).[14,15]

Penicillin-resistant enterococcal (susceptible to vancomycin and aminoglycoside): For native or prosthetic material, give 40 mg/kg/d divided q 8–12 h plus gentamicin (3 mg/kg/d divided q 8 h) for 6 weeks.[14,15]

Biologic warfare or bioterrorism: The CDC and other experts recommend that treatment of inhalational anthrax spores due to biologic warfare or bioterrorism should be started on a multiple-drug parenteral regimen that includes ciprofloxacin or doxycycline and one or two additional anti-infective agents (i.e., chloramphenicol, clindamycin, rifampin, vancomycin, clarithromycin, imipenem, penicillin, or ampicillin).[16,17]

Dosage *(cont.)*	**Central venous catheter infection:** 25 mg/L of vancomycin added to parenteral nutrition solution as a continuous infusion[18-20] or as a flush/lock.[21,22] Although this dose has been used for prophylaxis, to decrease catheter-related coagulase-negative staphylococcal sepsis, the Centers for Disease Control and Prevention discourage this practice.[19] **Ventricular shunt infection:** Most practitioners administer 10 mg/d (50 mg/mL diluted with NS to a final concentration of 5 mg/mL) directly into the ventricle (if the shunt is not externalized) or via the externalized shunt, which is then clamped for 1 h after administration.[23-26] Generally, given with concurrent systemic vancomycin 60 mg/kg/d divided q 6 h.
Dosage adjustment in organ dysfunction	Adjust dosage in renal dysfunction.[27,28] If CrCl is 10–50 mL/min, give a normal dose q 24–96 h; and if CrCl is <10 mL/min, give a normal dose q 4–7 d.[27] Adjust dosage based on serum concentrations. (See Comments section.)
Maximum dosage	15 mg/kg/dose when dosing interval is 6–12 h[6,11,12] or 60 or 80 mg/kg/d,[11] not to exceed *adult* dose of 4 g/d.[12] Patients on ECMO have an increased circulating volume and transiently altered renal function; therefore, a suggested dose is 20 mg/kg q 24 h.[29] Patients with malignancy may have increased clearance and require larger doses (i.e., mean dose of 71.5 mg/kg/d).[30,31] Although serum vancomycin concentration should not be routinely monitored, trough concentration may be helpful in patients who are not clinically responding.
IV push	Not recommended.[32]
Intermittent infusion	2.5–5 mg/mL in D5LR, D5NS, D5W, LR, NS, or SW.[33] Usually given over ≥60 min,[32,33] but has been given safely in 30 min.[9,11,34,35] ≤10 mg/min in *adults*.[32] (See Cautions related to IV administration and Comments sections.)
Continuous infusion	Dilute in 24 mL of D5W, or dilute in a sufficient volume of NS to infuse over 24 h.[33,36]
Other routes of administration	IM administration is not recommended because it may cause local necrosis.[32,33] Has been given by inhalation[37,38] and intraventricular routes[23-26] for the treatment of methicillin-resistant *Staphylococcus aureus*. No information available to support administration by other routes.
Maximum concentration	<5 mg/mL.[12]
Cautions related to IV administration	Administration rates over <60 min may be associated with Red-man syndrome. (See Comments section.) Tissue necrosis may occur following extravasation.[32] Thrombophlebitis can be minimized by using dilute solutions (e.g., 2.5–5 mg/mL) and rotating injection sites.[32] For PN compatibility information, please see Appendix C.
Other additives	None.

Vancomycin HCl

Comments

Rapid IV administration may result in Red-man syndrome. This syndrome may be accompanied by flushing and/or a maculopapular rash or erythematous rash on the face, neck, chest, and upper extremities. Severe hypotension and cardiac arrest have occurred in *adults* and children after rapid administration.[39,40] Symptoms usually begin minutes after start of the infusion, but they may present later. Symptoms usually resolve spontaneously after discontinuation of the infusion. Lengthen the infusion time to 2 h and/or pretreatment with an antihistamine (diphenhydramine HCl 1 mg/kg IV) or H-2 antagonist (cimetidine 4 mg/kg/IV) may prevent the syndrome.[41,42]

Studies have shown,[43,44] and the American Academy of Pediatrics[6] recommends, that routine monitoring of serum vancomycin concentrations is unnecessary.

Some fluorescence immunoassay and radioimmunoassay for vancomycin may overestimate serum vancomycin concentrations in patients with renal failure.[45] This occurs due to accumulation of vancomycin crystalline degradation products (CDP-1). Conversely, some assay do not suffer from this problem.[46] Practitioners should check with their clinical laboratory.

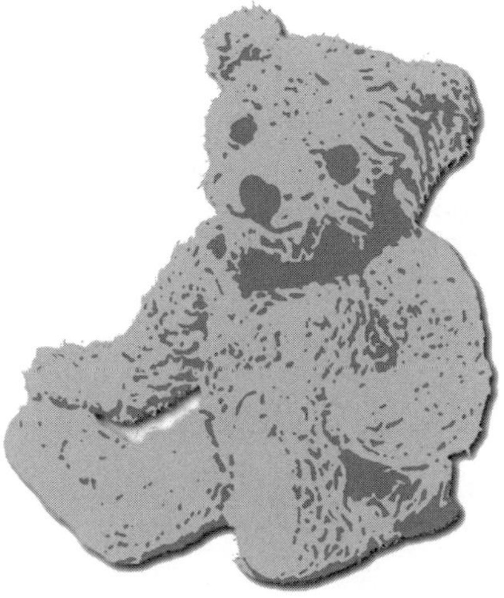

Vasopressin

Brand names	Pitressin
Dosage	**Central diabetes insipidus (DI):** A 3-day-old and a 3-year-old with DI were started on 0.003 unit/kg/h.[1] The polyuria resolved and the drug weaned over several days.[1] One source recommends a starting dose of 0.0005 unit/kg/h.[1,2] If no effect is seen, double the dose q 30 min until urine osmolality is twice that of plasma and urine output is <2 mL/kg/h.[2] The dosage required rarely exceeds 0.01 unit/kg/h.[2] **Shock:** Despite treatment with standard pressors, 11 children with continued hypotension following cardiac surgery (3 days–15 years of age) received 0.0003–0.002 unit/kg/min and had an increase in blood pressure and decrease in total inotrope score.[2] Three children with septic shock (ages 3 months, 2½ years, and 13 years) received a starting dose of 0.0002–0.0005 unit/kg/min that was increased gradually to 0.005–0.002 unit/kg/min to maintain a systolic blood pressure of 70, 80, and 90 mmHg, respectively.[4] In all *adults* with septic shock, use of continuous low-dose infusion of 0.01 and 0.04 unit/min (not titrated) in conjunction with other pressors is supported.[5] The Surviving Sepsis Campaign guidelines warn against the use of >0.04 unit/min because it has been associated with myocardial ischemia and cardiac arrest.[6] **Provocative testing for growth hormone and corticotropin release:** 0.3 unit/kg IM, then draw blood for hormone measurement.[7] **Gastrointestinal bleeding (other therapies have decreased the use of vasopressin for this indication)** **Age-based dosing:** 0.1 unit/min as a continuous infusion; increase by 0.05 unit/min each h up to a maximum of 0.2 unit/min in children <5 years, 0.3 unit/min in children 5–12 years, and 0.4 unit/min in adolescents >12 years.[8] **Weight-based dosing:** 0.07–0.6 unit/kg/h (0.001–0.01 unit/kg/min).[9,10] A bolus infusion of 0.3 unit/kg (up to 20 unit) may be used prior to a continuous infusion.[10] After gastrointestinal bleeding has been controlled for 12–24 h, gradually taper the dose over 24–36 h[8]; however, continued infusion may be needed for up to 3 weeks.[6] (See Comments section.) **Cardiac arrest:** A four-patient case series found evidence that vasopressin administration may be beneficial during prolonged pediatric cardiac arrest.[11] However, there is not enough evidence for the PALS guidelines for resuscitation to recommend for or against its use.[12]
Dosage adjustment in organ dysfunction	No dosage adjustment required in renal dysfunction.[7]
Maximum dosage	0.01 unit/kg/h for diabetes insipidus.[2] 0.01 unit/kg/min in children[9] or 0.9 unit/min in *adults*[7] for gastrointestinal bleeding.
IV push	Not recommended.[7]
Intermittent infusion	Usually not administered by this route.
Continuous infusion	0.1–1 unit/mL in D5W or NS.[13]
Other routes of administration	May be administered IM or SC.[7]

Maximum concentration	1 unit/mL.[7]
Cautions related to IV administration	Hypersensitivity reactions may occur.[7] Extravasation may result in tissue necrosis.[7]
Other additives	Chlorobutanol as a preservative.[7]
Comments	Endogenous vasopressin (antidiuretic hormone or ADH) maintains serum osmolality within the normal range. It is important that fluid status and electrolytes be monitored during treatment with this agent.[7] Hypersensitivity reactions have been reported.[7]

Vecuronium Bromide

Brand names	Norcuron
Dosage	Respiratory function must be supported during use. Concurrent administration of a sedative is necessary. Monitoring of neuromuscular transmission with a peripheral nerve stimulator is recommended during continuous infusion or with repeated dosing.[1] Because vecuronium does not cause histamine release, it is considered the neuromuscular blocking agent of choice in patients with allergies and/or asthma.[2] 0.08–0.1 mg/kg as required to maintain desired neuromuscular blockade[2-7] followed by a continuous infusion of 0.06–0.1 mg/kg/h titrated up to 0.17 mg/kg/h based on individual response.[2-7] One author suggests 0.06–0.09 mg/kg/h for infants and 0.09–0.15 mg/kg/h for children.[2]
Dosage adjustment in organ dysfunction	To avoid prolonged neuromuscular blockade, give smaller initial doses to anephric patients.[8] Patients with cirrhosis and cholestasis may experience prolonged recovery times.[8]
Maximum dosage	A single 0.4-mg/kg dose has been used safely in children 2–9 years old with normal renal and hepatic function.[6] The largest reported continuous infusion rate was 0.27 mg/kg/h for 21 h.[5] In a study of 11 infants and children, the mean infusion rate was 0.14 mg/kg/h (range= 0.1–0.27 mg/kg/h).[5] One neonate required 0.18 mg/kg/h.[5]
IV push	1 mg/mL in D5NS, D5W, LR, or NS administered rapidly over seconds.[8,9]
Intermittent infusion	Not administered by this method.
Continuous infusion	0.1–0.2 mg/mL in D5NS, D5W, LR, or NS.[4,5,9] A concentrated 1-mg/mL solution may be used in fluid restricted patients.
Other routes of administration	Should not be given IM.[9] No information available to support administration by other routes.
Maximum concentration	1 mg/mL for IV push or infusion.[9,10]
Cautions related to IV administration	Flushing, erythema, pruritus, urticaria, bronchospasm, and hypotension are uncommon but may occur.[10-12] For PN compatibility information, please see Appendix C.

Other additives

Benzyl alcohol: Multidose vials contain benzyl alcohol 0.9% as a preservative.[8] Administration of flushes containing benzyl alcohol (bacteriostatic water for injection) was associated with a fatal gasping syndrome, intraventricular hemorrhage, metabolic acidosis, and increased mortality in preterm infants.[13] While benzyl alcohol in small doses as a preservative in drugs is considered safe in newborns,[14] a 3-week-old, very low birth weight (710 g) infant experienced a profound desaturation that required resuscitation after receiving clindamycin (third and fourth doses), which was subsequently related to the benzyl alcohol preservative.[15]

Hypersensitivity reactions to benzyl alcohol in parenteral products have been reported in *adults*.[16,17]

Comments

Prolonged paralysis has been reported in several patients after long-term infusion of vecuronium.[18-20] Acute quadriplegic myopathy resulted when a 17-month-old infant was intubated for 24 days and treated with vecuronium bromide and high-dose methylprednisolone.[21]

Sinus node exit block occurred in a 14-year-old after administration of 0.08 mg/kg.[22]

Concomitant administration of corticosteroids[23,24] and certain antibiotics (e.g., aminoglycosides and polymyxin B)[25,26] with neuromuscular blockers has been shown to be a risk factor for prolonged paralysis.

Reduce vecuronium dose to 0.04–0.06 mg/kg in patients receiving succinylcholine, enflurane, or isoflurane.[10] Concomitant use of atracurium in an equipotent dose is more potent than either agent alone.[7]

Disruption of the blood brain barrier in critical illness may cause penetration of vecuronium into the CNS, resulting in dilated, nonreactive pupils. Three such cases were reported in a pediatric oncology unit.[27]

Verapamil HCl

Brand names	Isoptin, various generic
Dosage	The Pediatric Advance Life Support (PALS) guidelines state that during cardiopulmonary resuscitation verapamil, should not be used in infants because it may cause refractory hypotension and cardiac arrest, and it should be used cautiously in children because it may cause hypotension and myocardial depression.[1] **Tachyarrhythmias** **Neonates and infants:** 0.1–0.2 mg/kg (usually 0.75–2 mg) with continuous ECG monitoring.[2,8-12] If necessary, repeat dose one time 15–30 min after initial bolus.[2,8] (See Cautions related to IV administration section.) **Children 1–15 years:** Initially, 0.1–0.3 mg/kg[2,8-10,12-14] up to 5 mg/dose.[2] If necessary, repeat dose one time 15–30 min after initial bolus, not to exceed a single 10-mg dose.[2] Continuous ECG monitoring should be performed and IV calcium chloride 10% (10 mg/kg) should be available at bedside to treat hypotension and atropine to treat bradycardia.[2,14]
Dosage adjustment in organ dysfunction	None required.[15-17]
Maximum dosage	In neonates and infants, 0.2 mg/kg, not to exceed 5 mg/dose.[2] In children 1–15 years, 0.3 mg/kg, not to exceed 10 mg/dose.[2] An 18-year-old patient with anticholinergic-induced torsades de pointes and prolonged QT interval unresponsive to standard therapies was successfully treated with three 5-mg (0.1 mg/kg) bolus doses of verapamil followed by an infusion of 5 mcg/kg/min.[18]
IV push	Usually over 2–3 min.[2,19]. However, 0.5 mg/mL in D5W[13] and 2.5[2] mg/mL (available commercially) has been given over 30–60 sec.[8,9,12-14]
Intermittent infusion	Not indicated.
Continuous infusion	Usually administered IV push. However, verapamil is compatible in D5W, D½NS, NS, RL, D5½NS, D5NS, and D5RL.[19] A concentration of 0.4 mg/mL in D5W[20] infused at 2.5–5 mcg/kg/min for 5 days has been used in *adults*.[20-22]
Other routes of administration	No information available to support administration by other routes.
Maximum concentration	2.5 mg/mL (undiluted) for IV push.[2]
Cautions related to IV administration	Hypotension, bradycardia, tachycardia, asystole, and arrhythmias may occur, particularly in patients with sinus node dysfunction or impaired atrioventricular conduction.[12] Verapamil should not be used in children with Wolff-Parkinson-White syndrome.[7,23]

Other additives

Each mL contains 8.5 mg sodium chloride.[19]

Comments

Apnea, cardiovascular collapse, and respiratory arrest have been reported in pediatric patients, particularly those <1 year of age.[3-6]

Brief myoclonic seizures developed in an 18-month-old patient following intravenous verapamil.[24]

A 15-year-old with Duchenne's muscular dystrophy was given seven 5-mg doses of verapamil over 20 h and had resolution of the tachyarrhythmia.[25] Four hours after the last dose, severe bradycardia and hypotension occurred and the child was not able to be resuscitated.[25] The death was not felt to be related to the verapamil because of the length of time since the last dose and verapamil's short half-life.[25] A 17-year-old with Duchenne's muscular dystrophy developed irreversible respiratory failure felt to be related to verapamil.[26]

Concomitant use with digoxin (and other cardiac glycosides) results in increased digoxin concentrations; therefore, reduce digoxin dosage and monitor concentrations. Because of possible additive effects on atrioventricular nodal conduction, patients receiving verapamil and a cardiac glycoside concomitantly should undergo periodic ECG monitoring for atrioventricular block.[2]

Vinblastine Sulfate

Brand names	Velban
Dosage	Consult institutional protocol for complete dosing information. Vinblastine is used alone and in combination with a variety of antineoplastic agents for the treatment of Hodgkin's lymphoma, non-Hodgkin's lymphoma, histiocytic lymphoma, testicular cancer, Kaposi's sarcoma, histiocytosis X, and others. While it can be used as monotherapy, it is often part of a multidrug regimen, and the timing of doses for all drugs is critical to achieve the optimal outcome. Vinblastine is usually dosed once a week; however, there are specific protocols that vary. Some regimens that have been used in children are listed below: **Histiocytosis X:** 6.5 mg/m^2 weekly for 24 weeks.[1] **Hodgkin's disease (combined with other agents):** 6 mg/m^2 on protocol day 7.[2] **Testicular cancer (combined with other agents):** 3 mg/m^2 on two separate days[3] or on protocol days 22 and 23 or days 1 and 2.[4] In *adults*, the initial dose is usually 3.7 mg/m^2 and this is increased by 1.8 mg/m^2 weekly until the WBC is 3000/m^2 or a maximum dose of 18.5 mg/m^2 is reached. Once the dose that suppresses the WBC to <3000/m^2 is reached, the maintenance dose should be decreased by one step (1.8 mg/m^2). Usual weekly range of doses in *adults* is 5.5–7.4 mg/m^2.[5]
Dosage adjustment in organ dysfunction	No dose reduction is needed in patients with renal dysfunction.[6] Vinblastine doses should be reduced in patients with hepatic insufficiency.[7] The manufacturer recommends a 50% dose reduction in patients with a direct serum bilirubin >3 mg/dL.[8]
Maximum dosage	Maximum weekly dose should not exceed 18.5 mg/m^2 in *adults*.[8] Refer to treatment protocols for maximum-dose guidelines.
IV push	1 mg/mL administered via an intact, free-flowing IV needle or catheter over 1 min.[9]
Intermittent infusion	Although vinblastine has been administered by this method, it is not recommended because of the risk of infiltration.[9]
Continuous infusion	Not recommended.[9]
Other routes of administration	Contraindicated.[9]
Maximum concentration	1 mg/mL has an osmolality of 278 mOsm/kg and a pH of 3.5–5.[9]
Cautions related to IV administration	Vinblastine is only administered IV. IT administration of vinblastine is fatal.[9] Extravasation of vinblastine can cause considerable local tissue irritation.[8,10] The infusion should be stopped if the patient complains of discomfort. Because of extravasation and infiltration risk, small veins in the dorsum of the hand or foot and scalp veins should be avoided if at all possible. (See Comments section.)

Other additives

May contain benzyl alcohol 0.9%.[9]

Benzyl alcohol in small doses as a preservative in drugs is considered safe in newborns.[11] However, a 3-week-old, very low birth weight (710 g) infant who received clindamycin experienced a profound desaturation that required resuscitation after the third and fourth doses, which was subsequently related to the benzyl alcohol preservative.[12]

Administration of saline flushes containing benzyl alcohol (bacteriostatic water for injection) was associated with a fatal gasping syndrome, intraventricular hemorrhage, metabolic acidosis, and increased mortality in preterm infants.[13] This should not be used in neonates.

Hypersensitivity reactions to benzyl alcohol in parenteral products have been reported in *adults*.[14,15]

Comments

Vinblastine is contraindicated in patients with granulocytopenia that is not secondary to the disease being treated and in patients with bacterial infection.[5]

Vinblastine should not be given if the WBC is <4000/m^3.[5]

Extravasation injuries can be treated with either (1) local injection of hyaluronidase and application of moderate heat or (2) cold compresses, dilution with 0.9% sodium chloride injection, and/or local injection of hydrocortisone.[5]

Concurrent administration of vinblastine and medications that inhibit cytochrome P450 3A, such as azole antifungals, cyclosporine, and macrolide antibiotics, may increase vinca alkaloid-associated neurotoxicity.[16] Consult appropriate resources for dosing recommendations before combining any drug with vinblastine.

Neurotoxicity has been observed following vinblastine administration, but this adverse effect is much less common than with vincristine.[17]

Dyspnea has not been observed with vinblastine alone,[18] but there have been numerous case reports of an acute, temporally related, respiratory distress syndrome that occurs within 1–5 h following the combination of vinblastine and mitomycin C. Some of these acute reactions have been fatal.[19-24] The incidence of this toxic pulmonary reaction has been estimated to be as high as 3% to 6%.[20]

Vinblastine is associated with a minimal (<10%) risk of emesis.[25,26] Generally, prophylaxis for acute and delayed emesis is not needed. Patients may receive one-time prophylaxis with a phenothiazine (e.g., prochlorperazine) or a butyrophenone (e.g., droperidol). Breakthrough medications may be offered, such as a phenothiazine (e.g., prochlorperazine), a butyrophenone (e.g., droperidol), a substituted benzamide (e.g., metoclopramide), or a benzodiazepine (e.g., lorazepam). Selection should be based on what the patient is currently receiving for acute antiemesis prophylaxis.

Vincristine Sulfate

Brand names	Oncovin, Vincristine Sulfate Injection, USP
Dosage	Please consult institutional protocol for complete dosing information. Vincristine is used as a component of combination therapy to treat childhood acute lymphocytic (lymphoblastic) leukemia, Hodgkin's disease, non-Hodgkin's lymphoma, neuroblastoma, rhabdomyosarcoma, Wilms' Tumor, Kaposi's sarcoma, brain tumors, small cell lung cancer, and other neoplastic diseases. One protocol for high-risk acute lymphoblastic leukemia included vincristine on induction days 8, 15, 22, and 29; during block 1 of therapy on days 1 and 8; and as part of reinduction on days 8, 15, 22, and 29.[1] A protocol for treating Hodgkin's disease included doses of vincristine on day 0 (with the complete schedule of chemotherapies repeated q 28 days) or on day 42 of a 63-day multiple chemotherapy regimen.[2] Usual doses given no more frequently than weekly[3,5,6]: **<10 kg or BSA <1 m^2:** 0.05 mg/kg (up to 2 mg). **≥10 kg:** 1.5–2 mg/m^2 (up to 2 mg). **Adults:** 1.4 mg/m^2 (up to 2 mg). In infants, vincristine clearance is more closely related to body weight than BSA.[4]
Dosage adjustment in organ dysfunction	Dose should be reduced in patients with hepatic insufficiency.[7] A 50% reduction in dose is recommended if direct serum bilirubin is >3 mg/dL.[3] No dose reduction is needed in patients with renal dysfunction.[8]
Maximum dosage	Most, but not all, clinical trials and treatment protocols have maximum-dose guidelines of 2 mg in order to minimize neurotoxicity.[5,6,9] However, some clinicians have questioned the appropriateness of the 2-mg maximum vincristine dose.[10] Refer to treatment protocols for maximum-dose guidelines.
IV push	1 mg/mL administered via an intact, free-flowing IV needle or catheter over 1 min.[11]
Intermittent infusion	Can dilute in D5W or NS and infuse over 4–8 h.[11]
Continuous infusion	Can dilute in D5W or NS and infuse by this method if necessary.[11]
Other routes of administration	Not recommended; for IV infusion only.
Maximum concentration	1 mg/mL.[11] Osmolality is 610 mOsm/kg.[11]

Cautions related to IV administration

Vincristine is only administered IV.[11] IT administration of vincristine is fatal.[12,13]

Affix provided sticker ("Fatal if given intrathecally. For IV use only.") directly to the container of the individual dose. Dispense in overwrap with the following text, "Do not remove covering until moment of injection. Fatal if given intrathecally. For IV use only."[11]

Because extravasation may cause tissue sloughing and necrosis, the infusion should be stopped if the patient complains of discomfort.[3,14] Because of extravasation and infiltration risk, small veins in the dorsum of the hand or foot and scalp veins should be avoided if at all possible.

Other additives

None.

Comments

The dose-limiting effect of vincristine is neurotoxicity.[3] Severe vincristine-associated neurotoxicity has been observed with concurrent administration of drugs that inhibit hepatic cytochrome P4503A isoenzymes (e.g., azole antifungals, cyclosporine, and macrolide antibiotics).[15] Consult appropriate resources for dosing recommendations before combining any drug with vincristine.

Extravasation injuries can be treated with either (1) local injection of hyaluronidase and application of moderate heat or (2) cold compresses, dilution with 0.9% sodium chloride injection or infiltration of sodium bicarbonate (5 mL of 8.4%), and/or local injection of hydrocortisone.[3]

Vincristine should not be given to patients receiving radiation through ports that include the liver.[16]

In overdose, treatment includes fluid restriction due to likelihood of syndrome of inappropriate antidiuretic hormone (SIADH), prophylactic phenobarbital, enemas to prevent ileus, daily hemoglobin and hematocrit to evaluate need for transfusion, and monitoring the cardiovascular system. Some have suggested that leucovorin calcium 100 mg IV q 3 h for 24 h and then q 6 h for at least 48 h may be of value.[3]

Vincristine is contraindicated in patients with the demyelinating form of Charcot-Marie-Tooth syndrome, a hereditary motor and sensory neuropathy type I disease.[17-19]

Protection from light is recommended because vincristine is light sensitive.[11]

Vincristine is associated with a minimal (<10%) risk of emesis.[20,21] Generally, prophylaxis for acute and delayed emesis is not needed. Patients may receive one time prophylaxis with a phenothiazine (e.g., prochlorperazine) or a butyrophenone (e.g., droperidol). Breakthrough medications should be offered, such as a phenothiazine (e.g., prochlorperazine), a butyrophenone (e.g., droperidol), a substituted benzamide (e.g., metoclopramide), or a benzodiazepine (e.g., lorazepam). Selection should be based on what the patient is currently receiving for acute antiemesis prophylaxis.

Vitamin A

Brand names	Aquasol A Parenteral (water-miscible vitamin A palmitate)
Dosage	Not for IV infusion. **Vitamin A deficient children with xerophthalmia:** 5000–15,000 units IM for 10 days.[1] **Decrease morbidity from bronchopulmonary dysplasia in preterm infants:** 2000 international units (n = 20) or placebo (n = 20) IM was given to infants with increased risk for bronchopulmonary dysplasia (BPD) on day 1 of life and then every other day for 28 days. Vitamin A status was improved and morbidity associated with BPD was decreased.[2] In a follow-up multicenter study, either 5000 international units (n = 405) or placebo (n = 402) was given IM three times weekly for 4 weeks in premature infants as small as 770 ± 135 g. Vitamin A serum concentrations improved and the risk of chronic lung disease decreased compared to controls (55% vs. 62%, respectively).[3] This regimen continues to be recommended.[4] As a result of these studies and others, the following guidelines for dosing have been recommended[5]: 2000 international units IM on day of life 1 and every other day until enteral feedings are established. Once 75% of enteral feedings is attained, the route is changed to enteral and the dose increased to 4000 international units given enterally until discharge from the neonatal intensive care unit. Should the patient be placed NPO, the IM dose and route are resumed. Plasma concentrations of vitamin A and retinol binding protein should be measured weekly. (See Comments section.)
Dosage adjustment in organ dysfunction	Elevated serum retinol concentrations accompanied by clinical toxicity have been reported in patients with renal failure.[1,5]
Maximum dosage	15,000 international units in children,[1] 5000 international units in neonates.[2]
IV push	Not for IV use.[1,4,7]
Intermittent infusion	Not for IV use.[1,4,7]
Continuous infusion	Not for IV use.[1,4,7]
Other routes of administration	50,000 international units/mL for IM administration.[1,4,7]
Maximum concentration	50,000 international units/mL for IM administration.[1,4,7]
Cautions related to IV administration	Not for IV use.[1,4,7]
Other additives	Each mL contains 12% polysorbate 80, 0.5% chlorobutanol, and 0.1% citric acid.[7] Intravenous polysorbate 80 was associated with the E-Ferol syndrome (thrombocytopenia, renal insufficiency, hepatomegally, cholestasis, ascites, hypotension, and metabolic acidosis) in low birth weight infants.[8]

Comments

The target serum concentration range is 30–60 mcg/dL. Concentrations >100 mcg/dL are potentially toxic.[4,5] In particular, measuring serum concentrations is recommended in patients receiving glucocorticoids because steroids increase plasma concentrations of vitamin A.[4] This confounds the assessment of adequacy of vitamin A intake.

Vitamin K_1–Phytonadione

Brand names	AquaMEPHYTON; various manufacturers
Dosage	**Neonatal hemorrhagic disease** **Prophylaxis:** Usually given within 1 h of birth.[1] **≤1500 g:** 0.5 mg IM.[2-7] **>1500 g:** 1 mg IM.[2-7] **Treatment:** Usually 1 mg; however, doses up to 5 mg may be needed if the mother was receiving anticoagulant therapy.[2,3,7-11] **Prothrombin deficiency (malabsorption syndromes, broad spectrum antibiotics, etc.)** **Infants:** 2 mg.[1] **Older children:** 5–10 mg.[1] **Reversal of over-warfarinization in children (use not established):** 30 mcg/kg IV (0.35–1 mg) was used in seven children (age not reported).[12]
Dosage adjustment in organ dysfunction	No adjustment required in organ dysfunction. However, children with liver dysfunction may require more than one dose and measurement of the INR should be used to guide dosing.[12]
Maximum dosage	2 mg in infants and 5–10 mg in children.[1] In *adults* with anticoagulant-induced hypoprothrombinemia, doses are usually 2.5–10 mg; however, doses up to 50 mg may be needed.[1] It is prudent to limit the dose to the lowest effective amount so the patient can resume anticoagulation at the appropriate level.[1] Failure to respond may indicate that the underlying disease may be unresponsive to vitamin K.[2]
IV push	Over >1 mg/min in *adults*.[1] IV administration should be restricted due to the potential for severe adverse reactions.[1]
Intermittent infusion	2 or 10 mg/mL (undiluted)[1] or dilute in preservative-free D5NS, D5W, or NS[1,6,13] given over 15–30 min.[14] Concentrations of 50 mg/L are physically compatible in dextrose or dextrose and saline combinations.[15] During prothrombin deficiency, there is the increased risk of bleeding or hematoma formation at the IM or SC injection site and in this situation, IV administration may be preferred.[1]
Continuous infusion	Specified dose can be added to PN solutions and administered by this method.[16]
Other routes of administration	Undiluted. SC is the referred route of administration.[2] During prothrombin deficiency, there is the increased risk of bleeding or hematoma formation at the IM or SC injection site and IV administration may be preferred.[1]
Maximum concentration	10 mg/mL (undiluted).[1]
Cautions related to IV administration	Severe hypersensitivity-type reactions including death may occur.[1,2,13,14,17] For PN compatibility information, please see Appendix C.

Other additives

Each mL (2 mg or 10 mg) benzyl alcohol 0.9%.[1,2]

Benzyl alcohol in small doses as a preservative in drugs is considered safe in newborns.[18] However, a 3-week-old, very low birth weight (710 g) infant who received clindamycin experienced a profound desaturation that required resuscitation after the third and fourth doses, which was subsequently related to the benzyl alcohol preservative.[19]

Administration of saline flushes containing benzyl alcohol (BW) was associated with a fatal gasping syndrome, intraventricular hemorrhage, metabolic acidosis, and increased mortality in preterm infants.[20] This should not be used in neonates.

Hypersensitivity reactions to benzyl alcohol in parenteral products have been reported in *adults*.[21,22]

Comments

Improvement in hemostasis will not be seen for at least 1–2 h after administration.[1,2] Patients receiving vitamin K for reversal of over-warfarinization should have INR measured 4–6 h after the dose in those at high risk of bleeding or 12 h after the dose in less severe cases.[12]

Hyperbilirubinemia and severe hemolytic anemia have occurred in neonates receiving 10–20 mg doses.[1]

Two neonates who received IV phytonadione for prophylaxis developed late-onset hemorrhagic disease.[23]

Voriconazole

Brand names	Vfend
Dosage	**Neonates and infants:** Experience with voriconazole in neonates and infants is limited.[1] One report of two cases of VLBW infants receiving 3 mg/kg IV q 12 h for two doses, then 2 mg/kg IV q 12 h documented serum concentrations below that seen in *adults*; therapy was successful in both infants.[2] Two reports in infants (one preterm) utilized initial dosing of 6 mg/kg IV q 12 h.[3,4] The dose in the preterm infant was increased to 6 mg/kg IV q 8 h to obtain serum concentrations similar to that seen in *adults*.[3] A 3-month-old received 6 mg/kg IV q 12 h for two doses, then 4 mg/kg IV q 12 h.[5] One reference suggests a dosing regimen of 8 mg/kg IV q 12 h for two doses, then 6 mg/kg IV q 12 h.[6] **Children**[1,6-11] **Loading dose:** 6–8 mg/kg IV q 12 h for two doses. **Maintenance dose:** 4–7 mg/kg IV q 12 h. Children have required larger doses than *adults* to maintain similar concentrations.[7,10,11]
Dosage adjustment in organ dysfunction	**Hepatic impairment:** Patients with mild-to-moderate hepatic cirrhosis (Child-Pugh Class A or B) should receive a standard loading dose and 50% of maintenance dose.[12] Dosing has not been evaluated in patients with severe hepatic cirrhosis (Child-Pugh Class C) or chronic hepatitis B or C.[12] **Renal impairment:** Oral voriconazole is preferred in patients with CrCl <50 mL/min due to accumulation of the vehicle, sulfobutyl ether beta-cyclodextrin sodium (SBECD).[12] Peritoneal dialysis or hemodialysis does not remove a sufficient amount of voriconazole to warrant dose adjustment.[12,13]
Maximum dosage	No specific maximum dosage has been defined.
IV push	Not recommended.[12]
Intermittent infusion	Dilute reconstituted product to a final concentration of 0.5–5 mg/mL with appropriate diluent (NS, ½NS, LR, D5LR, D5NS, D5½NS, D5W, D5W + 20 mEq/L potassium chloride) and infuse over 1–2 h at a maximum rate of 3 mg/kg/h.[12]
Continuous infusion	No information available to support administration by this method.
Other routes of administration	No information available to support administration by other routes.

Maximum concentration	5 mg/mL.[12]
Cautions related to IV administration	Anaphylactic-type reactions have occurred uncommonly.[12] Do not administer through the same catheter or admix with other drugs, blood products, or PN.[12]
Other additives	Each 200-mg vial contains 160 mg/mL sulfobutyl ether beta-cyclodextrin sodium (SBECD).[12]
Comments	Visual adverse effects are commonly reported with voriconazole therapy.[12] Prolonged therapy should be used with caution in infants and children who are unable to vocalize visual effects.[7,12] Therapy has been associated with uncommon cases of hepatotoxicity, including liver failure and death.[12] Liver function should be monitored before and during therapy. Therapy has been associated with prolongation of QT interval.[12] Serum electrolytes (potassium, magnesium, calcium) should be within range before starting therapy to reduce risk of arrhythmias.[12] Stevens Johnson syndrome has been reported rarely.[12] Because voriconazole and its major metabolite inhibit CYP2C9/19 and 3A4, there are numerous drug interactions.[12] Consult appropriate resources for dosing recommendations before combining any drug with voriconazole. Patients on concomitant phenytoin therapy may require an increase in voriconazole maintenance dosing to 5 mg/kg.[12]

Zidovudine

Brand names	Retrovir (formerly called Azidothymidine, AZT)

Dosage

HIV-infected children should receive aggressive antiretroviral therapy with at least three drugs. Refer to www.aidsinfo.nih.gov or 1-800-TRIALS-A for the most up-to-date information regarding HIV treatment protocols in children.

Antiretroviral therapy[1-11]

Premature neonates[3]

<30 weeks GA: 1.5 mg/kg IV q 12 h, then 1.5 mg/kg IV q 8 h at 4 weeks of age.

≥30 weeks GA: 1.5 mg/kg IV q 12 h, then 1.5 mg/kg IV q 8 h at 2 weeks of age.

Term neonates and infants <6 weeks of age[3]: 1.5 mg/kg IV q 6 h.

Infants and children (6 weeks to 12 years of age)[3]: 120 mg/m^2 IV q 6 h or 20 mg/m^2/h continuous infusion.

Continuous infusion of 0.5–1.4 mg/kg/h (360–1000 mg/m^2/d) has been beneficial in children as young as 6 months with symptomatic HIV infection, especially those with encephalopathy.[8,10,11]

Prevention of perinatal transmission[1,2]: Maternal zidovudine (ZDV) 100 mg five times a day beginning at 14–34 weeks gestation and continued through pregnancy. During labor, 2 mg/kg ZDV IV over 1 h followed by continuous infusion of 1 mg/kg/h until delivery. Begin treatment in newborn as soon as possible after delivery (see recommended doses above), preferably within 6–12 h, and continue for the first 6 weeks of life. Continuation of therapy determined by virologic test results.

Dosage adjustment in organ dysfunction

Adjust dosage in patients with severe renal dysfunction.[3,12] If CrCl is <10 mL/min, give 50% of a normal dose.[12] May also be necessary to adjust dose or interrupt therapy in patients with significant anemia and/or neutropenia.[5,6,8,11,13] Insufficient data suggest a reduction in dose may be needed in patients with liver disease; these patients should be monitored for hematologic toxicity.[13]

Maximum dosage

640 mg/m^2/d for intermittent infusion.[5,9] 1.8 mg/kg/h (1300 mg/m^2/d) for continuous infusion.[10,11]

IV push

Not recommended.[13,14]

Intermittent infusion

≤4 mg/mL in D5W infused over 60 min.[13,14]

Continuous infusion

Although concentration and solution type were not specified, has been given by this method.[8,10,11]

Other routes of administration

No information available to support administration by other methods.[13,14]

Maximum concentration	4 mg/mL.[13,14]
Cautions related to IV administration	May cause pain or irritation at injection site.[13] For PN compatibility information, please see Appendix C.
Other additives	None.
Comments	Initiation of zidovudine postexposure prophylaxis therapy in the infant should begin as soon as possible after delivery and preferably within 6–12 h. Therapy initiating after 48 h is not likely to be effective.[2] Anemia necessitating treatment with partial volume exchange transfusion was reported in a 36-week-gestation infant born via emergent c-section (secondary to decreased fetal movement) to an HIV-positive woman receiving zidovudine, lamivudine, and nevirapine who developed macrocytic anemia at 29 weeks gestation (treated with packed red blood cell transfusion).[15] Severe lactic acidosis has been reported in a neonate receiving zidovudine; symptoms resolved following zidovudine discontinuation.[16] For conversion from IV to oral dosing, the oral dose is one–third greater than the IV dose.[5,7,13] Because zidovudine is associated with numerous drug interactions,[13] consult appropriate resources for dosing recommendations before combining any drug with zidovudine.

Appendix A

Nomogram for Determining Body Surface of Children from Height and Mass

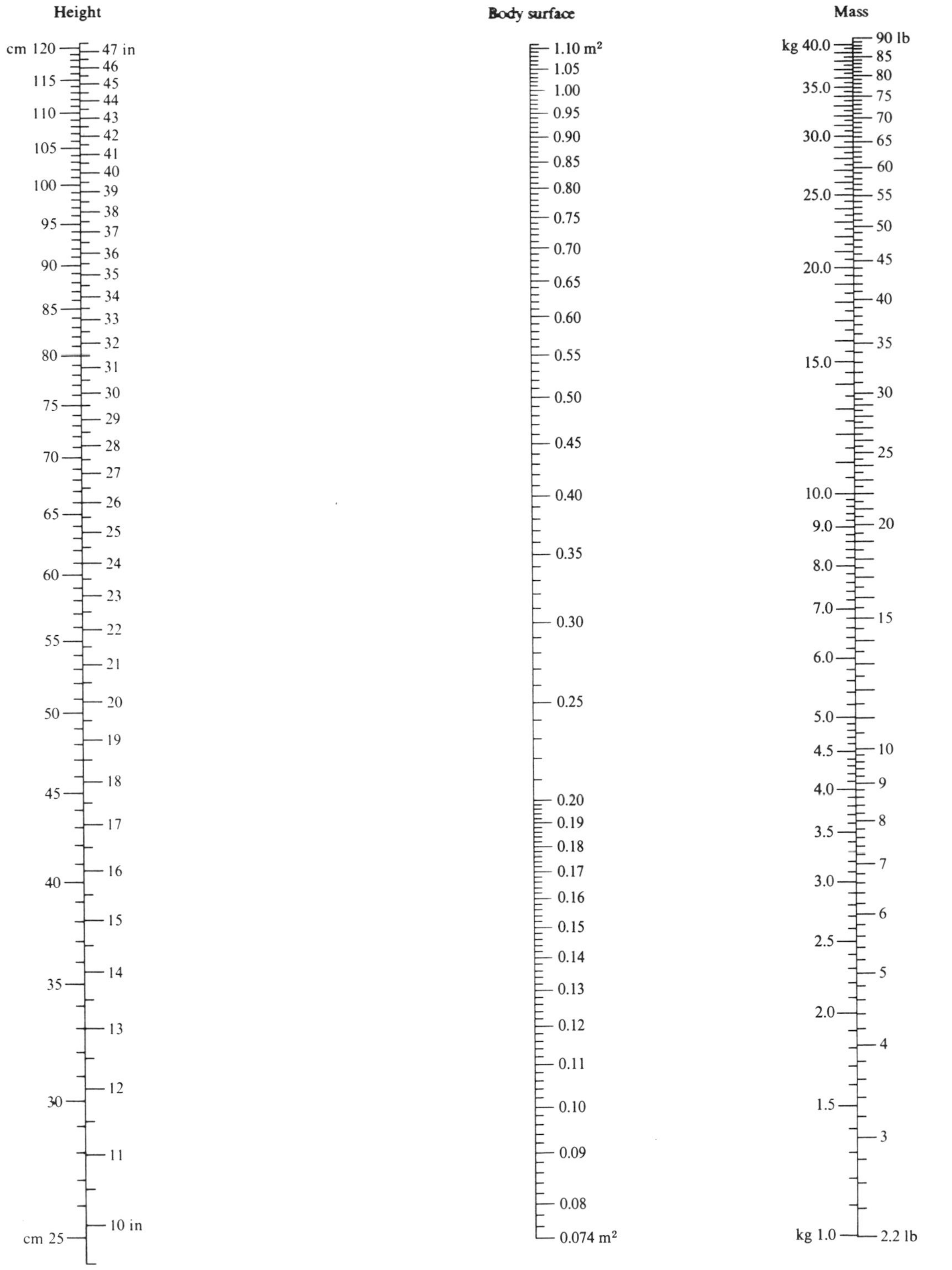

From the formula of Du Bois and Du Bois, *Arch. intern. Med.*, **17**, 863 (1916): $S = M^{0.425} \times H^{0.725} \times 71.84$, or $\log S = \log M \times 0.425 + \log H \times 0.725 + 1.8564$ (S: body surface in cm², M: mass in kg, H: height in cm).

Reproduced with permission, from Geigy scientific tables, volume 1. 8th ed. Lentner C, ed. Basie, Switzerland: CIBA-GEIGY Limited; 1993:226.

Appendix B

Nomogram for Estimating Ideal Body Mass in Children

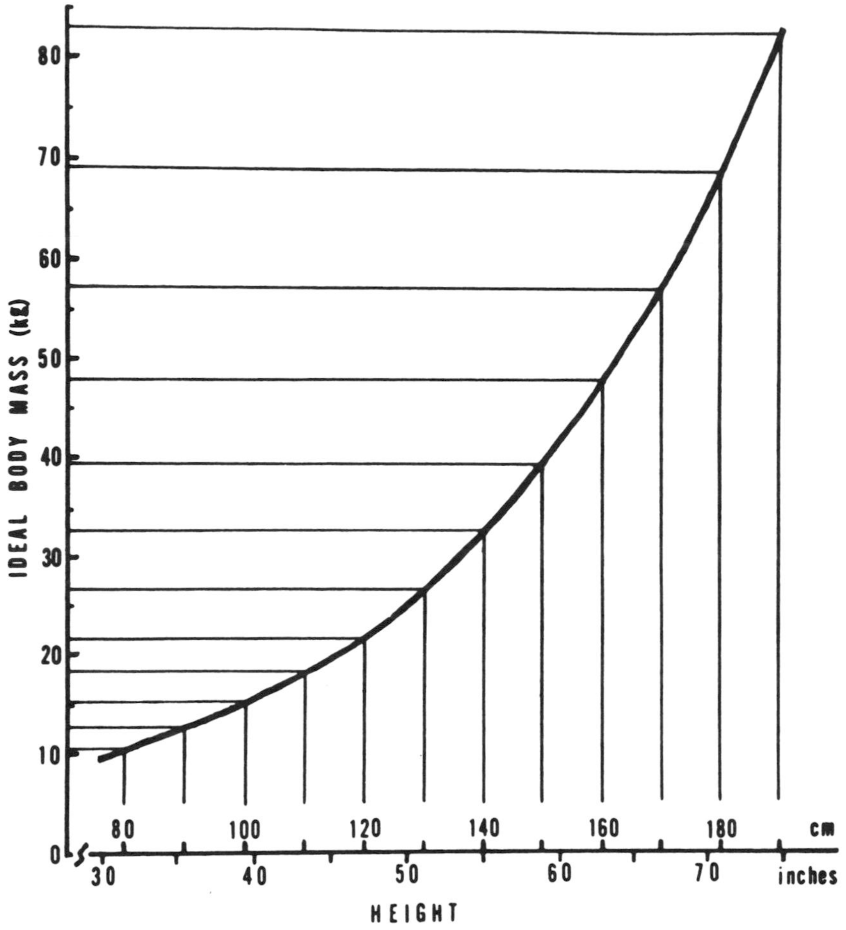

$$\text{IBM (kg)} = 2.396\, e^{0.01863(\text{height in cm})}$$

Appendix C

Y-Site Compatibility of Medications with Parenteral Nutrition

Christine A. Robinson, Pharm.D. and Jaclyn E. Lee, Pharm.D.

Many pediatric conditions such as abdominal wall defects of the newborn and short bowel syndrome warrant the use of parenteral nutrition. Obtaining and maintaining venous access in pediatric patients complicates the administration of this form of nutrition. Many patients require multiple treatment modalities to be administered intravenously including, medications, fluids, blood products, and nutrition. Clinicians must optimize available access to ensure appropriate and timely administration of all products prior to establishing additional access. This may require simultaneous administration of medications and parenteral nutrition; therefore, compatibility considerations become essential. It is important to recognize that compatibility only reflects the physical interactions such as formation of a precipitate and does not necessarily address stability or pharmacologic activity of the products. Published data may report both compatibility and stability; however, most evaluate compatibility alone. Currently there are multiple resources to use when answering the question of compatibility with parenteral nutrition. We strove to evaluate and present the available published data as a comprehensive and practical reference. We sought out primary literature regarding Y-site compatibility of multiple drugs commonly used in pediatric patients with three different parenteral nutrition formulas, 3-in-1, 2-in-1, and lipids alone. When conflicting results were encountered, the clinical strength was considered. When published data was not accessible, Lawrence Trissel's *Handbook on Injectable Drugs*[1] was used. Below please find each of the classifications utilized in this reference:

C Compatibility has been demonstrated. When Y-site compatibility was not available, medications compatible in solution for 24 hours were assumed to be Y-site compatible. Medications compatible with 3-in-1 admixtures were assumed to be compatible with lipids alone.[1]

I Incompatibility has been demonstrated

— Compatibility data not available

C/I Conflicting compatibility has been demonstrated and strength of the evidence supports compatible

I/C Conflicting compatibility has been demonstrated and strength of the evidence supports incompatible

Medication	Admixture Type			Comments	References	
	2-in-1	*Lipids*	*3-in-1*		C	I
Acetazolamide	I	—	—	White precipitate forms immediately		2
Acyclovir	I	I	I	White precipitate forms immediately		2,3,4
Amikacin	C	C/I	C/I	Visual breaking of emulsion within 1 h in select formulations	2,3,4,5,6,7	8
Aminophylline	C/I	C	C		3,4,9,10	2
Amphotericin B	I	I	I	Yellow precipitate formed immediately		3,4
Ampicillin sodium	C/I	C	C		3,4,11	2,5,7,12
Ampicillin sodium–Sulbactam sodium	C	C	C		3,4	
Atracurium besylate	C	—	—		13	
Aztreonam	C	C	C		3,4	
Bumetanide	C	C	C		3,4	
Caffeine	C	—	—		14	
Cefazolin Sodium	C/I	C	C	Incompatible at a dextrose concentration of 25%	3,4,5,14	3
Cefepime	C	—	—		15	
Cefoperazone sodium	C	C	C		3,4,5	
Cefotaxime sodium	C	C	C		2,3,4,5	
Cefotetan disodium	C	C	C		3,4	

Cefoxitin sodium	**C**	**C**	**C**		3,4,5,11	
Ceftazidime	**C**	**C**	**C**		2,3,4,16	
Ceftriaxone sodium	**C**	**C**	**C**		3,4,13	
Cefuroxime sodium	**C**	**C**	**C**		3,4	
Chloramphenicol sodium succinate	**C**	**C**	—		1,5	
Chlorpromazine HCl	**C**	**C**	**C**		3,4	
Cimetidine HCl	**C**	**C**	**C**		3,4,17	
Ciprofloxacin lactate	**I**	**C**	**C**	Amber discoloration in 1 to 4 h	4	3
Cisplatin	**I**	**C**	**C**	Amber discoloration in 1 to 4 h	4	3
Clindamycin phosphate	**C**	**C**	**C**		4,5,11	
Co-Trimoxazole	**C**	**C**	**C**		3,4	
Cyclophosphamide	**C**	**C**	**C**		3,4	
Cyclosporine	**C/I**	**C/I**	**C/I**	For 2:1, found to be compatible with Dextrose 5%/Amino Acids 4.25%, but not compatible with Dextrose 25%/Amino Acid 3.5%	3,4,18	3,4
Dexamethasone sodium phosphate	**C**	**C**	**C**		2,3,4	
Digoxin	**C**	**C**	**C**		3,4,19	
Diphenhydramine HCl	**C**	**C**	**C**		3,4	
Dobutamine HCl	**C**	**C**	**C**		2,3,4,6	
Dopamine HCl	**C**	**C/I**	**C/I**		2,3,4,19	4
Doxycycline hyclate	**C**	**I**	**I**	Emulsion disruption occurs immediately	3,5	4
Droperidol	**C**	**I**	**I**	Emulsion disruption occurs in 1 to 4 h	3	4
Enalaprilat	**C**	**C**	**C**		3,4	
Epinephrine HCl	**C**	—	—		13	
Epoetin alfa	**C**	—	—		20	
Erythromycin lactobionate	**C**	**C**	**C**		5,11,13	
Famotidine	**C**	**C**	**C**		3,4,17,21,22, 23,24,25	
Fentanyl citrate	**C**	**C**	**C**		2,3,4,26	
Fluconazole	**C**	**C**	**C**		3,4,27	
Foscarnet	**C**	—	—		28	
Furosemide	**C/I**	**C**	**C**	Small amount of precipitate formed in 4 h in select formulations	2,4,13,19	3
Ganciclovir sodium	**I/C**	**I**	**I**	Concentrations of ≥10 mg/mL resulted in precipitation within 0 to 30 min	29,30	3,4,29
Gentamicin sulfate	**C**	**C**	**C**		2,3,4,5,6,7, 8,11,12,13	
Granisetron HCl	**C**	**C**	**C**		3,4	
Haloperidol lactate	**C**	**I**	**I**	Emulsion disruption occurs immediately	3,13	4
Heparin sodium	**C**	**I**	**I**	Emulsion disruption occurs immediately with heparin 100 units/mL	3,13	4

Hydrochloric Acid	C	—	—		31	
Hydrocortisone sodium/phosphate/ succinate	C	C	C		3,4,13	
Ifosfamide	C	C	C		3,4	
Imipenem-Cilastatin Sodium	C	C	C		3,4	
Immune Globulin	—/C	—	—	Only supportive of Gammagard® 2.5%; not recommended to infuse with other drugs or solutions	32	
Indomethacin sodium trihydrate	I	—	—			33
Insulin, regular human	C	C	C		3,4,13	
Iron dextran	C/I	—	I/C	For 2:1, found to be compatible in solution at amino acid concentrations of 2% or greater	34,35,36	35,37
Isoproterenol HCl	C	C	C	For 2:1, compatible with dextrose 25%/amino acids 4.25% (electrolytes were not added)	19,38	
Kanamycin sulfate	C	C	C		11,12,38,39	
Lidocaine HCl	C	C	C	For 2:1, compatible with dextrose 25%/amino acids 4.25% (electrolytes were not added)	19,38	
Linezolid	C	—	—	Compatible with dextrose 20%/ amino acids 4.9%; electrolytes were not added	40	
Lorazepam	C	I	I	Partial emulsion disruption occurs in 1 h	3	4
Magnesium sulfate	C	C	C		3,4	
Mannitol	C	C	C		3,4	
Meperidine HCl	C	C	C		3,4,41	
Meropenem	—	C	C		4	
Methotrexate	I	C	C	For 2:1, hazy precipitate formed in 0 to 1 h	4	3
Methyldopate HCl	C	C/I	C/I	For 2:1, compatible with dextrose 25%/amino acids 4.25% (electrolytes were not added); cracked the lipid emulsion in select formulations	19,38	20
Methylprednisolone sodium succinate	C	C	C		3,4	
Metoclopramide HCl	I/C	C	C	Substantial loss of natural turbidity occurred immediately in select formulations	1,4	3
Metronidazole HCl	C	C	C		2,3,4,13	
Midazolam HCl	I/C	I	I	White precipitate forms immediately in select formulations	42	3,4,13
Milrinone lactate	C	—	—		43,44	
Morphine sulfate	C	C/I	C/I	For 3:1, morphine 1 mg/mL compatible, but 15 mg/mL was not compatible; emulsion disruption occurs immediately in select formulations	3,4,13,41	4

Appendix C

Nafcillin sodium	**C**	**C**	**C**		3,4,5,7	
Nitroglycerin	**C**	**C**	**C**		3,4	
Norepinephrine bitartrate	**C**	**C**	**C**		3,19	
Octreotide acetate	**C**	**C**	**C**		3,4	
Ondansetron HCl	**C**	**I**	**I**	Emulsion disruption occurs immediately	3	4
Oxacillin sodium	**C**	**C**	**C**		5,7,11	
Penicillin G potassium	**C**	**C**	**C**		2,5,7,11,13	
Penicillin G sodium	**C**	—	—		5,7	
Pentobarbital sodium	**C**	**I**	**I**	Emulsion disruption occurs immediately	3	4
Phenobarbital sodium	**C**	**I**	**I**	Emulsion disruption occurs immediately	3	4
Phenytoin sodium	**I**	**I**	—	Heavy white precipitate forms immediately; incompatible with dextrose		1,13
Piperacillin sodium	**C**	**C**	**C**		3,4,5,7	
Piperacillin sodium/ Tazobactam sodium	**C**	**C**	**C**		3,4	
Potassium chloride	**C**	**C**	**C**		3,4	
Potassium phosphate	**I**	**I**	**I**	Emulsion disruption occurs immediately; increased turbidity occurs immediately		3,4
Promethazine HCl	**C/I**	**C**	**C**	Amber discoloration in 4 h in select formulations	3,4	3
Propofol	**C**	—	—	Propofol injection contains approximately 10 g fat/100 mL	45	
Ranitidine HCl	**C**	**C**	**C**		2,3,4,13,17	
Sargramostim	**C**	—	—		46	
Sodium bicarbonate	**I/C**	**C**	**C**	Small amount of precipitate formed in 1 h in select formulations	3,5	3
Sodium nitroprusside	**C**	**C**	**C**		3,4	
Tacrolimus	**C**	**C**	**C**		3,4	
Ticarcillin disodium	**C**	**C**	**C**		3,4,5,7,11	
Ticarcillin disodium–Clavulanate potassium	**C**	**C**	**C**		3,4,13	
Tobramycin sulfate	**C**	**C**	**C**		2,3,4,5,6,7,8,11	
Vancomycin HCl	**C**	**C**	**C**		2,3,4,5,6,13	
Vecuronium bromide	**C**	—	—		13	
Vitamin K_1–phytonadione	**C**	**C**	—		12,47	
Zidovudine	**C**	**C**	**C**		2,3,4	

Source: Adapted with permission from Robinson CA, Lee JE. Y-Site compatibility of medications with parenteral nutrition. *J Pediatr Pharmacol Ther.* 2007;12 (In Press).

Appendix C

References

1. Trissel LA. *Handbook on Injectable Drugs.* 13th ed. Bethesda, MD: American Society of Health-System Pharmacists; 2005.
2. Veltri M, Lee CKK. Compatibility of neonatal parenteral nutrient solutions with selected intravenous drugs. *Am J Health-Syst Pharm.* 1996;53:2611-2613.
3. Trissel LA, Gilbert DL, Martinez JF, et al. Compatibility of parenteral nutrient solutions with selected drugs during simulated Y-site administration. *Am J Health-Syst Pharm.* 1997;54:1295-1300.
4. Trissel LA, Gilbert DL, Martinez JF, et al. Compatibility of medications with 3-in-1 parenteral nutrition admixtures. *J Parenter Enteral Nutr.* 1999;23:67-74.
5. Watson D. Piggyback compatibility of antibiotics with pediatric parenteral nutrition solutions. *J Parenter Enteral Nutr.* 1985;9:220-224.
6. Schilling CG. Compatibility of drugs with a heparin-containing neonatal total parenteral nutrient solution. *Am J Hosp Pharm.* 1988;45:313-314.
7. Kamen BA, Gunther N, Sowinsky N, et al. Analysis of antibiotic stability in a parenteral nutrition solution. *Pediatr Infect Dis.* 1985;4:387-389.
8. Bullock L, Clark JH, Fitzgerald JF, et al. The stability of amikacin, gentamicin, and tobramycin in total nutrient admixtures. *J Parenter Enteral Nutr.* 1989;13:505-509.
9. Andreu A, Cardona D, Pastor C, et al. Itravenous aminophylline: in vitro stability of fat-containing TPN. *Ann Pharmacother.* 1992;26:127-128.
10. Niemiec PW Jr, Vanderveen TW, Hohenwarter MW, et al. Stability of aminophylline injection in three parenteral nutrient solutions. *Am J Hosp Pharm.* 1983;40:428-432.
11. Baptisa RJ, Lawrence RW. Compatibility of total nutrient admixtures and secondary antibiotic infusions. *Am J Hosp Pharm.* 1985;42:362-363.
12. Schuetz DH, King JC. Compatibility and stability of electrolytes, vitamins and antibiotics in combination with 8% amino acids solutions. *Am J Hosp Pharm.* 1978;35:33-44.
13. Gilbar PJ, Groves CF. Visual compatibility of total parenteral nutrition solution (Synthamin 17 premix) with selected drugs during simulated Y-site injection. *Aust J Hosp Pharm.* 1994;24:167-170.
14. Nahata MC, Zingarelli J, Durrell DE. Stability of caffeine citrate injection in intravenous admixtures and parenteral nutrition solutions. *J Clin Pharm Ther.* 1989;14:53-55.
15. Maxipime® (Cefepime) [package insert]. Princeton, NJ: Bristol Meyers Squibb Company; revised December 2003.
16. Wade CS, Lampasona V, Mullins RE, et al. Stability of ceftazidime and amino acids in parenteral nutrient solutions. *Am J Hosp Pharm.* 1991;48:1515-1519.
17. Hatton J, Luer M, Hirsch J, et al. Histamine receptor antagonists and lipid stability in total nutrient admixtures. *J Parenter Enteral Nutr.* 1994;18:308-312.
18. Jacobson PA, Maksym CJ, Landvay A, et al. Compatibility of cyclosporine with fat emulsion. *Am J Hosp Pharm.* 1993;50:687-690.
19. Baptisa RJ, Dumas GJ, Bistrian BR, et al. Compatibility of total nutrient admixtures and secondary cardiovascular medications. *Am J Hosp Pharm.* 1985;42:777-778.
20. Ohls RK, Christensen RD. Stability of human recombinant epoetin alfa in commonly used neonatal intravenous solutions. *Ann Pharmacother.* 1996;30:466-468.
21. DiStefano JE, Mitrano JE, Baptista FP, et al. Long-term stability of famotidine 20 mg/mL in a total parenteral nutrient solution. *Am J Hosp Pharm.* 1989;46:2333-2335.
22. Bullock L, Fitzgerald JF, Glick MR, et al. Stability of famotidine 20 and 40 mg/L and amino acids in total parenteral nutrient solutions. *Am J Hosp Pharm.* 1989;46:2321-2325.
23. Bullock L, Fitzgerald JF, Glick MR. Stability of famotidine 20 and 50 mg/L in total nutrient admixtures. *Am J Hosp Pharm.* 1989;46:2326-2329.
24. Montoro JB, Pou L, Salvador P, et al. Stability of famotidine 20 and 40 mg/L in total nutrient admixtures. *Am J Hosp Pharm.* 1989;46:2329-2332.
25. Shea BF, Souney PF. Sability of famotidine in a 3-in-1 total nutrient admixture. *DCIP.* 1990;24:232-235.
26. Moshfeghi M, Ciuffo J. Visual compatibility of fentanyl citrate with parenteral nutrient solutions [Letters]. *Am J Health Sys Pharm.* 1998;55:1194-1197.
27. Couch P, Jacobson P, Johnson CE. Stability of fluconazole and amino acids in parenteral nutrient solutions. *Am J Hosp Pharm.* 1992;49:1459-1462.
28. Baltz JK, Kennedy P, Minor JR, et al. Visual compatibility of foscarnet with other injectable drugs during simulated Y-site administration. *Am J Hosp Pharm.* 1990;47:2075-2077.
29. Outman WR, Mitrano FP, Baptista RJ. Visual compatibility of ganciclovir sodium and parenteral nutrient solution during simulated Y-site injection. *Am J Hosp Pharm.* 1991;48:1538-1539.
30. Johnson CE, Jacobson PA, Chan E. Stability of ganciclovir sodium and amino acids in parenteral nutrient solutions. *Am J Hosp Pharm.* 1994;51:503-508.
31. Mirtallo JM, Rogers KR, Johnson JA, et al. Stability of amino acids and the availability of acid in total parenteral nutrition solutions containing hydrochloric acid. *Am J Hosp Pharm.* 1981;38:1729-1731.
32. Lindsay CA, Dang K, Adams JM, et al. Stability and activity of intravenous immunoglobulin with neonatal dextrose and total parenteral nutrient solutions. *Ann Pharmacother.* 1994;28:1014-1017.
33. Ishisaka DY, VanVleet J, Marquardt E. Visual compatibility of indomethacin sodium trihydrate with drugs given to neonates by continuous infusion. *Am J Hosp Pharm.* 1991;48:2442-2443.
34. Wan KK, Tsallas G. Dilute iron dextran formulation for addition to parenteral nutrient solutions. *Am J Hosp Pharm.* 1980;37:206-210.
35. Mayhew SL, Quick MW. Compatibility of iron dextran with neonatal parenteral nutrient solutions. *Am J Health-Syst Pharm.* 1997;54:570-571.
36. Tu YH, Knox NL, Biringer JM, et al. Compatibility of iron dextran with total nutrient admixtures. *Am J Hosp Pharm.* 1992;49:2233-2235.
37. Vaughan LM, Small C, Plunkett V. Incompatibility of iron dextran and a total nutrient admixture. *Am J Hosp Pharm.* 1990;47:1745-1746.
38. Athanikar N, Boyer B, Deamer R, et al. Visual compatibility of 30 additives with a parenteral nutrient solution. *Am J Hosp Pharm.* 1979;36:511-513.
39. Feigin RD. Moss KS. Shackelford PG Antibiotic stability in solutions used for intravenous nutrition and fluid therapy. *Pediatrics.* 1973;51:1016-1026.
40. Trissel LA, Williams KY, Gilbert DL. Compatibility screening of linezolid injection during simulated Y-site administration with other drugs and infusion solutions. *J Am Pharm Assoc.* 2000;40:515-519.
41. Pugh CB, Pabis DJ, Rodriguez C. Visual compatibility of morphine sulfate and meperidine hydrochloride with other injectable drugs during simulated Y-site injection. *Am J Hosp Pharm.* 1991;48:123-125.
42. Bhatt-Mehta V, Rosen DA, King RS, et al. Stability of midazolam hydrochloride in parenteral nutrient solutions. *Am J Hosp Pharm.* 1993;50:285-288.
43. Akkerman SR, Zhang H, Mullins RE, et al. Stability of milrinone lactate in the presence of 29 critical care drugs and 4 i.v. solutions. *Am J Health-Syst Pharm.* 1999;56:63-68.
44. Veltri MA, Conner KG. Physical compatibility of milrinone lactate injection with intravenous drugs commonly used in the pediatric intensive

45. Bhatt-Mehta V, Paglia RE, Rosen DA. Stability of propofol with parenteral nutrient solutions during simulated Y-site injection. *Am J Health-Syst Pharm.* 1995;52:192-196.
46. Trissel LA, Bready BB, Kwan JW, et al. Visual compatibility of sargramostim with selected antineoplastic agents, anti-infectives, or other drugs during simulated Y-site injection. *Am J Hosp Pharm.* 1992;49:402-406.
47. Dahl GB, Svensson L, Kinnander NJ, et al. Stability of multivitamins in soybean oil fat emulsion under conditions simulating intravenous feeding of neonates and children. *J Parenter Enteral Nutr.* 1994;18:234-239.

References

Acetazolamide

1. Thomson Healthcare Inc. USP DI® drug information for the health care professional. Available at: http://www.thomsonhc.com. MICROMEDEX® Healthcare Series [database online]. Accessed May 26, 2006.
2. Guignard JP. Diuresis. In: Yaffe SJ, Aranda JV, eds. *Neonatal and Pediatric Pharmacology.* 3rd ed. Philadelphia, PA: Lippincott Williams & Wilkins; 2005:595-611.
3. Manzi SF, Arnold A, Patterson A. Pediatric drug formulary. In: Yaffe SJ, Aranda JV, eds. *Neonatal and Pediatric Pharmacology.* 3rd ed. Philadelphia, PA: Lippincott Williams & Wilkins; 2005:890.
4. Shirkey JC, ed. *Pediatric Therapy.* 4th ed. St. Louis, MO: Mosby; 1972.
5. International PHVD Drug Trial Group. International randomized controlled trial of acetazolamide and furosemide in posthemorrhagic ventricular dilatation in infancy. *Lancet.* 1998;352:433-440.
6. Kennedy CR, Ayers S, Campbell MJ, et al. Randomized, controlled trial of acetazolamide and furosemide in posthemorrhagic ventricular dilation in infancy: follow-up at 1 year. *Pediatrics.* 2001;108:597-607.
7. Lieh-Lai M, Sarnaik AP. Therapeutic applications in pediatric intensive care. In: Yaffe SJ, Aranda JV, eds. *Neonatal and Pediatric Pharmacology.* 3rd ed. Philadelphia, PA: Lippincott Williams & Wilkins; 2005:261-277.
8. Aronoff A, Brier M, Bennett W. *The Renal Book, 2002.* Available at: http://www.kdp-baptist.louisville.edu/renalbook/. Accessed May 26, 2006.
9. Acetazolamide [package insert]. Bedford, OH: Ben Venue Laboratories Inc; December 2002.
10. Trissel LA, ed. *Handbook on Injectable Drugs.* 13th ed. [CD-ROM version 1.5]. Bethesda, MD: American Society of Health-System Pharmacists; 2005.

Acetylcysteine (NAC)

1. Acetadote [package insert]. Nashville, TN: Cumberland Pharmaceuticals Inc; February 2006.
2. American Society of Health-System Pharmacists. American Hospital Formulary System. Available at: http://ahfsfirst.firstdatabank.com/AHFSfirst/NSAHFSFirstSearchmain.asp. Accessed July 2, 2006.
3. Ahola T, Lapatto R, Raivio KO, et al. N-acetylcysteine does not prevent bronchopulmonary dysplasia in immature infants: a randomized controlled trial. *J Pediatr.* 2003;143:713-719.
4. Tepel M, van der Giet M, Schwarzfeld C et al. Prevention of radiographic-contrast-agent-induced reductions in renal function by acetylcysteine. *N Engl J Med.* 2000;343:180-184.
5. Safirstein R, Andrade L, Vieira JM. Acetylcysteine and nephrotoxic effects of radiographic contrast agents—a new use for an old drug. *N Engl J Med.* 2000;343:210-212.
6. Marenzi G, Assanelli E, Marana I, et al. N-Acetylcysteine and contrast-induced nephropathy in primary angioplasty. *N Engl J Med.* 2006;354:2773-2782.
7. Aronoff A, Brier M, Bennett W. *The Renal Book, 2002.* Available at: http://www.kdp-baptist.louisville.edu/renalbook/. Accessed July 2, 2006.
8. N-acetylcysteine. In: Goldfrank LR, Flomenbaum NE, Lewin NA, et al., eds. *Goldfrank's Toxicologic Emergencies.* 7th ed. New York, NY: McGraw-Hill; 2002:502-506.
9. Ahola T, Fellman V, Laaksonen R, et al. Pharmacokinetics of intravenous N-acetylcysteine in pre-term newborn infants. *Eur J Clin Pharmacol.* 1999;55:645-550.
10. Borgstrom L, Kagedal B, Paulsen O. Pharmacokinetics of N-acetylcysteine in man. *Eur J Clin Pharmacol.* 1986;31:217-222.
11. Horowitz RS, Dart RC, Jarvie DR, et al. Placental transfer of N-acetylcysteine following human maternal acetaminophen toxicity. *J Toxicol Clin Toxicol.* 1997;35:447-451.

Acyclovir Sodium

1. Zovirax [package insert]. Research Triangle Park, NC: GlaxoSmithKline; 2003.
2. Bacigalupo A, Frassoni F, Van Lint MT. Acyclovir for the treatment of severe aplastic anemia. *N Engl J Med.* 1984;310:1606-1607.
3. Yeager AS. Use of acyclovir in premature and term neonates. *Am J Med.* 1982;73:205-209.
4. Meyers JD, Reed EC, Shepp DH, et al. Acyclovir for prevention of cytomegalovirus infection and disease after allogeneic marrow transplantation. *N Engl J Med.* 1988;318:70-75.
5. Mitchell CD, Gentry SR, Boen JR, et al. Acyclovir therapy for mucocutaneous herpes simplex infections in immunocompromised patients. *Lancet.* 1981;1:1389-1392.
6. O'Meara A, Hillary IB. Acyclovir in the management of herpes virus infections in immunosuppressed children. *Ir J Med Sci.* 1981;150:73-77.
7. Gould JM, Chessells JM, Marshall WC, et al. Acyclovir in herpes virus infections in children: experience in an open study with particular reference to safety. *J Infect.* 1982;5:283-289.
8. Balfour HH. Intravenous acyclovir therapy for varicella in immunocompromised children. *J Pediatr.* 1984;104:134-136.
9. Balfour HH, Bean B, Laskin OL, et al. Acyclovir halts progression of herpes zoster in immunocompromised patients. *N Engl J Med.* 1983;308:1448-1453.
10. Prober CG, Kirk LE, Keeney RE. Acyclovir therapy of chickenpox in immunosuppressed children. A collaborative study. *J Pediatr.* 1982;101:622-625.
11. American Academy of Pediatrics. In: Pickering LK, ed. *Red Book: 2006 Report of the Committee on Infectious Diseases.* 27th ed. Elk Grove Village, IL: American Academy of Pediatrics; 2006.
12. Kimberlin DW, Lin CY, Jacobs RF, et al. Safety and efficacy of high-dose intravenous acyclovir in the management of neonatal herpes simplex virus infections. *Pediatrics.* 2001;108:230-238.
13. Balfour HH Jr. Antiviral drugs. *N Engl J Med.* 1999;340:1255-1268.
14. Carcao MD, Lau RC, Gupta A, et al. Sequential use of intravenous and oral acyclovir in the therapy of varicella in immunocompromised children. *Pediatr Infect Dis J.* 1998;17:626-631.
15. Kashtan CE, Cook M, Chavers BM, et al. Outcome of chickenpox in 66 pediatric renal transplant recipients. *J Pediatr.* 1997;131:874-877.
16. Prentice HG, Gluckman E, Powles RL, et al. Impact of long-term acyclovir on cytomegalovirus infection and survival after allogeneic bone marrow transplantation. *Lancet.* 1994;343:749-753.
17. Laskin OL, Longstreth JA, Whelton A, et al. Acyclovir kinetics in end-stage renal disease. *Clin Pharmacol Ther.* 1982;31:594-601.
18. Aronoff GR, Berns JS, Brier ME, et al. *Drug Prescribing in Renal Failure: Dosing Guidelines for Adults.* 4th ed. Philadelphia, PA: American College of Physicians; 1999.
19. Englund JA, Fletcher CV, Balfour HH. Acyclovir therapy in neonates. *J Pediatr.* 1991;119:129-135.
20. Baker KL, Baker DS, Morgan DL. Largest dose of acyclovir inadvertently administered to a neonate. *Pediatr Infect Dis J.* 2003;22:842.
21. Brigden D, Rosling AE, Woods NC. Renal function after acyclovir intravenous injection. *Am J Med.* 1982;73:182-185.
22. Trissel LA. *Handbook on Injectable Drugs.* 13th ed. Bethesda, MD: American Society of Health-System Pharmacists; 2005.
23. Van der Meer JW, Versteeg J. Acyclovir in severe herpes virus infections. *Am J Med.* 1982;73:271-274.
24. Rosenberry KR, Bryan CK, Sohn CA. Acyclovir: evaluation of a new antiviral agent. *Clin Pharm.* 1982;1:399-406.
25. Robbins MS, Stromquist C, Tan LH. Acyclovir pH—possible cause of extravasation tissue injury. *Ann Pharmacother.* 1993;27:238.
26. Buck ML, Vittone SB, Zaglul HF. Vesicular eruptions following acyclovir administration. *Ann Pharmacother.* 1993;27:1458-1459.
27. Feder HM, Goyal RK, Krause PJ. Acyclovir-induced neutropenia in an infant with herpes simplex encephalitis: case report. *Clin Infect Dis.* 1995;20:1557-1559.

References

28. Vachvanichsanong, Patamasucon P, Malagon M, Moore ES. Acute renal failure in a child associated with acyclovir. *Pediatr Nephrol.* 1995;9:346-347.

Adenosine

1. American Academy of Pediatrics Committee on Drugs. Emergency drug doses for infants and children. *Pediatrics.* 1998;101:e1-e11.
2. Konduri GG, Garcia DC, Kazzi NJ, et al. Adenosine infusion improves oxygenation in term infants with respiratory failure. *Pediatrics.* 1996;97:295-300.
3. Praghu AS, Singh TP, Morrow WR, et al. Safety and efficacy of intravenous adenosine for pharmacologic stress testing in children with aortic valve disease or Kawasaki disease. *Am J Cardiol.* 1999;83:284-286.
4. Overholt ED, Rheuban KS, Gutgesell HP, et al. Usefulness of adenosine for arrhythmias in infants and children. *Am J Cardiol.* 1988;61:336-340.
5. Till J, Shinebourne EA, Rigby ML, et al. Efficacy and safety of adenosine in the treatment of supraventricular tachycardia in infants and children. *Br Heart J.* 1989;62:204-211.
6. Muller G, Deal BJ, Benson DW Jr. Vagal maneuvers and adenosine for termination of atrioventricular reentrant tachycardia. *Am J Cardiol.* 1994;74:500-503.
7. Paret G, Steinmetz D, Kuint J, et al. Adenosine for the treatment of paroxysmal supraventricular tachycardia in full-term and preterm newborn infants. *Am J Perinatol.* 1996;13:343-346.
8. McDeed-Breault C, McClean TL. Case reviews: supraventricular tachycardia in an infant. *J Emer Nurs.* 1992;18:494-496.
9. DeWolf D, Rondia G, Verhaaren H, et al. Adenosine-tri-phosphate treatment for supraventricular tachycardia in infants. *Eur J Pediatr.* 1994;153:793-796.
10. American Heart Association. Guidelines 2005 for cardiopulmonary resuscitation and emergency cardiovascular care. Part 12: Pediatric advanced life support. *Circulation.* 2005;112:167-187.
11. Rossi AF, Steinburg LG, Kipel G, et al. Use of adenosine in the management of perioperative arrhythmias in the pediatric cardiac intensive care unit. *Crit Care Med.*1992;20:1107-1111.
12. Ralston MA, Knilans TK, Hannon DW, et al. Use of adenosine for diagnosis and treatment of tachyarrhythmias in pediatric patients. *J Pediatr.* 1994;24:139-143.
13. Luedtke SA, Kuhn RJ, McCaffrey FM. Pharmacologic management of supraventricular tachycardias in children. Part 1: Wolff-Parkinson-White and atrioventricular nodal reentry. *Ann Pharmacother.* 1997;31:1227-1242.
14. Losek JD, Endom E, Dietrich A, et al. Adenosine and pediatric supraventricular tachycardia in the emergency department: multicenter study and review. *Ann Emer Med.* 1999;33:85-191.
15. Kugler JD, Danford DA. Management of infants, children, and adolescents with paroxysmal supraventricular tachycardia. *J Pediatr.* 1996;129:324-338.
16. Dixon J, Foster K, Wyllie J, et al. Guidelines and adenosine dosing in supraventricular tachycardia. *Arch Dis Child.* 2005;90:1190-1191.
17. Rosenthal E. Pitfalls in the use of adenosine. *Arch Dis Child.* 2005;91:451.
18. Clarke B, Rowland E, Barnes PJ, et al. Rapid and safe termination of supraventricular tachycardia in children by adenosine. *Lancet.* 1987;1:299-301.
19. Aronoff A, Brier M, Bennett W. *The Renal Book, 2002.* Available at: http://www.kdp-baptist.louisville.edu/renalbook/. Accessed July 4, 2006.
20. Berul CI. Higher adenosine dosage required for supra-ventricular tachycardia in infants treated with theophylline. *Clin Pediatr.* 1993;32:167-168.
21. Fitzsimmons CL, Withington DE. Use of andeosine in multiple doses for supraventricular tachycardia in an infant. *Pediatr Cardiol.* 1997;18:432-433.
22. *Physicians' Desk Reference.* 60th ed. Montvale, NJ: Medical Economics Company; 2006.
23. DeGroff CG, Silka MJ. Bronchospasm after intravenous administration of adenosine in a patient with asthma. *J Pediatr.* 1994;125:822-823.
24. Burkhart KK. Respiratory failure following adenosine administration. *Am J Emer Med.* 1993;11:249-250.
25. Aggarwal A, Farber NE, Warltier DC. Intraoperative bronchospasm caused by adenosine. *Anesthesiology.* 1993;79:1132-1135.
26. Watt AH, Bernard MS, Webster J, et al. Intravenous adenosine in the treatment of supraventricular tachycardia: a dose-ranging study and interaction with dipyridamole. *Br J Clin Pharmacol.* 1986;21:227-230.

Albumin (Normal Human Serum)

1. Medical Economics, ed. *Physicians' Desk Reference.* 60th ed. Oradell, NJ: Medical Economics Company; 2006.
2. Lambert HJ, Baylis PH, Coulthard MG. Central-peripheral temperature difference, blood pressure, and arginine vasopressin in preterm neonates undergoing volume expansion. *Arch Dis Child Fetal Neonatal Ed.* 1998;78:F43-F45.
3. Ruelas-Orozco G, Varga-Origel A. Assessment of therapy for arterial hypotension in critically ill preterm infants. *Am J Perinatol.* 2000;17:95-99.
4. Lay KS, Bancalari E, Malkus H, et al. Acute effects of albumin infusion on blood volume and renal function in premature infants with respiratory distress syndrome. *J Pediatr.* 1980;97:619-623.
5. Greissman A, Silver P, Nimkoff L, et al. Albumin bolus administration versus continuous infusion in critically ill hypoalbuminemic pediatric patients. *Intensive Care Med.* 1996;22:495-499.
6. Hardin TC, Page CP, Schwesinger WH. Rapid replacement of serum albumin in patients receiving total parenteral nutrition. *Surg Gynecol Obstet.* 1986;163:359-362.
7. Cochran EB, Hogue SL. Prediction of serum albumin concentration after albumin supplementation in pediatric patients receiving parenteral nutrition. *Clin Pharm.* 1991;10:704-706.
8. Weiss RA, Schoeneman M, Greifer I. Treatment of severe nephrotic edema with albumin and furosemide. *NY State J Med.* 1984;84:384-386.
9. Haws RM, Baum M. Efficacy of albumin and diuretic therapy in children with nephrotic syndrome. *Pediatrics.* 1993;91:1142-1146.
10. Roth KS, Amaker BG, Chan JCM. Nephrotic syndrome: pathogenesis and management. *Pediatr Rev.* 2002;23:237-247.
11. Dixon H, Hawkins K, Stephenson T. Comparison of albumin versus bicarbonate treatment for neonatal acidosis. *Eur J Pediatr.* 1999;158:414-415.
12. McEvoy GK, ed. *AHFS Drug Information Essentials 2005–06.* Bethesda, MD: American Society of Health-System Pharmacists; 2005.
13. Trissel LA. *Handbook on Injectable Drugs.* 13th ed. Bethesda, MD: American Society of Health-System Pharmacists; 2005.
14. Goldberg RN, Chung D, Goldman SL, et al. The association of rapid volume expansion and intraventricular hemorrhage in the preterm infant. *J Pediatr.* 1980;96:1060-1063.
15. Stafford CT, Lobel SA, Fruge BC, et al. Anaphylaxis to human serum albumin. *Ann Allergy.* 1988;61:85-88.
16. Snyder RL. Filter clogging caused by albumin in I.V. nutrient solution. *Am J Hosp Pharm.* 1993;50:63-64.
17. Feldman F, Bergman G. Filter clogging caused by albumin in I.V. nutrient solution (response). *Am J Hosp Pharm.* 1993;50:64.

Alfentanil

1. Prostaphlin [package insert]. Evansville, IN: Bristol Laboratories; November 1984.
2. Marlow N, Weindling AM, Van Peer A, et al. Alfentanil pharmacokinetics in preterm infants. *Arch Dis Child.* 1990;65;349-351.
3. Pokela ML, Ryhanen PT, Koivisto ME, et al. Alfentanil-induced rigidity in newborn infants. *Anesth Analg.* 1992;75:252-257.

4. Killian A, Davis PJ, Stiller RL, et al. Influence of gestational age on pharmacokinetics of alfentanil in neonates. *Dev Pharmacol Ther.* 1990;15:82-85.
5. Leoni F, Benni F, Iacobucci T, et al. Pain control with low-dose alfentanil in children undergoing minor abdominal and genitor-urinary surgery. *Eur J Anaesth.* 2004;21:738-742.
6. Meistelman C, Saint-Maurice C, LePaul M, et al. A comparison of alfentanil pharmacokinetics in children and adults. *Anesthesiology.* 1987;66:13-16.
7. Davis PJ, Lerman J, Suresh S, et al. A randomized multicenter study of remifentanil compared with alfentanil, isoflurane, or propofol in anesthetized pediatric patients undergoing elective strabismus surgery. *Anesth Analg.* 1997;84:982-989.
8. Mulroy JJ, Davis PJ, Rymer DB, et al. Safety and efficacy of alfentanil and halothane in paediatric surgical patients. *Can J Anesth.* 1991;38(4 pt 1):445-449.
9. den Hollander JM, Hennis PJ, Burm AG, et al. Alfentanil in infants and children with congenital heart defects. *J Cardiothorac Anesth.* 1988;2:1-7.
10. Klemola U, Mennander S, Saarnivaara L. Tracheal intubation without the use of muscle relaxants: remifentanil or alfentanil in combination with propofol. *Acta Anaesthesthiol Scand.* 2000;44:465-469.
11. Aronoff A, Brier M, Bennett W. *The Renal Book, 2002.* Available at: http://www.kdp-baptist.louisville.edu/renalbook/. Accessed July 6, 2006.
12. Trissel LA, ed. *Handbook on Injectable Drugs.* 13th ed. [CD-ROM version 1.5]. Bethesda, MD: American Society of Health-System Pharmacists; 2005.
13. Keene DL, Roberts D, Splinter WM, et al. Alfentanil mediated activation of epileptiform activity in the electrocorticogram during resection of epileptogenic foci. *Can J Neurol Sci.* 1997;24:37-39.
14. Cascino GD, So EL, Sharbrough FW, et al. Alfentanil-induced epileptiform activity in patients with partial epilepsy. *J Clin Neurophysiol.* 1993;10:520-525.

Allopurinol Sodium

1. McEvoy GK, ed. *AHFS Drug Information Essentials 2005–06.* Bethesda, MD: American Society of Health-System Pharmacists; 2005.
2. *Physicians' Desk Reference.* 60th ed. Montvale, NJ: Thomson PDR; 2006.
3. Donnenberg A, Holton CP, Mayer CM, et al. Evaluation of intravenous allopurinol (NSC-1390) in pediatric neoplasia. *Cancer Chemother Rep.* 1974;58:737-739.
4. Brown CH, Stashick E, Carbone PP. Clinical efficacy and lack of toxicity of allopurinol (NSC-1390) given intravenously. *Cancer Chemother Rep.* 1970;54:125-129.
5. Van Bel F, Shadid M, Moison RM, et al. Effect of allopurinol on postasphyxial free radical formation, cerebral hemodynamic, and electrical brain activity. *Pediatrics.* 1998;101:185-193.
6. Marro PJ, Baumgart S, Delivoria-Papadopoulos M, et al. Purine metabolism and inhibition of xanthine oxidase in severely hypoxic neonates going onto extracorporeal membrane oxygenation. *Pediatr Res.* 1997;41:513-521.
7. McGaurn SP, Davis LE, Krawczeniuk MM, et al. The pharmacokinetics of injectable allopurinol in newborns with the hypoplastic left heart syndrome. *Pediatrics.* 1994;94:820-823.
8. Clancy RR, McGaurn SA, Goin JE, et al. Allopurinol neurocardiac protection trial in infants undergoing heart surgery using deep hypothermic circulatory arrest. *Pediatrics.* 2001;108:61-70.
9. Aronoff A, Brier M, Bennett W. *The Renal Book, 2002.* Available at: http://www.kdp-baptist.louisville.edu/renalbook/. Accessed June 29, 2006.
10. Smalley RV, Guaspari A, Haase-Statz S, et al. Allopurinol: intravenous use for prevention and treatment of hyperuricemia. *J Clin Oncol.* 2000;18:1758-1763.
11. Trissel LA, ed. *Handbook on Injectable Drugs.* 13th ed. Bethesda, MD: American Society of Health-System Pharmacists; 2005.
12. Breithaupt H, Tittel M. Kinetics of allopurinol after single intravenous and oral doses. *Eur J Clin Pharmacol.* 1982;22:77-84.
13. Appelbaum SJ, Mayersohn M, Dorr RT, et al. Allopurinol kinetics and bioavailability. *Cancer Chemother Pharmacol.* 1982;8:93-98.
14. Lin YW, Okazaki S, Hamahata K, et al. Acute pure red cell aplasia associated with allopurinol therapy. *Am J Hematol.* 1999;61:209-211.

Alprostadil

1. Schlegel PG, Haber HP, Beck J, et al. Hepatic veno-occlusive disease in pediatric stem cell recipients: successful treatment with continuous infusion of prostaglandin E1 and low-dose heparin. *Ann Hematol.* 1998;76:37-41.
2. Neutze JM, Starling MB, Elliott RB, et al. Palliation of cyanotic congenital heart disease in infancy with E-type prostaglandins. *Circulation.* 1977;55:238-241.
3. Lewis AB, Takahashi M, Lurie PR. Administration of prostaglandin E1 in neonates with critical congenital cardiac defects. *J Pediatr.* 1978;93:481-485.
4. Graham TP, Atwood GF, Boucek RJ. Pharmacologic dilatation of the ductus arteriosus with prostaglandin E1 in infants with congenital heart disease. *South Med J.* 1978;71:1238-1241, 1246.
5. Benson LN, Olley PM, Patel RG, et al. Role of prostaglandin E1 infusion in the management of transposition of the great arteries. *Am J Cardiol.* 1979;44:691-696.
6. Lang P, Freed MD, Bierman FZ, et al. Use of prostaglandin E1 in infants with d-transposition of the great arteries and intact ventricular septum. *Am J Cardiol.* 1979;44:76-81.
7. Freed MD, Heymann MA, Lewis AB, et al. Prostaglandin E1 in infants with ductus arteriosus-dependent congenital heart disease. *Circulation.* 1981;64:809-905.
8. Host A, Halken S, Kamper J, et al. Prostaglandin E1 treatment in ductus dependent congenital cardiac malformation: a review of 34 neonates. *Dan Med Bull.* 1988:35:81-84.
9. Heymann MA, Clyman RI. Evaluation of alprostadil (prostaglandin E1) in the management of congenital heart disease in infancy. *Pharmacotherapy.* 1982;2:148-155.
10. Von Planta M, Fasnacht M, Holm C, et al. Atypical Kawasaki disease with peripheral gangrene and myocardial infarction: therapeutic implications. *Eur J Pediatr.* 1995;154:830-834.
11. Kwan CM, Chang WC, Chen JH, Wang MY. The effect of intravenous infusion of prostaglandin E1 on cutaneous microcirculation in black foot disease. *J Formos Med Assoc.* 1993;92:603-608.
12. Bauer J, Dapper F, Demirakea S, et al. Perioperative management of pulmonary hypertension after heart transplantation in childhood. *J Heart Lung Transplant.* 1997;16:1238-1247.
13. Radovancevic B, Vrtovec B, Thomas CD, et al. Nitric oxide versus prostaglandin E1 for reduction of pulmonary hypertension in heart transplant candidates. *J Heart Lung Transplant.* 2005;24:690-695.
14. Zimmerman AA, Howard TK, Huddleston BC. Combined lung and liver transplantation in a girl with cystic fibrosis. *Can J Anesth.* 1999;46:571-575.
15. Giostra E, Chen H, Deng H, et al. Prophylactic administration of prostaglandin E1 in liver transplantation: results of a pilot trial. *Transplant Proc.* 1997;29:2381-2384.
16. Tancharoen S, Jones RM, Angus PW, et al. Prostaglandin E1 therapy in orthotopic liver transplantation recipients: indications and outcome. *Transplant Proc.* 1992;24:2248-2249.
17. Mollison LC, Angus PW, Jones RM. Prostaglandin E1 for the treatment of primary non-function of the donor organ in liver transplantation. *Med J Aust.* 1991;155:51-53.

References

18. Gaber AO, Thistlethwaite JR Jr, Busse-Henry S, et al. Improved results of preservation of hepatic grafts preflushed with albumin and prostaglandins. *Transplant Proc.* 1988;20:992-993.
19. Prostin VR pediatric (alprostadil) [product information]. Bedford, OH: Ben Venue Laboratories Inc, 2005.
20. Eades, S. Pharmacotherapy of congenital heart disease. *J Pediatri Pharmacol Ther.* 2004;9:160-178.
21. Ernst JA, Williams JM, Glick MR, et al. Osmolality of substances used in the intensive care nursery. *Pediatrics.* 1983;72:347-352.
22. American Society of Health-System Pharmacists. American Hospital Formulary System. Available at: http://ahfsfirst.firstdatabank.com/AHFSfirst/NSAHFSFirstSearchmain.asp. Accessed June 25, 2006.
23. Trissel LA, ed. *Handbook on Injectable Drugs.* 13th ed. [CD-ROM version 1.5]. Bethesda, MD: American Society of Health-System Pharmacists; 2005.
24. Carter EL, Garzon MC. Neonatal urticaria due to prostaglandin E1. *Pediatr Dermatol.* 2000;17:58-61.
25. Rao J, Campbell ME, Krol A. The harlequin color change and association with prostaglandin E1. *Pediatr Dermatol.* 2005;21:573-576.
26. Vanhaesebrouck S, Allegaert K, Vanhole C, et al. Pseudo-Bartter syndrome in a neonate on prostaglandin infusion. *Eur J Pediatr.* 2003;162:569-571.
27. Arav-Boger R, Baggett HC, Spevak PJ, et al. Leukocytosis caused by prostaglandin E1 in neonates. *J Pediatr.* 2001;138:263-265.
28. Kaufman MB, El-Chaar GM. Bone and tissue changes following prostaglandin therapy in neonates. *Ann Pharmacother.* 1996;20:269-274.
29. NadrooAm, Shringari S, Garg M, et al. Prostaglandin induced cortical hyperostosis in neonates with cyanotic heart disease. *J Perinat Med.* 2000;28:447-452.
30. Velaphi S, Cilliers A, Beckh-Arnold E, et al. Corticol hyperostosis in an infant on prolonged prostaglandin infusion: case report and literature review. *J Perinatol.* 2004;24:263-265.
31. Jureidine S, Chase NA, Alpert BS, et al. Soft-tissue swelling in two neonates during prostaglandin E1 therapy. *Pediatr Cardiol.* 1986;7:157-160.
32. Peled N, Dagan O, Babyn P, et al. Gastric-outlet obstruction induced by prostaglandin therapy in neonates. *N Engl J Med.* 1992;327:505-510.
33. Merkus JFM, Cromme-Dijkhuis AH, Robben SGF, et al. Prostaglandin E1 and gastric outlet obstruction in infants. *Lancet.* 1993;342:747.
34. Raboi CA, Smith W. Brown fat necrosis in the setting of congenital heart disease and prostaglandin E1 use: a case report. *Pediatr Radiol.* 1999;29:61-63.

Amikacin Sulfate

1. Schwartz SN, Pazin GJ, Lyon JA, et al. A controlled investigation of the pharmacokinetics of gentamicin and tobramycin in obese subjects. *J Infect Dis.* 1978;138:499-505.
2. Bauer LA, Blouin RA, Griffen WO, et al. Amikacin pharmacokinetics in morbidly obese patients. *Am J Hosp Pharm.* 1980;37:519-522.
3. Amikacin [package insert]. Irvine, CA: Sicor Pharmaceuticals; November 2003.
4. American Society of Health-System Pharmacists. American Hospital Formulary System. Available at: http://ahfsfirst.firstdatabank.com/AHFSfirst/NSAHFSFirstSearchmain.asp. Accessed May 26, 2006.
5. American Academy of Pediatrics. In: Pickering LK, ed. *2003 Red Book: Report of the Committee on Infectious Diseases.* 26th ed. Elk Grove Village, IL: American Academy of Pediatrics; 2003.
6. Amikacin. In: Kucer A, Crowe SM, Grayson ML, et al., eds. *The Use of Antibiotics: A Clinical Review of Antibacterial, Antifungal and Antiviral Drugs.* 5th ed. Boston, MA: Butterworth Heinemann; 1997;504-521.
7. Prober CG, Yeager AS, Arvin AM. The effect of chronologic age on the serum concentrations of amikacin in sick term and premature infants. *J Pediatr.* 1981;98:636-640.
8. Yow M. An overview of pediatric experience with amikacin. *Am J Med.* 1977;62:954-958.
9. Marik PE, Lipman J, Kobilski S, et al. A prospective randomized study comparing once- versus twice-daily amikacin dosing in critically ill adult and paediatric patients. *J Antimicrob Chemother.* 1991;28:753-764.
10. Myers MG, Roberts RJ, Mirhij NJ. Effects of gestational age, birth weight, and hypoxemia on pharmacokinetics of amikacin in serum of infants. *Antimicrob Agents Chemother.* 1977;11:1027-1032.
11. Sanderman H, Colding H, Hendel J, et al. Kinetics and dose calculations of amikacin in the newborn. *Clin Pharmacol Ther.* 1976;20:59-66.
12. Prober CG, Stevenson DK, Benitz WE. The use of antibiotics in neonates weighing less than 1200 grams. *Pediatr Infect Dis J.* 1990;9:111-121.
13. Nelson JS, Bradley JS. *Nelson's Pocketbook of Pediatric Antimicrobial Therapy.* 14th ed. Philadelphia, PA: Lippincott Williams & Wilkins; 2000.
14. Young TE, Mangum B, eds. *Neofax®.* 18th ed. Raleigh, NC: Acorn Publishing Inc; 2005.
15. Vogelstein B, Kowarski AA, Lietman PS. The pharmacokinetics of amikacin in children. *J Pediatr.* 1977;91:333-339.
16. Contopoulos-Ioannidis DG, Giotis ND, Baliatsa DV, et al. Extended-interval aminoglycoside administration for children: a meta-analysis. *Pediatrics.* 2004;114:e111-e118.
17. Kafetzis DA, Sianidou L, Vlachos E, et al. Clinical and pharmacokinetic study of a single daily dose of amikacin in paediatric patients with severe gram-negative infections. *J Antimicrob Chemother.* 1991;27:105-112.
18. Trujillo H, Robledo J, Robledo C, et al. Single dose amikacin in paediatric patients with severe gram-negative infections. *J Antimicrob Chemother.* 1991;27:141-147.
19. Langhendries JP, Battisti O, Bertrand JM, et al. Once-a-day administration of amikacin in neonates: assessment of nephrotoxicity and ototoxicity. *Dev Pharmacol Ther.* 1993;20:220-230.
20. Viscoli C, Dudley M, Ferrea G, et al. Serum concentration and safety of a single daily dose of amikacin in children undergoing bone marrow transplantation. *J Antimicrob Chemother.* 1991;27:113-120.
21. Bouffet E, Fuhrmann C, Frappaz D, et al. Once daily antibiotic regimen in paediatric oncology. *Arch Dis Child.* 1994;70:484-487.
22. International Antimicrobial Therapy Cooperative Group of the European Organization for Research and Treatment of Cancer. Efficacy and toxicity of single daily doses of amikacin and ceftriaxone versus multiple daily doses of amikacin and ceftazidime for infection in patients with cancer and granulocytopenia. *Ann Intern Med.* 1993;119:584-593.
23. Krivoy N, Postovsky S, Elhasid R, et al. Pharmacokinetic analysis of amikacin twice and single daily dosage in immunocompromised pediatric patients. *Infection.* 1998;26:396-398.
24. Gauthier M, Chevalier I, Sterescu A, et al. Treatment of urinary tract infections among febrile young children with daily intravenous antibiotic therapy at a day treatment center. *Pedaitrics.* 2002;114:e469-e476.
25. Chicella M. Once-daily aminoglycoside dosing in pediatrics. What is its role? *J Pediatr Pharm Pract.* 2000:5;98-103.
26. Aronoff A, Brier M, Bennett W. *The Renal Book, 2002.* Available at: http://www.kdp-baptist.louisville.edu/renalbook/. Accessed May 6, 2006.
27. Pea F, Viale P, Furlanut M. Antimicrobial therapy in critically ill patients: a review of pathophysiological conditions responsible for altered disposition and pharmacokinetic variability. *Clin Pharmacokinet.* 2005;44:1009-1034.
28. Kelly HB, Menendez R, Fan L, et al. Pharmacokinetics of tobramycin in cystic fibrosis. *J Pediatr.* 1982;100:318-321.
29. Loirat P, Rohan J, Baillet A, et al. Increased glomerular filtration rate in patients with major burns and its effect on the pharmacokinetics of tobramycin. *N Engl J Med.* 1978;299:915-919.
30. Kopcha RG, Fant WK, Warden GD. Increased dosing requirements for amikacin in burned children. *J Antimicrob Chemother.* 1999;28:747-752.
31. Buck ML. Pharmacokinetic changes during extracorporeal membrane oxygenation. *Clin Pharmacokinet.* 2003;42:403-417.
32. Gillett AP, Falk RH, Andrews J, et al. Rapid intravenous injection of tobramycin: suggested dosage schedule and concentrations in serum. *J Infect Dis.* 1976;134:S110-S113.
33. Dobbs SM, Mawer GE. Intravenous injection of gentamicin and tobramycin without impairment of hearing. *J Infect Dis.* 1976;134 (suppl): S114-S117.
34. Mendelson J, Portnoy J, Dick V, et al. Safety of the bolus administration of gentamicin. *Antimicrob Agents Chemother.*1976;9:633-638.

35. Bodey GP, Chang HY, Rodriguez V, et al. Feasibility of administering aminoglycoside antibiotics by continuous intravenous infusion. *Antimicrob Agents Chemother.* 1975;8:328-333.
36. Powell SH, Thompson WL, Luthe MA, et al. Once daily vs. continuous aminoglycoside dosing: efficacy and toxicity in animal and clinical studies of gentamicin, netilmicin and tobramycin. *J Infect Dis.* 1983;147:918-932.
37. Giacoia GP, Schentag JJ. Pharmacokinetics and nephrotoxicity of continuous intravenous infusion of gentamicin in low birth weight infants. *J Pediatr.* 1986;109:715-719.
38. Pagliaro LA, Pagliaro AM, eds. *Problems in Pediatric Drug Therapy.* 2nd ed. Hamilton, IL: Drug Intelligence Publications Inc; 1987.
39. Trissel LA, ed. *Handbook on Injectable Drugs.* 13th ed. Bethesda, MD: American Society of Health-System Pharmacists; 2005.
40. American Academy of Pediatrics Committee on Drugs. "Inactive" ingredients in pharmaceutical products: update. *Pediatrics.* 1997;99:268-278.
41. Lester MR. Sulfite sensitivity: significance in human health. *J Am Col Nutr.* 1995;14:229-232.
42. Franson TR, Ritch PS, Quebbeman EJ. Aminoglycoside serum concentration sampling via central venous catheters: a potential source of clinical error. *JPEN J Parenter Enteral Nutr.* 1987;11:77-79.
43. Massey KL, Hendeles L, Neims A. Identification of children for whom routine monitoring of aminoglycoside serum concentrations is not cost effective. *J Pediatr.* 1986;109:897-901.
44. Logsdon BA, Phelps SJ. Routine monitoring of gentamicin serum concentrations in pediatric patients with normal renal function is unnecessary. *Ann Pharmacother.* 1997;31:1514-1518.
45. Beaubien AR, Desjardins S, Ormsby E, et al. Incidence of amikacin ototoxicity: a sigmoid function of total drug exposure independent of plasma levels. *Am J Otolaryngol.* 1989;10:234-243.
46. Beaubien AR, Ormsby E, Bayne A, et al. Evidence that amikacin ototoxicity is related to total perilymph area under the concentration-time curve regardless of concentration. *Antimicrob Agents Chemother.* 1991;35:1070-1074.
47. Snavely SR, Hodges GR. The neurotoxicity of antibacterial agents. *Ann Intern Med.* 1984;101;92-104.
48. Manian FA, Stone WJ, Alford RH. Adverse antibiotic effects associated with renal insufficiency. *Rev Infect Dis.* 1990;12:236-249.

Aminocaproic Acid

1. Thomson Healthcare, Inc. *USP DI® Drug Information for the Health Care Professional.* Available at: http://www.thomsonhc.com-MICROMEDEX® Healthcare Series [database on the Internet]. Accessed April 10, 2006.
2. Florentino-Pineda I, Thompson GH, et al. The effect of Amicar on perioperative blood loss in idiopathic scoliosis: the results of a prospective, randomized double-blind study. *Spine.* 2004;29:233-238.
3. Downard CD, Betit P, Chang RW, et al. Impact of Amicar on hemorrhagic complications of ECMO: a ten-year review. *J Pediatr Surg.* 2003;38:1212-1216.
4. Wilson JM, Bower LK, Fackler JC, et al. Aminocaproic acid decreases the incidence of intracranial hemorrhage and other hemorrhagic complications of ECMO. *J Pediatr Surg.* 1993;28:536-541.
5. Horwitz JR, Cofer BR, Warner BW, et al. A multicenter trial of 6-aminocaproic acid (Amicar) in the prevention of bleeding in infants on ECMO. *J Pediatr Surg.* 1998; 33:1610-1613.
6. Williams GD, Bratton SI, Riley EC, et al. Efficacy of ε-aminocaproic acid in children undergoing cardiac surgery. *J Cardiothorac Vasc Anesth.* 1999; 13:304-308.
7. Haidet KK. Aminocaproic acid (epsilon aminocaproic acid) (Amicar). *Neonatal Netw.* 1995;14:75-77.
8. Florentino-Pineda I, Blakemore LC, Thompson GH, et al. The effect of epsilon-aminocaproic acid on perioperative blood loss in patients with idiopathic scoliosis undergoing posterior spinal fusion: a preliminary prospective study. *Spine.* 2001;26:1147-1151.
9. Chauhan S, Kumar BA, Rao BH, et al. Efficacy of aprotinin, epsilon aminocaproic acid, or combination in cyanotic heart disease. *Ann Thorac Surg.* 2000;70:1308-1312.
10. Taketomo CK, Hodding JH, Kraus DM. *Pediatric Dosage Handbook.* 12th ed. Hudson, OH: Lexi-Comp Inc; 2005:85-87.
11. AHFSfirst™ Web version 2.03. American Society of Health-System Pharmacists, First Databank, Inc. 2002. Accessed June 26, 2006.
12. Amicar injection [package insert]. Newport, KY: Xanodyne Pharmaceuticals Inc; April 2005.
13. Winter SS, Chaffee S, Kahler SG, et al. e-Aminocaproic acid-associated myopathy in a child. *J Pediatr Hematol Oncol.* 1995;17:53-55.
14. Trissel LA. *Handbook on Injectable Drugs.* 13th ed. Bethesda, MD: American Society of Health-System Pharmacists; 2005.
15. American Academy of Pediatrics Committee on Drugs. "Inactive" ingredients in pharmaceutical products: update. *Pediatrics.* 1997;99:268-278.
16. Hall CM, Milligan DWA, Berrington J. Probably adverse reaction to a pharmaceutical excipient. *Arch Dis Child Fetal Neonatal Ed.* 2004;89: F184.
17. Hiller JL, Benda GI, Rahatzad M, et al. Benzyl alcohol toxicity: impact on mortality and intraventricular hemorrhage among very low birth weight infants. *Pediatrics.* 1986;77:500-506.
18. Grant JA, Bilodeau PA, Guernsey BG, et al. Unsuspected benzyl alcohol hypersensitivity. *N Engl J Med.* 1982;306:108.
19. Wilson JP, Solimando DA, Edwards MS. Parenteral benzyl alcohol-induced hypersensitivity reaction. *Drug Intell Clin Pharm.* 1986;20:689-691.
20. Ririe DG, James RL, O'Brien JJ, et al. The pharmacokinetics of epsilon-aminocaproic acid in children undergoing surgical repair of congenital heart defects. *Anesth Analg.* 2002;94:44-49.

Aminophylline

1. Siberry GK, Iannone R, ed. *The Harriet Lane Handbook: A Manual for Pediatric House Officers.* 17th ed. Chicago, IL: Mosby Inc; 2005.
2. Taketomo CK, Hodding JH, Kraus DM. *Pediatric Dosage Handbook.* 11th ed. Hudson, OH: Lexi-Comp Inc; 2004–2005.
3. Al-Omran A, Al-Alaiyan S. Theophylline concentration following equal doses of intravenous aminophylline and oral theophylline in preterm infants. *Amer J Perinatol.* 1997;14:147-149.
4. Young TE, Mangum B. *Neofax®: A Manual of Drugs Used in Neonatal Care.* 18th ed. Raleigh, NC: Acorn Publishing; 2005:190.
5. Aminophylline [package insert]. Lake Forest, IL: Hospira Inc; June 2004.
6. Bada HS, Khanna NN, Somani SM, et al. Interconversion of theophylline and caffeine in newborn infants. *J Pediatr.* 1979;94:993-995.
7. Aranda JV, Sitar DS, Parsons WD, et al. Pharmacokinetic aspects of theophylline in premature newborns. *N Engl J Med.* 1976;295:413-416.
8. Bairam A, Boutroy M-J, Badonnel Y, et al. Theophylline versus caffeine: comparative effects in treatment of idiopathic apnea in the preterm infant. *J Pediatr.* 1987;110:636-639.
9. Tserng K-Y, King KC, Takieddine FN. Theophylline metabolism in premature infants. *Clin Pharmacol Ther.* 1981;29:594-600.
10. Tserng KY, Takieddine FN, King KC. Developmental aspects of theophylline metabolism in premature infants. *Clin Pharmacol Ther.* 1983;33:522-528.
11. Latini R, Assael BM, Bonati M, et al. Kinetics and efficacy of theophylline in the treatment of apnea of prematurity in the premature newborn. *Eur J Clin Pharmacol.* 1978;13:203-207.
12. Gilman JT, Gal P, Levine RS, et al. Factors influencing theophylline disposition in 179 newborns. *Ther Drug Monit.* 1986;8:4-10.
13. Anon. *National Asthma Education Program Expert Panel Report. Guidelines for the diagnosis and management of asthma, August 1991.* Bethesda, MD: NIH; publication no. 91–3042.
14. Carpenter TC, Dobyns EL, Mateev SN, et al. Critical care. In: Hay WW, Levin MJ, Sondheimer JM, et al., eds. *Current Pediatric Diagnosis and Treatment.* 17th ed. New York, NY: Lange Medical Books/McGraw-Hill; 2005.

References

15. Weinberger M, Hendeles L. Theophylline in asthma. *New Engl J Med.* 1996;334:1380-1388.
16. Huang D, O'Brien RG, Harman E, et al. Does aminophylline benefit adults admitted to the hospital for acute exacerbation of asthma? *Ann Intern Med.*1993;119:1155-1160.
17. Zainudin BM, Ismail O, Yusoff K. Effect of adding aminophylline infusion to nebulized salbutamol in severe acute asthma. *Thorax.* 1994;49:267-269.
18. Rodrigo C, Rodrigo G. Lack of therapeutic benefit and increase of the toxicity from aminophylline given in addition to high doses of salbutamol delivered by metered-dose inhaler with a spacer. *Chest.* 1994;106:1071-1076.
19. Murphy DG, McDermott MF, Rydman RJ, et al. Aminophylline in the treatment of acute asthma when 2-adrenergics and steroids are provided. *Arch Intern Med.* 1993;153:1784-1788.
20. Self TH, Abou-Shala N, Burns R, et al. Inhaled albuterol and oral prednisone therapy in hospitalized adult asthmatics. *Chest.* 1990;98:1317-1321.
21. Strauss RE, Wertheim DL, Bonagura VR, et al. Aminophylline therapy does not improve outcome and increases adverse effects in children hospitalized with acute asthmatic exacerbation. *Pediatrics.* 1994;93:205-210.
22. Needleman JP, Kaifer MC, Nold JT, et al. Theophylline does not shorten hospital stay for children admitted for asthma. *Arch Pediatr Adolesc Med.* 1995;149:206-209.
23. Carter E, Cruz M, Chesrown S, et al. Efficacy of intravenously administered theophylline in children hospitalized with severe asthma. *J Pediatr.* 1993;122:470-476.
24. DiGiulio GA, Kercsmar CM, Krug SE, et al. Hospital treatment of asthma: lack of benefit from theophylline given in addition to nebulized albuterol and intravenously administered corticosteroids. *J Pediatr.* 1993;122:464-469.
25. Mitra A, Bassler D, Goodman K, et al. Intravenous aminophylline for acute severe asthma in children over two years receiving inhaled bronchodilators. *The Cochrane Database of Systematic Reviews.* 2005, Issue 2. Art. No.: CD001276. DOI: 10.1002/14651858.CD001276.pub2.
26. Self TH, Redmond AM, Nguyen WT. Reassessment of theophylline use for severe asthma exacerbation: is it justified in critically ill hospitalized patients? *J Asthma.* 2002;39:677-686.
27. Hendeles L, Weinberger M. Theophylline: a state of the art review. *Pharmacotherapy.* 1983;3:2-44.
28. Hendeles L, Weinberger M. Guidelines for avoiding theophylline overdose. *N Engl J Med.* 1979;300:1217.
29. I.V. dosage guidelines for theophylline products. *FDA Drug Bull.* 1980;(Feb):4-6.
30. Hogue SL, Phelps SJ. Evaluation of three theophylline dosing equations for use in infants up to one year of age. *J Pediatr.* 1993;123:651-656.
31. Weinberger M, Hendeles L. Theophylline. In: Middleton E Jr, Reed CE, Ellis EF, et al., eds. *Allergy: Principles and Practice.* 4th ed. St. Louis, MO: Mosby-Yearbook Inc; 1993:816-855
32. Goldberg P, Leffert F, Gonzalez M, et al. Intravenous aminophylline therapy for asthma: a comparison of two methods of administration in children. *Am J Dis Child.* 1980;134:596-599.
33. Weinberger MW, Matthay RA, Ginchansky EJ, et al. Intravenous aminophylline dosage: use of serum theophylline measurement for guidance. *JAMA.* 1976;235:2110-2113.
34. Gal P, Boer HR, Toback J, et al. Effect of asphyxia on theophylline clearance in newborns. *South Med J.* 1982;75:836-838.
35. Weinberger M. The pharmacology and therapeutic use of theophylline. *J Allergy Clin Immunol.* 1984;73:525-540.
36. Wells TG, Kearns GL, Stillwell PC, et al. Rapid estimation of serum theophylline clearance in children with acute asthma. *Ther Drug Monit.* 1984;6:402-407.
37. Kubo M, Odajima Y, Ishizaki T, et al. Intraindividual changes in theophylline clearance during constant aminophylline infusion in children with acute asthma. *J Pediatr.* 1986;108:1011-1015.
38. Ellis EF, Koysooko R, Levy G. Pharmacokinetics of theophylline in children with asthma. *Pediatrics.* 1976;58:542-547.
39. Jones RAK, Baillie E. Dosage schedule for intravenous aminophylline in apnea of prematurity based on pharmacokinetic studies. *Arch Dis Child.* 1979;54:190-193.
40. Trissel LA. *Handbook on Injectable Drugs.* 13th ed. Bethesda, MD: American Society of Health-System Pharmacists; 2005.
41. McEvoy GK, ed. *AHFS Drug Information Essentials 2005–06.* Bethesda, MD: American Society of Health-System Pharmacists; 2005.
42. Mitenko PA, Ogilvie RI. Rational intravenous doses of theophylline. *N Engl J Med.* 1973;289:600-603.
43. American Academy of Pediatrics. Section on Allergy and Immunology. Management of asthma. *Pediatrics.* 1981;68:874-879.
44. LaFarce CF, Miller MF, Chai H. Effect of erythromycin on theophylline clearance in asthmatic children. *J Pediatr.* 1981;99:153-156.
45. Fenje PC, Isles AF, Baltodano A, et al. Interaction of cimetidine and theophylline in two infants. *Can Med Assoc J.* 1982;126:1178.
46. Jackson JE, Powell JR, Wandell M, et al. Cimetidine decreases theophylline clearance. *Am Rev Respir Dis.* 1981;123:615-617.
47. Thomson AH, Thomson GD, Hepburn M, et al. A clinically significant interaction between ciprofloxacin and theophylline. *Eur J Clin Pharmacol.* 1987;33:435-436.

Amphotericin B

1. Antifungal drugs for systemic fungal infections. In: Pickering LK, ed. *2003 Red Book. Report of the Committee on Infectious Diseases.* 26th ed. Elk Grove Village, IL: American Academy of Pediatrics; 2003:719-725.
2. Pappas PG, Rex JH, Sobel JD, et al. Guidelines for treatment of candidiasis. *Clin Infect Dis.* 2004;38:161-189.
3. Chapman RL. Candida infections in the neonate. *Curr Opin Pediatr.* 2003;15:97-102.
4. Fernandez M, Moylett EH, Noyola DE, et al. Candidal meningitis in neonates: a 10-year review. *Clin Infect Dis.* 2000;31:458-463.
5. Driessen M, Ellis JB, Cooper PA, et al. Fluconazole vs. amphotericin B for the treatment of neonatal fungal septicemia: a prospective randomized trial. *Pediatr Infect Dis J.* 1996;15:1107-1112.
6. Van Den Anker JN, Van Popele NML, Sauer PJJ. Antifungal agents in neonatal systemic candidiasis. *Antimicrob Agents Chemother.* 1995;39:1391-1397.
7. Donowitz LG, Hendley JO. Short-course amphotericin B therapy for candidemia in pediatric patients. *Pediatrics.* 1995;95:888-891.
8. Baley JE, Meyers C, Kliegman RM, et al. Pharmacokinetics, outcome of treatment, and toxic effects of amphotericin B and 5-fluorocytosine in neonates. *J Pediatr.* 1990;116:791-797.
9. Sanchez PJ, Siegel JD, Fishbein J. Candida endocarditis: successful medical management in three preterm infants and review of the literature. *Pediatr Infect Dis J.* 1991;10:239-243.
10. Zenker PN, Rosenberg EM, Van Dyke RB, et al. Successful medical treatment of presumed Candida endocarditis in critically ill infants. *J Pediatr.* 1991;119:472-477.
11. Butler KM, Rench MA, Baker CJ. Amphotericin B as a single agent in the treatment of systemic candidiasis in neonates. *Pediatr Infect Dis J.* 1990;9:51-56.
12. Sanchez PJ, Cooper BH. Candida lusitaniae: sepsis and meningitis in a neonate. *Pediatr Infect Dis J.* 1987;6:758-759.
13. Turner RB, Donowitz LG, Hendley JO. Consequences of candidemia for pediatric patients. *Am J Dis Child.* 1985;139:178-180.
14. Smego RA, Devoe PW, Sampson HA, et al. Candida meningitis in two children with severe combined immunodeficiency. *J Pediatr.* 1984;104:902-904.
15. Chesney PJ, Teets KC, Mulvihill JJ, et al. Successful treatment of Candida meningitis with amphotericin B and 5-fluorocytosine in combination. *J Pediatr.* 1976;89:1017-1019.
16. Medoff G, Kobayashi GS. Strategies in the treatment of systemic fungal infections. *N Engl J Med.* 1980;302:145-155.
17. Adler S, Randall J, Plotkin SA. Candidal osteomyelitis and arthritis in a neonate. *Am J Dis Child.* 1972;123:595-596.
18. Turner DJ, Wadlington WB. Blastomycosis in childhood: treatment with amphotericin B and a review of the literature. *J Pediatr.* 1969;75:708-717.

19. Cherry JD, Lloyd CA, Quilty JF, et al. Amphotericin B therapy in children. *J Pediatr.* 1969;75:1063-1069.
20. Hill HR, Mitchell TG, Masten JM, et al. Recovery from disseminated candidiasis in a premature neonate. *Pediatrics.* 1974;53:748-752.
21. Fosson AR, Wheeler WE. Short-term amphotericin B treatment of severe childhood histoplasmosis. *J Pediatr.* 1975;86:32-36.
22. Keller MA, Sellers BB, Melish ME, et al. Systemic candidiasis in infants: a case presentation and literature review. *Am J Dis Child.* 1977;131:1260-1263.
23. Ward RM, Sattler FR, Dalton AS. Assessment of antifungal therapy in an 800-gram infant with candidal arthritis and osteomyelitis. *Pediatrics.* 1983;72:234-238.
24. Faix RG. Systemic candida infections in infants in intensive care nurseries: high incidence of central nervous system involvement. *J Pediatr.* 1984;105:616-622.
25. Loke HL, Verber I, Szymonowicz W, et al. Systemic candidiasis and pneumonia in preterm infants. *Aust Paediatr J.* 1988;24:138-142.
26. Leibovitz E, Iuster-Reicher A, Amitai M, et al. Systemic candidal infections associated with use of peripheral venous catheters in neonates: a 9-year experience. *Clin Infect Dis.* 1992;14:485-491.
27. Grasela TH, Goodwin SD, Walawander MK, et al. Prospective surveillance of intravenous amphotericin B use patterns. *Pharmacotherapy.* 1990;10:341-348.
28. McEvoy GK, ed. *AHFS Drug Information Essentials 2005–06.* Bethesda, MD: American Society of Health-System Pharmacists; 2005.
29. Amphocin [package insert]. New York, NY: Pfizer; September 2003.
30. Starke JR, Mason EO, Kramer WG, et al. Pharmacokinetics of amphotericin B in infants and children. *J Infect Dis.* 1987;155:766-774.
31. Bennett JE. Chemotherapy of systemic mycoses (first of two parts). *N Engl J Med.* 1974;290:30-32.
32. Koren G, Lau A, Klein J, et al. Pharmacokinetics and adverse effects of amphotericin B in infants and children. *J Pediatr.* 1988;113:559-563.
33. Johnson DE, Thompson TR, Green TP, et al. Systemic candidiasis in very low-birth-weight infants (<1,500 grams). *Pediatrics.* 1984;73:138-143.
34. Baley JE, Kliegman RM, Fanaroff AA. Disseminated fungal infections in very low-birth-weight infants: therapeutic toxicity. *Pediatrics.* 1984;73:153-157.
35. Glick C, Graves GR, Feldman S. Neonatal fungemia and amphotericin B. *South Med J.* 1993;86:1368-1371.
36. Aronoff A, Brier M, Bennett W. *The Renal Book, 2002.* Available at: http://www.kdp-baptist.louisville.edu/renalbook/. Accessed June 26, 2006.
37. Weber ML, Abela A, de Repentigny L, et al. Myeloperoxidase deficiency with extensive candidal osteomyelitis of the base of the skull. *Pediatrics.* 1987;80:876-879.
38. Butler WT, Bennett JE, Alling DW, et al. Nephrotoxicity of amphotericin B: early and late effects in 81 patients. *Ann Intern Med.* 1964;61:175-187.
39. Maddux MS, Barriere SL. A review of complications of amphotericin-B therapy: recommendations for prevention and management. *Drug Intell Clin Pharm.* 1980;14:177-181.
40. Graybill JR. Is there a correlation between serum antifungal drug concentration and clinical outcome? *J Infect.* 1994;28(S1):17-24.
41. Cleary JD, Hayman J, Sherwood J, et al. Amphotericin B overdose in pediatric patients with associated cardiac arrest. *Ann Pharmacother.* 1993;27:715-718.
42. Wiest DB, Maish WA, Garner SS, et al. Stability of amphotericin B in four concentrations of dextrose injection. *Am J Hosp Pharm.* 1991;48:2430-2433.
43. Trissel LA. *Handbook on Injectable Drugs.* 13th ed. Bethesda, MD: American Society of Health-System Pharmacists; 2005.
44. Moreau P, Milpied N, Fayette N, et al. Reduced renal toxicity and improved clinical tolerance of amphotericin B in neutropenic patients. *J Antimicrob Chemother.* 1992;30:535-541.
45. Chavanet PY, Garry I, Charlier N, et al. Trial of glucose versus fat emulsion in preparation of amphotericin for use in HIV infected patients with candidiasis. *Br Med J.* 1992;305:921-925.
46. Taketomo CK, Hodding JH, Kraus DM, eds. *Pediatric Dosage Handbook.* 12th ed. Hudson, OH: Lexi-Comp; 2006.
47. Utz JP, Bennett JE, Brandriss MW, et al. Amphotericin B toxicity. General side effects. *Ann Intern Med.* 1964;61:340-343.
48. Lee MD, Hess MM, Boucher BA, et al. Stability of amphotericin B in 5% dextrose injection stores at 4 or 25°C for 120 hours. *Am J Hosp Pharm.* 1994;51:394-396.
49. Murray H. Allergic reactions to amphotericin B. *N Engl J Med.* 1974;290:693.
50. Wilson R, Feldman S. Toxicity of amphotericin B in children with cancer. *Am J Dis Child.* 1979;133:731-734.
51. Butler WT, Bennett JE, Hill GJ. Electrocardiographic and electrolyte abnormalities caused by amphotericin B in dog and man. *Proc Soc Exp Biol Med.* 1964;116:857-863.
52. Fields BT, Bates JH, Abernathy RS. Effect of rapid intravenous infusion on serum concentrations of amphotericin B. *Appl Microbiol.* 1971;22:615-617.
53. Barreuther AD, Dodge RR, Blondeaux AM. Administration of amphotericin B. *Drug Intell Clin Pharm.* 1977;11:368-369.
54. Tarala RA, Smith JD. Cryptococcosis treated by rapid infusion of amphotericin B. *Br Med J.* 1980;281:28.
55. Googe JH, Walterspiel JN. Arrhythmia caused by amphotericin B in a neonate. *Pediatr Infect Dis J.* 1988;7:73.
56. Aronoff GR, Berns JS, Brier ME, et al., eds. *Drug Prescribing in Renal Failure: Dosing Guidelines for Adults.* 4th ed. Philadelphia, PA: American College of Physicians; 1999.
57. Holler B, Omar SA, Farid MD, et al. Effects of fluid and electrolyte management on amphotericin B-induced nephrotoxicity among extremely low birth weight infants. *Pediatrics.* 2004;113:e608-e616.
58. Christenson JC, Shalit I, Welch DF, et al. Synergistic action of amphotericin B and rifampin against *Rhizopus* species. *Antimicrob Agents Chemother.* 1987;31:1775-1778.
59. Labadie EL, Hamilton RH. Survival improvement in coccidioidal meningitis by high-dose intrathecal amphotericin B. *Arch Intern Med.* 1986;146:2013-2018.
60. Tyler EM, Salamone FR, Brown AE. Management and prevention of amphotericin B-induced side effects. *Hosp Pharm.* 1988;23:254-259.
61. Arbuthnot R, Dullea A, Rippel S. Controlling thrombophlebitis from amphotericin B. *Am J Hosp Pharm.* 1978;35:129.

Amphotericin B Cholesteryl Sulfate Complex

1. American Academy of Pediatrics. In: Pickering LK, ed. *Red Book: 2006 Report of the Committee on Infectious Diseases.* 27th ed. Elk Grove Village, IL: American Academy of Pediatrics; 2006.
2. Janknegt R, de Marie S, Bakker-Woudenberg I, et al. Liposomal and lipid complex formulations of amphotericin B: clinical pharmacokinetics. *Clin Pharmacokinet.* 1992;23:279-291.
3. Henry N, Hoeker JL, Rhodes KH. Antimicrobial therapy for infants and children: guidelines for the inpatient and outpatient practice of pediatric infectious disease. *Mayo Clinic Proceed.* 2000;75:86-97.
4. Quilitz R. The use of lipid formulations of amphotericin B in cancer patients. *Cancer Control.* 1998;5:439-449.
5. Sandler ES, Mustafa MM, Tkaczewski I, et al. Use of amphotericin B colloidal dispersion in children. *J Pediatr Hematol Oncol.* 2000;22:242-246.
6. Bowden R, Chandrasekar P, White MH, et al. A double-blind, randomized, controlled trial of amphotericin B colloidal dispersion versus amphotericin B for treatment of invasive aspergillosis in immunocompromised patients. *Clin Infect Dis.* 2002;35:359-366.
7. Linder N, Klinger G, Shalit I, et al. Treatment of candidaemia in premature infants: comparison of three amphotericin B preparations. *J Antimicrob Chemother.* 2003;52:663-667.
8. Amphotec [prescribing information]. Cranberry Township, PA: Three Rivers Pharmaceuticals LLC; July 2005.
9. Trissel LA, ed. *Handbook on Injectable Drugs.* 13th ed. [CD-ROM version 1.5]. Bethesda, MD: American Society of Health-System Pharmacists; 2005.

References

10. White MH, Bowden RA, Sandler ES, et al. Randomized, double-blind, clinical trial of amphotericin B colloidal dispersion vs amphotericin B in the empiric treatment of fever and neutropenia. *Clin Infect Dis.* 1998;27:296-302.

Amphotericin B Lipid Complex

1. Wingard JR, White MH, Anaissie E. A randomized, double blind comparative trial evaluating the safety of liposomal amphotericin B versus amphotericin B lipid complex in the empirical treatment of febrile neutropenia. *CID.* 2000;31:1155-1163.
2. American Academy of Pediatrics. In: Pickering LK, ed. *Red Book: 2006 Report of the Committee on Infectious Diseases.* 27th ed. Elk Grove Village, IL: American Academy of Pediatrics; 2006.
3. *Physicians' Desk Reference.* 60th ed. Montvale, NJ: Thomson PDR; 2006.
4. Wurthwein G, Groll AH, Hempel G, et al. Population pharmacokinetics of amphotericin B lipid complex in neonates. *Antimicrob Agent Chemother.* 2005;5092-5098.
5. Janknegt R, de Marie S, Bakker-Woudenberg I, et al. Liposomal and lipid complex formulations of amphotericin B: clinical pharmacokinetics. *Clin Pharmacokinet.* 1992;23:279-291.
6. Wiley JM, Seibel NL, Walsh TJ. Efficacy and safety of amphotericin B lipid complex in 548 children and adolescents with invasive fungal infections. *Pediatr Infect Dis J.* 2005;24:167-174.
7. Herbrecht R, Auvrignon A, Andres E, et al. Efficacy of amphotericin B lipid complex in the treatment of invasive fungal infections in immunosuppressed paediatric patients. *Eur J Clin Microbiol Infect Dis.* 2001;20:77-82.
8. Adler-Shohet F, Waskin H, Lieberman JM. Amphotericin B lipid complex for neonatal invasive candidiasis. *Arch Dis Child Fetal Neonatal Ed.* 2001;84:131-133.
9. Alexander BD, Wingard JR. Study of renal safety in amphotericin B lipid complex-treated patients. *Clin Infect Dis.* 2005;40:S414-S421.
10. Hooshmand-Rad R, Reed MD, Chu A, et al. Retrospective study of the renal effects of amphotericin B lipid complex when used at higher-than recommended dosages and longer durations compared with lower dosages and shorter durations in patients with systemic fungal infections. *Clin Ther.* 2004;26:1652-1662.
11. Rowles DM, Fraser SL. Amphotericin B Lipid complex (ABLC)-associated hypertension: case report and review of the literature. *Clin Infect Dis.* 1999;29:1564-1565.

Amphotericin B Liposomal

1. Walsh TJ, Finberg RW, Arndt C, et al. Liposomal amphotericin B for empirical therapy in patients with persistent fever and neutropenia. National Institute of Allergy and Infectious Diseases Mycoses Study Group. *N Engl J Med.* 1999;340:764-771.
2. Wingard JR, White MH, Anaissie E. A randomized, double blind comparative trial evaluating the safety of liposomal amphotericin B versus amphotericin B lipid complex in the empirical treatment of febrile neutropenia. *CID.* 2000;31:1155-1163.
3. Pasic S, Flannagan L, Cant AJ. Liposomal amphotericin (AmBisome) is safe in bone marrow transplantation for primary immunodeficiency. *Bone Marrow Transplant.* 1997;19:1229-1232.
4. Tollemar J, Hockerstedt K, Ericzon BG, et al. Liposomal amphotericin B prevents invasive fungal infections in liver transplant recipients. A randomized, placebo-controlled study. *Transplantation.* 1995;59:45-50.
5. Noskin G, Gurwith M, Bowden R. Treatment of invasive fungal infections with amphotericin B colloidal dispersion in bone marrow transplant recipients. *Bone Marrow Transplant.* 1999;23:697-703.
6. Ringden O, Andstrom EE, Remberger M, et al. Prophylaxis and therapy using liposomal amphotericin B (AmBisome) for invasive fungal infections in children undergoing organ or allogenic bone-marrow transplantation. *Pediatr Transplant.* 1997;1:124-129.
7. Mehta P, Vinks A, Filipovich A, et al. High-dose weekly AmBisome antifungal prophylaxis in pediatric patients undergoing hematopoietic stem cell transplantation: a pharmacokinetic study. *Biol Blood Marrow Transplant.* 2006;12:235-240.
8. American Academy of Pediatrics. In: Pickering LK, ed. *Red Book: 2006 Report of the Committee on Infectious Diseases.* 27th ed. Elk Grove Village, IL: American Academy of Pediatrics; 2006.
9. Scarcella A, Pasquariello MB, Giugliano B, et al. Liposomal amphotericin B treatment for neonatal fungal infections. *Pediatr Inf Dis J.* 1998;146-148.
10. Weitkamp JH, Poets CF, Sievers R, et al. Candida infection in very low birth-weight infants: outcome and nephrotoxicity of treatment with liposomal amphotericin B (AmBisome). *Infection.* 1998;26:11-15.
11. Dornbusch HJ, Urban CE, Pinter H, et al. Treatment of invasive pulmonary aspergillosis in severely neutropenic children with malignant disorders using liposomal amphotericin B (AmBisome), granulocyte colony-stimulating factor, and surgery: report of five cases. *Pediatr Hemat Oncol.* 1995;12:577-586.
12. Seaman J, Boer C, Wilkinson R, et al. Liposomal amphotericin B (AmBisome) in the treatment of complicated kala-azar under field conditions. *Clin Infect Dis.* 1995;21:188-193.
13. Ng TT, Denning DW. Liposomal amphotericin B (AmBisome) therapy in invasive fungal infections. Evaluation of United Kingdom compassionate use data. *Arch Intern Med.* 1995;155:1093-1098.
14. Linder N, Klinger G, Shalit I, et al. Treatment of candidaemia in premature infants: comparison of three amphotericin preparations. *J Antimicrob Chemother.* 2003;52:663-667.
15. Juster-Reicher A, Flidel-Rimon O, Amitay M, et al. High-dose liposomal amphotericin B in the therapy of systemic candidiasis in neonates. *Eur J Clin Microbiol Infect Dis.* 2003;22:603-607.
16. Juster-Reicher A, Leibovitz E, Linder N, et al. Liposomal amphotericin B (AmBisome) in the treatment of neonatal candidiasis in very low birth weight infants. *Infection.* 2000;28:223-226.
17. Walsh TJ, Goodman JL, Pappas P, et al. Safety, tolerance, and pharmacokinetics of high-dose liposomal amphotericin B (AmBisome) in patients infected with Aspergillus species and other filamentous fungi: Maximum tolerated dose study. *Antimicrob Agent Chemother.* 2001;45:3487-3496.
18. *Physicians' Desk Reference.* 60th ed. Montvale, NJ: Thomson PDR; 2006.
19. Davidson RN, di Martino L, Gradoni L, et al. Short-course treatment of visceral leishmaniasis with liposomal amphotericin B (AmBisome). *Clin Infect Dis.* 1996;22:938-943.
20. Minodier P, Retornaz K, Horelt A, et al. Liposomal amphotericin B in the treatment of visceral leishmaniasis in immunocompetent patients. *Fundam Clin Pharm.* 2003;17:183-188.
21. Syriopoulou V, Daikos GL, Theodoridou M, et al. Two doses of a lipid formulation of amphotericin B for the treatment of Mediterranean visceral leishmaniasis. *Clin Infect Dis.* 2003;36:560-566.
22. Roden MM, Nelson LD, Knudsen TA, et al. Triad of acute infusion-related reactions associated with liposomal amphotericin B: analysis of clinical and epidemiological characteristics. *Clin Infect Dis.* 2003;36:1213-1220.
23. Johnson MD, Drew RH, Perfect JR. Chest discomfort associated with liposomal amphotericin B: report of three cases and review of the literature. *Pharmacotherapy.* 1998;18:1053-1061.

References

Ampicillin Sodium

1. Prober CG, Stevenson DK, Benitz WE. The use of antibiotics in neonates weighing less than 1200 grams. *Pediatr Infect Dis J.* 1990;9:111-121.
2. American Academy of Pediatrics. In: Pickering LK, ed. *2003 Red Book: Report of the Committee on Infectious Diseases.* 26th ed. Elk Grove Village, IL: American Academy of Pediatrics; 2003:701,708.
3. Nelson JD, Bradley JS, eds. *Pocketbook of Pediatric Antimicrobial Therapy.* 14th ed. Baltimore, MD: Williams & Wilkins; 2000–2001.
4. Baddour LM, Wilson WR, Bayer AS, et al. Infective endocarditis: diagnosis, antimicrobial therapy, and management of complications: a statement for healthcare professionals from the Committee on Rheumatic Fever, Endocarditis, and Kawasaki Disease, Council on Cardiovascular Disease in the Young, and the Councils on Clinical Cardiology, Stroke, and Cardiovascular Surgery and Anesthesia, American Heart Association: endorsed by the Infectious Diseases Society of America. *Circulation.* 2005;111:e394-e434.
5. Feigin RD, McCracken GH, Klein JO. Diagnosis and management of meningitis. *Pediatr Infect Dis J.* 1992;11:785-814.
6. Klein JO, Feigin RD, McCracken GH. Report of American Academy of Pediatrics task force on diagnosis and management of meningitis. *Pediatrics.* 1986;78(suppl):959-982.
7. American Academy of Pediatrics. Committee on Infectious Diseases. Treatment of bacterial meningitis. *Pediatrics.* 1988;6:904-907.
8. Fleming PC, Murray JDM, Fujiwara MW, et al. Ampicillin in the treatment of bacterial meningitis. *Antimicrob Agents Chemother.* 1966;47-52.
9. Odio CM, Faingezicht I, Salas JL, et al. Cefotaxime vs. conventional therapy for the treatment of bacterial meningitis of infants and children. *Pediatr Infect Dis J.* 1986;5:402-407.
10. Jadavji T, Biggar WD, Gold R, et al. Sequelae of acute bacterial meningitis in children treated for seven days. *Pediatrics.* 1986;78:21-25.
11. Ampicillin [package insert]. Schaumburg, IL: American Pharmaceutical Partners; September 2004.
12. Aronoff A, Brier M, Bennett W. *The Renal Book, 2002*. Available at: http://www.kdp-baptist.louisville.edu/renalbook/. Accessed July 30, 2006.
13. American Academy of Pediatrics Committee on Infectious Diseases. Ampicillin-resistant strains of Hemophilus influenza type B. *Pediatrics.* 1975;55:145-146.
14. Fleming PC, Murray JDM, Fujiwara MW, et al. Ampicillin in the treatment of bacterial meningitis. *Antimicrob Agents Chemother.* 1966;47-52.
15. American Society of Health-System Pharmacists. American Hospital Formulary System. Available at: http://ahfsfirst.firstdatabank.com/AHFSfirst/NSAHFSFirstSearchmain.asp. Accessed July 31, 2006.
16. Trissel LA, ed. *Handbook on Injectable Drugs.* 13th ed. [CD-ROM version 1.5]. Bethesda, MD: American Society of Health-System Pharmacists; 2005.
17. Colding H, Moller S, Andersen GE. Continuous intravenous infusion of ampicillin and gentamicin during parenteral nutrition in 88 newborn infants. *Arch Dis Child.* 1982;57:602-606.
18. Leff RD, Roberts RJ. Effect of intravenous fluid and drug solution coadministration on final-infusate osmolality, specific gravity, and pH. *Am J Hosp Pharm.* 1982;39:468-471.
19. Pagliaro LA, Pagliaro AM, eds. *Problems in Pediatric Drug Therapy*. 2nd ed. Hamilton, IL: Drug Intelligence Publications Inc; 1987.
20. Savello DR, Shangraw RF. Stability of sodium ampicillin solutions in the frozen and liquid states. *Am J Hosp Pharm.* 1971;28:754-759.
21. McLaughlin JE, Reeves DS. Clinical and laboratory evidence for inactivation of gentamicin by carbenicillin. *Lancet.* 1971;1(7693):261-264.
22. Riff LJ, Jackson GG. Laboratory and clinical conditions for gentamicin inactivation by carbenicillin. *Arch Intern Med.* 1972;130:887-891.
23. Manian FA, Stone WJ, Alford RH. Adverse antibiotic effects associated with renal insufficiency. *Rev Infect Dis.* 1990;12:236-249.
24. Davies M, Morgan JR, Anand C. Interactions of carbenicillin and ticarcillin with gentamicin. *Antimicrob Agents Chemother.* 1975;7:431-434.
25. Weibert R, Keane W, Shapiro F. Carbenicillin inactivation of aminoglycosides in patients with severe renal failure. *Trans Amer Soc Artif Int Organs.* 1976;22:439-443.
26. Shaffer CL, Davey AM, Ransom JL, et al. Ampicillin-induced neurotoxicity in very-low-birth-weight neonates. *Ann Pharmacother.* 1998;32:482-484.

Ampicillin Sodium–Sulbactam Sodium

1. Unasyn [package insert]. New York, NY: Pfizer Inc; September 2003.
2. American Academy of Pediatrics. In: Pickering LK, ed. *2003 Red Book: Report of the Committee on Infectious Diseases.* 26th ed. Elk Grove Village, IL: American Academy of Pediatrics; 2003.
3. Bassetti D, Solbiati M, Ravelli A, et al. Clinical evaluation of sulbactam plus ampicillin in the treatment of general pediatric infections. *APMIS.* 1989;5:41-44.
4. Kanra G, Secmeer G, Akalin E, et al. Sulbactam/ampicillin in the treatment of pediatric infections. *Diagn Microbiol Infect Dis.* 1989;12:185S-187S.
5. Azimi PH, Barson WJ, Janner D, et al. Efficacy and safety of ampicillin/sulbactam and cefuroxime in the treatment of serious skin and skin structure infections in pediatric patients. *Pediatr Infect Dis J.* 1999;18:609-613.
6. Wald E, Reilly JS, Bluestone CD, et al. Sulbactam/ampicillin in the treatment of acute epiglottitis in children. *Rev Infect Dis.* 1986;8:6617-6619.
7. Bluestone CD. Role of sulbactam/ampicillin and sultamicillin in the treatment of bacterial infections of the upper respiratory tract of children. *APMIS.* 1989;5:35-40.
8. Collins MD, Dajani AS, Kim KS, et al. Comparison of ampicillin/sulbactam plus aminoglycoside vs. ampicillin plus clindamycin plus aminoglycosides in the treatment of intra-abdominal infections in children. *Pediatr Infect Dis J.* 1998;17:S15-S18.
9. Foulds G, McBride TJ, Knirsch AK, et al. Penetration of sulbactam and ampicillin into cerebrospinal fluid of infants and young children with meningitis. *Antimicrob Agents Chemother.* 1987;31:1703-1705.
10. Kulhanjian J, Dunphy MG, Hamstra S, et al. Randomized comparative study of ampicillin/sulbactam vs. ceftriaxone for treatment of soft tissue and skeletal infections in children. *Pediatr Infect Dis J.* 1989;8:605-610.
11. Meier H, Springsklee M, Wildfeuer A. Penetration of ampicillin and sulbactam into human costal cartilage. *Infection.* 1994;22:152-155.
12. Aronoff SC, Scoles PV, Makley JT, et al. Efficacy and safety of sequential treatment with parenteral sulbactam/ampicillin and oral sultamicillin for skeletal infections in children. *Rev Infect Dis.* 1986;8:S639-S643.
13. Syriopoulou V, Bitsi M, Theodoridis C, et al. Clinical efficacy of sulbactam/ampicillin in pediatric infections caused by ampicillin-resistant or penicillin-resistant organisms. *Rev Infect Dis*. 1986;8:S630-S633.
14. Baddour LM, Wilson WR, Bayer AS, et al. Infective endocarditis: diagnosis, antimicrobial therapy, and management of complications: a statement for healthcare professionals from the Committee on Rheumatic Fever, Endocarditis, and Kawasaki Disease, Council on Cardiovascular Disease in the Young, and the Councils on Clinical Cardiology, Stroke, and Cardiovascular Surgery and Anesthesia, American Heart Association: endorsed by the Infectious Diseases Society of America. *Circulation.* 2005;111:e394-e434.
15. American Society of Health-System Pharmacists. American Hospital Formulary System. Available at: http://ahfsfirst.firstdatabank.com/AHFSfirst/NSAHFSFirstSearchmain.asp. Accessed August 3, 2006.
16. Foulds G, McBride TJ, Knirsch AK, et al. Penetration of sulbactam and ampicillin into cerebrospinal fluid of infants and young children with meningitis. *Antimicrob Agents Chemother.* 1987;31:1703-1705.
17. Foster MC, Morris DL, Legan C, et al. Perioperative prophylaxis with sulbactam and ampicillin compared with metronidazole and cefotaxime in the prevention of wound infection in children undergoing appendectomy. *J Pediatr Surg.* 1987;22:869-872.
18. Syriopoulou V, Bitsi M, Theodoridis C, et al. Clinical efficacy of sulbactam/ampicillin in pediatric infections caused by ampicillin-resistant or penicillin-resistant organisms. *Rev Infect Dis.* 1986;8:S630-S633.
19. Trissel LA, ed. *Handbook on Injectable Drugs.* 13th ed. [CD-ROM version 1.5]. Bethesda, MD: American Society of Health-System Pharmacists; 2005.

References

20. McLaughlin JE, Reeves DS. Clinical and laboratory evidence for inactivation of gentamicin by carbenicillin. *Lancet.* 1971;1(7693):261-264.
21. Riff LJ, Jackson GG. Laboratory and clinical conditions for gentamicin inactivation by carbenicillin. *Arch Intern Med.* 1972;130:887-891.
22. Manian FA, Stone WJ, Alford RH. Adverse antibiotic effects associated with renal insufficiency. *Rev Infect Dis.* 1990;12:236-249.
23. Weibert R, Keane W, Shapiro F. Carbenicillin inactivation of aminoglycosides in patients with severe renal failure. *Trans Amer Soc Artif Int Organs.* 1976;22:439-443.
24. Davies M, Morgan JR, Anand C. Interactions of carbenicillin and ticarcillin with gentamicin. *Antimicrob Agents Chemother.* 1975;7:431-434.
25. Leong CF, Cheong SK, Fadilah SA, et al. Positive direct antiglobulin test with Unasyn. A case report. *Med J Malaysia.* 1999;54:517-519.

Anidulafungin

1. American Academy of Pediatrics. In: Pickering LK, ed. *Red Book: 2006 Report of the Committee on Infectious Diseases.* 27th ed. Elk Grove Village, IL: American Academy of Pediatrics; 2006.
2. Pannaraj PS, Walsh TJ, Baker CJ. Advances in antifungal therapy. *Pediatr Infect Dis J.* 2005;24:921-922.
3. Benjamin DK, Driscoll T, Seibel NL, et al. Safety and pharmacokinetics of intravenous anidulafungin in children with neutropenia at high risk for invasive fungal infections. *Antimicrob Agents Chemother.* 2006;50:632-638.
4. Eraxis [prescribing information]. New York, NY: Pfizer Inc; March 2006.
5. Steinbach WJ, Benjamin DK. New Antifungal agents under development in children and neonates. *Curr Opin Infect Dis.* 2005;18:484-489.

Aprotinin

1. Trasylol [prescribing information]. West Haven, CT: Bayer Pharmaceuticals Corporation; December 2003.
2. McEnvoy GK, ed. *AHFS Drug Information Essentials 2005-06.* Bethesda, MD: American Society of Health-System Pharmacists; 2005.
3. Dietrich W, Spath P, Zuhlsdorf M, et al. Anaphylactic reactions to aprotinin re-exposure in cardiac surgery. *Anesthesiol.* 2001;95:64-71.
4. D'Errico CC, Munro HM, Buchman SR, et al. Efficacy of aprotinin in children undergoing craniofacial surgery. *J Neurosurg.* 2003;99:287-290.
5. Jaquiss RDB, Ghanayem NS, Zacharisen MC, et al. Safety of aprotinin use and re-use in pediatric cardiothoracic surgery. *Circulation.* 2002;1069(suppl I):I90-I94.
6. Mossinger H, Dietrich W, Braun SL, et al. High-dose aprotinin reduces activation of hemostasis, allogenic blood requirement, and duration of postoperative ventilation in pediatric cardiac surgery. *Ann Thorac Surg.* 2003;75:430-437.
7. Chauhan S, Kumar BA, Heramba B, et al. Efficacy of aprotinin, epsilon aminocaproic acid, or a combination in cyanotic heart disease. *Ann Thorac Surg.* 2000;70:1308-1312.
8. Dietrich W, Mossinger H, Spannagl M, et al. Hemostatic activation during cardiopulmonary bypass with different aprotinin dosages in pediatric patients having cardiac operations. *J Thorac Cardiovasc Surg.* 1993;105:712-720.
9. Boldt J, Knothe C, Zickmann B, et al. Comparison of two aprotinin dosage regimens in pediatric patients having cardiac operations. *J Thorac Cardiovasc Surg.* 1993;105:705-711.
10. Miller BE, Tosone SR, Tan VKH, et al. Hematologic and economic impact of aprotinin in reoperative pediatric cardiac operations. *Ann Thorac Surg.* 1998;66:535-541.
11. Oliver WC, Fass DN, Nuttall GA, et al. Variability of plasma aprotinin concentrations in pediatric patients undergoing cardiac surgery. *J Thorac Cardiovasc Surg.* 2004;127:1670-1677.
12. Carrel TP, Schwanda M, Vogt PR, et al. Aprotinin in pediatric cardiac operations: a benefit in complex malformations wand with high-dose regimen only. *Ann Thorac Surg.* 1998;66:153-158.
13. Arnold DM, Fergusson DA, Chan AKC, et al. Avoiding transfusions in children undergoing cardiac surgery: a meta-analysis of randomized trial of aprotinin. *Anesth Analg.* 2006;102:731-737.
14. Davies MJ, Allen A, Kort H, et al. Prospective, randomized, double-blind study of high-dose in pediatric cardiac operations. *Ann Thorac Surg.* 1997;63:497-503.
15. Mangano DT, Tudor I, et al. The risk associated with aprotinin in cardiac surgery. *N Engl J Med.* 2006;354:353-365.
16. Cohen DM, Norberto J, Cartabuke, et al. Severe anaphylactic reaction after primary exposure to aprotinin. *Ann Thorac Surg.* 1999;67:837-838.
17. Garcia-Huete L, Domenech P, Sabate A, et al. The prophylactic effect of aprotinin on intraoperative bleeding in liver transplantation: a randomized clinical study. *Hepatology.* 1997;26:1143-1148.

Argatroban

1. Hursting MJ, Dubb J, Verme-Gibboney CN. Argatroban anticoagulation in pediatric patients: a literature analysis. *J Pediatr Hematol Oncol.* 2006;28:4-10.
2. John TE, Hallisey RK. Argatroban and lepirudin requirements in a 6-year old. *Pharmacotherapy.* 2005;25:1383-1388.
3. Dyke PC 2nd, Russo P, Mureebe L, et al. Argatroban for anticoagulation during cardiopulmonary bypass in an infant. *Paediatr Anaesth.* 2005;15:328-333.
4. McCullen CH. [personal communication]. GlaxoSmithKline; April 14, 2006.
5. *Physicians' Desk Reference.* 60th ed. Montvale, NJ: Thomson PDR; 2006.
6. McEvoy GK, ed. *AHFS Drug Information Essentials 2005–06.* Bethesda, MD: American Society of Health-System Pharmacists; 2005.
7. Tcheng WY, Wong WY. Successful use of argatroban in pediatric patients requiring anticoagulant alternatives to heparin. *Blood.* 2004;104:107b-108b. Abstract.
8. Trissel LA. *Handbook on Injectable Drugs.*13th ed. Bethesda, MD: American Society of Health-System Pharmacists; 2005.
9. Monagle P, Chan A, Massicotte P, et al. Antithrombotic therapy in children: the seventh ACCP conference on antithrombotic and thrombolytic therapy. *Chest.* 2004;126:645S-687S. Available at: http://www.chestjournal.org/cgi/content/full/126/3_suppl/645S.

Arginine HCl

1. American Hospital Formulary Service Drug Information. Arginine Hydrochloride, AHFS Class: Pituitary Function (36:66). Available at: http// www.ashp.org/ahfs/d_agents/a382240.cfm. Accessed March 3, 2006.
2. Root AW, Saenz-Rodriguez C, Bongiovanni AM, et al. The effect of arginine infusion on plasma growth hormone and insulin in children. *J Pediatr.* 1969;74:187-197.
3. Taketomo CK, Hodding JH, Kraus DM. *Pediatric Dosage Handbook.* 11th ed. Cleveland, OH: Lexi-Comp Inc; 2004–2005.
4. Thomson PDR, ed. *Physicians' Desk Reference.* 60th ed. Montvale, NJ: Thomson Healthcare; 2006.
5. Summar MS. Current strategies for the management of neonatal urea cycle disorders. *J Pediatr.* 2001;138:S30-S39.
6. Batshaw ML, MacArthur RB, Mendel Tuchman. Alternative pathway therapy for urea cycle disorders: twenty years later. *J Pediatr.* 2001;138: S46-S55.
7. McCaffrey MJ, Bose CL, Reiter PD, et al. Effect of L-Arginine infusion on infants with persistent pulmonary hypertension of the newborn. *Biol Neonate.* 1995;67:240-243.

8. Mehta S, Stewart DJ, Langleben D et al. Short-term pulmonary vasodilation with L-arginine in pulmonary hypertension. *Circulation.* 1995;92:1539-1545.
9. Schulze-Nick I, Penny DJ, Rigby ML et al. L-arginine and substance P reverse the pulmonary endothelial dysfunction caused by congenital heart surgery. *Circulation.* 1999;100:749-755.
10. Martin WF, Matzke GR. Treating severe metabolic alkalosis. *Clin Pharm.* 1982;1:42-48.
11. Sher GD, Ginder GD, Little J, et al. Extended therapy with intravenous arginine butyrate in patients with beta-hemoglobinopathies. *N Engl J Med.* 1995;332:1606-1610.
12. Gerard JM, Luisiri A. A fatal overdose of arginine hydrochloride. *Clin Toxicol.* 1997;35:621-625.
13. Tiwary CM, Rosenbloom AI, Julius RL. Anaphylactic reactions to arginine infusion. *N Engl J Med.* 1973;288:218. Letter.
14. Resnick DJ, Softness B, Murphy AR et al. Case report of an anaphylactoid reaction to arginine. *Ann Allergy Asthma Immunol.* 2002;88:67-68.
15. Nelin LD, Hoffman GM. L-arginine infusion lowers blood pressure in children. *J Pediatr.* 2001;139:747-749.
16. Bowlby HA, Elanjian SI. Necrosis caused by extravasation of arginine hydrochloride. *Ann Pharmacother.* 1992;26:263-264.
17. Baker GL, Franklin JD. Management of arginine mono-hydrochloride extravasation in the forearm. *S Med J.* 1991;84:381-384.
18. Salameh Y, Shoufani A. Full-thickness skin necrosis after arginine extravasation—a case report and review of literature. *J Pediatr Surg.* 2004;39(4):E9-E11.
19. Bushinsky DA, Gennari FJ. Life-threatening hyperkalemia induced by arginine. *Ann Intern Med.* 1978;89:632-634.
20. Hertz P, Richardson JA. Arginine-induced hyperkalemia in renal failure patients. *Arch Intern Med.* 1972;130:778-780.

Asparaginase

1. *Physicians' Desk Reference.* 60th ed. Montvale, NJ: Thomson PDR; 2006.
2. Kung FH, Nythan WL, Cuttner J, et al. Vincristine, prednisone, and L-asparaginase in the induction of remission in children with acute lymphoblastic leukemia following relapse. *Cancer.* 1979;41(2):428-434.
3. Jones B, Holland JF, Glidewell O. Optimal use of asparaginase in acute lymphocytic leukemia. *Med Pediatr Oncol.* 1979;3(4):387-400.
4. Ertel IJ, Nesbit ME, Hammond D, et al. Effective dose of L-asparaginase for induction of remission in previously treated children with acute lymphoblastic leukemia: a report from Children's Cancer Study Group. *Cancer Res.* 1979;39(10):3893-3896.
5. Ortega JA, Nesbit ME, Donaldson MH, et al. L-asparaginase, vincristine, and prednisone for induction of first remission in acute lymphocytic leukemia. *Cancer Res.* 1977;37(2):535-540.
6. Pession A, Valsecchi MG, Masera G, et al. Long-term results of a randomized trial on extended use of high dose L-asparaginase for standard risk childhood acute lymphoblastic leukemia. *J Clin Oncol.* 2005;23(28):7161-7167.
7. Haskell CM, Canellos GP, Leventhal BG, et al. L-asparaginase: therapeutic and toxic effects in patients with neoplastic disease. *N Engl J Med.* 1969;281(19):1028-1034.
8. Trissel LA, ed. *Handbook on Injectable Drugs.* 13th ed. [CD-ROM version 1.5]. Bethesda, MD: American Society of Health-System Pharmacists; 2005.
9. Rodriguez T, Baumgarten E, Fengler R, et al. Long-term infusion of L-asparaginase—an alternative to intramuscular injection? *Klin Pediatr.* 1995;207(4):207-210.
10. Nesbit M, Chard R, Evans A. Evaluation of intramuscular versus intravenous administration of L-asparaginase in childhood leukemia. *Am J Pediatr Hematol Oncol.* 1979;1(1):9-13.
11. Tan C, Oettgen H. Clinical experience with L-asparaginase administered intrathecally. *Proc Am Assoc Cancer Res.* 1969;10:92 (abstract 365).
12. Dorr RT, Fritz WL. *Cancer Chemotherapy Handbook*. New York, NY: Elsevier; 1980:230-239.
13. Taketomo CK, Hodding JH, Kraus DM, eds. *Pediatric Dosage Handbook.* 12th ed. [CD-ROM version 2006.1] Hudson, OH: Lexi-Comp; 2006.
14. American Society of Health-System Pharmacists. American Hospital Formulary System. Available at: http://ahfsfirst.firstdatabank.com/AHFSfirst/NSAHFSFirstSearchmain.asp. Accessed September 26, 2006.

Asparaginase–pegylated (Pegaspargase)

1. Oncaspar [package insert]. Bridgewater, NJ: Enzon Pharmaceuticals Inc; April, 2005.
2. Abshire TC, Pollock BH, Billett AL, et al. Weekly polyethylene glycol conjugated L-asparaginase compared with biweekly dosing produces superior induction remission rates in childhood relapsed acute lymphoblastic leukemia: a pediatric oncology group study. *Blood.* 2000;96:1709-1715.
3. Avramis AI, Sencer S, Periclou, et al. A randomized comparison of native *Escherichia coli* asparaginase and polyethylene glycol conjugated asparaginase for treatment of children with newly diagnosed standard-risk acute lymphoblastic leukemia: a Children's Cancer Group study. *Blood.* 2002;99:1986-1994.
4. Hawkins DS, Park JR, Thomson BG, et al. Asparaginase pharmacokinetics after intensive polyethylene glycol-conjugated L-asparaginase therapy for children with relapsed acute lymphoblastic leukemia. *Clin Cancer Res.* 2004;10:5335-5341.
5. McEvoy GK, ed. *AHFS Drug Information Essentials 2005–06.* Bethesda, MD: American Society of Health-System Pharmacists; 2005.
6. Solimando DA, ed. *Lexi-Comp's Drug Information Handbook for Oncology.* 4th ed. Hudson, OH: Lexi-Comp; 2004:651-654.

Atenolol

1. National High Blood Pressure Education Program Working Group on High Blood Pressure in Children and Adolescents. The fourth report on the diagnosis, evaluation, and treatment of high blood pressure in children and adolescents. *Pediatrics.* 2004 Aug;114(2 suppl 4th Report):555-576.
2. Kay JD, Sinaiko AR, Daniels SR. Pediatric hypertension. *Am Heart J.* 2001;142:422-432.
3. Buck ML, Wiest D, Gillette PC, et al. Pharmacokinetics and pharmacodynamics of atenolol in children. *Clin Pharmacol Ther.* 1989;46:629-633.
4. *Physicians' Desk Reference*. 60th ed. Montvale, NJ: Thomson PDR; 2006.
5. Aronoff A, Brier M, Bennett W. *The Renal Book, 2002.* Available at: http://www.kdp-baptist.louisville.edu/renalbook/. Accessed May 6, 2006.
6. American Society of Health-System Pharmacists. American Hospital Formulary System. Available at: http://ahfsfirst.firstdatabank.com/AHFSfirst/NSAHFSFirstSearchmain.asp. Accessed June 10, 2006.
7. Ramsdale DR, Faragher EB, Bennett DH, et al. Ischemic pain relief in patients with acute myocardial infarction by intravenous atenolol. *Am Heart J.* 1982;103:459-467.
8. Trissel LA, ed. *Handbook on Injectable Drugs.* 13th ed. [CD-ROM version 1.5]. Bethesda, MD: American Society of Health-System Pharmacists; 2005.

References

Atracurium Besylate

1. Rowlee SC. Monitoring neuromuscular blockade in the intensive care unit: the peripheral nerve stimulator. *Heart Lung.* 1999;28:352-362.
2. American Society of Health-System Pharmacists. American Hospital Formulary System. Available at: http://ahfsfirst.firstdatabank.com/AHFSfirst/NSAHFSFirstSearchmain.asp. Accessed July 10, 2006.
3. Meakin G, Shaw EA, Baker RD, et al. Comparison of atracurium-induced neuromuscular blockade in neonates, infants and children. *Br J Anaesth.* 1988;60:171-175.
4. Piotrowski A. Comparison of atracurium and pancuronium in mechanically ventilated neonates. *Intensive Care Med.* 1993;19:401-405.
5. Martin LD, Bratton SL, O'Rourke PP. Clinical uses and controversies of neuromuscular blocking agents in infants and children. *Crit Care Med.* 1999;27:1358-1368.
6. Meretoja OA, Wirtavori K. Influence of age on the dose-response relationship of atracurium in paediatric patients. *Acta Anaesthesiol Scand.* 1988;32:614-618.
7. Nightingale DA, Bush GH. Atracurium in paediatric anaesthesia. *Br J Anaesth.* 1983;55:115S.
8. Brandom BW, Rudd GD, Cook DR. Clinical pharmacology of atracurium in paediatric patients. *Br J Anaesth.* 1983;55:117S-121S.
9. Brandom BW, Woelfel SK, Cook DR, et al. Clinical pharmacology of atracurium in infants. *Anesth Analg.* 1984;63:309-312.
10. Goudsouzian NG, Liu LM, Cote CJ, et al. Safety and efficacy of atracurium in adolescents and children anesthetized with halothane. *Anesthesiology.* 1983;59:459-462.
11. Goudsouzian NG, Liu LM, Gionfriddo M, et al. Neuromuscular effects of atracurium in infants and children. *Anesthesiology.* 1985;62:75-79.
12. Brandom BW, Stiller RL, Cook DR, et al. Pharmacokinetics of atracurium in anaesthetized infants and children. *Br J Anaesth.* 1986;58:1210-1213.
13. Eagar BM, Flynn P, Hughes R. Infusion of atracurium for long surgical procedures. *Br J Anaesth.* 1984;56:447-452.
14. Wait CM, Goat VA. Atracurium infusion during paediatric craniofacial surgery. *Anaesthesia.* 1989;44:567-570.
15. Brandom BW, Cook DR, Woelfel SK, et al. Atracurium infusion requirements in children during halothane, isoflurane, and narcotic anesthesia. *Anesth Analg.* 1985;64:471-476.
16. Playfor SD, Thomas DA, Choonara I. Duration of action of atracurium when given by infusion to critically ill children. *Paediatr Anaesth.* 2000;10:77-81.
17. Kushimo OT, Darowski MJ, Hollis S, et al. Dose requirements of atracurium in paediatric intensive care patients. *Br J Anaesth.* 1991;67:781-783.
18. Ridley SA, Hatch DJ. Post-tetanic count and profound neuromuscular blockade with atracurium infusion in paediatric patients. *Br J Anaesth.* 1988;60:3135.
19. Aronoff A, Brier M, Bennett W. *The Renal Book, 2002.* Available at: http://www.kdp-baptist.louisville.edu/renalbook/. Accessed July 17, 2006.
20. Simpson DA, Green DW. Use of atracurium during major abdominal surgery in infants with hepatic dysfunction from biliary atresia. *Br J Anaesth.* 1986;58:1214-1217.
21. Kalli I, Metetoja OA. Infusion of atracurium in neonates, infants, and children. *Br J Anaesth.* 1988;60:651-654.
22. Branney SW, Haenel JB, Moore FA, et al. Prolonged paralysis with atracurium infusion: a case report. *Crit Care Med.* 1994;22:1699-1701.
23. Goudsouzian NG, Young ET, Moss J, et al. Histamine release during the administration of atracurium or vecuronium in children. *Br J Anaesth.* 1986;58:1229-1233.
24. Basta SJ, Savarese JJ, Ali HH, et al. Histamine-releasing potencies of atracurium, dimethyltubocurarine and tubocurarine. *Br J Anaesth.* 1983; 55:105S-106S.
25. McHutchon A, Lawler PG. Bradycardia following atracurium. *Anaesthesia.* 1983;38:597-598.
26. Carter ML. Bradycardia after the use of atracurium. *BMJ.* 1983;287:247-248.
27. Hiller JL, Benda GI, Rahatzad M, et al. Benzyl alcohol toxicity: impact on mortality and intraventricular hemorrhage among very low birth weight infants. *Pediatrics.* 1986;77:500-506.
28. American Academy of Pediatrics Committee on Drugs. "Inactive" ingredients in pharmaceutical products: update. *Pediatrics.*1997;99:268-278.
29. Hall CM, Milligan DWA, Berrington J. Probably adverse reaction to a pharmaceutical excipient. *Arch Dis Child Fetal Neonatal Ed.* 2004;89:F184.
30. Grant JA, Bilodeau PA, Guernsey BG, et al. Unsuspected benzyl alcohol hypersensitivity. *N Engl J Med.* 1982;306:108.
31. Wilson JP, Solimando DA, Edwards MS. Parenteral benzyl alcohol-induced hypersensitivity reaction. *Drug Intell Clin Pharm.* 1986;20:689-691.
32. Watling SM, Dasta JF. Prolonged paralysis in intensive care unit patients after the use of neuromuscular blocking agents: a review of the literature. *Crit Care Med.* 1994;22:884-893.
33. Brandom BW, Woelfel SK, Cook DR, et al. Relative potency of atracurium in children during halothane, isoflurane, or thiopental–fentanyl anesthesia. *Anesthesiology.* 1983;59:A442.
34. Fahey MR, Rupp SM, Canfell C, et al. Effect of renal failure on laudansoine excretion in man. *Br J Anaesth.* 1985;576:1049-1051.
35. Grigore AM, Brusco L, Kuroda M, et al. Laudanosine and atracurium in a patient receiving long-term atracurium infusion. *Crit Care Med.* 1998;26:180-183.

Atropine Sulfate

1. The International Liaison Committee on Resuscitation (ILCOR) Consensus on Science with Treatment Recommendations for Pediatric and Neonatal Patients: Neonatal Resuscitation. *Pediatrics.* 2006;117:e955-e977.
2. Sims DG, Heal CA, Bartle SM. Use of adrenaline and atropine in neonatal resuscitation. *Arch Dis Child.* 1994;70:F3-F10.
3. Standards and guidelines for cardiopulmonary resuscitation (CPR) and emergency cardiac care (ECC). Part VI: Neonatal advanced life support. *JAMA.* 1986;255:2969-2973.
4. Leuthner SR, Jansen RD, Hageman JR. Cardiopulmonary resuscitation of the newborn. An update. *Pediatr Clin North Am.* 1994;41:893-907.
5. 2005 American Heart Association guidelines for cardiopulmonary resuscitation and emergency cardiovascular care. Part 12: Pediatric advanced life support. *Circulation.* 2005;112(24 suppl):IV-167–IV-187.
6. American Academy of Pediatrics Committee on Drugs. Emergency drug doses for infants and children. *Pediatrics.* 1998;101:e1-e11.
7. Gaviotaki A, Smith RM. Use of atropine in pediatric anesthesia. *Int Anesthesiol Clin.* 1962;1:97-113.
8. Bachman L, Freeman A. The cardiac rate and rhythm in infants during anesthesia induction with cyclopropane. Atropine versus scopolamine as preanesthetic medication. *J Pediatr.* 1961;59:922-927.
9. Wark HJ, Overton JH, Marian P. The safety of atropine premedication in children with Down's syndrome. *Anaesthesia.* 1983;38:871-874.
10. Hofley MA, Hofley PM, Keom TP, et al. A placebo-controlled trial using intravenous atropine as an adjunct to conscious sedation in pediatric esophagogastroduodenoscopy. *Gastrointest Endosc.* 1995;42:457-460.
11. McEvoy GK, ed. *AHFS Drug Information Essentials 2005–06.* Bethesda, MD: American Society of Health-System Pharmacists; 2005.
12. Thomson Healthcare, Inc., POISINDEX® Managements Available at: http://www.thomsonhc.com-MICROMEDEX® Healthcare Series[database on the Internet]. Accessed April 27, 2006.
13. Rotenberg JS, Newmark J. Nerve agent attacks on children: Diagnosis and management. *Pediatrics.* 2003;112;648-658.
14. Zwiener RJ, Ginsburg CM. Organophosphate and carbamate poisoning in infants and children. *Pediatrics.* 1988;81:121-125.
15. Trissel LA, ed. *Handbook on Injectable Drugs.* 13th ed. Bethesda, MD: American Society of Health-System Pharmacists; 2005.

16. LeBlanc FN, Benson BE, Gilig AD. A severe organophosphate poisoning requiring the use of an atropine drip. *J Toxicol Clin Toxicol.* 1986;24:69-76.
17. Sullivan KJ, Berman LS, Koska J, et al. Intramuscular atropine sulfate in children: comparison of injection sites. *Anesth Analg Paris.* 1997;84:54-58.
18. Soni MG, Taylor SL, Greenberg NA, et al. Evaluation of the health aspects of methyl paraben: a review of the published literature. *Food Chem Toxicol.* 2002;40:1335-1373.
19. Nagel JE, Fuscaldo JT, Firemen P. Paraben allergy. *JAMA.* 1977;237:1594-1595.
20. American Academy of Pediatrics Committee on Drugs. "Inactive" ingredients in pharmaceutical products: update. *Pediatrics.* 1997;99:268-278.
21. Hall CM, Milligan DWA, Berrington J. Probably adverse reaction to a pharmaceutical excipient. *Arch Dis Child Fetal Neonatal Ed.* 2004;89: F184.
22. Grant JA, Bilodeau PA, Guernsey BG, et al. Unsuspected benzyl alcohol hypersensitivity. *N Engl J Med.* 1982;306:108.
23. Wilson JP, Solimando DA, Edwards MS. Parenteral benzyl alcohol-induced hypersensitivity reaction. *Drug Intell Clin Pharm.* 1986;20:689-691.
24. Chhabra A, Mishra S, Kumar A, et al. Atropine-induced lens extrusion in an open eye surgery. *Pediatr Anesthesia.* 2006;16:59-62.

Azithromycin

1. Zithromax® (azithromycin) for injection for IV infusion only [prescribing information]. New York, NY: Pfizer Labs; October 2003.
2. Plouffe J, Schwartz DB, Kolokathis A, et al. Clinical efficacy of intravenous followed by oral azithromycin monotherapy in hospitalized patients with community-acquired pneumonia. *Antimicrob Agents Chemother.* 2000;44:1796-1802.
3. Vergis EN, Indorf A, File TM, et al. Azithromycin vs. cefuroxime plus erythromycin for empirical treatment of community-acquired pneumonia in hospitalized patients: a prospective, randomized, multicenter trial. *Arch Intern Med.* 2000;160:1294-1300.
4. Bartlett JG, Dowell SF, Mandell LA, et al. Practice guidelines for the management of community-acquired pneumonia in adults. *Clin Infect Dis.* 2000;31:347-382.
5. Aronoff A, Brier M, Bennett W. *The Renal Book, 2002.* Available at: http://www.kdp-baptist.louisville.edu/renalbook/. Accessed August 12, 2006.
6. American Society of Health-System Pharmacists. American Hospital Formulary System. Available at: http://ahfsfirst.firstdatabank.com/AHFSfirst/NSAHFSFirstSearchmain.asp. Accessed August 12, 2006.
7. Jacobs RF, Maples HD, Aranda JV, et al. Pharmacokinetics of intravenously administered azithromycin in pediatric patients. *Pediatr Infect Dis J.* 2005;24:34-39.
8. Luke DR, Foulds G, Cohen SF, Levy B. Safety, toleration, and pharmacokinetics of intravenous azithromycin. *Antimicrob Agents Chemother.* 1996;40:2577-2581.
9. Trissel LA, ed. *Handbook on Injectable Drugs.* 13th ed [CD-ROM version 1.5]. Bethesda, MD: American Society of Health-System Pharmacists; 2005.
10. Bizjak ED, Haug MT, Schilz RJ, et al. Intravenous azithromycin-induced ototoxicity. *Pharmacotherapy.* 1999;19:245-248.

Aztreonam

1. American Academy of Pediatrics. In: Pickering LK, ed. *2003 Red Book: Report of the Committee on Infectious Diseases.* 26th ed. Elk Grove Village, IL: American Academy of Pediatrics; 2003.
2. Nelson JD, Bradley JS, eds. *Pocketbook of Pediatric Antimicrobial Therapy.* 14th ed. Baltimore, MD: Williams & Wilkins; 2000-2001.
3. Stutman HR. Clinical experience with aztreonam for treatment of infections in children. *Rev Infect Dis.* 1991;13:S582-S585.
4. Bosso JA, Black PG. The use of aztreonam in pediatric patients: a review. *Pharmacotherapy.* 1991;11:20-25.
5. Stutman HR, Chartrand SA, Tolentino T, et al. Aztreonam therapy for serious gram-negative infections in children. *Am J Dis Child.* 1986;140:1147-1151.
6. Kline MW, Kaplan SL, Mason EO. Aztreonam therapy of gram-negative infections predominantly of the urinary tract in children. *Curr Ther Res.* 1986;39:625-631.
7. Bosso JA, Black PG, Matsen JM. Efficacy of aztreonam in pulmonary exacerbations of cystic fibrosis. *Pediatr Infect Dis J.* 1987;6:393-397.
8. Bosso JA, Black PG. Controlled trial of aztreonam vs. tobramycin and azlocillin for acute pulmonary exacerbations of cystic fibrosis. *Pediatr Infect Dis J.* 1988;7:171-176.
9. Aronoff A, Brier M, Bennett W. *The Renal Book, 2002.* Available at: http://www.kdp-baptist.louisville.edu/renalbook/. Accessed August 7, 2006.
10. American Society of Health-System Pharmacists. American Hospital Formulary System. Available at: http://ahfsfirst.firstdatabank.com/AHFSfirst/NSAHFSFirstSearchmain.asp. Accessed August 7, 2006.
11. Trissel LA, ed. *Handbook on Injectable Drugs.* 13th ed. [CD-ROM version 1.5]. Bethesda, MD: American Society of Health-System Pharmacists; 2005.
12. Azactam [package insert]. Princeton, NJ: Bristol-Myers Squibb Co; January 2004.
13. de la Fuente PR, Armentia MA, Sanchez PP, et al. Urticaria caused by sensitization to aztreonam. *Allergy.* 1993;8:634-636.

Baclofen

1. McEvoy GK, ed. *AHFS Drug Information Essentials 2005–06.* Bethesda, MD: American Society of Health-System Pharmacists; 2005.
2. Disabato J, Ritchie A. Intrathecal baclofen for the treatment of spasticity of cerebral origin. *JSPN.* 2003;8:31-34.
3. Campbell WM, Ferrel A, McLaughlin JF, et al. Long-term safety and efficacy of continuous intrathecal baclofen. *Dev Med Child Neurol.* 2002;44:660-665.
4. Buonaguro V, Scelsa B, Curci D, et al. Epilepsy and intrathecal baclofen therapy in children with cerebral palsy. *Pediatr Neurol.* 2005;33:110-113.
5. Stokic DS, Yablon SA, Hayes A. Comparison of clinical and neurophysiologic responses to intrathecal baclofen bolus administration in moderate-to-severe spasticity after acquired brain injury. *Arch Phys Med Rehabil.* 2005;86:1801-1806.
6. Stempien L, Tsai T. Intrathecal baclofen pump use for spasticity. *Am J Phys Med Rehabil.* 2000;79:536-541.
7. Ward LAC. Spasticity in kids: an intrathecal option. *RN.* 2001;64(1):39-41.
8. Van Schaeybroeck P, Nuttin B, Lagae L, et al. Intrathecal baclofen for intractable cerebral spasticity: a prospective, placebo-controlled, double-blind study. *Neurosurgery.* 2000;46:603-612.
9. Bjornson KF, McLaughlin JF, Loeser JD, et al. Oral motor, communication, and nutritional status of children during intrathecal baclofen therapy: a descriptive pilot study. *Arch Phys Med Rehabil.* 2003;84:500-506.
10. Armstrong RW, Steinbok P, Cochrane DD, et al. Intrathecally administered baclofen for treatment of children with spasticity of cerebral origin. *J Neurosurg.* 1997;87:409-414.
11. Pohl M, Rockstroh G, Rückriem S, et al. Time course of the effect of a bolus dose of intrathecal baclofen on severe cerebral spasticity. *J Neurol.* 2003;250:1195-2000.
12. Trissel LA, ed. *Handbook on Injectable Drugs.* 13th ed. Bethesda, MD: American Society of Health-System Pharmacists; 2005.

References

13. Coffey RJ, Edgar TS, Francisco GE, et al. Abrupt withdrawal from intrathecal baclofen: recognition and management of a potentially life-threatening syndrome. *Arch Phys Med Rehabil.* 2002;83:735-741.
14. Kao LW, Amin Y, Kirk MA, et al. Intrathecal baclofen withdrawal mimicking sepsis. *J Emerg Med.* 2003;24:423-427.
15. Bardutzky J, Tronnier V, Schwab S, et al. Intrathecal baclofen for stiff-person syndrome: life-threatening intermittent catheter leakage. *Neurology.* 2003;60:1976-1978.
16. Samson-Fang L, Gooch J, Norlin C. Intrathecal baclofen withdrawal simulating neuroleptic malignant syndrome in a child with cerebral palsy. *Dev Med Child Neurol.* 2000;42:561-565.
17. Douglas AF, Weiner HL, Schwartz DR. Prolonged intrathecal baclofen withdrawal syndrome. *J Neurosurg.* 2005;102:1133-1136.
18. Green LB, Nelson VS. Death after acute withdrawal of intrathecal baclofen: case report and literature review. *Arch Phys Med Rehabil.* 1999;80:1600-1604.
19. Colachis SC, Rea GL. Monitoring of creatinine kinase during weaning of intrathecal baclofen and with symptoms of early withdrawal. *Am J Phys Med Rehabil.* 2003;82:489-492.
20. Meythaler JM, Roper JF, Brunner RC. Cyproheptadine for intrathecal baclofen withdrawal. *Arch Phys Med Rehabil.* 2003;84:638-642.
21. Khorasani A, Peruzzi WT. Dantrolene treatment for abrupt intrathecal baclofen withdrawal. *Anesth Analg.* 1995;80:1054-1056.
22. Greenberg MI, Hendrickson RG. Baclofen withdrawal following removal of an intrathecal baclofen pump despite oral baclofen replacement. *J Toxicol Clin Toxicol.* 2003;41:83-85.
23. Dickerman RD, Schneider SJ. Recurrent intrathecal baclofen pump catheter leakage: a surgical observation with recommendations. *J Pediatr Surg.* 2002;37:E17-E19.
24. Al-Khodairy AT, Vuagnat H, Uebelhart D. Symptoms of recurrent intrathecal baclofen withdrawal resulting from drug delivery failure: a case report. *Am J Phys Med Rehabil.* 1999;78:272-277.
25. Vaidyanathan S, Soni BM, Oo T, et al. Bladder stones—red herring for resurgence of spasticity in a spinal cord injury patient with implantation of Medtronic Synchromed pump for intrathecal delivery of baclofen—a case report. *BMC Urology.* 2003;3:1-7.
26. Albright AL, Ferson S, Carlos S. Occult hydrocephalus in children with cerebral palsy. *Neurosurgery.* 2005;56:93-97.
27. Schuele SU, Kellinghaus C, Shook SJ, et al. Incidence of seizures in patients with multiple sclerosis treated with intrathecal baclofen. *Neurology.* 2005;64:1086-1087.
28. Schuele SU, Ahrens CL, Kellinghaus C, et al. Incidence of seizures in patients with multiple sclerosis treated with intrathecal baclofen. *Neurology.* 2006;66:784-785.
29. Segal LS, Wallach DM, Kanev PM. Potential complications of posterior spine fusion and instrumentation in patients with cerebral palsy treated with intrathecal baclofen infusion. *Spine.* 2005;30:E219-E224.
30. Sansone JM, Mann D, Noonan K, et al. Rapid progression of scoliosis following insertion of intrathecal baclofen pump. *J Pediatr Orthop.* 2006;26:125-128.
31. Dressnandt J, Knostanzer A, Weinzierl FX, et al. Intrathecal baclofen in tetanus: four cases and a review of reported cases. *Intensive Care Med.* 1997;23:896-902.
32. Engrand N, Guerot E, Alexis R, et al. The efficacy of intrathecal baclofen in severe tetanus. *Anesthesiology.* 1999;90:1773-1776.

Bretylium Tosylate

1. American Heart Association. Guidelines 2005 for cardiopulmonary resuscitation and emergency cardiovascular care. Part 12: Pediatric advanced life support. *Circulation.* 2005;112:167-187.
2. Kudenchuk PJ. Advanced cardiac life support antiarrhythmic drugs. *Cardiol Clin.* 2002;20:79-87.
3. United States Food and Drug Administration, U.S. Department of Heath and Human Services. Summary of the safety related drug labeling changes approved by the FDA April 1999; Bretylium tosylate in 5% dextrose injection (April 16, 1999:Abbott). Available at: http://www.fda.gov/medwatch/safety/1999/apr99.htm#bretyl. Accessed May 10, 2006.
4. American Heart Association in collaboration with the International Liaison Committee on Resuscitation. Guidelines 2000 for cardiopulmonary resuscitation and emergency cardiovascular care. Part 10: Pediatric advanced life support. *Circulation.* 2000;128(suppl 1):1291-1342.
5. Gelman CR, Rumack BH, Hess AJ, eds. *DRUGDEX(R) System.* Englewood, CO: MICROMEDEX Inc. Accessed May 15, 2006.
6. Mongkolsmai C, Dove JT, Kyrouac JT. Bretylium tosylate for ventricular fibrillation in a child. *Clin Pediatr.* 1984;23:696–698.
7. Castaneda AR, Bacaner MB. Effect of bretylium tosylate on the prevention and treatment of postoperative arrhythmias. *Am J Cardiol.* 1970;25:461-466.
8. Robertson J, Shilkofski N, eds. *The Harriet Lane Handbook.* 17th ed. Philadelphia, PA: Elsevier Mosby; 2005:493.
9. Zaritsky A. Drug therapy of cardiopulmonary resuscitation in children. *Drugs.* 1989;37:356-374.
10. Strasburger JF. Cardiac arrhythmias in childhood. Diagnostic considerations and treatment. *Drugs.* 1991;42:974-983.
11. Serratto M. Diagnosis and management of heart failure in infants and children. *Comprehensive Ther.* 1992;18:11-19.
12. Ushay HM, Notterman DA. Pharmacology of pediatric resuscitation. *Pediatr Clin North Am.* 1997;44:207-233.
13. Koch-Weser J. Bretylium. *N Engl J Med.* 1979;300:473-477.
14. Adir J, Narang PK, Josselson J, et al. Pharmacokinetics of bretylium in renal insufficiency. *N Engl J Med.* 1979;300:1390-1391.
15. Aronoff A, Brier M, Bennett W. The Renal Book. 2002. Available at: http://www.kdp-baptist.louisville.edu/renalbook/. Accessed May 15, 2006.
16. Trissel LA, ed. *Handbook on Injectable Drugs.* 13th ed. [CD-ROM version 1.5]. Bethesda, MD: American Society of Health-System Pharmacists; 2005.
17. Thibaukt J. Hyperthermia associated with bretylium tosylate injection. *Clin Pharm.* 1989;8:145-146.
18. Thompson AE, Sussmane JB. Bretylium intoxication resembling clinical brain death. *Crit Care Med.* 1989;17:194-195.

Bumetanide

1. Wells TG. The pharmacology and therapeutics of diuretics in the pediatric patient. *Pediatr Clin North Am.* 1990;37:463-504.
2. Sullivan JE, Witte MK, Yamashita TS, et al. Dose-ranging evaluation of bumetanide pharmacodynamics in critically ill infants. *Clin Pharmacol Ther.* 1996;60:424-434.
3. Ward OC, Lam LK. Bumetanide in heart failure in infancy. *Arch Dis Child.* 1977;52:877-882.
4. Shankaran S, Ilagan N, Liang KC, et al. Bumetanide pharmacokinetics in preterm neonates. *Pediatr Res.* 1989;25:72A. Abstract.
5. Gale R, Armon Y, Aranda JV. Pharmacodynamic profile of bumetanide in newborn infants. *Pediatr Res.* 1988;23:257A. Abstract.
6. Wells TG, Fasules JW, Taylor BJ, et al. Pharmacokinetics and pharmacodynamics of bumetanide in neonates treated with extracorporeal membrane oxygenation. *J Pediatr.* 1992;121:974-980.
7. Witte MK, Rudloff AC, Yamashita TS, et al. Dose ranging pharmacokinetic and pharmacodynamic evaluation of bumetanide in infants with volume overload. *Pediatr Res.* 1986;20:210A. Abstract.
8. Lopez-Samblas AM, Adams JA, Goldberg RN, et al. The pharmacokinetics of bumetanide in the newborn infant. *Biol Neonate.* 1997;72:265-272.
9. Marshall JD, Wells TG, Letzig L, et al. Pharmacokinetics and pharmacodynamics of bumetanide in critically ill pediatric patients. *J Clin Pharmacol.* 1998;38:994-1002.
10. Sullivan JE, Witte MK, Yamashita TS, et al. Analysis of the variability in the pharmacokinetics and pharmacodynamics of bumetanide in critically ill infants. *Clin Pharmacol Ther.* 1996;60:414-423.
11. Sullivan JE, Witte MK, Yamashita TS, et al. Pharmacokinetics of bumetanide in critically ill infants. *Clin Pharmacol Ther.* 1996;60:405-413.
12. Rudy DW, Voelker JR, Greene PK, et al. Loop diuretics for chronic renal insufficiency: a continuous infusion is more efficacious than bolus therapy. *Ann Intern Med.* 1991;115:360-366.

13. Howard PA, Dunn MI. Severe musculoskeletal symptoms during continuous infusion of bumetanide. *Chest.* 1997;111:359-364.
14. Aronoff A, Brier M, Bennett W. The Renal Book, 2002. Available at: http://www.kdp-baptist.louisville.edu/renalbook/. Accessed May 18, 2006.
15. McEvoy GK, ed. *AHFS Drug Information Essentials 2005–06.* Bethesda, MD: American Society of Health-System Pharmacists; 2005.
16. Trissel LA. *Handbook on Injectable Drugs.* 13th ed. Bethesda, MD: American Society of Health-System Pharmacists; 2005.
17. American Academy of Pediatrics Committee on Drugs. "Inactive" ingredients in pharmaceutical products: update. *Pediatrics.* 1997;99:268-278.
18. Hall CM, Milligan DWA, Berrington J. Probable adverse reaction to a pharmaceutical excipient. *Arch Dis Child Fetal Neonatal Ed.* 2004;89: F184.
19. Hiller JL, Benda GI, Rahatzad M, et al. Benzyl alcohol toxicity: impact on mortality and intraventricular hemorrhage among very low birth weight infants. *Pediatrics.* 1986;77:500-506.
20. Grant JA, Bilodeau PA, Guernsey BG, et al. Unsuspected benzyl alcohol hypersensitivity. *N Engl J Med.* 1982;306:108.
21. Wilson JP, Solimando DA, Edwards MS. Parenteral benzyl alcohol-induced hypersensitivity reaction. *Drug Intell Clin Pharm.* 1986;20:689-691.
22. Turmen T, Thom P, Louridas AT, et al. Protein binding and bilirubin displacing properties of bumetanide and furosemide. *J Clin Pharmacol.* 1982;22:551-556.

Bupivacaine

1. McEvoy GK, ed. *AHFS Drug Information Essentials 2005–06.* Bethesda, MD: American Society of Health-System Pharmacists; 2005.
2. Taketomo CK, Hodding JH, Kraus DM. *Pediatric Dosage Handbook.* 12th ed. Hudson, OH: Lexi-Comp Inc; 2005.
3. Hansen TG, Henneberg SW, Walther-Larsen S, et al. Caudal bupivacaine supplemented with caudal or intravenous clonidine in children undergoing hypospadias repair: a double-blind study. *Br J Anaesth.* 2004;92:223-227.
4. Bozkurt P, Arslan I, Bakan M, et al. Free plasma levels of bupivacaine and ropivacaine when used for caudal block in children. *Eur J Anaesth.* 2005;22:634-643.
5. Brindley N, Taylor R, Brown S. Reduction of incarcerated inguinal hernia in infants using caudal epidural anaesthesia. *Pediatr Surg Int.* 2005;21:715-717.
6. Hansen TG, Morton NS, Cullen PM, et al. Plasma concentrations and pharmacokinetics of bupivacaine with and without adrenaline following caudal anaesthesia in infants. *Acta Anaesthesiol Scand.* 2001;45:42-47.
7. Khalil S, Campos C, Farag AM, et al. Caudal block in children: ropivacaine compared with bupivacaine. *Anesthesiology.* 1999;91:1279-1284.
8. Kumar P, Rudra A, Pan AK, et al. Caudal additives in pediatrics: a comparison among midazolam, ketamine, and neostigmine coadministered with bupivacaine. *Br J Anaesth.* 2005;101:69-73.
9. Meunier JF, Goujard E, Dubousset AM, et al. Pharmacokinetics of bupivacaine after continuous epidural infusion in infants with and without biliary atresia. *Anesthesiology.* 2001;95:87-95.
10. Larsson BA, Lonnqvist PA, Olsson GL. Plasma concentrations of bupivacaine in neonates after continuous epidural infusion. *Anesth Analg.* 1997;84:501-505.
11. Trissel LA. *Handbook on Injectable Drugs.* 13th ed. Bethesda, MD: American Society of Health-System Pharmacists; 2005.
12. Soni MG, Taylor SL, Greenberg NA, et al. Evaluation of the health aspects of methyl paraben: a review of the published literature. *Food Chem Toxicol.* 2002;40:1335-1373.
13. Nagel JE, Fuscaldo JT, Firemen P. Paraben allergy. *JAMA.* 1977;237:1594-1595.
14. American Academy of Pediatrics Committee on Drugs. "Inactive" ingredients in pharmaceutical products: update. *Pediatrics.* 1997;99:268-278.
15. Lester MR. Sulfite sensitivity: significance in human health. *J Am Col Nutr.* 1995;14:229-232.
16. Smolinske SC. Review of parenteral sulfite reactions. *J Toxicol Clin Toxicol.* 1992;30:597-606.
17. Shlizerman L, Ashkenazi D. Peripheral facial nerve paralysis after peritonsillar infiltration of bupivacaine: a case report. *Am J Otolaryngol.* 2005;26:406-407.

Caffeine Citrate

1. Schmidt B, Roberts RS, Davis P, et al. Caffeine therapy for apnea of prematurity. *N Engl J Med.* 2006;354:2112-2121.
2. Erenberg A, Leff RD, Haack DG. Caffeine citrate for the treatment of apnea of Prematurity: a double-blind, placebo-controlled study. *Pharmacotherapy.* 2000;20:644-652.
3. Bauer J, Maier K, Linderkamp O, et al. Effect of caffeine on oxygen consumption and metabolic rate in very low birth weight infants with idiopathic apnea. *Pediatrics.* 2001;107:660-663.
4. Thomson AH, Kerr S, Wright S. Population pharmacokinetics of caffeine in neonates and young infants. *Ther Drug Monit.* 1996;18:245-253.
5. Lee TC, Charles C, Steer P et al. Population pharmacokinetics of intravenous caffeine in neonates with apnea of prematurity. *Clin Pharmacol Ther.* 1997;61:628-640.
6. Erenberg A, Leff RD, Haack DG. Caffeine citrate for the treatment of apnea of prematurity: a double-blind, placebo-controlled study. *Pharmacotherapy.* 2000;20:644-652.
7. Young TE, Mangum B. *Neofax®: A Manual of Drugs Used in Neonatal Care.* 18th ed. Raleigh, NC: Acorn Publishing; 2005.
8. Taketomo CK, Hodding JH, Kraus DM. *Pediatric Dosage Handbook.* 11th ed. Hudson, OH: Lexi-Comp Inc; 2004–2005.
9. McEvoy GK, ed. *American Hospital Formulary Service Drug Information 2006.* Bethesda, MD: American Society of Health-System Pharmacists; 2006.
10. Thomson PDR, ed. *Physicians' Desk Reference.* 60th ed. Montvale, NJ: Thomson Healthcare; 2006.
11. Steer P, Flenady V, Shearman A, et al. High dose caffeine citrate for extubation of preterm infants: a randomized controlled trial. *Arch Dis Child Fetal Neonatal Ed.* 2004;89:F499-F503.
12. Trissel LA. *Handbook on Injectable Drugs.* 13th ed. Bethesda, MD: American Society of Health-System Pharmacists; 2005.

Calcitriol

1. Medical Economics, ed. *Physicians' Desk Reference.* 60th ed. Oradell, NJ: Medical Economics Company; 2006.
2. Greenbaum LA, Grenda R, Qiu P, et al. Intravenous calcitriol for treatment of hyperparathyroidism in children on hemodialysis. *Pediatr Nephrol.* 2005;20:622-630.
3. Salusky IB, Kuizon BD, Belin TR, et al. Intermittent calcitriol therapy in secondary hyperparathyroidism: a comparison between oral and intraperitoneal administration. *Kid Internat.* 1998;54:907-914.
4. Bellazzini MA, Howes DS. Pediatric hypocalcemic seizures: a case of rickets. *J Emerg Med.* 2005;28:161-164.
5. Venkataraman PS, Tsang RC, Steichen JJ, et al. Early neonatal hypocalcemia in extremely preterm infants. *Am J Dis Child.* 1986;140:1004-1008.
6. McEvoy GK, ed. *AHFS Drug Information Essentials 2005–06.* Bethesda, MD: American Society of Health-System Pharmacists; 2005.
7. Salusky IB, Goodman WG, Horst R, et al. Pharmacokinetics of calcitriol in continuous ambulatory and cycling peritoneal dialysis patients. *Am J Kidney Dis.* 1990;16:126-132.

References

8. Pecosky DA, Parasrampuria J, Luk CL, et al. Stability and sorption of calcitriol in plastic tuberculin syringes. *Am J Hosp Pharm.* 1992;49:1463-1466.
9. Mouser JF, Cochran EB, McKay CP, et al. Relationship between 1, 25 dihydroxyvitamin D (calcitriol) plasma concentrations and parathyroid hormone suppression in pediatric hemodialysis patients. *Pharmacotherapy.* 1994;14:366. Abstract.
10. Trachtman H, Gauthier B. Parenteral calcitriol for treatment of severe renal osteodystrophy in children with chronic renal insufficiency. *J Pediatr.* 1987;110:966-970.

Calcium Chloride

1. Calcium chloride [package insert]. Lake Forest, IL: Hospira Inc; October 2004.
2. McEvoy GK, ed. *AHFS Drug Information Essentials 2005–06.* Bethesda, MD: American Society of Health-System Pharmacists; 2005.
3. Broner CW, Stidham GL, Westerkirchner DF, et al. A prospective randomized, double-blind comparison of calcium chloride and calcium gluconate therapies for hypocalcemia in critically ill children. *J Pediatr.* 1990;117:986-989.
4. Cote CJ, Drop LJ, Hoaglin DC, et al. Ionized hypocalcemia after fresh frozen plasma administration to thermally injured children: effects of infusion rate, duration, and treatment with calcium chloride. *Anesth Analg.* 1988;67:152-160.
5. 2005 American Heart Association guidelines for cardiopulmonary resuscitation and emergency cardiovascular care: Part 12: Pediatric advanced life support. *Circulation.* 2005;112(24)(suppl1):IV167-IV187.
6. Young TE, Mangum B. *Neofax®: A Manual of Drugs Used in Neonatal Care.* 18th ed. Raleigh, NC: Acorn Publishing; 2005:224.
7. Trissel LA. *Handbook on Injectable Drugs.* 13th ed. Bethesda, MD: American Society of Health-System Pharmacists; 2005.
8. Upton J, Mulliken JB, Murray JE. Major intravenous extravasation injuries. *Am J Surg.* 1979;137:497-506.
9. Heckler FR, McCraw JB. Calcium-related cutaneous necrosis. *Surg Forum.* 1976;27:553-555.
10. Yosowitz P, Ekland DA, Shaw RC, et al. Peripheral intravenous infiltration necrosis. *Ann Surg.* 1975;182:553-556.
11. MacCara ME. Extravasation: a hazard of intravenous therapy. *Drug Intell Clin Pharm.* 1983;17:713–717.

Calcium EDTA (Edetate Calcium Disodium)

1. Piomelli S, Rosen JF, Chisolm JJ, et al. Management of childhood lead poisoning. *J Pediatr.* 1984;105:523-532.
2. Preventing lead poisoning in young children. Washington, DC: Centers for Disease Control, US Department of Health and Human Services; October 1991.
3. Calcium disodium versenate [package insert]. Northridge, CA: 3M Pharmaceuticals; July 2004.
4. American Academy of Pediatrics. Committee on Drugs. Treatment guidelines for lead exposure in children. *Pediatrics.* 1995;96:155-160.
5. Trissel LA. *Handbook on Injectable Drugs.* 13th ed. Bethesda, MD: American Society of Health-System Pharmacists; 2005.
6. Markowitz ME, Rosen JF. Need for the lead mobilization test in children with lead poisoning. *J Pediatr.* 1991;119:305-310.
7. Markowitz ME, Rosen JF. Assessment of lead stores in children: validation of an 8-hour $CaNa_2EDTA$ provocative test. *J Pediatr.* 1984;104:337-341.
8. Iniguez JL, Leverger G, Dollfus C, et al. Lead mobilization test in children with lead poisonings: validation of a 5-hours edetate calcium disodium provocation test. *Arch Pediatr Adolesc Med.* 1995;149:338-340.
9. Kassner J, Shannon M, Graef J. Role of forced diuresis on urinary lead excretion after the ethylenediaminetetraacetic acid mobilization test. *J Pediatr.* 1990;117:914-916.
10. Garrettson LK. Lead poisoning. In: Haddad LM, Winchester JF, eds. *Clinical Management of Poisoning and Drug Overdose.* Philadelphia, PA: WB Saunders Company; 1983:652-655.
11. Centers for Disease Control and Prevention (CDC). Deaths associated with hypocalcemia from chelation therapy—Texas, Pennsylvania, and Oregon, 2003-2005. *MMWR Morb Mortal Wkly Rep.* 2006;55:204-207.
12. Moel DI, Kumar K. Reversible nephrotoxic reactions to a combined 2,3-dimercapto-1-propanol and calcium disodium ethylenediaminetetraacetic acid regimen in asymptomatic children with elevated blood levels. *Pediatrics.* 1982;70:259-262.
13. Cory-Slechta DA, Weiss B, Cox C. Mobilization of lead over the course of calcium disodium ethylenediamine tetraacetate chelation therapy. *J Pharmacol Exp Ther.* 1987;243:804-813.
14. Mycyk MB, Leikin JB. Combined exchange transfusion and chelation therapy for neonatal lead poisoning. *Ann Pharmacother.* 2004;38:821-824.
15. Horowitz BZ, Mirkin DB. Lead poisoning and chelation in a mother-neonate pair. *J Toxicol Clin Toxicol.* 2001;39:727-731.
16. Chisolm JJ. The use of chelating agents in the treatment of acute and chronic lead intoxication in childhood. *J Pediatr.* 1968;73:1-38.
17. Taketomo CK, Hodding JH, Kraus DM, eds. *Pediatric Dosage Handbook.* 12th ed. Hudson, OH: Lexi-Comp; 2006.

Calcium Gluconate

1. Calcium gluconate injection [USP prescribing information]. Schaumburg, IL: American Pharmaceutical Partners Inc; November 2002.
2. McEvoy GK, ed. *AHFS Drug Information Essentials 2005–06.* Bethesda, MD: American Society of Health-System Pharmacists; 2005.
3. Bifano E, Kavey R, Pergolizzi J, et al. The cardiopulmonary effects of calcium infusion in infants with persistent pulmonary hypertension of the newborn. *Pediatr Res.* 1989;25:262-265.
4. Venkataraman PS, Wilson DA, Sheldon RE, et al. Effect of hypocalcemia on cardiac function in very-low-birth-weight preterm neonates: studies of blood ionized calcium, echocardiography, and cardiac effect of intravenous calcium therapy. *Pediatrics.* 1985;76:543-550.
5. Brown DR, Steranka BH, Taylor FH. Treatment of early onset neonatal hypocalcemia. *Am J Dis Child.* 1981;135:24-28.
6. Mizrahi A, London RD, Gribetz D. Neonatal hypocalcemia—its causes and treatment. *N Engl J Med.* 1968; 278:1163-1165.
7. Scott SM, Ladenson JH, Aguanna JJ, et al. Effect of calcium therapy in the sick premature infant with early neonatal hypocalcemia. *J Pediatr.* 1984;104:747-751.
8. Tsang RC, Steichen JJ, Chan GM. Neonatal hypocalcemia. Mechanism of occurrence and management. *Crit Care Med.* 1977;5:56-61.
9. Taketomo CK, Hodding JH, Kraus DM. *Pediatric Dosage Handbook.* 12th ed. Hudson, OH: Pediatric Lexi-Drugs; 2005.
10. Young TE, Mangum B. *Neofax®: A Manual of Drugs Used in Neonatal Care.* 18th ed. Raleigh, NC: Acorn Publishing; 2005:226.
11. Upton J, Mulliken JB, Murray JE. Major intravenous extravasation injuries. *Am J Surg.* 1979;137:497-506.
12. Heckler FR, McCraw JB. Calcium-related cutaneous necrosis. *Surg Forum.* 1976;27:553-555.
13. Lee FA, Gwinn JL. Roentgen patterns of extravasation of calcium gluconate in the tissues of the neonate. *J Pediatr.* 1975;86:598-601.
14. Weiss Y, Ackerman C, Shmilovitz L. Localized necrosis of scalp in neonates due to calcium gluconate infusions: a cautionary note. *Pediatrics.* 1975;56:1084-1086.
15. MacCara ME. Extravasation: a hazard of intravenous therapy. *Drug Intell Clin Pharm.* 1983;17:713-717.
16. Millard TP, Harris AJ, MacDonald DM. Calcinosis cutis following intravenous infusion of calcium gluconate. *Br J Derm.* 1999;140:184-186.
17. Book LS, Herbst JJ, Stewart D. Hazards of calcium gluconate therapy in the newborn infant: intra-arterial injection producing intestinal necrosis in rabbit ileum. *J Pediatr.* 1978;92:793-797.
18. Broner CW, Stidham GL, Westerkirchner DF, et al. A prospective randomized, double-blind comparison of calcium chloride and calcium gluconate therapies for hypocalcemia in critically ill children. *J Pediatr.* 1990;117:986-989.
19. Cote CJ, Drop LJ, Hoaglin DC, et al. Ionized hypocalcemia after fresh frozen plasma administration to thermally injured children: effects of infusion rate, duration, and treatment with calcium chloride. *Anesth Analg.* 1988;67:152-160.

20. Driscoll MB, Driscoll DF. Calculating aluminum content in total parenteral nutrition admixtures. *Am J Health-Syst Pharm.* 2005;62:312-315.
21. Frey OR, Maier L. Polyethylene vials of calcium gluconate reduce aluminum contamination of TPN. *Ann Pharmacother.* 2000;34:811-812.

Caspofungin

1. Odio CM, Araya R, Pinto LE, et al. Caspofungin therapy of neonates with invasive candidiasis. *Pediatr Infect Dis J.* 2004;23(12):1093-1097.
2. Manzar S, Kamat M, Pyati S. Caspofungin for Refractory Candidemia in Neonates. *Pediatr Infect Dis J.* 2006;25(3):282-283.
3. Pannaraj PS, Walsh TJ, Baker CJ. Advances in antifungal therapy. *Pediatr Infect Dis J.* 2005;24:921-922.
4. Yalaz M, Akisu M, Hilmioglu S, et al. Successful caspofungin treatment of multidrug resistant *Candida parapsilosis* septicaemia in an extremely low birth weight neonate. *Mycoses.* 2006;49:242-245.
5. American Academy of Pediatrics. In: Pickering LK, ed. *Red Book: 2006 Report of the Committee on Infectious Diseases.* 27th ed. Elk Grove Village, IL: American Academy of Pediatrics; 2006.
6. Walsh T, Adamson P, Seibel N, et al. Pharmacokinetics, Safety, and Tolerability of Caspofungin in Children and Adolescents. *Antimicrob Agents Chemother.* 2005;49:4536-4545.
7. Groll AH, Attarbaschi A, Schuster FR, et al. Treatment with caspofungin in immunocompromised paediatric patients: a multicentre survey. *J Antimicrob Chemother.* 2006;57:527-535.
8. Cesaro S, Toffolutti T, Messina C, et al. Safety and efficacy of caspofungin and liposomal amphotericin B, followed by voriconazole in young patients affected by refractory invasive mycosis. *Eur J Haematol.* 2004;73:50-55.
9. Pancham S, Hemmaway C, New H, et al. Caspofungin for invasive fungal infections: Combination treatment with liposomal amphotericin B in children undergoing hemopoietic stem cell transplantation. *Pediatr Transplantation.* 2005;9:254-257.
10. Elanjikal Z, Sorensen J, Schmidt H, et al. Combination therapy with caspofungin and liposomal amphotericin B for invasive aspergillosis. *Pediatr Infect Dis J.* 2003;22:653-656.
11. Pacctti SA, Gelone SP. Caspofungin acetate for treatment of invasive fungal infections. *Ann Pharmacother.* 2003 Jan;37(1):90-98.
12. *Physicians' Desk Reference.* 60th ed. Montvale, NJ: Thomson PDR; 2006.
13. Bliss JM, Wellington M, Gigliotti F. Antifungal Pharmacotherapy for Neonatal Candidiasis. *Semin Perinatol.* 2003;27:365-374.
14. Kontny U, Walsh TJ, Rossler J, et al. Successful Treatment of Refractory Chronic Disseminated Candidiasis After Prolonged Administration of Caspofungin in a Child With Acute Myeloid Leukemia. *Pediatr Blood Cancer.* 2006;Jan 26:Epub ahead of print.
15. Soni MG, Taylor SL, Greenberg NA, et al. Evaluation of the health aspects of methyl paraben: a review of the published literature. *Food Chem Toxicol.* 2002;40:1335-1373.
16. Nagel JE, Fuscaldo JT, Firemen P. Paraben allergy. *JAMA.* 1977;237:1594-1595.
17. American Academy of Pediatrics Committee on Drugs. "Inactive" ingredients in pharmaceutical products: update. *Pediatrics.* 1997;99:268-278.
18. Hall CM, Milligan DWA, Berrington J. Probably adverse reaction to a pharmaceutical excipient. *Arch Dis Child Fetal Neonatal Ed.* 2004;89: F184.
19. Hiller JL, Benda GI, Rahatzad M, et al. Benzyl alcohol toxicity: impact on mortality and intraventricular hemorrhage among very low birth weight infants. *Pediatrics.* 1986;77:500-506.
20. Grant JA, Bilodeau PA, Guernsey BG, et al. Unsuspected benzyl alcohol hypersensitivity. *N Engl J Med.* 1982;306:108.
21. Wilson JP, Solimando DA, Edwards MS. Parenteral benzyl alcohol-induced hypersensitivity reaction. *Drug Intell Clin Pharm.* 1986;20:689-691.
22. Castagnola E, Machetti M, Cappelli B. Caspofungin associated with liposomal amphotericin B or voriconazole for treatment of refractory fungal pneumonia in children with acute leukaemia or undergoing allogeneic bone marrow transplant. *Clin Microbiol Infect.* 2004;10:255-257.

Cefazolin Sodium

1. *Physicians' Desk Reference.* 60th ed. Montvale, NJ: Medical Economics Company; 2006.
2. Prober CG, Stevenson DK, Benitz WE. The use of antibiotics in neonates weighing less than 1200 grams. *Pediatr Infect Dis J.* 1990;9:111-121.
3. Nelson JD, Bradley JS, eds. *Pocketbook of Pediatric Antimicrobial Therapy.* 14th ed. Baltimore, MD: Williams & Wilkins; 2000–2001.
4. Dajani AS, Taubert KA, Wilson W, et al. Prevention of bacterial endocarditis: Recommendations by the American Heart Association. *JAMA.* 1997;277:1794–1801.
5. Baddour LM, Wilson WR, Bayer AS, et al. Infective endocarditis: diagnosis, antimicrobial therapy, and management of complications: a statement for healthcare professionals from the Committee on Rheumatic Fever, Endocarditis, and Kawasaki Disease, Council on Cardiovascular Disease in the Young, and the Councils on Clinical Cardiology, Stroke, and Cardiovascular Surgery and Anesthesia, American Heart Association: endorsed by the Infectious Diseases Society of America. *Circulation.* 2005;111:e394-e434.
6. Pickering LK, O'Connor DM, Anderson D, et al. Comparative evaluation of cefazolin and cephalothin in children. *J Pediatr.* 1974;85:842-847.
7. Pickering LK, O'Connor DM, Anderson D, et al. Clinical and pharmacologic evaluation of cefazolin in children. *J Infect Dis.* 1973;128:S407-S414.
8. American Academy of Pediatrics. In: Pickering LK, ed. *2003 Red Book: Report of the Committee on Infectious Diseases.* 26th ed. Elk Grove Village, IL: American Academy of Pediatrics; 2003.
9. Rhodes KH, Henry NK. Antibiotic therapy for severe infections in infants and children. *Mayo Clin Proc.* 1992;67:59-68.
10. Hiner LB, Baluarte HJ, Polinsky MS, et al. Cefazolin in children with renal insufficiency. *J Pediatr.* 1980;96:335-339.
11. Trissel LA, ed. *Handbook on Injectable Drugs.* 13th ed. [CD-ROM version 1.5]. Bethesda, MD: American Society of Health-System Pharmacists; 2005.
12. Pagliaro LA, Pagliaro AM, eds. Problems in pediatric drug therapy. 2nd ed. Hamilton, IL: Drug Intelligence Publications Inc; 1987.
13. Craig WA, Ebert SC. Continuous infusion of beta-lactam antibiotics. *Antimicrob Agents Chemother.* 1992;36:2577-2583.
14. Robinson DC, Cookson TL. Concentration guidelines for parenteral antibiotics in fluid-restricted patients. *Drug Intell Clin Pharm.* 1987;21:985-989.

Cefepime

1. Capparelli E, Hochwald C, Rasmussen M, et al. Population pharmacokinetics of cefepime in the neonate. *Antimicrob Agents Chemother.* 2005;49:2760-2766.
2. American Academy of Pediatrics. In: Pickering LK, ed. *2003 Red Book: Report of the Committee on Infectious Diseases.* 26th ed. Elk Grove Village, IL: American Academy of Pediatrics; 2003.
3. *Physicians' Desk Reference*. 60th ed. Montvale, NJ: Thomson PDR; 2006.
4. Baddour LM, Wilson WR, Bayer AS, et al. Infective endocarditis: diagnosis, antimicrobial therapy, and management of complications: a statement for healthcare professionals from the Committee on Rheumatic Fever, Endocarditis, and Kawasaki Disease, Council on Cardiovascular Disease in the Young, and the Councils on Clinical Cardiology, Stroke, and Cardiovascular Surgery and Anesthesia, American Heart Association: endorsed by the Infectious Diseases Society of America. *Circulation.* 2005;111:e394-e434.
5. Hamelin BA, Moore N, Knupp CA, et al. Cefepime pharmacokinetics in cystic fibrosis. *Pharmacotherapy.* 1993;465-470.

References

6. Arguedas AG, Stutman HR, Zaleska M, et al. Pharmacokinetics and clinical response in patients with cystic fibrosis. *Am J Dis Child.* 1992;146;797-802.
7. Chastagner P, Plouvier E, Eyer D, et al. Efficacy of cefepime and amikacin in the empiric treatment of febrile neutropenic children with cancer. *Med Ped Oncol.* 2000;34:306-308.
8. Mustafa MM, Carlson L, Tkaczewski I, et al. Comparative study of cefepime versus ceftazidime in the empiric treatment of pediatric cancer patients with fever and neutropenia. *Pediatr Infect Dis J.* 2001;20:362-369.
9. Borbolla JR, Lopez-Hernandez MA, Gonzalez-Avante M, et al. Comparison of cefepime versus ceftriaxone-amikacin as empirical regimens for the treatment of febrile neutropenia in acute leukemia patients. *Chemotherapy.* 2001;47:381-384.
10. Saez-Llorens X, Castano E, Garcia R, et al. Prospective randomized comparison of cefepime and cefotaxime for treatment of bacterial meningitis in infants and children. *Antimicrob Agents Chemother.* 1995;39:937-940.
11. Saez-Llorens X, O'Ryan M. Cefepime in the empiric treatment of meningitis in children. *Pediatr Infect Dis J.* 2001;20:356-361.
12. Schaad, UB, Eskola J, Kafetzis D, et al. Cefepime vs. ceftazidime treatment of pyelonephritis: a European randomized, controlled study of 300 pediatric cases. *Pediatr Infect Dis J.* 1998;17:639-644.
13. Reed MD, Yamashita TS, Knupp CK, et al. Pharmacokinetics of intravenously or intramuscularly administered cefepime in infants and children. *Antimicrob Agents Chemother.* 1997;41:1783-1787.
14. Henry N, Hoeker JL, Rhodes KH. Antimicrobial therapy for infants and children: guidelines for the inpatient and outpatient practice of pediatric infectious disease. *Mayo Clinic Proceed.* 2000;5:86-97.
15. Bradley JS, Arrieta A. Empiric use of cefepime in the treatment of lower respiratory tract infections in children. *Pediatr Infect Dis.* 2001;20:343-349.
16. Arrieta AC, Bradley JS. Empiric use of cefepime in the treatment of serious urinary tract infections in children. *Pediatr Infect Dis J.* 2001;20:350-355.
17. Arnoff GR, Berns JS, Brier ME, et al. *Drug Prescribing in Renal Failure: Dosing Guidelines for Adults.* 4th ed. Philadelphia, PA: American College of Physicians; 1999.
18. Sampol E, Jacquet A, Viggiano M, et al. Plama, urine, and skin pharmacokinetics of cefepime in burn patients. *J Antimicrob Chemother.* 2000;46:315-317.
19. Garrelts JC, Wagner DJ. The pharmacokinetics, safety, and tolerance of cefepime administered as an intravenous bolus or a rapid infusion. *Ann Pharmacother.* 1999;33:1258-1261.
20. Trissel LA, ed. *Handbook on Injectable Drugs.* 13th ed. [CD-ROM version 1.5]. Bethesda, MD: American Society of Health-System Pharmacists; 2005.
21. Burgess DS, Hastings RW, Hardin TC. Pharmacokinetic and pharmacodynamics of cefepime administration by intermittent and continuous infusion. *Clin Ther.* 2000;22:66-75.
22. McLaughlin JE, Reeves DS. Clinical and laboratory evidence for inactivation of gentamicin by carbenicillin. *Lancet.* 1971;1(7693):261-264.
23. Riff LJ, Jackson GG. Laboratory and clinical conditions for gentamicin inactivation by carbenicillin. *Arch Intern Med.* 1972;130:887-891.
24. Manian FA, Stone WJ, Alford RH. Adverse antibiotic effects associated with renal insufficiency. *Rev Infect Dis.* 1990;12:236-249.
25. Davies M, Morgan JR, Anand C. Interactions of carbenicillin and ticarcillin with gentamicin. *Antimicrob Agents Chemother.* 1975;7:431-434.
26. Weibert R, Keane W, Shapiro F. Carbenicillin inactivation of aminoglycosides in patients with severe renal failure. *Trans Amer Soc Artif Int Organs.* 1976;22:439-443.
27. American Society of Health-System Pharmacists. American Hospital Formulary System. Available at: http://ahfsfirst.firstdatabank.com/AHFSfirst/NSAHFSFirstSearchmain.asp. Accessed August 6, 2006.

Cefoperazone Sodium

1. Benitz WE, Tatro DS. *The Pediatric Drug Handbook.* Chicago, IL: Year Book; 1988:14.
2. Nelson JD, Bradley JS, eds. *Pocketbook of Pediatric Antimicrobial Therapy.* 14th ed. Baltimore, MD: Williams & Wilkins; 2000–2001.
3. American Academy of Pediatrics. In: Pickering LK, ed. *2003 Red Book: Report of the Committee on Infectious Diseases.* 26th ed. Elk Grove Village, IL: American Academy of Pediatrics; 2003.
4. Gordon AJ, Phyfferoen M. Cefoperazone sodium in the treatment of serious bacterial infections in 2,100 adults and children: multicentered trials in Europe, Latin America, and Australia. *Rev Infect Dis.* 1983;5(suppl Mar–Apr):S188-S199.
5. Motohiro T, Taechi, T, Sujima N, et al. Laboratory and clinical studies on cefoperazone in pediatrics treatment. *Jpn J Antibiot.* 1980;32:958.
6. Aronoff A, Brier M, Bennett W. *The Renal Book, 2002.* Available at: http://www.kdp-baptist.louisville.edu/renalbook/. Accessed August 13, 2006.
7. Cefobid [package insert]. New York, NY; Pfizer Roerig; January 2003.
8. Trissel LA, ed. *Handbook on Injectable Drugs.* 13th ed. [CD-ROM version 1.5]. Bethesda, MD: American Society of Health-System Pharmacists; 2005.
9. American Society of Health-System Pharmacists. American Hospital Formulary System. Available at: http://ahfsfirst.firstdatabank.com/AHFSfirst/NSAHFSFirstSearchmain.asp. Accessed August 13, 2006.
10. Nishimura T, Hiromatsu K, Takashidia T, et al. Laboratory and clinical studies of cefoperazone in pediatric field. *Jpn J Antibiot.* 1980;32:909.
11. Craig WA, Ebert SC. Continuous infusion of beta-lactam antibiotics. *Antimicrob Agents Chemother.* 1992;36:2577-2583.
12. Robinson DC, Cookson TL, Frisafe JA. Concentration guidelines for parenteral antibiotics in fluid-restricted patients. *Drug Intell Clin Pharm.* 1987;21:985-989.
13. Stewart GT. Cross allergenicity of penicillin G and related substances. *Lancet.* 1962;1:509-510.
14. Grieco MH. Cross-allergenicity of the penicillins and the cephalosporins. *Arch Intern Med.* 1967;119:141-146.
15. Sullivan TJ. Pathogenesis and management of allergic reactions to penicillin and other beta-lactam antibiotics. *Pediatr Infect Dis.* 1982;1:344-350.
16. Saxon A. Immediate hypersensitivity reactions to B-lactam antibiotics. *Rev Infect Dis.* 1983;5(suppl 2):S368-S378.
17. Sher TH. Penicillin hypersensitivity—a review. In: Symposium on anti-infective therapy I. Speck WT, Blummer JL, eds. *Pediatr Clin North Am.* 1983;30:161-177.
18. Williams KJ, Bax RP, Brown H, et al. Antibiotic treatment and associated prolonged prothrombin time. *J Clin Pathol.* 1991;44:738-741.

Cefotaxime Sodium

1. Prober CG, Stevenson DK, Benitz WE. The use of antibiotics in neonates weighing less than 1200 grams. *Pediatr Infect Dis J.* 1990;9:111-121.
2. American Academy of Pediatrics. In: Pickering LK, ed. *2003 Red Book: Report of the Committee on Infectious Diseases.* 26th ed. Elk Grove Village, IL: American Academy of Pediatrics; 2003.
3. Nelson JD, Bradley JS, eds. *Pocketbook of Pediatric Antimicrobial Therapy.* 14th ed. Baltimore, MD: Williams & Wilkins; 2000–2001.
4. McCracken GH, Threlkeld NE, Thomas ML. Pharmacokinetics of cefotaxime in newborn infants. *Antimicrob Agents Chemother.* 1982;21:683-684.
5. Kearns GL, Jacobs RF, Thomas BR, et al. Cefotaxime and desacetylcefotaxime pharmacokinetics in very low birth weight neonates. *J Pediatr.* 1989;114:461-467.
6. Gouyon JB, Pechinot A, Safran C, et al. Pharmacokinetics of cefotaxime in preterm infants. *Dev Pharmacol Ther.* 1990;14:29-34.
7. Claforan [package insert]. Bridgewater, NJ: Aventis Pharmaceuticals; May 2002.

8. Kafetzis DA, Brater DC, Kanarios J, et al. Clinical pharmacology of cefotaxime in pediatric patients. *Antimicrob Agents Chemother.* 1981;20:487-490.
9. Kearns GL, Young RA, Jacobs RF. Cefotaxime dosage in infants and children: pharmacokinetic and clinical rationale for an extended dosage interval. *Clin Pharmacokinet.* 1992;22:284-297.
10. Tunkel AR, Hartman BJ, Kaplan SL, et al. Practice guidelines for the management of bacterial meningitis. *Clin Infect Dis.* 2004;39:1267-1284.
11. Kaplan SL, Patrick CC. Cefotaxime and aminoglycoside treatment of meningitis caused by gram-negative enteric organisms. *Pediatr Infect Dis J.* 1990;9:810-814.
12. Trang JM, Jacobs RF, Kearns GL, et al. Cefotaxime and desacetylcefotaxime pharmacokinetics in infants and children with meningitis. *Antimicrob Agents Chemother.* 1985;28:791-795.
13. Odio CM, Faingezicht I, Salas JL, et al. Cefotaxime vs. conventional therapy for the treatment of bacterial meningitis of infants and children. *Pediatr Infect Dis* J. 1986;5:402-407.
14. Sexually Transmitted Diseases Treatment Guidelines—2006. Available at: http://www.cdc.gov/std/treatment. Accessed August 26, 2006.
15. Fillastre JP, Leroy A, Humbert G, et al. Pharmacokinetics of cefotaxime in subjects with normal and impaired renal function. *J Antimicrob Chemother.* 1980;6(suppl A):103-111.
16. Arnoff GR, Berns JS, Brier ME, et al. *Drug Prescribing in Renal Failure: Dosing Guidelines for Adults.* 4th ed. Philadelphia, PA: American College of Physicians; 1999.
17. American Society of Health-System Pharmacists. American Hospital Formulary System. Available at: http://ahfsfirst.firstdatabank.com/AHFSfirst/NSAHFSFirstSearchmain.asp. Accessed August 26, 2006.
18. Trissel LA, ed. *Handbook on Injectable Drugs.* 13th ed. [CD-ROM version 1.5]. Bethesda, MD: American Society of Health-System Pharmacists; 2005.
19. Robinson DC, Cookson TL, Frisafe JA. Concentration guidelines for parenteral antibiotics in fluid-restricted patients. *Drug Intell Clin Pharm.* 1987;21:985-989.

Cefotetan Disodium

1. American Academy of Pediatrics. In: Pickering LK, ed. *2003 Red Book: Report of the Committee on Infectious Diseases.* 26th ed. Elk Grove Village, IL: American Academy of Pediatrics; 2003.
2. Nelson JD, Bradley JS, eds. *Pocketbook of Pediatric Antimicrobial Therapy*. 14th ed. Baltimore, MD: Williams & Wilkins; 2000–2001.
3. Cefotan [package insert]. Deerfield, IL: Baxter Healthcare; January 2004.
4. Hemsell DL, Little BB, Faro S, et al. Comparison of three regimens recommended by the Centers for Disease Control and Prevention for the treatment of women hospitalized with acute pelvic inflammatory disease. *Clin Infect Dis.* 1994;19:720-727.
5. http://wonder.cdc.gov/wonder/prevguid/p0000133/p0000133.asp#head009000000000000. Accessed August 2006.
6. Trissel LA, ed. *Handbook on Injectable Drugs.* 13th ed. [CD-ROM version 1.5]. Bethesda, MD: American Society of Health-System Pharmacists; 2005.
7. Craig WA, Ebert SC. Continuous infusion of beta-lactam antibiotics. *Antimicrob Agents Chemother.* 1992;36:2577-2583.
8. Martin C, Thomachot L, Albanese J. Clinical Pharmacokinetics of cefotetan. *Clin Pharmacokinet.* 1994;26:248-258.
9. Williams KJ, Bax RP, Brown H, et al. Antibiotic treatment and associated prolonged prothrombin time. *J Clin Pathol.* 1991;44:738-741.

Cefoxitin Sodium

1. *Physicians' Desk Reference.* 60th ed. Montvale, NJ: Medical Economics Company; 2006.
2. Regazzi MB, Chirico G, Cristiani D, et al. Cefoxitin in newborn infants. A clinical and pharmacokinetic study. *Eur J Clin Pharmacol.* 1983;25:507-509.
3. Farmer K. Use of cefoxitin in the newborn. *N Z Med J.* 1982;95:398.
4. Yogev R, Delaplane D, Wiringa K. Cefoxitin in a neonate. *Pediatr Infect Dis.* 1983;2:342-343.
5. American Academy of Pediatrics. In: Pickering LK, ed. *2003 Red Book: Report of the Committee on Infectious Diseases.* 26th ed. Elk Grove Village, IL: American Academy of Pediatrics; 2003.
6. Nelson JD, Bradley JS, eds. *Pocketbook of Pediatric Antimicrobial Therapy.* 14th ed. Baltimore, MD: Williams & Wilkins; 2000–2001.
7. Gnehm HE, Seger RA, Boyle CM. The efficacy and tolerance of cefoxitin in the treatment of paediatric infections. *Curr Med Res Opin.* 1982;8:44-50.
8. Jacobson JA, Santos JI, Palmer WM. Clinical and bacteriological evaluation of cefoxitin in children. *Antimicrob Agents Chemother.* 1979;16:183-185.
9. Feldman WE, Moffitt S, Sprow N. Clinical and pharmacokinetic evaluation of parenteral cefoxitin in infants and children. *Antimicrob Agents Chemother.* 1980;17:669-674.
10. http://www.cdc.gov/std/treatment/. Accessed August 12, 2006.
11. Bennet R, Eriksson M, Nord CE, et al. Fecal bacterial microflora of newborn infants during intensive care management and treatment with five antibiotic regimens. *Pediatr Infect Dis.* 1986;5:533-539.
12. Gutierrez C, Vila J, Garcia-Sala C, et al. Study of appendicitis in children treated with four different antibiotic regimens. *J Pediatr Surg.* 1987;22:865-868.
13. Robinson DC, Cookson TL, Frisafe JA. Concentration guidelines for parenteral antibiotics in fluid-restricted patients. *Drug Intell Clin Pharm.* 1987;21:985-989.
14. American Society of Health-System Pharmacists. American Hospital Formulary System. Available at: http://ahfsfirst.firstdatabank.com/AHFSfirst/NSAHFSFirstSearchmain.asp. Accessed August 12, 2006.
15. Trissel LA, ed. *Handbook on Injectable Drugs.* 13th ed. [CD-ROM version 1.5]. Bethesda, MD: American Society of Health-System Pharmacists; 2005.
16. Craig WA, Ebert SC. Continuous infusion of beta-lactam antibiotics. *Antimicrob Agents Chemother.* 1992;36:2577-2583.
17. McLaughlin JE, Reeves DS. Clinical and laboratory evidence for inactivation of gentamicin by carbenicillin. *Lancet.* 1971;1(7693):261-264.
18. Riff LJ, Jackson GG. Laboratory and clinical conditions for gentamicin inactivation by carbenicillin. *Arch Intern Med.* 1972;130:887-891.
19. Manian FA, Stone WJ, Alford RH. Adverse antibiotic effects associated with renal insufficiency. *Rev Infect Dis.* 1990;12:236-249.
20. Davies M, Morgan JR, Anand C. Interactions of carbenicillin and ticarcillin with gentamicin. *Antimicrob Agents Chemother.* 1975;7:431-434.
21. Weibert R, Keane W, Shapiro F. Carbenicillin inactivation of aminoglycosides in patients with severe renal failure. *Trans Amer Soc Artif Int Organs.* 1976;22:439-443.

Ceftazidime

1. American Academy of Pediatrics. In: Pickering LK, ed. *2003 Red Book: Report of the Committee on Infectious Diseases.* 26th ed. Elk Grove Village, IL: American Academy of Pediatrics; 2003.
2. Nelson JD, Bradley JS, eds. *Pocketbook of Pediatric Antimicrobial Therapy.* 14th ed. Baltimore, MD: Williams & Wilkins; 2000–2001.
3. Mulhall A, de Louvois J. The pharmacokinetics and safety of ceftazidime in the neonate. *J Antimicrob Chemother.* 1985;15:97-103.
4. Tessin L, Trollfors B, Thiringer K, et al. Concentrations of ceftazidime, tobramycin, and ampicillin on the cerebrospinal fluid of newborn infants. *Eur J Pediatr.* 1989;148:679-681.

References

5. Tessin L, Thiringer K, Trollfors B, et al. Comparison of serum concentrations of ceftazidime and tobramycin in newborn infants. *Eur J Pediatr.* 1988;147:405-407.
6. McCracken GH, Threlkeld N, Thomas ML. The pharmacokinetics of ceftazidime in newborn infants. *Antimicrob Agents Chemother.* 1984;26:583-584.
7. Assael BM, Boccazi A, Caccamo ML, et al. Clinical pharmacology of ceftazidime in paediatrics. *J Antimicrob Chemother.* 1983;12(suppl A):341-346.
8. Prinsloo JG, Delport SD, Moncrieff J, et al. A preliminary pharmacokinetic study of ceftazidime in premature, newborn and small infants. *J Antimicrob Chemother.* 1983;12(suppl A):361-364.
9. Mulhall A, de Louvois J. The pharmacokinetics and safety of ceftazidime in the neonate. *J Antimicrob Chemother.* 1985;15:97-103.
10. van den Anker JN, Schoemaker RC, van der Heijden BJ. Once-daily versus twice-daily administration of ceftazidime in the premature infant. *Antimicrob Chemother.* 1995;39:2048-2050.
11. van den Anker JN, Schoemaker RC, Hop WC, et al. Ceftazidime pharmacokinetics in preterm infants: effect of renal function and gestational age. *Clin Pharmacol Ther.* 1995;58:650-659.
12. Rodriguez WJ, Khan WN, Gold B, et al. Ceftazidime in the treatment of meningitis in infants and children over one month of age. *Am J Med.* 1985;79(suppl 2A):52-55.
13. Hatch D, Overturf GD, Kovacs A, et al. Treatment of bacterial meningitis with ceftazidime. *Pediatr Infect Dis.* 1986;5:416-420.
14. Rodriguez WJ, Puig JR, Khan W, et al. Ceftazidime vs. standard therapy for pediatric meningitis: therapeutic, pharmacologic and epidemiologic observations. *Pediatr Infect Dis J.* 1986;5:408-415.
15. Viscoli C, Moroni C, Boni L, et al. Ceftazidime plus amikacin versus ceftazidime plus vancomycin as empiric therapy in febrile neutropenic children with cancer. *Rev Infect Dis.* 1991;13:397-404.
16. Granowetter L, Wells H, Lange BJ. Ceftazidime with or without vancomycin vs. cephalothin, carbenicillin and gentamicin as the initial therapy of the febrile neutropenic pediatric cancer patient. *Pediatr Infect Dis.* 1988;7:165-170.
17. Jacobs RF, Vats TS, Pappa KA, et al. Ceftazidime versus ceftazidime plus tobramycin in febrile neutropenic children. *Infection.* 1993;21:223-228.
18. Tunkel AR, Hartman BJ, Kaplan SL, et al. Practice guidelines for the management of bacterial meningitis. *Clin Infect Dis.* 2004;39:1267-1284.
19. *Physicians' Desk Reference.* 60th ed. Montvale, NJ: Thomson PDR; 2006.
20. Cullen RT, McCrae WM, Govan J, et al. Ceftazidime in cystic fibrosis: clinical, microbiological and immunological studies. *J Antimicrob Chemother.* 1983;12(suppl A):369-375.
21. Schadd UB, Wedgwood-Krucko J, Suter S, et al. Efficacy of inhaled amikacin as adjunct to intravenous combination therapy (ceftazidime and amikacin) in cystic fibrosis. *J Pediatr.* 1987;111:599-605.
22. Gold R, Carpenter S, Heurter H, et al. Randomized trial of ceftazidime versus placebo in the management of acute respiratory exacerbations in patients with cystic fibrosis. *J Pediatr.* 1987;111:907-913.
23. DeBoeck K, Breysem L. Treatment of pseudomonas aeruginosa lung infection in cystic fibrosis with high or conventional doses of ceftazidime. *J Antimicrob Chemother.* 1998;41:407-409.
24. Munzenberger PJ, Man-Ching J, Holliday SJ. Relationship of ceftazidime pharmacokinetics indices with therapeutic outcomes in patients with cystic fibrosis. *Pediatr Infect Dis J.* 1993;12:997-1001.
25. Bosso JA, Bonapace CR, Flume PA, et al. A pilot study of the efficacy of constant infusion ceftazidime in the treatment of endobronchial infections in adults with cystic fibrosis. *Pharmacotherapy.* 1999;19:620-626.
26. Chuang YY, Hung IJ, Yang CP, et al. Cefepime versus ceftazidime as empiric monotherapy for fever and neutropenia in children with cancer. *Pediatr Infect Dis J.* 2002;21:203-209.
27. Ohkawa M, Nakashima T, Shoda R, et al. Pharmacokinetics of ceftazidime in patients with renal insufficiency and in those undergoing hemodialysis. *Chemotherapy.* 1985;31:410-416.
28. Welage LS, Schultz RW, Schentag JJ. Pharmacokinetics of ceftazidime in patients with renal insufficiency. *Antimicrob Agents Chemother.* 1984;25:201-204.
29. Ackerman BH, Ross J, Tofte RW, et al. Effect of decreased renal function on the pharmacokinetics of ceftazidime. *Antimicrob Agents Chemother.* 1984;25:785-786.
30. Yost RL, Ramphal R. Ceftazidime review. *Drug Intell Clin Pharm.* 1985;19:509-513.
31. Scully BE, Neu HC. Clinical efficacy of ceftazidime: treatment of serious infection due to multiresistant Pseudomonas and other gram-negative bacteria. *Arch Intern Med.* 1984;144:57-62.
32. Trissel LA, ed. *Handbook on Injectable Drugs.* 13th ed. [CD-ROM version 1.5]. Bethesda, MD: American Society of Health-System Pharmacists; 2005.
33. Battersby NC, Patel L, David TJ. Increasing dose regimen in children with reactions to ceftazidime. *Clin Exp Allergy.* 1995;25:1211-1217.
34. Craig WA, Ebert SC. Continuous infusion of beta-lactam antibiotics. *Antimicrob Agents Chemother.* 1992;36:2577-2583.
35. Dalle JH, Gnansounou M, Husson MO, et al. Continuous infusion of ceftazidime in the empiric treatment of febrile neutropenic children with cancer. *J Pediatr Hem Onc.* 2002:24:714-716.
36. Robinson DC, Cookson TL, Frisafe JA. Concentration guidelines for parenteral antibiotics in fluid-restricted patients. *Drug Intell Clin Pharm.* 1987;21:985-989.
37. van den Anker JN, Hop WC, Schoemaker RC, et al. Ceftazidime pharmacokinetics in preterm infants: effect of postnatal age and postnatal exposure to indomethacin. *Br J Clin Pharmacol.* 1995;40:439-443.

Ceftriaxone Sodium

1. Robertson A, Fink S, Karp W. Effect of cephalosporins on bilirubin-albumin binding. *J Pediatr.* 1988;112:291-294.
2. American Academy of Pediatrics. In: Pickering LK, ed. *2003 Red Book: Report of the Committee on Infectious Diseases.* 26th ed. Elk Grove Village, IL: American Academy of Pediatrics; 2003.
3. Prober CG, Stevenson DK, Benitz WE. The use of antibiotics in neonates weighing less than 1200 grams. *Pediatr Infect Dis J.* 1990;9:111-121.
4. Nelson JD, Bradley JS, eds. *Pocketbook of Pediatric Antimicrobial Therapy.* 14th ed. Baltimore, MD: Williams & Wilkins; 2000–2001.
5. McCracken GH, Siegel JD, Threlkeld N, et al. Ceftriaxone pharmacokinetics in newborn infants. *Antimicrob Agents Chemother.* 1983;23:341-343.
6. Ceftriaxone [package insert]. Deerfield, IL: Baxter Healthcare Corporation; March 2005.
7. Higham M, Cunningham FM, Teele DW. Ceftriaxone administered once or twice a day for treatment of bacterial infections of childhood. *Pediatr Infect Dis.* 1985;4:22-26.
8. Chadwick EG, Connor EM, Shulman ST, et al. Efficacy of ceftriaxone in treatment of serious childhood infections. *J Pediatr.* 1983;103:141-145.
9. Tunkel AR, Hartman BJ, Kaplan SL, et al. Practice guidelines for the management of bacterial meningitis. *Clin Infect Dis.* 2004;39:1267-1284.
10. Congeni BL, Bradley J, Hammerschlag MR. Safety and efficacy of once daily ceftriaxone for the treatment of bacterial meningitis. *Pediatr Infect Dis.* 1986;5:293-297.
11. Lebel MH, Hoyt MJ, McCracken GH. Comparative efficacy of ceftriaxone and cefuroxime for treatment of bacterial meningitis. *J Pediatr.* 1989;114:1049-1054.
12. Kavaliotis J, Manios SG, Kansouzidou A, et al. Treatment of childhood bacterial meningitis with ceftriaxone once daily: open, prospective randomized, comparative study of short-course versus standard-length therapy. *Chemotherapy.* 1989;35:296-303.
13. Frenkel LD. Multicenter Ceftriaxone Pediatric Study Group. Once-daily administration of ceftriaxone for the treatment of selected serious bacterial infections in children. *Pediatrics.* 1988;82:486-491.

14. Peltola H, Anttila M, Renkonen O, et al. Randomized comparison of chloramphenicol, ampicillin, cefotaxime, and ceftriaxone for childhood bacterial meningitis. *Lancet.* 1989;i:1281-1287.
15. Grubbauer HM, Dornbusch HJ, Dittrich P, et al. Ceftriaxone monotherapy for bacterial meningitis in children. *Chemotherapy.* 1990;36:441-447.
16. Tuncer AM, Gur I, Ertem U, et al. Once daily ceftriaxone for meningococcemia and meningococcal meningitis. *Pediatr Infect Dis.* 1988;7:711-713.
17. Del Rio MA, Chrane D, Shelton S, et al. Ceftriaxone versus ampicillin and chloramphenicol for treatment of bacterial meningitis in children. *Lancet.* 1983;1:1241-1244.
18. Steele RW, Eyre LB, Bradsher RW, et al. Pharmacokinetics of ceftriaxone in pediatric patients with meningitis. *Antimicrob Agents Chemother.* 1983;23:191-194.
19. Steele RW, Bradsher RW. Comparison of ceftriaxone with standard therapy for bacterial meningitis. *J Pediatr.* 1983;103:138-140.
20. Chonmaitree T, Congeni BL, Munoz J, et al. Twice daily ceftriaxone therapy for serious bacterial infections in children. *J Antimicrob Chemother.* 1984;13:511-516.
21. Prado V, Cohen J, Banfi A, et al. Ceftriaxone in the treatment of bacterial meningitis in children. *Chemotherapy.* 1986;32:383-390.
22. Craig JC, Abbott GD, Mogridge NB. Ceftriaxone for pediatric bacterial meningitis: a report of 62 children and a review of the literature. *NZ Med J.* 1992;105:441-444.
23. Workowski KA, Berman SM. Sexually transmitted diseases treatment guidelines, 2008. *Morbid Mortal Weekly.* 2006;55:RR-11.
24. Green SM, Rothrock SG. Single-dose intramuscular ceftriaxone for acute otitis media in children. *Pediatrics.* 1993;91:23-30.
25. Chamberlain JM, Boenning DA, Waisman Y, et al. Single-dose ceftriaxone versus 10 days of cefaclor for otitis media. *Clin Pediatr.* 1994;33:642-646.
26. Barnett ED, Teele DW, Klein JO, et al. Comparison of ceftriaxone and trimethoprim-sulfamethoxazole for acute otitis media. Greater Boston Otitis Media Study Group. *Pediatrics.* 1997;99:23-28.
27. Aronoff A, Brier M, Bennett W. *The Renal Book, 2002.* http://www.kdp-baptist.louisville.edu/renalbook/. Accessed August 18, 2006.
28. Patel IH, Sugihara JG, Weinfeld RE, et al. Ceftriaxone pharmacokinetics in patients with various degrees of renal impairment. *Antimicrob Agents Chemother.* 1984;5:438-442.
29. Trissel LA, ed. *Handbook on Injectable Drugs.* 13th ed. [CD-ROM version 1.5]. Bethesda, MD: American Society of Health-System Pharmacists; 2005.
30. Baumgartner JD, Glauser MP. Single daily dose treatment of severe refractory infections with ceftriaxone. *Arch Intern Med.* 1983;143:1868-1873.
31. Lossos IS, Lossos A. Hazards of rapid administration of ceftriaxone. *Ann Pharmacother.* 1994;28:807. Letter.
32. Bonnet JP, Abid L, Dabhar A, et al. Early biliary pseudolithiasis during ceftriaxone therapy for acute pyelonephritis in children: a prospective study in 34 children. *Eur J Pediatr Surg.* 2000;10:368-371.
33. Prince JS, Senac MO Jr. Ceftriaxone-associated nephrolithiasis and biliary pseudolithiasis in a child. *Pediatr Radiol.* 2003;33:648-651. Epub 2003 Jun 26.
34. Mattis LE, Saavedra JM, Shan H, et al. Life-threatening ceftriaxone-induced immune hemolytic anemia in a child with Crohn's disease. *Clin Pediatr.* 2004;43:175-178.

Cefuroxime Sodium

1. *Physicians' Desk Reference.* 60th ed. Montvale, NJ: Thomson PDR; 2006.
2. Nelson JD, Bradley JS, eds. *Pocketbook of Pediatric Antimicrobial Therapy.* 14th ed. Baltimore, MD: Williams & Wilkins; 2000–2001.
3. Renlund M, Petty O. Pharmacokinetics and clinical efficacy of cefuroxime in the newborn period. *Proc R Soc Med.* 1977;70(suppl 9):179-182.
4. Wilkinson PJ, Belohradsky BH, Marget W. A clinical study of cefuroxime in neonates. *Proc R Soc Med.* 1977; 70(suppl 9):183-185.
5. American Academy of Pediatrics. In: Pickering LK, ed. *2003 Red Book: Report of the Committee on Infectious Diseases.* 26th ed. Elk Grove Village, IL: American Academy of Pediatrics; 2003.
6. Nelson JD. Cefuroxime: a cephalosporin with unique applicability to pediatric practice. *Pediatr Infect Dis.* 1983;2:394-396.
7. Barson WJ, Miller MA, Marcon MJ, et al. Cefuroxime therapy for bacteremic soft-tissue infections in children. *Am J Dis Child.* 1985;139:1141-1144.
8. Nelson JD, Kusmiesz H, Shelton S. Cefuroxime therapy for pneumonia in infants and children. *Pediatr Infect Dis.* 1982;1:159-163.
9. Nelson JD, Bucholz RW, Kusmiesz H, et al. Benefits and risks of sequential parenteral-oral cephalosporin therapy for suppurative bone and joint infections. *J Pediatr Orthop.* 1982;2:255-262.
10. Azimi PH, Barson WJ, Janner D, et al. Efficacy and safety of ampicillin/sulbactam and cefuroxime in the treatment of serious skin and skin structure infections in pediatric patients. *Pediatr Infect Dis J.* 1999;18:609-613.
11. Lebel MH, Hoyt MJ, Waagner DC, et al. Magnetic resonance imaging and dexamethasone therapy for bacterial meningitis. *Am J Dis Child.* 1989;143:301-306.
12. Lebel MH, Hoyt MJ, McCracken GH. Comparative efficacy of ceftriaxone and cefuroxime for treatment of bacterial meningitis. *J Pediatr.* 1989;114:1049-1054.
13. Trissel LA, ed. *Handbook on Injectable Drugs.* 13th ed. [CD-ROM version 1.5]. Bethesda, MD: American Society of Health-System Pharmacists; 2005.
14. Robinson DC, Cookson TL, Frisafe JA. Concentration guidelines for parenteral antibiotics in fluid-restricted patients. *Drug Intell Clin Pharm.* 1987;21:985-989.
15. Schaad UB, Suter S, Gianella-Borradori A, et al. A comparison of ceftriaxone and cefuroxime for the treatment of bacterial meningitis in children. *N Engl J Med.* 1990;322:141-147.

Chloramphenicol Sodium Succinate

1. American Academy of Pediatrics. In: Pickering LK, ed. *2006 Red Book: Report of the Committee on Infectious Diseases.* 27th ed. Elk Grove Village, IL: American Academy of Pediatrics; 2006.
2. Mulhall A, Berry DJ, de Louvois J. Chloramphenicol in paediatrics: current prescribing practice and the need to monitor. *Eur J Pediatr.* 1988;147:574-578.
3. Feder HM. Chloramphenicol: what we have learned in the last decade. *South Med J.* 1986;79:1129-1134.
4. Rajchgot P, Prober CG, Soldin S, et al. Initiation of chloramphenicol therapy in the newborn infant. *J Pediatr.* 1982;101:1018-1021.
5. Prober CG, Stevenson DK, Benitz WE. The use of antibiotics in neonates weighing less than 1200 grams. *Pediatr Infect Dis J.* 1990;9:111-121.
6. Glazer JP, Danish MA, Plotkin SA, et al. Disposition of chloramphenicol in low birth weight infants. *Pediatrics.* 1980; 66:573-578.
7. Meissner HC, Smith AL. The current status of chloramphenicol. *Pediatrics.* 1979;64:348-356.
8. Laferriere CI, Marks MI. Chloramphenicol: properties and clinical use. *Pediatr Infect Dis.* 1982;1:257-264.
9. Bartlett JG. Chloramphenicol. *Med Clin North Am.* 1982;66:91-102.
10. Smith AL, Weber A. Pharmacology of chloramphenicol. *Pediatr Clin North Am.* 1983;30:209-236.
11. Friedman CA, Lovejoy FC, Smith AL. Chloramphenicol disposition in infants and children. *J Pediatr.* 1979;95:1071-1077.
12. Sack CM, Koup JR, Smith AL. Chloramphenicol pharmacokinetics in infants and young children. *Pediatrics.* 1980;66:579-584.
13. Kauffman RE, Thirumoorthi MC, Buckley JA, et al. Relative bioavailability of intravenous chloramphenicol succinate and oral chloramphenicol palmitate in infants and children. *J Pediatr.* 1981;99:963-967.

14. Burckhart GJ, Barrett FF, Straughn AB, et al. Chloramphenicol clearance in infants. *J Clin Pharmacol.* 1982;22:49-52.
15. Rodriguez WJ, Puig JR, Khan W, et al. Ceftazidime vs. standard therapy for pediatric meningitis: therapeutic, pharmacologic and epidemiologic observations. *Pediatr Infect Dis J.* 1986;5:408-415.
16. Nahata MC. Serum concentrations and adverse effects of chloramphenicol in pediatric patients. *Chemotherapy*. 1987;33:322-327.
17. Craig JC, Abbott GD, Mogridge NB. Ceftriaxone for pediatric bacterial meningitis: a report of 62 children and a review of the literature. *NZ Med J.* 1992;105:441-444.
18. Mato SP, Robinson S, Begue RE. Vancomycin-resistant enterococcus faecium meningitis successfully treated with chloramphenicol. *Pediatr Infect Dis J.* 1999;18:483-484.
19. Marks WA, Stutman HR, Marks MI, et al. Cefuroxime versus ampicillin plus chloramphenicol in childhood bacterial meningitis: a multicenter randomized controlled trial. *J Pediatr*. 1986;109:123-130.
20. Odio CM, Faingezicht I, Salas JL, et al. Cefotaxime vs. conventional therapy for the treatment of bacterial meningitis of infants and children. *Pediatr Infect Dis J.* 1986;5:402-407.
21. Brasfield JH, Record KE, Griffen WO, et al. Chloramphenicol and chloramphenicol succinate concentrations in patients with renal impairment. *Clin Pharm.* 1983;2:355-358.
22. Phelps SJ, Tsiu W, Barrett FF, et al. Chloramphenicol-induced cardiovascular collapse in an anephric patient. *Pediatr Infect Dis J.* 1987;6:285-288.
23. Aronoff A, Brier M, Bennett W. *The Renal Book, 2002.* http://www.kdp-baptist.louisville.edu/renalbook/. Accessed August 11, 2006.
24. American Society of Health-System Pharmacists. American Hospital Formulary System. Available at: http://ahfsfirst.firstdatabank.com/AHFSfirst/NSAHFSFirstSearchmain.asp. Accessed August 11, 2006.
25. Weiss CF, Glazko AJ, Weston JK. Chloramphenicol in the newborn infant: a physiologic explanation of its toxicity when given in excessive doses. *N Engl J Med.* 1960;262:787-794.
26. Trissel LA, ed. *Handbook on Injectable Drugs.* 13th ed. [CD-ROM version 1.5]. Bethesda, MD: American Society of Health-System Pharmacists; 2005.
27. Rapp RP, Wermeling DP, Piecoro JJ Jr. Guidelines for the administration of commonly used intravenous drugs—1984 update. *Drug Intell Clin Pharm.* 1984;18:217-232.
28. Weber MW, Gatchalian SR, Ogunelesi O, et al. Chloramphenicol pharmacokinetics in infants less than three months of age in the Philippines and the Gambia. *Pediatr Infect Dis J.* 1999;18:896-901.
29. Scapellato PG, Ormazabal C, Scapellato JL, et al. Meningitis due to vancomycin-resistant *enterococcus faecium* successfully treated with combined intravenous and intraventricular chloramphenicol. *J Clin Microbiol.* 2005;43:3578-3579.
30. Brown RT. Chloramphenicol toxicity in an adolescent. *J Adolesc Health Care.* 1982;3:53-55.
31. Biancaniello T, Meyer RA, Kaplan S. Chloramphenicol and cardiotoxicity. *J Pediatr.* 1981;98:828-830.
32. Krasinski K, Perkin R, Rutledge J. Gray baby syndrome revisited. *Clin Pediatr.* 1982;21:571-572.
33. Wilkinson JD, Pollack MM, Costello J. Chloramphenicol toxicity: hemodynamic and oxygen utilization effects. *Pediatr Infect Dis J.* 1985;4:69-72.
34. Craft AW, Brocklebank JT, Hey EN, et al. The grey toddler: chloramphenicol toxicity. *Arch Dis Child.* 1974;49:235-237.
35. Evans LS, Kleiman MB. Acidosis as a presenting feature of chloramphenicol toxicity. *J Pediatr.* 1986;108:475-477.
36. Koup JR, Gibaldi M, McNamara P, et al. Interaction of chloramphenicol with phenytoin and phenobarbital. *Clin Pharmacol Ther.* 1978;24:571-575.
37. Bui LL, Huang DD. Possible interaction between cyclosporin and chloramphenicol. *Ann Pharmacother.* 1999;33:252-253.
38. Schulman SL, Shaw LM, Jabs K, et al. Interaction between tacrolimus and chloramphenicol in a renal transplant recipient. *Transplantation.* 1998;65:1397-1398.

Chlorpromazine HCl

1. Thorazine [prescribing information]. Research Triangle Park, NC: GlaxoSmithKline; April 2002.
2. Infants of drug-dependent mothers. In: Kagan BM, Gellis SS, eds. *Current Pediatric Therapy Eleven.* Philadelphia, PA: WB Saunders Company; 1984:653.
3. Larsson LE, Ekstrom-Jodal B, Hjalmarson O. The effect of chlorpromazine in severe hypoxia in newborn infants. *Acta Paediatr Scand.* 1982;71:399-402.
4. Marshall G, Kerr S, Vowels M, et al. Antiemetic therapy for chemotherapy-induced vomiting: metoclopramide, benztropine, dexamethasone, and lorazepam regimens compared with chlorpromazine alone. *J Pediatr.* 1989;115:156-160.
5. Mehta P, Gross S, Graham-Pole J, et al. Methylprednisolone for chemotherapy-induced emesis: a double-blind randomized trial in children. *J Pediatr.* 1986;108:774-776.
6. Graham-Pole J, Weare J, Engle S, et al. Antiemetics in children receiving cancer chemotherapy: a double-blind prospective randomized study comparing metoclopramide with chlorpromazine. *J Clin Oncol.* 1986;4:1110-1113.
7. Relling RV, Mulhern RK, Fairclough D, et al. Chlorpromazine with and without lorazepam as antiemetic therapy in children receiving uniform chemotherapy. *J Pediatr.* 1993;12:811-816.
8. Taketomo CK, Hodding JH, Kraus DM, eds. *Pediatric Dosage Handbook.* 12th ed. [CD-ROM version 2006.1] Hudson, OH: Lexi-Comp; 2006.
9. Nordeng H, Lindemann R, Perminov KV, et al. Neonatal withdrawal syndrome after *in utero* exposure to selective serotonin reuptake inhibitors. *Acta Paediatr.* 2001;90:288-291.
10. Miscellaneous drugs. In: Roberts RJ, ed. *Drug Therapy in Infants: Pharmacologic Principles and Clinical Experience*. Philadelphia, PA: WB Saunders Company; 1984:296-308.
11. Ruckman RN, Keane JF, Freed MD, et al. Sedation for cardiac catheterization: a controlled study. *Pediatr Cardiol.* 1980;1:263-268.
12. Aronoff A, Brier M, Bennett W. *The Renal Book, 2002.* Available at: http://www.kdp-baptist.louisville.edu/renalbook/. Accessed May 5, 2006.
13. Trissel LA. *Handbook on Injectable Drugs.* 13th ed. Bethesda, MD: American Society of Health-System Pharmacists; 2005.
14. Riemenschneider TA, Nielsen HC, Ruttenberg HD, et al. Disturbances of the transitional circulation: spectrum of pulmonary hypertension and myocardial dysfunction. *J Pediatr.* 1976;89:622-625.
15. American Academy of Pediatrics Committee on Drugs. "Inactive" ingredients in pharmaceutical products: update. *Pediatrics.* 1997;99:268-278.
16. Lester MR. Sulfite sensitivity: significance in human health. *J Am Col Nutr.* 1995;14:229-232.
17. Smolinske SC. Review of parenteral sulfite reactions. *J Toxicol Clin Toxicol.* 1992;30:597-606.
18. Hall CM, Milligan DWA, Berrington J. Probably adverse reaction to a pharmaceutical excipient. *Arch Dis Child Fetal Neonatal Ed.* 2004;89:F184.
19. Hiller JL, Benda GI, Rahatzad M, et al. Benzyl alcohol toxicity: impact on mortality and intraventricular hemorrhage among very low birth weight infants. *Pediatrics.* 1986;77:500-506.
20. Grant JA, Bilodeau PA, Guernsey BG, et al. Unsuspected benzyl alcohol hypersensitivity. *N Engl J Med.* 1982;306:108.
21. Wilson JP, Solimando DA, Edwards MS. Parenteral benzyl alcohol-induced hypersensitivity reaction. *Drug Intell Clin Pharm.* 1986;20:689-691.
22. Fixler DE, Carrell T, Browne R, et al. Oxygen consumption in infants and children during cardiac catheterization under different sedation regimens. *Circulation.* 1974;50:788-794.
23. Nahata MC, Clotz MA, Krogg EA. Adverse effects of meperidine, promethazine, and chlorpromazine for sedation in pediatric patients. *Clin Pediatr*. 1985;24:558-660.
24. Nahata MC. Sedation in pediatric patients undergoing diagnostic procedures. *Drug Intell Clin Pharm.* 1988;22:711-715.

25. Cook BA, Bass JW, Nomizu S, et al. Sedation of children for technical procedures: current standards of practice. *Clin Pediatr.* 1992;31:137-142.
26. American Academy of Pediatrics. Committee on Drugs. Reappraisal of lytic cocktail/demerol, phenergan, and thorazine (DPT) for the sedation of children. *Pediatrics.* 1995;95:598-602.
27. Snodgrass WR, Dodge WF. Lytic/DPT cocktail: time for rational and safer alternatives. *Pediatr Clin North Am.* 1989;36:1285-1291.
28. Brown ET, Corbett SW, Green SM. Iatrogenic cardiopulmonary arrest during pediatric sedation with meperidine, promethazine, and chlorpromazine. *Pediatr Emerg Care.* 2001;17:351-353.
29. Kelly AM, Ardagh M, Curry C, et al. Intravenous chlorpromazine versus intramuscular sumatriptan for acute migraine. *J Accid Emerg Med.* 1997;14:209-211.
30. Nakano T, Kado H, Shiokawa Y, et al. The low resistance strategy for the perioperative management of the Norwood procedure. *Ann Thorac Surg.* 2004;77:908-912.
31. Abajo FJ, Montero D, Madurga M, et al. Acute and clinically relevant drug induced liver injury: a population based case-control study. *Br J Clin Pharmacol.* 2004;58:71-80.
32. Isbister CK, Balit CR, Kilham HA. Antipsychotic poisoning in young children. *Drug Safety.* 2005;28:1029-1044.

Cimetidine

1. Aranda JV, Outerbridge EW, Schentag JJ. Pharmacodynamics and kinetics of cimetidine in a premature newborn. *Am J Dis Child.* 1983;137:1207.
2. Ziemniak JA, Wynn RJ, Aranda JV, et al. The pharmacokinetic and metabolism cimetidine in neonate. *Dev Pharmacol Ther.* 1984;7:30-38.
3. Chhattriwalla Y, Colon AR, Scanion JW. The use of cimetidine in the newborn. *Pediatrics.* 1980;65:301-302.
4. Vandenplas Y, Sacre L. Cimetidine influence on gastric emptying time in neonates. *Drug Intell Clin Pharm.* 1986;20:232-233.
5. Lloyd CW, Martin WJ, Taylor BD. The pharmacokinetics of cimetidine and metabolites in a neonate. *Drug Intell Clin Pharm.* 1985;19:203-205.
6. Vandenplas Y, Sacre L. The use of cimetidine in newborns. *Am J Perinatol.* 1987;4:131-133.
7. Agarwal AK, Saili A, Pandey KK, et al. Role of cimetidine in prevention and treatment of stress-induced gastric bleeding in neonates. *Indian Pediatr.* 1990;27:465-469.
8. Lacroix J, Infante-Rivard C, Gauthier M, et al. Upper gastrointestinal tract bleeding acquired in a pediatric intensive care unit: prophylaxis trial with cimetidine. *J Pediatr.* 1986;108:1015-1018.
9. Chin TWF, MacLeod SM, Fenje P, et al. Pharmacokinetics of cimetidine in critically ill children. *Pediatr Pharmacol.* 1982;2:285-292.
10. Somogyi A, Becker M, Gugler R. Cimetidine pharmacokinetics and dosage requirements in children. *Eur J Pediatr.* 1985;144:72-76.
11. Lloyd CW, Martin WJ, Taylor BD, et al. Pharmacokinetics and pharmacodynamics of cimetidine and metabolites in critically ill children. *J Pediatr.* 1985;107:295-300.
12. Martyn JAJ. Cimetidine and/or antacid for the control of gastric acidity in pediatric burn patients. *Crit Care Med.* 1985;13:1-3.
13. Kelly DA. Do H_2 receptor antagonists have a therapeutic role in childhood? *J Pediatr Gastroenterol Nutr.* 1994;19:270-276.
14. Crill CM, Hak EB. Upper gastrointestinal bleeding in critically ill pediatric patients. *Pharmacotherapy.* 1999;19:162-180.
15. Ostro MJ, Russell JA, Soldin SJ, et al. Control of gastric pH with cimetidine: boluses versus primed infusions. *Gastroenterology.* 1985;89:532-537.
16. Frank W, Karlstadt R, Rockhold F, et al. Comparison between continuous and intermittent infusion regimens of cimetidine in ulcer patients. *Clin Pharmacol Ther.* 1989;46:234-239.
17. Martin LF, Booth FV, Karlstadt RG, et al. Continuous intravenous cimetidine decreases stress-related upper gastrointestinal hemorrhage without promoting pneumonia. *Crit Care Med.* 1993;21:19-30.
18. Aronoff A, Brier M, Bennett W. *The Renal Book, 2002.* Available at: http://www.kdp-baptist.louisville.edu/renalbook/. Accessed August 9, 2006.
19. Larsson R, Erlanson P, Bodemar G, et al. The pharmacokinetics of cimetidine and its sulphoxide metabolite in patients with normal and impaired renal function. *Br J Clin Pharmacol.* 1982;13:163-170.
20. American Society of Health-System Pharmacists. American Hospital Formulary System. Available at: http://ahfsfirst.firstdatabank.com/AHFSfirst/NSAHFSFirstSearchmain.asp. Accessed August 9, 2006.
21. Martyn JA, Greenblatt DJ, Hagen J, et al. Alteration by burn injury of the pharmacokinetics and pharmacodynamics of cimetidine in children. *Eur J Clin Pharmacol.* 1989;36:361-367.
22. Ziemniak JA, Assael BM, Padoan R, et al. The bioavailability and pharmacokinetics of cimetidine and its metabolites in juvenile cystic fibrosis patients: age related differences as compared to adults. *Eur J Clin Pharmacol.* 1984;26:183-189.
23. Priebe HJ, Skillman JJ, Bushnell LS, et al. Antacid versus cimetidine in preventing acute gastrointestinal bleeding. *N Engl J Med.* 1980;302:426-430.
24. Morgan DJ, Uccellini DA, Raymond K, et al. The influence of duration of intravenous infusion of an acute dose on plasma concentrations of cimetidine. *Eur J Clin Pharmacol.* 1983;25:29-34.
25. Mahon WA, Kolton M. Hypotension after intravenous cimetidine. *Lancet.* 1978;1:828. Letter.
26. Shaw RG, Mashford ML, Desmond PV. Cardiac arrest after intravenous injection of cimetidine. *Med J Aust.* 1980;2:629-630.
27. Trissel LA, ed. *Handbook on Injectable Drugs.* 13th ed. [CD-ROM version 1.5]. Bethesda, MD: American Society of Health-System Pharmacists; 2005.
28. Hatton J, Leur M, Hirsch J, et al. Histamine receptor antagonists and lipid stability in total nutrient admixtures. *JPEN.* 1994;18:308-312.
29. Baptista RJ, Palombo JD, Tahan SR, et al. Stability of cimetidine hydrochloride in a total nutrient admixture. *Am J Hosp Pharm.* 1985;42:2208-2210.
30. Jefferys DB, Vale JA. Cimetidine and bradycardia. *Lancet.* 1978;1:828. Letter.
31. Smith CL, Bardgett DM, Hunter JM. Haemodynamic effects of the IV administration of cimetidine or ranitidine in the critically ill patient. A double-blind prospective study. *Br J Anaesth.* 1987;59:1397-1402.
32. Thompson J, Lilly J. Cimetidine-induced cerebral toxicity in children. *Lancet.* 1979;1:725.
33. Bale JF, Roberts C, Book LS. Cimetidine-induced cerebral toxicity in children. *Lancet.* 1979;1:725-726.
34. Kuint J, Linder N, Reichman B. Hypoxemia associated with cimetidine therapy in a newborn infant. *Am J Perinatol.* 1996;13:301-303.
35. Guillet R, Stoll BJ, Cotton CM, et al. Association of H2-blocker therapy and higher incidence of necrotizing enterocolitis in very low birth weight infants. *Pediatrics.* 2006;117:e137-e142.

Ciprofloxacin Lactate

1. *Physicians' Desk Reference.* 60th ed. Montvale, NJ: Thomson PDR; 2006.
2. Schaad UB, Stoupis C, Wedgewood J, et al. Clinical, radiologic and magnetic resonance monitoring for skeletal toxicity in pediatric patients with cystic fibrosis receiving a three-month course of ciprofloxacin. *Pediatr Infect Dis J.* 1991;10:723-729.
3. Orenstein DM, Pattishall EN, Noyes BE, et al. Safety of ciprofloxacin in children with cystic fibrosis. *Clin Pediatr.* 1993;32:504-506.
4. Schaad UB, Sander E, Wedgewood J, et al. Morphologic studies for skeletal toxicity after prolonged ciprofloxacin therapy in two juvenile cystic fibrosis patients. *Pediatr Infect Dis J.* 1992;11:1047-1049.
5. Schaad UB, Wedgewood J. Lack of quinolone-induced arthropathy in children. *J Antimicrob Chemother.* 1992;30:414-416.
6. Hampel B, Hullmann R, Schmidt H. Ciprofloxacin in pediatrics: worldwide clinical experience based on compassionate use-safety report. *Pediatr Infect Dis J.* 1997;16:127-129.

References

7. Jick S. Ciprofloxacin safety in a pediatric population. *Pediatr Infect Dis J.* 1997;16:130-134.
8. Camp KA, Miyagi SL, Schroeder DJ. Potential quinolone-induced cartilage toxicity in children. *Ann Pharmacother.* 1994;28:336-338.
9. American Academy of Pediatrics. In: Pickering LK, ed. *2003 Red Book: Report of the Committee on Infectious Diseases.* 26th ed. Elk Grove Village, IL: American Academy of Pediatrics; 2003.
10. Lumbiganon P, Pengsaa K, Sookpranee T, et al. Ciprofloxacin in neonates and its possible adverse effect on teeth. *Pediatr Infect Dis J.* 1991;10:619-620.
11. Wessalowski R, Thomas L, Kivit J, et al. Multiple brain abscesses caused by Salmonella enteritidis in a neonate: successful treatment with ciprofloxacin. *Pediatr Infect Dis J.* 1993;12:683-688.
12. Van den Oever HL, Versteegh FG, Thewessen EA, et al. Ciprofloxacin in preterm neonates: case report and review of the literature. *Eur J Pediat.* 1998;157:843-845.
13. Krcmery V, Filka J, Uher J, et al. Ciprofloxacin in treatment of nosocomial meningitis in neonates and in infants: report of 12 cases and review. *Diagn Microbiol Infect Dis.* 1999;35:75-80.
14. Drossou-Agakidou V, Roilides E, Papakyriakidou-Koliouska P, et al. Use of ciprofloxacin in neonatal sepsis: lack of adverse events up to one year. *Pediatr Infect Dis J.* 2004;23:346-349.
15. Lipman J, Gous AG, Mathivha LR, et al. Ciprofloxacin pharmacokinetic profiles in paediatric sepsis: how much ciprofloxacin is enough? *Intensive Care Med.* 2002;28:493-500.
16. Goepp JG, Lee CK, Anderson T, et al. Use of ciprofloxacin in an infant with ventriculitis. *J Pediatr.* 1992;121:303-305.
17. Inglesby TV, O'Toole T, Henderson DA, et al., for the Working Group on Civilian Biodefense. Anthrax as a biological weapon 2002: updated recommendations for management. *JAMA.* 2002;287:2236-2252.
18. Centers for Disease Control and Prevention. Update: Investigation of bioterrorism-related anthrax and interim guidelines for exposure management and antimicrobial therapy, October 2001. *MMWR Morb Mortal Wkly Rep.* 2001;50:909-919.
19. Heggers JP, Villarreal C, Edgar P, et al. Ciprofloxacin as a therapeutic modality in pediatric burn wound infections. *Arch Surg.* 1998;133:1247-1250.
20. Church DA, Kanga JF, Kuhn RJ, et al. Sequential ciprofloxacin therapy in pediatric cystic fibrosis: comparative study vs. ceftazidime/tobramycin in the treatment of acute pulmonary exacerbations. *Pediatr Infect Dis J.* 1997;16:97-105.
21. Schaefer HG, Stass H, Wedgwood J, et al. Pharmacokinetics of ciprofloxacin in pediatric cystic fibrosis patients. *Antimicrob Agents Chemother.* 1996;40:29-34.
22. Rubio TT, Miles MV, Lettieri JT, et al. Pharmacokinetic disposition of sequential intravenous/oral ciprofloxacin in pediatric cystic fibrosis patients with acute pulmonary exacerbation. *Pediatr Infect Dis J.* 1997;16:112-117.
23. Dutta P, Rasaily R, Saha R, et al. Ciprofloxacin for treatment of severe typhoid fever in children. *Antimicrob Agents Chemother.* 1993;37:1197-1199.
24. Thomsen LL, Paerregaard A. Treatment with ciprofloxacin in children with typhoid fever. *Scand J Infect Dis.* 1998;30:355-357.
25. Aronoff A, Brier M, Bennett W. *The Renal Book, 2002.* http://www.kdp-baptist.louisville.edu/renalbook/. Accessed September 6, 2006.
26. Gasser TC, Ebert SC, Graversen PH, et al. Ciprofloxacin pharmacokinetics in patients with normal and impaired renal function. *Antimicrob Agents Chemother.* 1987;31:709-712.
27. Gasser TC, Ebert SC, Graverson PH, et al. Pharmacokinetic study of patients with impaired renal function. *Am J Med.* 1987;82:139-141.
28. Esposito S, Miniero M, Barba D, et al. Pharmacokinetics of ciprofloxacin in impaired liver function. *Int J Clin Pharm Res.* 1989;9:37-41.
29. Chysky V, Kapila K, Hullman R, et al. Safety of ciprofloxacin in children: worldwide clinical experience based on compassionate use. Emphasis on joint evaluation. *Infection.* 1991;19:289-296.
30. Hussey G, Kibel M, Parker N, et al. Ciprofloxacin treatment of multiply drug-resistant extrapulmonary tuberculosis in a child. *Pediatr Infect Dis J.* 1992;11:408-409.
31. Trissel LA, ed. *Handbook on Injectable Drugs.* 13th ed. [CD-ROM version 1.5]. Bethesda, MD: American Society of Health-System Pharmacists; 2005.
32. Davis H, McGoodwin E, Reed TG. Anaphylactoid reactions reported after treatment with ciprofloxacin. *Ann Intern Med.* 1989;111:1041-1043.
33. Deamer RL, Prichard JG, Loman GJ. Hypersensitivity and anaphylactoid reactions to ciprofloxacin. *DICP Ann Pharmacother.* 1992;26:1081-1084.
34. Arcieri GM. Safety of intravenous ciprofloxacin: a review. *Am J Med.* 1989;87(suppl 5A):92-97.
35. Atasoy H, Erdem G, Ceyhan M, et al. Hypertension associated with ciprofloxacin use in an infant. *Ann Pharmacother.* 1995;29:1049.
36. Erdem G, Staat MA, Connelly BL, et al. Anaphylactic reaction to ciprofloxacin in a toddler: successful desensitization. *Pediatr Infect Dis J.* 1999;18:563-564.
37. Lantner RR. Ciprofloxacin desensitization in a patient with cystic fibrosis. *J Allergy Clin Immunol.* 1995;96:1001-1002.

Cisatracurium Besylate

1. *Physicians' Desk Reference.* 60th ed. Montvale; NJ: Thomson PDR; 2006.
2. Rowlee SC. Monitoring neuromuscular blockade in the intensive care unit: the peripheral nerve stimulator. *Heart Lung.* 1999;28:352-362.
3. Martin LD, Bratton SL, O'Rourke PP. Clinical uses and controversies of neuromuscular blocking agents in infants and children. *Crit Care Med.* 1999;27:1358-1368.
4. de Ruiter J, Crawford MW. Dose-response relationship and infusion requirements of cisatracurium besylate in infants and children during nitrous oxide-narcotic anesthesia. *Anesthesiology.* 2001;94:790-792.
5. Reich DL, Hollinger I, Harrington DJ, et al. Comparison of cisatracurium and vecuronium by infusion in neonates and small infants after congenital heart surgery. *Anesthesiology*. 2004;101:1122-1127.
6. Burmester M, Mok Q. Randomised controlled trial comparing cisatracurium and vecuronium infusions in a paediatric intensive care unit. *Intensive Care Med.* 2005;31;686-692.
7. Trissel LA, ed. *Handbook on Injectable Drugs*. 13th ed. [CD-ROM version 1.5]. Bethesda, MD: American Society of Health-System Pharmacists; 2005.
8. Legros CB, Oreliaguet GA, Mayer M, et al. Severe anaphylactic reaction to cisatracurium in a child. *Anesth Analg.* 2001;92:648-649.
9. American Academy of Pediatrics Committee on Drugs. "Inactive" ingredients in pharmaceutical products: update. *Pediatrics.* 1997;99:268-278.
10. Hall CM, Milligan DWA, Berrington J. Probably adverse reaction to a pharmaceutical excipient. *Arch Dis Child Fetal Neonatal Ed.* 2004;89:F184.
11. Hiller JL, Benda GI, Rahatzad M, et al. Benzyl alcohol toxicity: impact on mortality and intraventricular hemorrhage among very low birth weight infants. *Pediatrics.* 1986;77:500-506.
12. Grant JA, Bilodeau PA, Guernsey BG, et al. Unsuspected benzyl alcohol hypersensitivity. *N Engl J Med*. 1982;306:108.
13. Wilson JP, Solimando DA, Edwards MS. Parenteral benzyl alcohol-induced hypersensitivity reaction. *Drug Intell Clin Pharm.* 1986;20:689-691.
14. Davis NA, Rodgers JE, Gonzalez ER, et al. Prolonged weakness after cisatracurium infusion: a case report. *Crit Care Med.* 1998;26:1290-1292.
15. Watling SM, Dasta JF. Prolonged paralysis in intensive care unit patients after the use of neuromuscular blocking agents: a review of the literature. *Crit Care Med.* 1994;22:884-893.
16. Panacek EA, Sherman B. Hydrocortisone and pancuronium bromide: acute myopathy during status asthmaticus. *Crit Care Med.* 1988;16:732.

References

Cisplatin

1. American Society of Health-System Pharmacists. American Hospital Formulary System. Available at: http://ahfsfirst.firstdatabank.com/AHFSfirst/NSAHFSFirstSearchmain.asp. Accessed September 26, 2006.
2. Platinol-AQ [package insert]. Princeton, NJ: Bristol-Meyers Squibb; October 1999.
3. Kushner B, Helson L. Coordinated use of sequentially escalated cyclophosphamide and cell-cycle-specific chemotherapy (N4SE Protocol) for advanced neuroblastoma: experience with 100 patients. *J Clin Oncol*. 1987;5:1746-1751.
4. West DC, Shamberger RC, Macklis RM, et al. Stage III neuroblastoma over 1 year of age at diagnosis: improved survival with intensive multimodality therapy including multiple alkylating agents. *J Clin Oncol*. 1993;11:84-90.
5. McWilliams NB, Hayes FA, Green AA, et al. Cyclophosphamide/doxorubicin vs. cisplatin/teniposide in the treatment of children older than 12 months of age with disseminated neuroblastoma: a pediatric oncology group randomized phase II study. *Med Ped Onc*. 1995;24:176-180.
6. Gasparini M, Tondini C, Rottoli L, et al. Continuous cisplatin infusion in combination with vincristine and high-dose methotrexate for advanced osteogenic sarcoma. *Am J Clin Oncol*. 1987;10:152-155.
7. Uchida A, Myoui A, Araki N, et al. Neoadjuvant chemotherapy for pediatric osteosarcoma patients. *Cancer*. 1997;79:411-415.
8. Harris MB, Gieser P, Goorin AM, et al. Treatment of metastatic osteosarcoma at diagnosis: a pediatric oncology group study. *J Clin Onc*. 1998;16:3641-3648.
9. Walker RW, Allen, JC. Cisplatin in the treatment of recurrent childhood primary brain tumors. *J Clin Oncol*. 1988;6:62-66.
10. Nitsche R, Starling K, et al. Cis-diamminedichloroplatinum (NSC-119875) in childhood malignancies. A southwest oncology group study. *Med Ped Onc*. 1978;4:127-132.
11. Kamalakar P, Freeman A, Higby DJ, et al. Clinical response and toxicity with cis-dichlorodiammineplatinum(II) in children. *Cancer Treat Rep*. 1977; 61:835-839.
12. Aronoff GR, Berns JS, Brier ME, et al. *Drug Prescribing in Renal Failure: Dosing Guidelines for Adults.* 4th ed. Philadelphia, PA: American College of Physicians; 1999.
13. Taketomo CK, Hodding JH, Kraus DM, eds. *Pediatric Dosage Handbook.* 12th ed. [CD-ROM version 2006.1]. Hudson, OH: Lexi-Comp; 2006.
14. Trissel LA, ed. *Handbook on Injectable Drugs.* 13th ed. [CD-ROM version 1.5]. Bethesda, MD: American Society of Health-System Pharmacists; 2005.
15. MacCara ME. Extravasation: a hazard of intravenous therapy. *Drug Intell Clin Pharm*. 1983;17:713-717.
16. Gutierrez ML, Crooke ST. Pediatric cancer chemotherapy: an updated review I. Cis-diamminedichloroplatinum II (cisplatin), VM-26 (teniposide), VP-16 (etoposide), mitomycin C. *Cancer Treat Rev*. 1979;6:153-164.
17. Jaffe N, Keifer R III, Robertson R, et al. Renal toxicity with cumulative doses of cis-diamminedichloroplatinum II in pediatric patients with osteosarcoma. *Cancer*. 1987;59:1577-1581.
18. Marin AC, Rierson B. Peripheral neuropathy secondary to cis-Dichlorodiammino-platinum (II) (Platinol). Treatment for advanced ovarian cancer. *Ariz Med*. 1979;36:898-899.
19. Mollman JE. Cisplatin neurotoxicity. *N Engl J Med*. 1990;2:126-127.
20. Greenspan A, Treat J. Peripheral neuropathy and low dose cisplatin. *Am J Clin Onc*. 1988;11:660-662.
21. Blachley JD, Hill JB. Renal and electrolyte disturbances associated with cisplatin. *Ann Intern Med*. 1981;95:628-632.
22. Piel IJ, Meyer D, Perlia CP, et al. Effects of cis-diamminedichloroplatinum (NSC-119875) on hearing function in man. *Cancer Chemother Rep*. 1974;58:871.
23. Moroso MJ, Blair R. A review of cis-platinum ototoxicity. *J Otolaryngol*. 1983;12:365-369.
24. Reddel RR, Kefford RF, Grant JM, et al. Ototoxicity in patients receiving cisplatin: importance of dose and method of drug administration. *Cancer Treat Rep*. 1982;66:19.
25. National Comprehensive Cancer Network (NCCN) Antiemesis Panel Members. NCCN Clinical Practice Guidelines in Oncology. Antiemesis, v.1.2006. Available at www.nccn.org. Accessed March 29, 2006.
26. Roila F, Feyer P, Maranzamo E, et al. Antiemetics in children receiving chemotherapy. *Support Care Cancer*. 2005;13:129-131.

Clindamycin Phosphate

1. American Academy of Pediatrics. In: Pickering LK, ed. *Red Book: 2003 Report of the Committee on Infectious Diseases.* 26th ed. Elk Grove Village, IL: American Academy of Pediatrics; 2003.
2. Nelson JD, Bradley JS, eds. *Pocketbook of Pediatric Antimicrobial Therapy.* 14th ed. Baltimore, MD: Lippincott Williams & Wilkins; 2000–2001.
3. Koren G, Zarfin Y, Maresky D, et al. Pharmacokinetics of intravenous clindamycin in newborn infants. *Pediatr Pharmacol.* 1986;5:287-292.
4. Bell M, Shackelford P, Smith R, et al. Pharmacokinetics of clindamycin phosphate in the first year of life. *J Pediatr*. 1984;105:482-486.
5. Faix RG, Polley TZ, Grasela TH. A randomized controlled trial of parenteral clindamycin in neonatal necrotizing enterocolitis. *J Pediatr.* 1988;112:271-277.
6. Young TE, Mangum B, eds. *Neofax®*. 18th ed. Raleigh, NC: Acorn Publishing Inc; 2005.
7. Feigin RD, Pickering LK, Anderson D, et al. Clindamycin treatment of osteomyelitis and septic arthritis in children. *Pediatrics.* 1975;55:213-223.
8. Jacobson SJ, Griffiths K, Diamond S, et al. A randomized controlled trial of penicillin vs. clindamycin for the treatment of aspiration pneumonia in children. *Arch Pediatr Adolesc Med.* 1997;151:701-704.
9. Inglesby TV, O'Toole T, Henderson DA. et al for the Working Group on Civilian Biodefense. Anthrax as a biological weapon 2002: updated recommendations for management. *JAMA.* 2002;287:2236-2252.
10. Centers for Disease Control and Prevention. Update: Investigation of bioterrorism-related anthrax and interim guidelines for exposure management and antimicrobial therapy, October 2001. *MMWR Morb Mortal Wkly Rep.* 2001;50:909-919.
11. Ciftci AO, Tanyel FC, Buyukpamukcu N, et al. Comparative trial of four antibiotic combinations for perforated appendicitis in children. *Eur J Surg.* 1997;163:591-596.
12. Antimicrobial prophylaxis for surgery. *Treat Guidel Med Lett.* 2004;2:27–32.
13. Bratzler DW, Houck PM; et al. Antimicrobial prophylaxis for surgery: an advisory statement from the National Surgical Infection Prevention Project. *Clin Infect Dis.* 2004;38:1706-1715.
14. Aronoff A, Brier M, Bennett W. *The Renal Book, 2002.* Available at: http://www.kdp-baptist.louisville.edu/renalbook/. Accessed June 10, 2006.
15. Cleocin Phosphate® (clindamycin phosphate) injection and injection in 5% dextrose [prescribing information]. Kalamazoo, MI: Pharmacia & Upjohn Company; September 2003.
16. American Society of Health-System Pharmacists. American Hospital Formulary System. Available at: http://ahfsfirst.firstdatabank.com/AHFSfirst/NSAHFSFirstSearchmain.asp. Accessed June 10, 2006.
17. Trissel LA, ed. *Handbook on Injectable Drugs.* 13th ed. [CD-ROM version 1.5]. Bethesda, MD: American Society of Health-System Pharmacists; 2005.
18. American Academy of Pediatrics Committee on Drugs. "Inactive" ingredients in pharmaceutical products: update. *Pediatrics.* 1997;99:268-278.
19. Hall CM, Milligan DWA, Berrington J. Probably adverse reaction to a pharmaceutical excipient. *Arch Dis Child Fetal Neonatal Ed.* 2004;89: F184.
20. Hiller JL, Benda GI, Rahatzad M, et al. Benzyl alcohol toxicity: impact on mortality and intraventricular hemorrhage among very low birth weight infants. *Pediatrics.* 1986;77:500-506.

21. Grant JA, Bilodeau PA, Guernsey BG, et al. Unsuspected benzyl alcohol hypersensitivity. *N Engl J Med.* 1982;306:108.
22. Wilson JP, Solimando DA, Edwards MS. Parenteral benzyl alcohol-induced hypersensitivity reaction. *Drug Intell Clin Pharm.* 1986;20:689-691.
23. Beavers-May T, Jacobs RF. Clinical and laboratory issues in community-acquired MRSA. *J Pediatr Pharmacol Ther.* 2004;9:82-88.

Co-Trimoxazole (Trimethoprim-Sulfamethoxazole)

1. Sulfamethoxazole and trimethoprim injection [USP package insert]. Irvine, CA: Sicor Pharmaceuticals Inc; 2005.
2. American Academy of Pediatrics. In: Pickering LK, ed. *2003 Red Book: Report of the Committee on Infectious Diseases.* 26th ed. Elk Grove Village, IL: American Academy of Pediatrics; 2003.
3. Tunkel AR, Hartman BJ, Kaplan SL, et al. Practice guidelines for the management of bacterial meningitis. *Clin Infect Dis.* 2004;39:1267-1284.
4. Armstrong RW, Slater B. Listeria monocytogenes meningitis treated with trimethoprim–sulfamethoxazole. *Pediatr Infect Dis.* 1986;5:712-713.
5. Ferlauto JJ, Wells DH. Flavobacterium meningosepticum in the neonatal period. *South Med J.* 1981;74:757-759.
6. Murphy TF, Fernald GW. Trimethoprim–sulfamethoxazole therapy for relapses of Salmonella meningitis. *Pediatr Infect Dis.* 1983;2:465-468.
7. Tamer MA, Bray JD. Trimethoprim–sulfamethoxazole treatment of multiantibiotic-resistant staphylococcal endocarditis and meningitis. *Clin Pediatr.* 1982;21:125-126.
8. Hughes WT, Feldman S, Chaudhary SC, et al. Comparison of pentamidine isethionate and trimethoprim–sulfamethoxazole in the treatment of Pneumocystis carinii pneumonia. *J Pediatr.* 1978;92:285-291.
9. Sattler FR, Remington JS. Intravenous trimethoprim–sulfamethoxazole therapy for Pneumocystis carinii pneumonia. *Am J Med.* 1981;70:1215-1221.
10. Wharton JM, Coleman DL, Wofsy CB, et al. Trimethoprim–sulfamethoxazole or pentamidine for Pneumocystis carinii pneumonia in the acquired immunodeficiency syndrome: a prospective randomized trial. *Ann Intern Med.* 1986;105:37-44.
11. Small CB, Harris CA, Friedland GH, et al. The treatment of Pneumocystis carinii pneumonia in the acquired immunodeficiency syndrome. *Arch Intern Med.* 1985;145:837-840.
12. Hughes WT. Trimethoprim–sulfamethoxazole therapy for Pneumocystis carinii pneumonitis in children. *Rev Infect Dis.* 1982;4:602-607.
13. Lipson A, Marshall WC, Hayward AR. Treatment of Pneumocystis carinii pneumonia in children. *Arch Dis Child.* 1977; 52:314-319.
14. Larter WE, John TJ, Sieber OF, et al. Trimethoprim–sulfamethoxazole treatment of Pneumocystis carinii pneumonitis. *J Pediatr.* 1978;92:826-828.
15. Siegel SE, Wolff LJ, Baehner RL, et al. Treatment of Pneumocystis carinii pneumonitis. A comparative trial of sulfamethoxazole–trimethoprim vs. pentamidine in pediatric patients with cancer: report from the children's cancer study group. *Am J Dis Child.* 1984;138:1051-1054.
16. Hoppu K, Koskimies O, Tuomisto J. Trimethoprim pharmacokinetics in children with renal insufficiency. *Clin Pharmacol Ther.* 1987;42:181-186.
17. Siber GR, Gorham CC, Ericson JF, et al. Pharmacokinetics of intravenous trimethoprim–sulfamethoxazole in children and adults with normal and impaired renal function. *Rev Infect Dis.* 1982;4:566-578.
18. Welling PG, Craig WA, Amidon GL, et al. Pharmacokinetics of trimethoprim and sulfamethoxazole in normal subjects and in patients with renal failure. *J Infect Dis.* 1973;128(suppl):S556-S566.
19. Baumgartner TG, Russell WL. Intravenous trimethoprim–sulfamethoxazole administration alert. *Am J IV Ther Clin Nutr.* 1983;10:14-15.
20. Jarosinski PF, Kennedy PE, Gallelli JF. Stability on concentrated trimethoprim-sulfamethoxazole admixtures. *Am J Hosp Pharm.* 1989;46:732-737.
21. American Society of Health-System Pharmacists. American Hospital Formulary System. Available at: http://ahfsfirst.firstdatabank.com/AHFSfirst/NSAHFSFirstSearchmain.asp. Accessed September 9, 2006.
22. American Academy of Pediatrics Committee on Drugs. "Inactive" ingredients in pharmaceutical products: update. *Pediatrics.* 1997;99:268-278.
23. Smolinske SC. Review of parenteral sulfite reactions. *J Toxicol Clin Toxicol.* 1992;30:597-606.
24. Lester MR. Sulfite sensitivity: significance in human health. *J Am Col Nutr.* 1995;14:229-232.
25. Louis S, Kutt H, McDowell F. The cardiocirculatory changes caused by intravenous Dilantin and its solvent. *Am Heart J.* 1967;74:523-529.
26. Glasgow AM, Boeckx RL, Miller MK, et al. Hyper-osmolality in small infants due to propylene glycol. *Pediatrics.* 1983;72:353-355.
27. MacDonald MG, Getson PR, Glasgow AM, et al. Propylene glycol: increased incidence of seizures in low birth weight infants. *Pediatrics.* 1987;79:622-625.
28. Hall CM, Milligan DWA, Berrington J. Probably adverse reaction to a pharmaceutical excipient. *Arch Dis Child Fetal Neonatal Ed.* 2004;89:F184.
29. Hiller JL, Benda GI, Rahatzad M, et al. Benzyl alcohol toxicity: impact on mortality and intraventricular hemorrhage among very low birth weight infants. *Pediatrics.* 1986;77:500-506.
30. Grant JA, Bilodeau PA, Guernsey BG, et al. Unsuspected benzyl alcohol hypersensitivity. *N Engl J Med.* 1982;306:108.
31. Wilson JP, Solimando DA, Edwards MS. Parenteral benzyl alcohol-induced hypersensitivity reaction. *Drug Intell Clin Pharm.* 1986;20:689-691.

Coagulation Factor VIIa (Recombinant) (rFVIIa)

1. NovoSeven® (Coagulation Factor VIIa recombinant) [prescribing information]. Princeton, NJ: Novo Nordisk Inc; October 2005.
2. Gelman CR, Rumack BH, Hess AJ, eds. *DRUGDEX® System.* Englewood, CO: MICROMEDEX Inc. Accessed August 20, 2006.
3. Pirrello R, Siragusa S, Giambona C, et al. Bleeding prophylaxis in a child with cleft palate and factor VII deficiency: a case report. *Cleft Palate Craniofac J.* 2006;43:108-111.
4. O'Connell KA, Wood JJ, Wise RP, et al. Thromboembolic adverse events after use of recombinant human coagulation factor VIIa. *JAMA.* 2006;295:293-298.
5. Pychynska-Pokorska M, Moll JJ, Krajewski W, et al. The use of recombinant factor VIIa in uncontrolled postoperative bleeding in children undergoing cardiac surgery with cardiopulmonary bypass. *Pediatr Crit Care Med.* 2004;5:246-250.
6. Tobias JD, Berkenbosch JW, Russo P. Recombinant factor FIIa to treat bleeding after cardiac surgery in an infant. *Pediatr Crit Care Med.* 2003;4:49-51.
7. Al Douri M, Shafi T, Al Khudairi D, et al. Effect of the administration of recombinant factor VII (rFIIa; NovoSeven) in the management of severe uncontrolled bleeding in patients undergoing heart valve replacement surgery. *Blood Coagul Fibrinolysis.* 2000;11(suppl):S121-S127.
8. Malherbe S, Tsui BCH, Stobart K, et al. Argatroban as an anticoagulant in cardiopulmonary bypass in an infant and attempted reversal with recombinant activated factor VII. *Anesthesiol.* 2004;100:443-445.
9. Dominguez TE, Mitchell M, Friess SH, et al. Use of recombinant factor VIIa for refractory hemorrhage during extracorporeal membrane oxygenation. *Pediatr Crit Care Med.* 2005;6:348-351.
10. Wittenstein B, Ravn H, Goldman A. Recombinant factor VII for severe bleeding during extracorporeal membrane oxygenation following open heart surgery. *Pediatr Crit Care Med.* 2005;6:473-476.
11. Tofil NM, Winkler MK, Watts RG, et al. The use of recombinant factor VIIa in a patient with Noonan syndrome and life-threatening bleeding. *Pediatr Crit Care Med.* 2005;6:352-354.
12. Kurekci AE, Atay AA, Okutan V, et al. Recombinant activated factor VII for severe gastrointestinal bleeding after chemotherapy in an infant with acute megakaryoblastic leukemia. *Blood Coagul Fibrinolysis.* 2005;16:145-147.

13. Brown JB, Emerick KM, Brown DL, et al. Recombinant factor VIIa improves coagulopathy caused by liver failure. *J Pediatr Gastroenterol Nutr.* 2003;37:268-272.
14. Pettersson M, Fischler B, Petrini P, et al. Recombinant FVIIa in children with liver disease. *Thrombosis Res.* 2005;116:185-197.
15. Atkison PR, Jardine L, Williams S, et al. Use of recombinant factor VIIa in pediatric patients with liver failure and severe coagulopathy. *Transplant Proc.* 2005;37:1091-1093.
16. Barro C, Brobleski I, Piolat C, et al. Successful use of recombinant factor VIIa for severe surgical liver bleeding in a 5 month old baby. *Haemophilia.* 2004;10:183-185.
17. Kalicinski P, Kaminski A, Drewniak T, et al. Quick correction of hemostasis in two patients with fulminant liver failure undergoing liver transplantation by recombinant activated factor VII. *Transplant Proc.* 1999;31:378-379.
18. Markiewicz M, Kalicinski P, Kaminski A, et al. Acute coagulopathy after reperfusion of the liver graft in children correction with recombinant activated factor VII. *Transplant Proc.* 2003;35:2381-2391.
19. Pavese P, Bonodona A, Beaubien J, et al. FVIIa corrects the coagulopathy of fulminant hepatic failure but may be associated with thrombosis: a report of four cases. *Can J Anesth.* 2005;52:26-29.
20. Ozelo MC, Svirin P, Larina L. Use of recombinant factor VIIa in the management of severe bleeding episodes in patients with Bernard-Soulier syndrome. *Ann Hematol.* 2005;84:816-822.
21. Poon MC, Demers C, Jobin F, et al. Recombinant factor VIIa is effective for bleeding and surgery in patients with glanzmann thromboasthenia. *Blood.* 1999;94:3951-3953.
22. Almedia AM, Khair K, Hann I, et al. The use of recombinant factor VIIa in children with inherited platelet function disorders. *Br J Hematol.* 2003;121:477-481.
23. Olomu N, Kulkarni R, Manco-Johnson M. Treatment of severe pulmonary hemorrhage with activated recombinant factor VII (rFIIa) in very low birth weight infants. *J Perinatol.* 2002;22:672-674.
24. Duncan A, Benson L, Critz A, et al. Neonatal coagulopathy treatment with rFVIIa. *Pediatr Res.* 2001;49:290A.
25. Cetin H, Yalaz M, Akisu M, et al. The use of recombinant activated factor VII in the treatment of massive pulmonary hemorrhage in a preterm infant. *Blood Coagul Fibrinolysis.* 2006;17:213-216.
26. Veldman A, Josef J, Fischer D, et al. A prospective pilot study of prophylactic treatment of preterm neonates with recombinant activated factor VII during the first 72 hours of life. *Pediatr Crit Care Med.* 2006;7:34-39.
27. Filan PM, Mills JF, Clarnette TD, et al. Spontaneous liver hemorrhage during laparotomy for necrotizing enterocolitis: a potential role for recombinant factor VIIa. *J Pediatr.* 2005;147:857-859.
28. Schulman S. Safety, efficacy, and lessons from continuous infusion with rFVIIa. *Haemophilia.* 1998;4:564-567.
29. Schulman S. Continuous infusion of recombinant factor VIIa in hemophilic patients with inhibitors: safety, monitoring, and cost effectiveness. *Semin Thromb Hemost.* 2000;26:421-424.
30. Montoro JB, Altisent C, Pico M, et al. Recombinant factor VIIa in continuous infusion during central line insertion in a child with factor VIII high-titre inhibitor. *Haemophilia*. 1998;4:762-765.
31. Erhardtsen E. Pharmacokinetics of recombinant activated factor VII (rFVIIa). *Semin Thromb Hemost.* 2000;26:385-391.
32. Velik-Salchner C, Sergi C, Fries D, et al. Use of recombinant factor FVIIa (Novoseven®) in combination with other coagulation products led to a thrombotic occlusion of the truncus brachiocephalicus in a neonate supported by extracorporeal membrane oxygenation. *Anesth Analg.* 2005;101:920-929.

Cyclophosphamide

1. Cytoxan [package insert]. Deerfield, IL: Baxter; November 2003.
2. Solimando DA, ed. *Lexi-Comp's Drug Information Handbook for Oncology.* 4th ed. Hudson, OH: Lexi-Comp; 2004:210-218.
3. American Society of Health-System Pharmacists. American Hospital Formulary System. Available at: http://ahfsfirst.firstdatabank.com/AHFSfirst/NSAHFSFirstSearchmain.asp. Accessed May 10, 2006.
4. Taketomo CK, ed. *Lexi-comp's Pediatric Dosage Handbook.* 12th ed. Hudson, OH: Lexi-Comp; 2005:353-355.
5. Spunt SL, Smith LM, Ruymann FB, et al. Cyclophosphamide dose intensification during induction therapy for intermediate-risk pediatric rhabdomyosarcoma is feasible but does not improve outcome: a report from the soft tissue sarcoma committee of the children's oncology group. *Clin Cancer Res.* 2004;10(18 Pt 1):6072-6079.
6. Lehman TJ, Onel K. Intermittent intravenous cyclophosphamide arrests progression of the renal chronicity index in childhood systemic lupus erythematosus. *J Pediatr.* 2000;136(2):243-247.
7. Yee CS, Gordon C, Dostal C, et al. EULAR randomised controlled trial of pulse cyclophosphamide and methylprednisolone versus continuous cyclophosphamide and prednisolone followed by azathioprine and prednisolone in lupus nephritis. *Ann Rheum Dis.* 2004;63(5):525-529.
8. Cassileth PA, Harrington DP, Appelbaum FR, et al. Chemotherapy compared with autologous or allogeneic bone marrow transplantation in the management of acute myeloid leukemia in first remission. *N Engl J Med.* 1998;339(23):1649-1656.
9. Trissel LA, ed. *Handbook on Injectable Drugs.* 13th ed. [CD-ROM version 1.5]. Bethesda, MD: American Society of Health-System Pharmacists; 2005.
10. National Comprehensive Cancer Network (NCCN) Antiemesis Panel Members. NCCN Clinical Practice Guidelines in Oncology. Antiemesis, v.1.2006. Available at: www.nccn.org. Accessed March 29, 2006.
11. Roila F, Feyer P, Maranzamo E, et al. Antiemetics in children receiving chemotherapy. *Support Care Cancer.* 2005;13(2):129-131.

Cyclosporine

1. Margarit C, Ibanez VM, Potau N, et al. Cyclosporine in pediatric liver transplantation: is there a therapeutic blood level that abrogates rejection? *Transplant Proc.* 1988;20(suppl 3):369-374.
2. Burckart G, Starzl T, Williams L, et al. Cyclosporine monitoring and pharmacokinetics in pediatric liver transplant patients. *Transplant Proc.* 1985;17:1172-1175.
3. Wonigeit K, Brolsch C, Neuhaus P, et al. Special aspects of immunosuppression with cyclosporine in liver transplantation. *Transplant Proc.* 1983;15:2586-2591.
4. Yee GC, Lennon TP, Gmur DJ, et al. Age-dependent cyclosporine: pharmacokinetics in marrow transplant recipients. *Clin Pharmacol Ther.* 1986;40:438-443.
5. Clardy CW, Schroeder TJ, Myre SA, et al. Clinical variability of cyclosporine pharmacokinetics in adult and pediatric patients after renal, cardiac, hepatic, and bone-marrow transplants. *Clin Chem.* 1988;34:2012-2015.
6. Burckart GJ, Venkataramanan R, Ptachcinski RJ, et al. Cyclosporine absorption following orthotopic liver transplantation. *J Clin Pharmacol.* 1986;26:647-651.
7. Tzakis AG, Reyes J, Todo S, et al. FK506 versus cyclosporine in pediatric liver transplantation. *Transplant Proc.* 1991;23:3010-3015.
8. McDiarmid SV, Busuttil RW, Ascher NL, et al. FK506 (Tacrolimus) compared with cyclosporine for primary immunosuppression after pediatric liver transplantation. *Transplantation.* 1995;59:530-536.
9. Chiavarelli M, Boucek MM, Nehlsen-Cannarella SL, et al. Neonatal cardiac transplantation. *Arch Surg.* 1992;127:1072-1076.
10. Kahan BD, Conley S, Portman R, et al. Parent-to-child transplantation with cyclosporine immunosuppression. *J Pediatr.* 1987;111:1012-1016.
11. Conley SB, al-Urzi A, So S, et al. Prevention of rejection and graft loss with an aggressive quadruple immunosuppressive therapy regimen in children and adolescents. *Transplantation.* 1994;57:540-544.

References

12. Houtenbos I, Bracho F, Davenport V, et al. Autologous bone marrow transplantation for childhood acute lymphoblastic leukemia: a novel combined approach consisting of *ex vivo* marrow purging, modulation of multi-drug resistance, induction of autograft vs. leukemia effect, and post-transplant immuno- and chemotherapy (PTIC). *Bone Marrow Transplant.* 2001;27:145-153.
13. Alvarez F, Atkinson PR, Grant DR, et al. NOF-11: A one-year pediatric randomized double-blind comparison of neoral versus sandimmune in orthotopic liver transplantation. *Transplantation.* 2000;69:87-92.
14. Benfield MR, Tejani A, Harmon WE, et al. A randomized multicenter trial of OKT3 mAbs induction compared with intravenous cyclosporine in pediatric renal transplantation. *Pediatr Transplant.* 2005;9:282-292.
15. Salomon R, Gagnadoux M, Niaudet P. Intravenous cyclosporine therapy in recurrent nephrotic syndrome after renal transplantation in children. *Transplantation.* 2003;75:810-814.
16. Schwinghammer TL, Bloom EJ, Rosenfield CS, et al. High-dose cyclosporine and corticosteroids for prophylaxis of acute and chronic graft-versus-host disease. *Bone Marrow Transplant.* 1995;16:147-154.
17. Koga Y, Nagatoshi Y, Kawano Y, et al. Methotrexate *vs* Cyclosporin A as a single agent for graft-versus-host-disease prophylaxis in pediatric patients with hematological malignancies undergoing allogeneic bone marrow transplantation from HLA-identical siblings: a single-center analysis in Japan. *Bone Marrow Transplant.* 2003;32:171-176.
18. Ross M, Schmidt GM, Niland JC, et al. Cyclosporine, methotrexate, and prednisone compared with cyclosporine and prednisone for prevention of acute graft-vs.-host disease: effect on chronic gravt-vs.-host disease and long-term survival. *Biol Blood Marrow Transplant.* 1999;5:285-291.
19. Locatelli F, Zecca M, Rondelli R, et al. Graft versus host disease prophylaxis with low-dose cyclosporine-A reduces the risk of relapse in children with acute leukemia given HLA identical sibling bone marrow transplantation: results of a randomized trial. *Blood.* 2000;95:1572-1579.
20. Chao NJ, Snyder DS, Jain M, et al. Equivalence of 2 effective graft-versus-host disease prophylaxis regimens: results of a prospective double-blind randomized trial. *Biol Blood Marrow Transplant.* 2000;6:254-261.
21. Locatelli F, Bruno B, Zecca M, et al. Cyclosporin A and short-term methotrexate versus cyclosporine A as graft versus host disease prophylaxis in patients with severe aplastic anemia given allogeneic bone marrow transplantation from an HLA-identical sibling: results of a GITMO/EBMT randomized trial. *Blood.* 2000;96:1690-1697.
22. Dahl GV, Lacayo NJ, Brophy N, et al. Mitoxantrone, etoposide, and cyclosporine therapy in pediatric patients with recurrent or refractory acute myeloid leukemia. *J Clin Oncol.* 2000;18:1867-1875.
23. Santos JV, Baudat JA, Casellas FJ, et al. Intravenous cyclosporine for steroid-refractory attacks of Crohn's Disease. *J Clin Gastroenterol.* 1995;20:207-210.
24. Santos J, Baudat S, Casellas FJ, et al. Efficacy of intravenous cyclosporine for steroid refractory attacks of ulcerative colitis. *J Clin Gastroenterol.* 1995;20:285-289.
25. Gurudu SR, Griffel LH, Gialanella RJ, et al. Cyclosporine therapy in inflammatory bowel disease. *J Clin Gastroenterol.* 1999;29:151-154.
26. Carbonnel F, Boruchowicz A, Duclos B, et al. Intravenous cyclosporine in attacks of ulcerative colitis. *Dig Diseases and Sciences.* 1996;41:2471-2476.
27. Egan LJ, Sandborn WJ, Tremaine WJ. Clinical outcome following treatment of refractory inflammatory and fistulizing Crohn's Disease with intravenous cyclosporine. *Am J Gastroenterol.* 1998; 93:442-447.
28. Cohen RD, Stein R, Hanauer SB. Intravenous cyclosporin in ulcerative colitis: a five-year experience. *Am J Gastroenterol.* 1999;94:1587-1592.
29. Bernstein EF, Whitington PF. Successful treatment of atypical sprue in an infant with cyclosporine. *Gastroenterology.* 1988;95:199-204.
30. Aronoff A, Brier M, Bennett W. *The Renal Book, 2002.* Available at: http://www.kdp-baptist.louisville.edu/renalbook/. Accessed May 6, 2006.
31. McEvoy GK, ed. *American Hospital Formulary Service Drug Information 2004.* Bethesda, MD: American Society of Health-System Pharmacists; 2004.
32. Medical Economics, ed. *Physicians' Desk Reference.* 60th ed. Oradell, NJ: Medical Economics Company; 2006.
33. Ptachcinski RJ, Logue LW, Burckart GJ, et al. Stability and availability of cyclosporine in 5% dextrose injection or 0.9% sodium chloride injection. *Am J Hosp Pharm.* 1986;43:94-97.
34. Kahan BD. Cyclosporine. *N Engl J Med.* 1989;321:1725-1738.
35. Friedman LS, Dienstag JL, Nelson PW, et al. Anaphylactic reaction and cardiopulmonary arrest following intravenous cyclosporine. *Am J Med.* 1985;78:343-345.
36. Howrie DL, Ptachcinski RJ, Griffith BP, et al. Anaphylactoid reactions associated with parenteral cyclosporine use: possible role of Cremophor EL. *Drug Intell Clin Pharm.* 1985;19:425-427.
37. Chapuis B, Helg C, Jeannet M, et al. Anaphylactic reaction to intravenous cyclosporine. *N Engl J Med.* 1985;312:1259. Letter.
38. Theis JG, Liau-Chu M, Chan HS, et al. Anaphylactoid reactions in children receiving high-dose intravenous cyclosporine for reversal of tumor resistance: the causative role of improper dissolution of cremophor EL. *J Clin Oncol.* 1995;13:2508-2516.
39. Bisogno G, Cowie F, Boddy A, et al. High-dose cyclosporin with etoposide- toxicity and pharmacokinetic interaction in children with solid tumours. *Br J Cancer.* 1998;77:2304-2309.
40. Napoli KL, Kahan BD. Nonselective measurement of cyclosporine for therapeutic drug monitoring by fluorescence polarization immunoassay with a rabbit polyclonal antibody: I. Evaluation of the serum methodology and comparison with a sheep polyclonal antibody in an ^{3}H tracer-mediated radioimmunoassay. *Transplant Proc.* 1990;22:1175-1181.
41. Napoli KL, Kahan BD. Nonselective measurement of cyclosporine for therapeutic drug monitoring by fluorescence polarization immunoassay with a sheep polyclonal antibody: II. Evaluation of the whole blood methodology and comparison with an ^{3}H tracer-mediated radioimmunoassay with a sheep polyclonal antibody. *Transplant Proc.* 1990;22:1181-1185.
42. Bertault-Peres P, Berland Y, Mucke MK, et al. A novel technique for plasma CSA determination-application to drug monitoring during transplantation. *Transplant Proc.* 1989;21:904-905.
43. Strologo LD, Campagnano P, Federici G, et al. Cyclosporine A monitoring in children: abbreviated area under curve formulas and C2 level. *Pediatr Nephrol.* 1999;13:95-97.
44. Weber LT, Armstrong VW, Shipkova M, et al. Cyclosporin A absorption profiles in pediatric renal transplant recipients predict the risk of acute rejection. *Ther Drug Monit.* 2004;26:415-424.
45. Bowers LD, Canafax DM. Cyclosporine: experience with therapeutic monitoring. *Ther Drug Monit.* 1984;6:142-147.
46. Rodriguez E, Delucchi MA, Cano F. Comparison of cyclosporine concentrations 2 hours post-dose determined using 3 different methods and trough level in pediatric renal transplantation. *Transplant Proc.* 2005;37:3354-3357.
47. Leson CL, Bryson SM, Giesbrecht EE, et al. Therapeutic monitoring if cyclosporine following pediatric bone marrow transplantation: problems with sampling from silicone central venous lines. *DICP Ann Pharmacother.* 1989;23:300-303.
48. Duffner U, Bergstraesser E, Sauter S, et al. Spuriously raised cyclosporin concentrations drawn through polyurethane central venous catheter. *Lancet.* 1998;352:1442.
49. Senner AM, Johnston K, McLachlan AJ. A comparison of peripheral and centrally collected cyclosporine A blood levels in pediatric patients undergoing stem cell transplant. *Oncol Nurs Forum.* 2005;32:73-77.
50. Venkataramanan R, Burckart GJ, Ptachcinski RJ, et al. Leaching of diethylhexyl phthalate from polyvinyl chloride bags into intravenous cyclosporine solution. *Am J Hosp Pharm.* 1986;43:2800-2802.
51. Gotardo MA, Monteiro M. Migration of diethylhexyl phthalate from PVC bags into intravenous cyclosporine solutions. *J Pharm Biomed Anal.* 2005;38:709-713.

References

Cytomegalovirus Immunoglobulin

1. Gungor T, Funk M, Linde R, et al. Combined therapy in human immunodeficiency virus infected children: a four year experience. *Eur J Pediatr.* 1993;152:650-654.
2. Snydman DR, Werner BG, Meissner HC, et al. Use of cytomegalovirus immunoglobulin in multiply transfused premature neonates. *Pediatr Infect Dis J.* 1995;14:34-40.
3. Bowden RA, Fisher LD, Rogers K, et al. Cytomegalovirus (CMV)-specific intravenous immunoglobulin for the prevention of primary CMV infection and disease after marrow transplant. *J Infect Dis.* 1991;164:483-487.
4. CytoGam [package insert]. Gaithersburg, MD: MedImmune Inc; June 2004.
5. Falagas ME, Syndman DR, Ruthazer R, et al. Cytomegalovirus immune globulin (CMVIG) prophylaxis is associated with increased survival after orthotopic liver transplantation. *Clin Transplant.* 1997;11:432-437.
6. Tzakis AG. Cytomegalovirus prophylaxis with ganciclovir and cytomegalovirus immune globulin in liver and intestinal transplantation. *Transpl Infect Dis.* 2001;3:35-39.
7. Fontana I, Verrina E, Timitilli A, et al. Cytomegalovirus infection in pediatric kidney transplantation. *Transplant Proc.* 1994;26:18-19.
8. Snydman DR, Werner BG, Heinze-Lacey B, et al. Use of cytomegalovirus immune globulin to prevent cytomegalovirus disease in renal-transplant recipients. *N Engl J Med.* 1987;317:1049-1054.
9. Murray JC, Bernini JC, Bijou HL, et al. Infantile cytomegalovirus-associated autoimmune hemolytic anemia. *J Pediatr Hematol Oncol.* 2001;23:318-320.
10. Atkinson WL, Pickering LK, Schwartz B, et al. General recommendations on immunization. Recommendations of the Advisory Committee on Immunization Practices (ACIP) and the American Academy of Family Physicians (AAFP). *MMWR Recomm Rep.* 2002;51(RR-2):1-35.

Dactinomycin

1. Cosmegen [package insert]. Whitehouse Station, NJ: Merck & Co Inc; June, 2005.
2. Green DM, Norkool P, Breslow NE, et al. Severe hepatic toxicity after treatment with vincristine and dactinomycin using single-dose or divided-dose schedules: a report from the National Wilms' Tumor Study. *J Clin Oncol.* 1990;8(9):1525-1530.
3. de Carmargo B, Franco EL. A randomized clinical trial of single-dose versus fractionated-dose dactinomycin in the treatment of Wilms' tumor. Results after extended follow-up. Brazilian Wilms' Tumor Study Group. *Cancer.* 1994;73(12):3081-3086.
4. D'Angio GJ, Breslow N, Beckwith JB, et al. Treatment of Wilms' tumor. Results of the Third National Wilms' Tumor Study. *Cancer.* 1989;64(2):349-360.
5. Craft AW, Cotterill SJ, Bullimore JA, et al. Long-term results from the first UKCCSG Ewing's Tumour Study (ET-1). United Kingdom Children's Cancer Study Group (UKCCSG) and the medical research council bone sarcoma working party. *Eur J Cancer.* 1997;33(7):1061-1069.
6. Vugrin D, Herr HW, Whitmore WF, et al. VAB-6 combination chemotherapy in disseminated cancer of the testis. *Ann Intern Med.* 1981;95(1):59-61.
7. Osathanondh R, Goldstein DP, Pastorfide GB, et al. Actinomycin D as the primary agent for gestational trophoblastic disease. *Cancer.* 36(3):863-866.
8. Newlands ES, Bagshawe KD, Begent RH, et al. Results with the EMA/CO (etoposide, methotrexate, actinomycin D, cyclophosphamide, vincristine) regimen in high risk gestational trophoblastic tumours, 1979 to 1989. *Br J Obstet Gynaecol.* 1991;98(6):550-557.
9. Trissel LA, ed. *Handbook on Injectable Drugs.* 13th ed. [CD-ROM version 1.5]. Bethesda, MD: American Society of Health-System Pharmacists; 2005.
10. Arndt C, Hawkins D, Anderson JR, et al. Age is a risk factor for chemotherapy-induced hepatopathy with vincristine, dactinomycin, and cyclophosphamide. *J Clin Oncol.* 2004;22(10):1894-1901.
11. National Comprehensive Cancer Network (NCCN) Antiemesis Panel Members. NCCN Clinical Practice Guidelines in Oncology. Antiemesis, v.1.2006. Available at www.nccn.org. Accessed March 29, 2006.
12. Roila F, Feyer P, Maranzamo E, et al. Antiemetics in children receiving chemotherapy. *Support Care Cancer.* 2005;13:129-131.

Darbepoietin

1. Aranesp [package insert]. Thousand Oaks, CA: Amgen Inc; March 24, 2006.
2. Lerner G, Kale AS, Warady BA, et al. Pharmacokinetics of darbepoetin alfa in pediatric patients with chronic kidney disease. *Pediatr Nephrol.* 2002;17:933-937.
3. Geary DF, Keating LE, Vigneux A, et al. Darbepoetin alfa (Aranesp™) in children with chronic renal failure. *Kidney International.* 2005;68:1759-1765.
4. De Palo T, Giordano M, Palumbo F, et al. Clinical experience with darbepoietin alfa (NESP) in children undergoing hemodialysis. *Pediatr Nephrol.* 2004;19:337-340.
5. Durkan AM, Keating LE, Vigneux A, et al. The use of darbepoetin in infants with chronic renal impairment. *Pediatr Nephrol.* 2006;21:694-697.
6. Joy MS. Darbepoetin alfa: a novel erythropoiesis-stimulating protein. *Ann Pharmacother.* 2002;36:1183-1192.
7. McEvoy GK, ed. *American Hospital Formulary Service Drug Information 2006.* Bethesda, MD: American Society of Health-System Pharmacists; 2006.
8. Thomson PDR, ed. *Physicians' Desk Reference.* 60th ed. Montvale, NJ: Thomson Healthcare; 2006.
9. Pirker R, Vansteenkiste J, Gateley J, et al. A phase III, double-blind, placebo-controlled, randomized study of novel erythropoiesis stimulating protein (NESP) in patients undergoing platinum-treatment for lung cancer. *Eur J Cancer.* 2001;37 (suppl 6)abstract:254.
10. Smith RE Jr, Tchekmedyian NS, Chan D, et al. A dose- and schedule-finding study of darbepoetin alpha for the treatment of chronic anaemia of cancer. *Cancer.* 2003;88:1851-1858
11. Glaspy J, Jadeja J, Justice G, et al. Darbepoetin alfa given every 1 or 2 weeks alleviates anaemia associated with cancer chemotherapy. *Br J Cancer.* 2002;87:268-276.
12. Kotasek D, Steger G, Faught W, et al. Darbepoetin alfa administered every 3 weeks alleviates anaemia in patients with solid tumours receiving chemotherapy; results of a double-blind, placebo-controlled, randomised study. *Eur J Cancer.* 2003;39:2026-2034.
13. Ohls RK, Dai A. The effect of Aranesp on the growth of fetal and neonatal erythroid progenitors. *Blood.* 2003;102:18b (abstract).
14. Warwood TL, Ohls RK, Wiedmeier SE, et al. Single-dose darbepoietin administration to anemic preterm neonates. *J Perinatol.* 2005;25:725-730.
15. Warwood TL, Ohls RK, Lambert DK, et al. Intravenous administration of darbepoetin to NICU patients. *J Perinatol.* 2006;26:296-300.

Deferoxamine Mesylate

1. *Physicians' Desk Reference.* 60th ed. Montvale, NJ: Medical Economics Company; 2006.
2. Mills KC, Cury SC. Acute iron poisoning. *Emerg Med Clin North Am.* 1994;12:397-413.
3. Cohen AR, Mizanin J, Schwartz E. Rapid removal of excessive iron with daily, high-dose intravenous chelation therapy. *Pediatrics.* 1989;115:151-155.
4. Peck MG, Rogers JF, Rivenbark JF. Use of high doses of deferoxamine (Desferal) in an adult patient with acute iron overdosage. *J Toxicol Clin Toxicol.* 1982;19:865-869.

References

5. Banner W Jr, Tong TG. Iron poisoning. *Pediatr Clin North Am.* 1986;33:393-409.
6. American Society of Health-System Pharmacists. American Hospital Formulary System. Available at: http://ahfsfirst.firstdatabank.com/AHFSfirst/NSAHFSFirstSearchmain.asp. Accessed July 14, 2006.
7. Gallant T, Mizanin J, Schwartz E, et al. Serial studies of auditory neurotoxicity in patients receiving deferoxamine therapy. *Am J Med.* 1987;83:1085-1090.
8. Graziano JH, Markensen A, Miller DR, et al. Chelation therapy in ß-thalassemia major. I. Intravenous and subcutaneous deferoxamine. *J Pediatr.* 1978;92:648-652.
9. Porter JB, Jaswon MS, Huehns ER, et al. Desferrioxamine ototoxicity: evaluation of risk factors in thalassemic patients and guidelines for safe dosage. *Br J Haematol.* 1989;73:403-409.
10. National Kidney Foundation. K/DOQI clinical practice guidelines for bone metabolism and disease in chronic kidney disease. *Am J Kidney Dis.* 2003;42:S1-S201.
11. Aronoff A, Brier M, Bennett W. *The Renal Book, 2002.* Available at: http://www.kdp-baptist.louisville.edu/renalbook/. Accessed July 14, 2006.
12. Propper RD, Shurin SB, Nathan DG. Reassessment of the use of desferrioxamine B in iron overload. *N Engl J Med.* 1976;294:1421-143.
13. Cohen AR, Martin M, Mizanin J, et al. Vision and hearing during deferoxamine therapy. *J Pediatr.* 1990;117:326-330.
14. Scanderberg AC, Izzi GC, Butturini A, et al. Pulmonary syndrome and intravenous high-dose desferrioxamine. *Lancet.* 1990;336:1511.
15. Davies SC, Hungerford JL, Arden GB, et al. Ocular toxicity of high-dose intravenous desferrioxamine. *Lancet.* 1983;23:181-184.
16. Bentur Y, Koren G, Tesoro A, et al. Comparison of deferoxamine pharmacokinetics between asymptomatic thalassemic children and those exhibiting severe neurotoxicity. *Clin Pharmacol Ther.* 1990;47:478-482.
17. Miller KB, Rosenwasser LJ, Bessette JM, et al. Rapid desensitization for desferrioxamine anaphylactic reaction. *Lancet.* 1981;1:1059.
18. Dickerhoff R. Acute aphasia and loss of vision with deferoxamine overdose. *Am J Pediatr Hematol Oncol.* 1987;9:287-288.
19. Bentur Y, McGuigan M, Koren G. Deferoxamine (desferrioxamine). New toxicities for an old drug. *Drug Safety.* 1991;6:37-46.
20. Eisen TF, Lacouture PG, Woolf A. Visual detection of ferrioxamine color changes in urine. *Vet Hum Toxicol.* 1988;30:369-70.
21. Freedman MH, Grisaru D, Olivieri N, et al. Pulmonary syndrome in patients with thalassemia major receiving intravenous deferoxamine infusions. *Am J Dis Child.* 1990;144:565-569.
22. Koren G, Bentur Y, Strong D, et al. Acute changes in renal function associated with deferoxamine therapy. *Am J Dis Child.* 1989;143:1077-1080.
23. Adamson IY, Sienko A, Tenenbein M. Pulmonary toxicity of deferoxamine in iron poisoned mice. *Toxicol Appl Pharm.* 1993;120:13-19.
24. Tenenbein M, Kowalski S, Sienko A, et al. Pulmonary toxic effects of continuous desferrioxamine administration in acute poisoning. *Lancet.* 1992;339:699-701.
25. Chan KW, Bond M, Fernandez W. Desferrioxamine in acute iron poisoning. *Lancet.* 1992;339:1601-1602
26. Anderson KJ, Rivers RPA. Desferrioxamine in acute iron poisoning. *Lancet.* 1992;339:1602.
27. Macarol V, Yawalkar SH. Desferrioxamine in acute iron poisoning. *Lancet.* 1992;339:1601.
28. Shannon M. Desferrioxamine in acute iron poisoning. *Lancet.* 1992;339:1601.
29. Cheney K, Gumbiner C, Blaine B, et al. Survival after a severe iron poisoning treated with intermittent infusions of deferoxamine. *Clin Toxicol.* 1995;33:61-66.

Dexamethasone Sodium Phosphate

1. Gross SJ, Anbar RD, Mettelman BB. Follow-up at 15 years of preterm infants from a controlled trial of moderately early dexamethasone for the prevention of chronic lung disease. *Pediatrics.* 115;681-687.
2. LeFlore JL, Salhab WA, Broyles RS, et al. Association of antenatal and postnatal dexamethasone exposure with outcomes in extremely low birth weight neonates. *Pediatrics.* 2002;110:275-279.
3. Durand M, Sardesai S, McEvoy C. Effects of early dexamethasone therapy on pulmonary mechanics and chronic lung disease in very low birth weight infants: a randomized, controlled trial. *Pediatrics.* 1995;95:584-590.
4. The Vermont Oxford Network Steroid Study Group. Early postnatal dexamethasone therapy for the prevention of chronic lung disease. *Pediatrics.* 2001;108:741-748.
5. American Academy of Pediatrics, Canadian Paediatric Society: Postnatal corticosteroids to treat or prevent chronic lung disease in preterm infants. *Pediatrics.* 2002;109:330-338.
6. Couser RJ, Ferrara B, Falde B, et al. Effectiveness of dexamethasone in preventing extubation failure in preterm infants at increased risk for airway edema. *J Pediatr.* 1992;121:591-596.
7. Doyle LW, Davis PG, Morley CJ, et al. Low-dose dexamethasone facilitates extubation among chronically ventilator dependent infants: a multicenter, international, randomized, controlled. *Pediatrics.* 2006;117:75-83.
8. Anene O, Meert KL, Uy H, et al. Dexamethasone for the prevention of post-extubation airway obstruction: a prospective, randomized, double-blind, placebo-controlled trial. *Crit Care Med.* 1996;24:1666-1669.
9. Alvarez O, Freeman A, Bedros A, et al. Randomized double-blind crossover ondansetron-dexamethasone versus ondansetron-placebo study for the treatment of chemotherapy-induced nausea and vomiting in pediatric patients with malignancies. *J Pediatr Hematol Oncol.* 1995;17:145-150.
10. Holdsworth MT, Raisch DW, Frost J. Acute and delayed nausea and emesis control in pediatric oncology patients. *Cancer.* 2006;106:931-940.
11. Madan R, Bhatia A, Chakithandy S, et al. Prophylactic dexamethasone for postoperative nausea and vomiting in pediatric strabismus surgery: a dose ranging and safety evaluation study. *Anesth Analg.* 2005;100:1622-1666.
12. Subramaniam B, Madan R, Sadhasivam S, et al. Dexamethasone is a cost-effective alternative to ondansetron in preventing PONV after paediatric strabismus repair. *Br J Anaesthesia.* 2001;86:84-89.
13. Elhakim M, Ali NM, Rashed I, et al. Dexamethasone reduces postoperative vomiting and pain after pediatric tonsillectomy. *Can J Anesth.* 2003;50:392-397.
14. Hanasono MM, Lalakea L, Mikulec AA, et al. Perioperative steroids in tonsillectomy using electrocautery and sharp dissection techniques. *Arch Otolaryngol Head Neck Surg.* 2004;130:917-921.
15. Super DM, Cartelli NA, Brooks LJ, et al. A prospective randomized double-blind study to evaluate the effect of dexamethasone in acute laryngotracheitis. *J Pediatr.* 1989;115:323-329.
16. Fitzgerald DA, Kilham HA. Croup: assessment and evidence-based management. *Med J Austral.* 2003;179:372-377.
17. Arditi M, Mason EO, Bradley JS, et al. Three-year multicenter surveillance of pneumococcal meningitis in children: clinical characteristics, and outcome related to penicillin susceptibility and dexamethasone use. *Pediatrics.* 1998;102:1087-1097.
18. Molyneux EM, Walsh AL, Forsyth H, et al. Dexamethasone treatment in childhood bacterial meningitis in Malawi: a randomized controlled trial. *Lancet.* 2002;360:211-218.
19. Tunkel AR, Hartman BJ, Kaplan SL, et al. Practice guidelines for the management of bacterial meningitis. *Clin Infect Dis.* 2004;39:1267-1284.
20. National Asthma Education and Prevention Program Expert Panel Report 2: Guidelines for the diagnosis and management of asthma. Update on Selected Topics. National Institutes of Health Publication No. 02-5074, Bethesda, MD. June 2003.
21. Ghajar J, Hariri RJ. Management of pediatric head injury. In: Pediatric emergency medicine. *Pediatr Clin North Am.* 1992;39:1093-1124.
22. Dexamethasone sodium phosphate injection, USP. Shirley, NY: American Regent Laboratories; August 1998.
23. Trissel LA. *Handbook on Injectable Drugs.* 13th ed. Bethesda, MD: American Society of Health-System Pharmacists; 2005.
24. Rittichier KK, Ledwith CA. Outpatient treatment of moderate croup with dexamethasone: intramuscular versus oral dosing. *Pediatrics.* 2000;106:1344-1348.

25. Klassen T. Croup: a current perspective. *Pediatr Clin North Am.* 1999;46:1167-1178.
26. American Academy of Pediatrics Committee on Drugs. "Inactive" ingredients in pharmaceutical products: update. *Pediatrics.* 1997;99:268-278.
27. Smolinske SC. Review of parenteral sulfite reactions. *J Toxicol Clin Toxicol.* 1992;30:597-606.
28. Lester MR. Sulfite sensitivity: significance in human health. *J Am Col Nutr.* 1995;14:229-232.
29. Soni MG, Taylor SL, Greenberg NA, et al. Evaluation of the health aspects of methyl paraben: a review of the published literature. *Food Chem Toxicol.* 2002;40:1335-1373.
30. Nagel JE, Fuscaldo JT, Firemen P. Paraben allergy. *JAMA.* 1977;237:1594-1595.
31. Hall CM, Milligan DWA, Berrington J. Probable adverse reaction to a pharmaceutical excipient. *Arch Dis Child Fetal Neonatal Ed.* 2004;89:F184.
32. Hiller JL, Benda GI, Rahatzad M, et al. Benzyl alcohol toxicity: impact on mortality and intraventricular hemorrhage among very low birth weight infants. *Pediatrics.* 1986;77:500-506.
33. Grant JA, Bilodeau PA, Guernsey BG, et al. Unsuspected benzyl alcohol hypersensitivity. *N Engl J Med.* 1982;306:108.
34. Wilson JP, Solimando DA, Edwards MS. Parenteral benzyl alcohol-induced hypersensitivity reaction. *Drug Intell Clin Pharm.* 1986;20:689-691.
35. Stark AR, Carlo WA, Tyson JE, et al. Adverse effects of early dexamethasone treatment in extremely-low-birth-weight infants. *N Engl J Med.* 2001;344:95-101.
36. Kaempf JW, Campbell B, Sklar RS, et al. Implementing potentially better practices to improve neonatal outcomes after reducing postnatal dexamethasone use in infants born between 501 and 1250 grams. *Pediatrics.* 2003;111:e534-e541.
37. Tellez DW, Galvis AG, Storgion SA, et al. Dexamethasone in the prevention of postextubation stridor in children. *J Pediatr.* 1991;118:289-294.
38. Chamberlin P, Meyer WJ. Management of pituitary-adrenal suppression secondary to corticosteroid therapy. *Pediatrics.* 1981;67:245-251.
39. Atkinson WL, Pickering LK, Schwartz B, et al. General recommendations on immunization. Recommendations of the Advisory Committee on Immunization Practices (ACIP) and the American Academy of Family Physicians (AAFP). *MMWR Recomm Rep.* 2002;51(RR-2):1-35.

Dexmedetomidine HCl

1. Berkenbosch JW, Wankum PC, Tobias JD. Prospective evaluation of dexmedetomidine for noninvasive procedural sedation in children. *Pediatr Crit Care Med.* 2005;6:435-439.
2. Koroglu A, Demirbilek S, Teksan H, et al. Sedative, haemodynamic and respiratory effects of dexmedetomidine in children undergoing magnetic resonance imaging examination: preliminary results. *Br J Anaesth.* 2005;94:821-824.
3. Tobias JD, Berkenbosch JW. Sedation during mechanical ventilation in infants and children: dexmedetomidine versus midazolam. *S Med J.* 2004;97:451-455.
4. Chrysostomou C, Di Filippo S, Manrique AM, et al. Use of dexmedetomidine in children after cardiac and thoracic surgery. *Pediatr Crit Care Med.* 2006;7:126-131.
5. Finkel JC, Johnson YJ, Quezado ZMN. The use of dexmedetomidine to facilitate acute discontinuation of opioids after cardiac transplantation in children. *Crit Care Med.* 2005;33:2110-2112.
6. Precedex [package insert]. North Chicago, IL: Abbott Laboratories; February 2001.
7. McEvoy GK, ed. *AHFS Drug Information Essentials 2005–06.* Bethesda, MD: American Society of Health-System Pharmacists; 2005.
8. Trissel LA. *Handbook on Injectable Drugs.* 13th ed. Bethesda, MD: American Society of Health-System Pharmacists; 2005.
9. Berkenbosch JW, Tobias JD. Development of bradycardia during sedation with dexmedetomidine in an infant concurrently receiving digoxin. *Pediatr Crit Care Med.* 2004;4:203-205.

Dextrose

1. Polk DH. Disorders of carbohydrate metabolism. In: Tauesch HW, Ballard RA, eds. *Avery's Diseases of the Newborn.* 7th ed. Philadelphia, PA: WB Saunders Company; 1998:1235-1241.
2. Sperling MA. Hypoglycemia. In: Behrman RE, Kliegman RM, Jenson HB, eds. *Nelson Textbook of Pediatrics.* 17th ed. Philadelphia, PA: WB Saunders Company; 2004:505-508.
3. Frankel L, Stevenson DK. Metabolic emergencies of the newborn: hypoxemia and hypoglycemia. *Compr Ther.* 1987;13:14-19.
4. Pryds O, Christensen NJ, Friis-Hansen B. Increased cerebral blood flow and plasma epinephrine in hypoglycemic, preterm neonates. *Pediatrics*. 1990;85:172-176.
5. LaFranchi S. Hypoglycemia of infancy and childhood. *Pediatr Clin North Am.*1987;34:961-982.
6. Lilien LD, Grajwer LA, Pildes RS. Treatment of neonatal hypoglycemia with continuous intravenous glucose infusion. *J Pediatr.* 1977;91:779-782.
7. Lilien LD, Pildes RS, Srinivasan G, et al. Treatment of neonatal hypoglycemia with minibolus and intravenous glucose infusion. *J Pediatr.* 1980;97:295-298.
8. Mehta A. Prevention and management of neonatal hypoglycemia. *Arch Dis Child.* 1994;70:F54-65.
9. Taketomo CK, Hodding JH, Kraus DM. *Pediatric Dosage Handbook* [CD-ROM]. Hudson, OH: Lexi-Comp, Inc; 2006.
10. Lui K, Thungappa U, Nair A, et al. Treatment with hypertonic dextrose and insulin in severe hyperkalemia of immature infants. *Acta Paediatr.* 1992;81:213-216.
11. AHFSfirst™ Web version 2.03. Bethesda, MD: American Society of Health-System Pharmacists, First Databank, Inc; 2002. Accessed May 15, 2006.
12. Collins JE, Leonard JV. Hyperinsulinism in asphyxiated and small-for-dates infants with hypoglycemia. *Lancet.* 1984;2:311-313.
13. Aynsley-Green A, Polak JM, Bloom SR, et al. Nesidioblastosis of the pancreas: definition of the syndrome and the management of the severe neonatal hyperinsulinaemic hypoglycaemia. *Arch Dis Child.* 1981;56:496-508.
14. 50% Dextrose Injection [USP package insert]. North Chicago, IL: Abbott Laboratories; February 2000.
15. Okada A, Imura K. Parenteral nutrition in neonates. In: Rombeau JL, Caldwell MD, eds. *Clinical Nutrition: Parenteral Nutrition.* 2nd ed. Philadelphia, PA: WB Saunders Company; 1993:756-769.

Diazepam

1. Shankar V, Deshpande JK. Procedural sedation in the pediatric patient. *Anesthesiol Clin N Am.* 2005;23:635-654, viii.
2. Flood RG, Krauss B. Procedural sedation and analgesia for children in the emergency department. *Emerg Med Clin North Am.* 2003;21:121-139.
3. Krauss B, Green S. Procedural sedation and analgesia in children. *Lancet.* 2006;367:766-780.
4. Taketomo CK, Hodding JH, Kraus DM, eds. *Pediatric Dosage Handbook.* 12th ed. [CD-ROM version 2006.1] Hudson, OH: Lexi-Comp; 2006.
5. Bavdekar SB, Mahajan MD, Chandu KV. Analgesia and sedation in paediatric intensive care unit. *J Postgrad Med.* 1999;45:95-102.
6. Wheless JW, Clarke DF, Carpenter D. Treatment of pediatric epilepsy: expert opinion, 2005. *J Child Neurol.* 2005;20(suppl 1):1-57.
7. Maytal J, Novak GP, King KC. Lorazepam in the treatment of refractory neonatal seizures. *J Child Neurol.* 1991;6:319-323.
8. Zupanc ML. Neonatal seizures. *Pediatr Clin N Amer.* 2004;51:961-978.

References

9. Chamberlain JM, Altieri MA, Futterman C, et al. A prospective randomized study comparing intramuscular midazolam with intravenous diazepam for the treatment of seizures in children. *Pediatr Emerg Care.* 1997;13:92-94.
10. Giang DW, McBride MC. Lorazepam versus diazepam for the treatment of status epilepticus. *Pediatr Neurol.* 1988;4:358-361.
11. American Academy of Pediatrics Committee on Drugs. Emergency drug doses for infants and children. *Pediatrics.* 1998;101:e1-11.
12. *Camfield PR. Treatment of status epilepticus in children. Can Med Assoc J.* 1983;128:671-672.
13. Eriksson K, Kalviainen R. Pharmacologic management of convulsive status epilepticus in childhood. *Expert Rev Neurotherapeutics.* 2005;5:777-783.
14. Khoo BH, Lee EL, Lam KL. Neonatal tetanus treated with high dosage diazepam. *Arch Dis Child.* 1978;53:737-739.
15. Tekur U, Gupta A, Tayal G, et al. Blood concentrations of diazepam and its metabolites in children and neonates with tetanus. *J Pediatr.* 1983;102:145-147.
16. American Society of Health-System Pharmacists. American Hospital Formulary System. Available at: http://ahfsfirst.firstdatabank.com/AHFSfirst/NSAHFSFirstSearchmain.asp. Accessed May 19, 2006.
17. Bennett W. *The Renal Book, 2002.* Available at: http://www.kdp-baptist.louisville.edu/renalbook/. Accessed May 19, 2006.
18. Smith BT, Masotti RE. Intravenous diazepam in the treatment of prolonged seizure activity in neonates and infants. *Dev Med Child Neurol.* 1971;13:630-634.
19. Thong YH, Abramson DC. Continuous infusion of diazepam in infants with severe recurrent convulsions. *Med Ann DC.* 1974;43:63-65.
20. Lopez-Herce J, Bonet C, Meana A, et al. Benzyl alcohol poisoning following diazepam intravenous infusion. *Ann Pharmacother.* 1995;29:632.
21. Okstein CJ, Odal M, Kelly RW. Emergency drug dosage guides. *Pediatrics.* 1988;82:119-121.
22. Delgado-Escueta AV, Wasterlain C, Treiman DM, et al. Current concepts in neurology. Management of status epilepticus. *N Engl J Med.* 1982;306:1337-1340.
23. Trissel LA, ed. *Handbook on Injectable Drugs.* 13th ed. [CD-ROM version 1.5]. Bethesda, MD: American Society of Health-System Pharmacists; 2005.
24. Bell HE, Bertino JS. Constant diazepam infusion in the treatment of continuous seizure activity. *Drug Intell Clin Pharm.* 1984;18:965-970.
25. Singhi S, Banerjee S, Singhi P. Refractory status epilepticus in children: role of continuous diazepam infusion. *J Child Neurol.* 1998;13:23-26.
26. Upton J, Mulliken JB, Murray JE. Major intravenous extravasation injuries. *Am J Surg.* 1979;137:497-506.
27. Sillers BR. Irritant properties of diazepam. *Br Dent J.* 1968;124:295.
28. American Academy of Pediatrics Committee on Drugs. "Inactive" ingredients in pharmaceutical products: update. *Pediatrics.* 1997;99:268-278.
29. Hall CM, Milligan DWA, Berrington J. Probably adverse reaction to a pharmaceutical excipient. *Arch Dis Child Fetal Neonatal Ed.* 2004;89:F184.
30. Walker JE, Homan RW, Vasko MR, et al. Lorazepam in status epilepticus. *Ann Neurol.* 1979;6:207-213.
31. Grant JA, Bilodeau PA, Guernsey BG, et al. Unsuspected benzylalcohol hypersensitivity. *N Engl J Med.* 1982;306:108.
32. Wilson JP, Solimando DA, Edwards MS. Parenteral benzyl alcohol-induced hypersensitivity reaction. *Drug Intell Clin Pharm.* 1986;20:689-691.
33. Louis S, Kutt H, McDowell F. The cardiocirculatory changes caused by intravenous ilantin and its solvent. *Am Heart J.* 1967;74:523-529.
34. Glasgow AM, Boeckx RL, Miller MK, et al. Hyperosmolality in small infants due to propylene glycol. *Pediatrics.* 1983;72:353-355.
35. MacDonald MG, Getson PR, Glasgow AM, et al. Propylene glycol: increased incidence of seizures in low birth weight infants. *Pediatrics*. 1987;79:622-625.
36. Straaten HL, Rademaker CM, de Vries LS. Comparison of the effect of midazolam or vecuronium on blood pressure and cerebral blood flow velocity in premature newborns. *Dev Pharmacol Ther.* 1992;19:191-195.
37. Young TE, Mangum B, eds. *Neofax®.* 18th ed. Raleigh, NC: Acorn Publishing Inc; 2005.
38. Tobias JD. Sedation analgesia in paediatric intensive care units. *Pediatr Drugs.*1999;1:109-126.
39. Cronin CM. Neurotoxicity of lorazepam in a premature infant. *Pediatrics.* 1992;89:1129.
40. Reiter PD, Stiles AD. Lorazepam toxicity in a premature infant. *Ann Pharmacother.* 1993;27:727-729.
41. Chess PR, D'Angio CT. Clonic movement following lorazepam administration in full-term infants. *Arch Pediatr Adolesc Med.* 1998;152:98-99.
42. Sugarman JM, Paul RI. Flumazenil: a review. *Pediatr Emerg Care.* 1994;10:37-43.

Diazoxide

1. McEvoy GK, ed. *Drug Information Essentials 2005–06.* Bethesda, MD: American Society of Health-System Pharmacists; 2005.
2. Deal JE, Barratt TM, Dillon MJ. Management of hypertensive emergencies. *Arch Dis Child.* 1992;67:1089-1092.
3. Adelman RD, Coppo R, Dillon MJ. The emergency management of severe hypertension. *Pediatr Nephrol.* 2000;14:422-427.
4. *Physicians' Desk Reference*. 60th ed. Montvale, NJ: Thomson PDR; 2006.
5. American Academy of Pediatrics Committee on Drugs. Emergency drug doses for infants and children. *Pediatrics*. 1998;101:e1-e11.
6. Boerth RC, Long WR. Dose response relation of diazoxide in children with hypertension. *Circulation*. 1977;56:1062-1066.
7. McNair A, Andreasen F, Nielsen PE. Antihypertensive effect of diazoxide given intravenously in small repeated doses. *Eur J Clin Pharmacol*. 1983;24:151-156.
8. Hanna JD, Chan JC, Gill JR. Hypertension and the kidney. *J Pediatr*. 1991;118:327-340.
9. Fivush B, Neu A, Furth S. Acute hypertensive crises in children: emergencies and urgencies. *Curr Opin Pediatr.* 1997;9:233-236.
10. Aronoff A, Brier M, Bennett W. *The Renal Book, 2002.* Available at: http://www.kdp-baptist.louisville.edu/renalbook/. Accessed August 1, 2006.
11. Thien TA, Huysmans FTM, Gerlag PGG, et al. Diazoxide infusion in severe hypertension and hypertensive crisis. *Clin Pharmacol Ther.* 1979;25:795-799.
12. Huysmans FT, Thien T, Koene RA. Acute treatment of hypertension with slow infusion of diazoxide. *Arch Intern Med*. 1983;143:882-884.
13. Grossman E, Ironi AN, Messerli FH. Comparative tolerability profile of hypertensive crisis treatments. *Drug Safety*. 1998;19:99-122. Review.
14. Trissel LA. *Handbook on Injectable Drugs.* 13th ed. Bethesda, MD: American Society of Health-System Pharmacists; 2005.
15. Jacobs RF, Nix RA, Paulus TE, et al. Intravenous infusion of diazoxide in the treatment of chlorpropamide-induced hypoglycemia. *J Pediatr*. 1978;93:801-803.
16. McCrory WW, Kohaut EC, Lewy JE, et al. Safety of intravenous diazoxide in children with severe hypertension. *Clin Pediatr*. 1979;18:661-671.

Digoxin

1. Lanoxin injection pediatric [prescribing information]. Research Triangle Park, NC: GlaxoSmithKline; July 2002.
2. Halkin H, Radomsky M, Blieden L, et al. Steady state serum digoxin concentrations in relation to digitalis toxicity in neonates and infants. *Pediatrics.* 1978;61:184-188.
3. Bendayan R, McKenzie MW. Digoxin pharmacokinetics and dosage requirements in pediatric patients. *Clin Pharm.* 1983;2:224-235.
4. Pinsky WW, Jacobsen JR, Gillette PC, et al. Dosage of digoxin in premature infants. *J Pediatr.* 1979;96:639-642.
5. Park MK. Use of digoxin in infants and children, with specific emphasis on dosage. *J Pediatr.* 1986;108:871-877.
6. Lang D, von Bernuth G. Serum concentrations and serum half-life of digoxin in premature and mature newborns. *Pediatrics.* 1977;59:902-906.
7. Berman W, Dubynsky O, Whitman V, et al. Digoxin therapy in low-birth-weight infants with patent ductus arteriosus. *J Pediatr.* 1978;93:652-655.

8. Gortner L, Hellenbrecht D. Estimation of digoxin dosage in VLBW infants using serum creatinine concentrations. *Acta Paediatr Scand.* 1986;75:433-438.
9. Johnson GL, Desai NS, Pauly TH, et al. Complications associated with digoxin therapy in low-birth weight infants. *Pediatrics.* 1982;69:463-465.
10. Nyberg L, Wettrell G. Pharmacokinetics and dosage of digoxin in neonates and infants. *Eur J Clin Pharmacol.* 1980;18:69-74.
11. Rutkowski MM, Cohen SN, Doyle EF. Drug therapy of heart disease in pediatric patients II. The treatment of congestive heart failure in infants and children with digitalis preparations. *Am Heart J.* 1973;86:270-275.
12. Hastreiter AR, van der Horst RL, Voda C, et al. Maintenance digoxin dosage and steady-state plasma concentration in infants and children. *J Pediatr.* 1985;107:140-146.
13. Bakir M, Bilgic A. Single daily dose of digoxin for maintenance therapy of infants and children with cardiac disease: is it reliable? *Pediatr Cardiol.* 1994;15:229-232.
14. Aronoff A, Brier M, Bennett W. *The Renal Book, 2002.* Available at: http://www.kdp-baptist.louisville.edu/renalbook/. Accessed July 5, 2006.
15. American Academy of Pediatrics. Committee on Drugs. Emergency drug doses for infants and children. *Pediatrics.* 1988;81:462-465.
16. Nyberg L, Wettrell G. Digoxin dosage schedules for neonates and infants based on pharmacokinetic considerations. *Clin Pharmacokinet.* 1978;3:453-461.
17. Trissel LA, ed. *Handbook on Injectable Drugs.* 13th ed. Bethesda, MD: American Society of Health-System Pharmacists; 2005.
18. Berman W, Whitman V, Marks KH, et al. Inadvertent overadministration of digoxin to low-birth-weight infants. *J Pediatr.* 1978;92:1024-1025.
19. Lanoxin injection [prescribing information]. Research Triangle Park, NC: GlaxoSmithKline; February 2002.
20. Bhambhani V, Beri RS, Puliyel JM. Inadvertent overdosing of neonates as a result of the dead space of the syringe hub and needle. *Arch Dis Child Fetal Neonatol Ed.* 2005;90:F444-F446.
21. Louis S, Kutt H, McDowell F. The cardiocirculatory changes caused by intravenous Dilantin and its solvent. *Am Heart J.* 1967;74:523-529.
22. American Academy of Pediatrics Committee on Drugs. "Inactive" ingredients in pharmaceutical products: update. *Pediatrics.* 1997;99:268-278.
23. Glasgow AM, Boeckx RL, Miller MK, et al. Hyper-osmolality in small infants due to propylene glycol. *Pediatrics.* 1983;72:353-355.
24. MacDonald MG, Getson PR, Glasgow AM, et al. Propylene glycol: increased incidence of seizures in low birth weight infants. *Pediatrics.* 1987;79:622-625.
25. Zenk KE, Sills JH, Koeppel RM. *Neonatal Medications & Nutrition.* 2nd ed. Santa Rosa, CA: NICU Ink; 2000.
26. Young TE, Mangum B, eds. *Neofax.* 18th ed. Raleigh, NC: Acorn Publishing Inc; 2005.
27. Lemon M, Andrews DJ, Binks AM, et al. Concentrations of free serum digoxin after treatment with antibody fragments. *Br Med J.* 1987;295:1520-1521.
28. Phelps SJ, Kamper CA, Bottorff MB, et al. Effect of age and serum creatinine on endogenous digoxin-like substances in infants and children. *J Pediatr.* 1987;110:136-139.
29. Pudek MR, Seccombe DW, Whitfield MF, et al. Digoxin-like immunoreactivity in premature and full-term infants not receiving digoxin therapy. *N Engl J Med.* 1983;308:904-905.
30. Valdes R, Graves SW, Brown BA, et al. Endogenous substance in newborn infants causing false positive digoxin measurements. *J Pediatr.* 1983;102:947-950.
31. Ebara H, Suzuki S, Nagashima K, et al. Digoxin-like immunoreactive substances in urine and serum from preterm and term infants: relationship to renal excretion of sodium. *J Pediatr.* 1986;108:760-762.
32. Graves SW, Brown B, Valdes R. An endogenous digoxin-like substance in patients with renal impairment. *Ann Intern Med.* 1983;99:604-608.
33. Greenway DC, Nanji AA. Falsely increased results of digoxin sera from patients with liver disease: ten immunoassay kits compared. *Clin Chem.* 1985;31:1078-1079.

Digoxin Immune Fab

1. Digibind [prescribing information]. Research Triangle Park, NC: GlaxoSmithKline; September 2003.
2. Woolf AD, Wenger T, Smith TW, et al. The use of digoxin-specific Fab fragments for severe digitalis intoxication in children. *N Engl J Med.* 1992;326:1739-1744.
3. Martiny SS, Phelps SJ, Massey KL. Treatment of severe digitalis intoxication with digoxin-specific antibody fragments: a clinical review. *Crit Care Med.* 1988;16:629-635.
4. Zucker AR, Lacina SJ, DasGupta DS, et al. Fab fragments of digoxin-specific antibodies used to reverse ventricular fibrillation induced by digoxin ingestion in a child. *Pediatrics.* 1982;70:468-471.
5. Murphy DJ, Bremner WF, Haber E, et al. Massive digoxin poisoning treated with Fab fragments of digoxin-specific antibodies. *Pediatrics.* 1982;70:472-473.
6. Presti S, Friedman D, Saslow J, et al. Digoxin toxicity in a premature infant: treatment with Fab fragments of digoxin-specific antibodies. *Pediatr Cardiol.* 1985;6:91-94.
7. Hursting MF, Raisys VA, Opheim KE, et al. Determination of free digoxin concentrations in serum for monitoring Fab treatment of digoxin overdose. *Clin Chem.*1987;33:1652-1655.
8. Kaufman J, Leikin J, Kendzierski D, et al. Use of digoxin Fab immune fragments in a seven-day-old infant. *Pediatr Emerg Care.* 1990;6:118-121.
9. Allen NM, Dunham GD. Treatment of digitalis intoxication with emphasis on the clinical use of digoxin immune FAB. *DICP Ann Pharmacother.* 1990;24:991-998.
10. American Academy of Pediatrics Committee on Drugs. Emergency drug doses for infants and children. *Pediatrics.* 1998;101:e1-e11.
11. Fazio A. Fab fragments in the treatment of digoxin overdose: pediatric considerations. *South Med J.* 1987;80:1553-1556.
12. Lemon M, Andrews DJ, Binks AM, et al. Concentrations of free serum digoxin after treatment with antibody fragments. *Br Med J.* 1987;295:1520-1521.
13. Butler VP, Smith TW. Immunologic treatment of digitalis toxicity: a tale of two prophecies. *Ann Intern Med.* 1986;105:613-614.
14. Ujhelyi MR, Green PJ, Cummings DM, et al. Determination of free serum digoxin concentrations in digoxin toxic patients after administration of digoxin Fab antibodies. *Ther Drug Monitor.* 1992;14:147-154.
15. Ujhelyi MR, Colucci RD, Cummings DM, et al. Monitoring serum digoxin concentrations during digoxin immune Fab therapy. *DICP Ann Pharmacother.* 1991;25:1047-1049.
16. Ujhelyi MR, Robert S, Cummings DM, et al. Influence of digoxin immune Fab therapy and renal dysfunction on the disposition of total and free digoxin. *Ann Intern Med.* 1993;119:273-277.
17. Phillips SD. Digoxin immune Fab therapy for digoxin toxicity. *Ann Intern Med.* 1994;120:247.
18. Ocal IT, Green TR. Serum digoxin in the presence of digibind: determination of digoxin by the Abbott AxSYM and Baxter Stratus II immunoassays by direct analysis without pretreatment of serum samples. *Clin Chem.* 1998;44:1947-1950.
19. Wenger TL, Butler VP Jr, Haber E, et al. Treatment of 63 severely digoxin-specific Fab patients with digoxin-specific antibody fragments. *J Am Coll Cardiol.* 1985;5:118A-123A.

References

Dihydroergotamine Methanesulfonate

1. American Society of Health-System Pharmacists. American Hospital Formulary System. Available at: http://ahfsfirst.firstdatabank.com/AHFSfirst/NSAHFSFirstSearchmain.asp. Accessed July 10, 2006.
2. Kabbouche MA, Linder SL. Acute treatment of pediatric headache in the emergency department and inpatient settings. *Pediatr Ann.* 2005;34:466-471.
3. Linder SL. Treatment of childhood headaches with dihydroergotamine mesylate. *Headache.* 1994;34:578-580.
4. Evers S. Drug treatment of migraines in children: a comparative review. *Paediatric Drugs.* 1999;1:7-18.
5. Raskin NH. Repetitive intravenous dihydroergotamine as therapy for intractable migraine. *Neurology.* 1986;3:995-997.
6. Ford RG, Ford KT. Continuous intravenous dihydroergotamine in the treatment of intractable headache. *Headache.* 1997;37:129-136.
7. Edwards KR, Norton J, Behnke M. Comparison of intravenous valproate versus intramuscular dihydroergotamine and metoclopramide for acute treatment of migraine headache. *Headache.* 2001;41:976-980.
8. Winner P, Dalessio D, Mathew N, et al. Concomitant administration of antiemetics is not necessary with intramuscular dihydroergotamine. Concomitant administration of antiemetics is not necessary with intramuscular dihydroergotamine. *Am J Emerg Med.* 1994;12:138-141.
9. Padon A, Ostadian M, Wright C, et al. Dihydroergotamine-associated intestinal ischemia in a child with cyclic vomiting syndrome. *J Pediatr Gastroenterol Nutr.* 2006;42:573-575.

Diltiazem HCl

1. Flynn JT, Pasko DA. Calcium channel blockers: pharmacology and place in therapy of pediatric hypertension. *Pediatr Nephrol.* 2000;15:302-316.
2. Pass RH, Libermam L, Al-Fayadd HM, et al. Continuous intravenous diltiazem infusion for short-term ventricular rate control in children. *Am J Cardiol.* 2000; 86:559-562.
3. Islam S, Masiakos P, Schnitzer JJ, et al. Diltiazem reduces pulmonary arterial pressures in recurrent pulmonary hypertension associated with pulmonary hypoplasia. *J Pediatr Surg.* 1999;34:712-714.
4. Houde C, Bohn DJ, Freedom RM, et al. Profile of paediatric patients with pulmonary hypertension judged by responsiveness to vasodilators. *Br Heart J.* 1993;70:461-468.
5. Diltiazem hydrochloride injection [package insert]. Bedford, OH: Bedford Laboratories; May 2005.
6. American Society of Health-System Pharmacists. American Hospital Formulary System. Available at: http://ahfsfirst.firstdatabank.com/AHFSfirst/NSAHFSFirstSearchmain.asp. Accessed August 7, 2006.
7. American Academy of Pediatrics Committee on Drugs. "Inactive" ingredients in pharmaceutical products: update. *Pediatrics.* 1997;99:268-278.
8. Hall CM, Milligan DWA, Berrington J. Probably adverse reaction to a pharmaceutical excipient. *Arch Dis Child Fetal Neonatal Ed.* 2004;89:F184.
9. Hiller JL, Benda GI, Rahatzad M, et al. Benzyl alcohol toxicity: impact on mortality and intraventricular hemorrhage among very low birth weight infants. *Pediatrics.* 1986;77:500-506.
10. Grant JA, Bilodeau PA, Guernsey BG, et al. Unsuspected benzyl alcohol hypersensitivity. *N Engl J Med.* 1982;306:108.
11. Wilson JP, Solimando DA, Edwards MS. Parenteral benzyl alcohol-induced hypersensitivity reaction. *Drug Intell Clin Pharm.* 1986;20:689-691.
12. Porter CJ, Garson A, Gillette PC. Verapamil: an effective calcium blocking agent for pediatric patients. *Pediatrics.* 1983;71:748-755.

Diphenhydramine HCl

1. Benadryl injection [package insert]. New York, NY: Parke Davis, Division of Pfizer Inc; May 2001.
2. American Society of Health-System Pharmacists. American Hospital Formulary System. Available at: http://ahfsfirst.firstdatabank.com/AHFSfirst/NSAHFSFirstSearchmain.asp. Accessed July 17, 2006.
3. American Academy of Pediatrics Committee on Drugs. Emergency drug doses for infants and children. *Pediatrics.* 1998;101:e1-e11.
4. Gupta JM, Lovejoy FH Jr. Acute phenothiazine toxicity in childhood: a five-year survey. *Pediatrics.* 1967;39:771-774.
5. American Academy of Pediatrics. Committee on Drugs. Anaphylaxis. *Pediatrics.* 1973;51:136-140.
6. Cohen GH, Casta A, Sapire DW, et al. Decorticate posture following cardiac cocktail. *Pediatr Cardiol.* 1982;2:251-253.
7. Knight ME, Roberts RJ. Phenothiazine and butyrophenone intoxication in children. *Pediatr Clin North Am.* 1986;33:298-309.
8. Relling RV, Mulhern RK, Fairclough D, et al. Chlorpromazine with and without lorazepam as antiemetic therapy in children receiving uniform chemotherapy. *J Pediatr.* 1993;12:811-816.
9. Aronoff A, Brier M, Bennett W. *The Renal Book, 2002*. Available at: http://www.kdp-baptist.louisville.edu/renalbook/. Accessed July 17, 2006.
10. Rapp RP, Wermeling DP, Piecoro JJ Jr. Guidelines for the administration of commonly used intravenous drugs—1984 update. *Drug Intell Clin Pharm.* 1984;18:217-232.
11. Trissel LA, ed. *Handbook on Injectable Drugs.* 13th ed. [CD-ROM version 1.5]. Bethesda, MD: American Society of Health-System Pharmacists; 2005.
12. Hestand HE, Teske DW. Diphenhydramine hydrochloride intoxication. *J Pediatr.* 1977;90:1017-1018.
13. Santiago-Palma J, Fischberg D, Kornick C, et al. Diphenhydramine as an analgesic adjuvant in refractory cancer pain. *J Pain Symptom Manage.* 2001;22:699-703.

Dobutamine HCl

1. DOBUTamine Injection USP [package insert]. Bedford, OH: Bedford Laboratories Inc; June 2005.
2. McEvoy GK, ed. *American Hospital Formulary Service Drug Information 2006*. Bethesda, MD: American Society of Health-System Pharmacists; 2006.
3. Driscoll DJ, Gillette PC, Duff DF, et al. The hemodynamic effect of dobutamine in children. *Am J Cardiol.* 1979;43:581-585.
4. Bohn DJ, Poirier CS, Edmonds JF, et al. Hemodynamic effects of dobutamine after cardiopulmonary bypass in children. *Crit Care Med.* 1980;8:367-371.
5. Jose JB, Niguidula F, Botros S, et al. Hemodynamic effects of dobutamine in children. *Anesthesiology.* 1981;55:A61.
6. Schranz D, Stopfkuchen H, Jungst BK, et al. Hemodynamic effects of dobutamine in children with cardiovascular failure. *Eur J Pediatr.* 1982;139:4-7.
7. Perkin RM, Levin DL, Webb R, et al. Dobutamine: a hemodynamic evaluation in children with shock. *J Pediatr.* 1982;100:977-983.
8. Martinez AM, Padbury JF, Thio S. Dobutamine pharmacokinetics and cardiovascular responses in critically ill neonates. *Pediatr.* 1992;89:47-51.
9. Greenough A, Emery EF. Randomized trial comparing dopamine and dobutamine in preterm infants. *Eur J Pediatr.* 1993;152:925-927.
10. Roze JC, Tohier C, Maingueneau C, et al. Response to dobutamine and dopamine in the hypotensive very preterm infant. *Arch Dis Child.* 1993;69:59-63.

11. Berg RA, Donnerstein RL, Padbury JF, et al. Dobutamine infusions in stable, critically ill children: pharmacokinetics and hemodynamic actions. *Crit Care Med.* 1993;21:678-686.
12. Klarr JM, Faix RG, Pryce CJE, et al. Randomized, blind trial of dopamine versus dobutamine for treatment of hypotension in preterm infants with respiratory distress syndrome. *J Pediatr.* 1994;125:117-122.
13. Hentschel R, Hensel D, Brune T, et al. Impact on blood pressure and intestinal perfusion of dobutamine or dopamine in hypotensive preterm infants. *Biol Neonate.* 1995;68:318-324.
14. Ruelas-Orozco G, Vargas-Origel A. Assessment of therapy for arterial hypotension in critically ill preterm infants. *Am J Perinatol.* 2000;17:95-99.
15. Committee on Drugs. Drugs for pediatric emergencies. *Pediatrics.* 1998;101:e13
16. American Heart Association guidelines for cardiopulmonary resuscitation and emergency Cardiovascular care. Part 12: pediatric advanced life support. *Circulation.* 2005;112(suppl 1):167-187.
17. Banner W, Vernon DD, Minton SD, et al. Nonlinear dobutamine pharmacokinetics in a pediatric population. *Crit Care Med.* 1991;19:871-873.
18. Berg RA, Padbury JF, Donnerstein RL, et al. Dobutamine pharmacokinetics and pharmacodynamics in normal children and adolescents. *J Pharmacol Experiment Ther.* 1993;265:1232-1238.
19. Aronoff A, Brier M, Bennett W. *The Renal Book, 2002*. Available at: http://www.kdp-baptist.louisville.edu/renalbook/. Accessed July 18, 2006.
20. Trissel LA. *Handbook on Injectable Drugs*. 13th ed. Bethesda, MD: American Society of Health-System Pharmacists; 2005.
21. JCAHO's compliance expectations for standardized concentrations. Rule of Six in pediatrics does not meet requirements. *Jt Comm Perspect.* 2004 May;24(5):11.
22. American Academy of Pediatrics Committee on Drugs. "Inactive" ingredients in pharmaceutical products: update. *Pediatrics* .1997;99:268-278.
23. Smolinske SC. Review of parenteral sulfite reactions. *J Toxicol Clin Toxicol.* 1992;30:597-606.
24. Lester MR. Sulfite sensitivity: significance in human health. *J Am Col Nutr.* 1995;14:229-232.
25. Allen EM, Van Boerum DH, Olsen AF, et al. Difference between the measured and ordered dose of catecholamine infusion. *Ann Pharmacother.* 1995;29:1095-1100.
26. Unverferth DV, Blanford M, Kates RE, et al. Tolerance to dobutamine after a 72-hour continuous infusion. *Am J Med.* 1980;69:262–266.

Dolasetron Mesylate

1. McEvoy GK, ed. *AHFS Drug Information Essentials 2005–06.* Bethesda, MD: American Society of Health-System Pharmacists; 2005.
2. Thomson PDR, ed. *Physicians' Desk Reference.* 60th ed. Montvale, NJ: Thomson Healthcare; 2006.
3. Coppes MJ, Lau R, Ingram LC, et al. Open-label comparison of the antiemetic efficacy of single intravenous doses of dolasetron mesylate in pediatric cancer patients receiving moderately to highly emetogenic chemotherapy. *Med Pediatr Onco.* 1999;33:99-105.
4. ASHP Therapeutic guidelines on the pharmacologic management of nausea and vomiting in adult and pediatric patients receiving chemotherapy or radiation therapy or undergoing surgery. *Am J Health Syst Pharm.* 1999;56:729-764.
5. Wagner D, Pandit U, Voepel-Lewis T, et al. Dolasetron for the prevention of postoperative vomiting in children undergoing strabismus surgery. *Paediatr Anaesth.* 2003;13:522-526.
6. Sukhani R, Pappas AL, Lurie J, Ondansetron and dolasetron provide equivalent postoperative vomiting control after ambulatory tonsillectomy in dexamethasone-pretreated children. *Anesth Analg.* 2002;95:1230-1235.
7. Trissel LA. *Handbook on Injectable Drugs.* 13th ed. Bethesda, MD: American Society of Health-System Pharmacists; 2005.

Dopamine HCl

1. Dopamine hydrochloride injection USP [package insert]. Shirley, NY: American Reagent Laboratories Inc; April 2001.
2. McEvoy GK, ed. *American Hospital Formulary Service Drug Information 2006*. Bethesda, MD: American Society of Health-System Pharmacists; 2006.
3. American Heart Association Guidelines for Cardiopulmonary Resuscitation and Emergency Cardiovascular Care. Part 12: Pediatric Advanced Life Support. *Circulation.* 2005;112(suppl 1):167-187.
4. Driscoll DJ, Gillette PC, McNamara DG. The use of dopamine in children. *J Pediatr.* 1978;92:309-314.
5. Bhatt-Mehta V, Nahata MC, McClead RE, et al. Dopamine pharmacokinetics in critically ill newborn infants. *Eur J Clin Pharmacol.* 1991;40:593-597.
6. Greenough A, Emery EF. Randomized trial comparing dopamine and dobutamine in preterm infants. *Eur J Pediatr.* 1993;152:925-927.
7. Hentschel R, Hensel D, Brune R, et al. Impact on blood pressure and intestinal perfusion of dobutamine or dopamine in hypotensive preterm infants. *Biol Neonate*. 1995;68:318-324.
8. Lang P, Williams RG, Norwood WI, et al. The hemodynamic effects of dopamine in infants after corrective cardiac surgery. *J Pediatr.* 1980;96:630-634.
9. DiSessa TG, Leitner M, Ti CC, et al. The cardiovascular effects of dopamine in the severely asphyxiated neonate. *J Pediatr*. 1981;99:772-776.
10. Fiddler GI, Chatrath R, Williams GJ, et al. Dopamine infusion for the treatment of myocardial dysfunction associated with a persistent transitional circulation. *Arch Dis Child*. 1980;55:194-198.
11. Seri I, Rudas G, Bors Z, et al. Effects of low-dose dopamine infusion on cardiovascular and renal functions, cerebral blood flow, and plasma catecholamine levels in sick preterm neonates. *Pediatr Res.* 1993;34:742-749.
12. Klarr JM, Faix RG, Pryce C, et al. Randomized, blind trial of dopamine versus dobutamine for treatment of hypotension in preterm infants with RDS. *J Pediatr*. 1994;125:117-122.
13. Roze JC, Tohier C, Maingueneau, et al. Response to dobutamine and dopamine in the hypotensive very preterm infant. *Arch Dis Child.* 1993;69:59-63.
14. Rennie JM. Cerebral blood flow velocity variability after cardiovascular support in premature babies. *Arch Dis Child*. 1989;64:897-901.
15. Ruelas-Orozco G, Vargas-Origel A. Assessment of therapy for arterial hypotension in critically ill preterm infants. *Am J Perinatol.* 2000;17:95-99.
16. Valverde E, Pellicer A, Madero R, et al. Dopamine versus epinephrine for cardiovascular support in low birth weight infants: analysis of systemic effects and neonatal clinical outcomes. *Pediatrics.* 2006;117:e1213-e1222.
17. Guller B, Fields AI, Coleman MG, et al. Changes in cardiac rhythm in children treated with dopamine. *Crit Care Med*. 1978;6:151-154.
18. Han YY, Carcillo JA, Dragotta MA. Early reversal of pediatric-neonatal septic shock by community physicians is associated with improved outcome. *Pediatrics.* 2003;112:793-799.
19. Zaritsky A, Lotze A, Stull R, et al. Steady-state dopamine clearance in critically ill infants and children. *Crit Care Med*. 1988;16:217-220.
20. Trissel LA. *Handbook on Injectable Drugs*. 13th ed. Bethesda, MD: American Society of Health-System Pharmacists; 2005.
21. Rich DS. New JCAHO medication management standards for 2004. *Am J Health-Syst Pharm.* 2004;61:1349-1358.
22. Taketomo CK, Hodding JH, Kraus DM. *Pediatric Dosage Handbook*. 11th ed. Hudson, OH: Lexi-Comp Inc; 2004-2005.
23. Gaze NR. Tissue necrosis caused by commonly used intravenous infusions. *Lancet*. 1978;2:417-419.
24. Stier PA, Bogner MP, Webster K, et al. Use of subcutaneous terbutaline to reverse peripheral ischemia. *Am J Emerg Med*. 1999;17:91-94.
25. Maggi JC, Angelats J, Scott JP. Gangrene in a neonate following dopamine therapy. *J Pediatr*. 1982;100:323-325.
26. Koerber RK, Haven GT, Cohen SM, et al. Peripheral gangrene associated with dopamine infusion in a child. *Clin Pediatr*. 1984;23:106-107.

References

27. Goenka S, Mehta AV, Powers PJ. An unusual peripheral vascular response to dopamine in a neonate. *Tenn Med*. 1999;92;375-376.
28. Zenk KE, Noerr B, Ward R. Severe sequelae from umbilical arterial catheter administration of dopamine. *Neonatal Network*. 1994;13:89-91.
29. American Academy of Pediatrics Committee on Drugs. "Inactive" ingredients in pharmaceutical products: update. *Pediatrics*. 1997;99:268-278.
30. Smolinske SC. Review of parenteral sulfite reactions. *J Toxicol Clin Toxicol*. 1992;30:597-606.
31. Lester MR. Sulfite sensitivity: significance in human health. *J Am Col Nutr*. 1995;14:229-232.
32. Holmes CL, Walley KR. Bad medicine: low-dose dopamine in the ICU. *Chest*. 2003;123(4):1266-1275.
33. Seri I. Cardiovascular, renal, and endocrine actions of dopamine in neonates and children. *J Pediatr*. 1995;126:333-344.
34. Allen EM, Van Boerum DH, Olsen AF, et al. Difference between the measured and ordered dose of catecholamine infusion. *Ann Pharmacother*. 1995;29:1095-1100.
35. Driscoll DJ, Gillette PC, Duff DF, et al. The hemodynamic effect of dopamine in children. *J Thorac Cardiovasc Surg*. 1979;78:765-768.
36. Booker PD, Evans C, Franks R. Comparison of haemodynamic effects of dopamine and dobutamine in young children undergoing cardiac surgery. *Br J Anaesth*. 1995;74:419-423.
37. Hoffman TM, Bush DM, Wernovsky G, et al. Postoperative junctional ectopic tachycardia in children: incidence, risk factors, and treatment. *Ann Thorac Surg*. 2002;74:1607-1611.
38. Padbury JF, Agata Y, Baylen BG, et al. Dopamine pharmacokinetics in critically ill newborn infants. *J Pediatr*. 1986;110:293-298.
39. Banner W, Vernon DD, Dean JM, et al. Nonlinear dopamine pharmacokinetics in a pediatric population. *J Pharmacol Exp Ther*. 1989;249:131-133.
40. Notternan DA, Greenwald BM, Moran F, et al. Dopamine clearance in critically ill infants and children: effect of age and organ system dysfunction. *Clin Pharmacol Ther*. 1990;48:138-147.

Doxapram HCl

1. Doxapram hydrochloride injection [USP package insert]. Bedford, OH: Bedford Laboratories; January 2005.
2. Peliowski A, Finer NN. A blinded, randomized, placebo-controlled trial to compare theophylline and doxapram for the treatment of apnea of prematurity. *J Pediatr*. 1990;116:648-653.
3. Kumita H, Mizuno S, Shinohara M, et al. Low-dose doxapram therapy in premature infants and its CSF and serum concentrations. *Acta Paediatr Scand*. 1991;80:786-791.
4. Eyal F, Alpan G, Sagi E, et al. Aminophylline versus doxapram in idiopathic apnea of prematurity: a double-blind controlled study. *Pediatrics*. 1985;75:709-713.
5. Barrington KJ, Finer NN, Torok-Both G, et al. Dose- response relationship of doxapram in the therapy of refractory idiopathic apnea of prematurity. *Pediatrics*. 1987;80:22-27.
6. Barrington KJ, Finer NN, Peters KL, et al. Physiologic effects of doxapram in idiopathic apnea of prematurity. *J Pediatr*. 1986;108:125-129.
7. Eyal FG, Sagi EF, Alpan G, et al. Aminophylline versus doxapram in weaning premature infants from mechanical ventilation: preliminary report. *Crit Care Med*. 1985;13:124-125.
8. Trissel LA. *Handbook on Injectable Drugs*. 13th ed. Bethesda, MD: American Society of Health-System Pharmacists; 2005.
9. Ruggins NR. Pathophysiology of apnoea in preterm infants. *Arch Dis Child*. 1991;66:70-73.
10. American Academy of Pediatrics Committee on Drugs. "Inactive" ingredients in pharmaceutical products: update. *Pediatrics*. 1997;99:268-278.
11. Hall CM, Milligan DWA, Berrington J. Probable adverse reaction to a pharmaceutical excipient. *Arch Dis Child Fetal Neonatal Ed*. 2004;89: F184.
12. Grant JA, Bilodeau PA, Guernsey BG, et al. Unsuspected benzyl alcohol hypersensitivity. *N Engl J Med*. 1982;306:108.
13. Wilson JP, Solimando DA, Edwards MS. Parenteral benzyl alcohol-induced hypersensitivity reaction. *Drug Intell Clin Pharm*. 1986;20:689-691.
14. Sreenam C, Etches PC, Demianczuk N, et al. Isolated mental developmental delay in very low birth weight infants: association with prolonged doxapram therapy for apnea. *J Pediatr*. 2001;139:832-837.
15. Dani C, Bertini G, Pezzati M, et al. Brain hemodynamic effects of doxapram in preterm infants. *Biol Neonate*. 2006;98:69-74.
16. Maillard C, Boutroy MJ, Fresson J et al. QT interval lengthening in premature infants treated with doxapram. *Clin Pharmacol Ther*. 2001;70:540-545.

Doxycycline Hyclate

1. Smith MW, Unkel JH, Fenton SJ, et al. The use of tetracyclines in pediatric patients. *J Pediatr Pharmacol Ther*. 2001;6:66-71.
2. Medical Economics, ed. *Physicians' Desk Reference*. 54th ed. Oradell, NJ: Medical Economics Company; 2000.
3. Nelson JD, Bradley JS, eds. *Pocketbook of Pediatric Antimicrobial Therapy*. 14th ed. Baltimore, MD: Williams & Wilkins; 2000–2001.
4. McEvoy GK, ed. *Drug Information Essentials 2005–06*. Bethesda, MD: American Society of Health-System Pharmacists; 2005.
5. Wilson WR, Cockerill FR III. Tetracyclines, chloramphenicol, erythromycin, and clindamycin. *Mayo Clin Proc*. 1983;58:92-98.
6. Heaney D, Eknoyan G. Minocycline and doxycycline kinetics in chronic renal failure. *Clin Pharmacol Ther*. 1978;24:233-239.
7. Aronoff A, Brier M, Bennett W. *The Renal Book, 2002*. Available at: http://www.kdp-baptist.louisville.edu/renalbook/. Accessed July 7, 2006.
8. Whelton A. Tetracyclines in renal insufficiency: resolution of a therapeutic dilemma. *Bull NY Acad Med*. 1978;54:223-237.
9. Whelton A, von Wittenau MS, Twomey TM, et al. Doxycycline pharmacokinetics in the absence of renal function. *Kidney International*. 1974;5:365-371.
10. Trissel LA, ed. *Handbook on Injectable Drugs*. 13th ed. CD-ROM version 1.5]. Bethesda, MD: American Society of Health-System Pharmacists; 2005.
11. Leibowitz BJ, Hakes JL, Cahn MM, et al. Doxycycline blood levels in normal subjects after intravenous and oral administration. *Curr Ther Res*. 1972;14:820-832.
12. Holloway WJ. Preliminary report on intravenous doxycycline. *Del Med J*. 1971;43:394-397.
13. Beneventi FA. Intravenously administered doxycycline in urological and surgical infections. *Curr Ther Res*. 1972;14:367-371.
14. Hackett E, Axelrod M. Intravenous doxycycline (Vibramycin I.V.): a clinical evaluation. *Curr Ther Res*. 1972;14:626-637.
15. McCracken GH Jr, Nelson JD, eds. *Antimicrobial Therapy for Newborns: Practical Application*. 2nd ed. New York, NY: Grune and Stratton; 1983.
16. Robertson J, Shilkofski N, eds. *The Harriet Lane Handbook*. 17th ed. Philadelphia, PA: Elsevier Mosby; 2005.
17. American Academy of Pediatrics. Committee on Drugs. Requiem for tetracyclines. *Pediatrics*. 1975;55:142-143.
18. American Academy of Pediatrics. In: Pickering LK, ed. *2003 Red Book: Report of the Committee on Infectious Diseases*. 26th ed. Elk Grove Village, IL: American Academy of Pediatrics; 2003.
19. Taketomo CK, Hodding JH, Kraus DM, eds. *Pediatric Dosage Handbook*. 12th ed. [CD-ROM version 2006.1] Hudson, OH: Lexi-Comp; 2006.
20. St. Clair EW, Wilkinson WE, Pisetsky DS, et al. The effects of intravenous doxycycline therapy for rheumatoid arthritis. *Arthritis and Rheumatism*. 2001;44:1043-1047.
21. Nguyen VX, Nix DE, Gillikin S, et al. Effect of oral antacid administration on the pharmacokinetics of intravenous doxycycline. *Antimicrobial Agents and Chemotherapy*. 1989;33:434-436.
22. Akcam M, Artan R, Akcam FY, et al. Nail discoloration induced by doxycycline. *Pediatr Infect Dis J*. 2005;9:845-846.

References

Droperidol

1. http://www.fda.gov/medwatch/SAFETY/2001/inapsine.htm. Accessed July 16, 2006.
2. Lin DM, Furst ST, Rodarte A. A double-blinded comparison of metoclopramide and droperidol for prevention of emesis following strabismus surgery. *Anesthesiol.* 1992;76:357-361.
3. Watcha MF, Simeon RM, White PF, et al. Effect of propofol on the incidence of postoperative vomiting after strabismus surgery in pediatric outpatients. *Anesthesiology.* 1992;75:204-209.
4. Larsson S, Jonmarker C. Postoperative emesis after pediatric strabismus surgery: the effect of dixyrazine compared to droperidol. *Anaesthesiol Scand.* 1990;34:227-230.
5. Abramowitz MD, Oh TH, Epstein BS, et al. The antiemetic effect of droperidol following outpatient strabismus surgery in children. *Anesthesiology.* 1983;59:579-583.
6. Lerman J, Eustis S, Smith DR. Effect of droperidol pretreatment on postanesthetic vomiting in children undergoing strabismus surgery. *Anesthesiology.* 1986;65:322-325.
7. Christensen S, Farrow-Gillespie A, Lerman J. Incidence of emesis and postanesthetic recovery after strabismus surgery in children: a comparison of droperidol and lidocaine. *Anesthesiology.* 1989;70:251-254.
8. ASHP Commission on Therapeutics. ASHP therapeutic guidelines on the pharmacologic management of nausea and vomiting in adult and pediatric patients receiving chemotherapy or radiation therapy or undergoing surgery. *Am J Health-Syst Pharm.* 1999;56:729-764.
9. Blanc VF. Antiemetic prophylaxis with promethazine or droperidol in paediatric outpatient strabismus surgery. *Can J Anaesth.* 1991;38:54-60.
10. Taketomo CK, Hodding JH, Kraus DM, eds. *Pediatric Dosage Handbook.* 12th ed. [CD-ROM version 2006.1] Hudson, OH: Lexi-Comp; 2006.
11. Droperidol injection [package insert]. Shirley, NY: American Regent Laboratories Inc; January 2002.
12. Park CK, Choi HY, In YO, et al. Acute dystonia by droperidol during intravenous patient-controlled analgesia in young patients. *J Korean Med Sci.* 2002;17:715-717.

Edrophonium Chloride

1. American Society of Health-System Pharmacists. American Hospital Formulary System. Available at: http://ahfsfirst.firstdatabank.com/AHFSfirst/NSAHFSFirstSearchmain.asp. Accessed July 22, 2006.
2. Leih-Lai m, Sarnaik AP. Therapeutic applications in pediatric intensive care. In: Yaffe SJ, Aranda JV, eds. *Neonatal and Pediatric Pharmacology.* 3rd ed. Philadelphia, PA: Lippincott Williams & Wilkins; 2005:264.
3. Fisher DM, Cronnelly R, Sharma M, et al. Clinical pharmacology of edrophonium in infants and children. *Anesthesiology.* 1984;61:428-433.
4. Gwinnutt CL, Walker RW, Meakin G. Antagonism of intense atracurium-induced neuromuscular block in children. *Br J Anaesth.* 1991;67;13-16.
5. Kirkegaard-Nielsen H, Meretoja OA, Wirtavuori K. Reversal of atracurium-induced neuromuscular block in paediatric patients. *Acta Anaesthesiol Scand.* 1995;39:906-911.
6. Abdulatif M, El-Sanabary M. Edrophonium antagonism of cisatracurium-induced neuromuscular block: dose requirements in children and adults. *Anaesth Intensive Care.* 2001;29:364-370.
7. Suzuki T, Lien CA, Belmont MR, et al. Edrophonium effectively antagonizes neuromuscular block at the laryngeal adductors induced by rapacuronium, rocuronium and cisatracurium, but not mivacurium. *Can J Anaesth.* 2003;50:879-885.
8. American Academy of Pediatrics Committee on Drugs. "Inactive" ingredients in pharmaceutical products: update. *Pediatrics.* 1997;99:268-278.
9. Lester MR. Sulfite sensitivity: significance in human health. *J Am Col Nutr.* 1995;14:229-232.
10. Smolinske SC. Review of parenteral sulfite reactions. *J Toxicol Clin Toxicol.* 1992;30:597-606.
11. Trissel LA, ed. *Handbook on Injectable Drugs.* 13th ed. [CD-ROM version 1.5]. Bethesda, MD: American Society of Health-System Pharmacists; 2005.

Enalaprilat

1. Marcadis ML, Kraus DM, Hatzopoulos FK, et al. Use of enalaprilat for neonatal hypertension. *J Pediatr.* 1991;119:505. Letter.
2. Wells TG, Bunchman TE, Kearns GL. Treatment of neonatal hypertension with enalaprilat. *J Pediatr.* 1990;117:664-667.
3. Manzi SF, Arnold A, Patterson A. Pediatric drug formulary. In: Yaffe SJ, Aranda JV, eds. *Neonatal and Pediatric Pharmacology.* 3rd ed. Philadelphia, PA: Lippincott Williams & Wilkins; 2005:901.
4. Mason T, Polak MJ, Pyles L, et al. Treatment of neonatal renovascular hypertension with intravenous enalapril. *Am J Perinatol.* 1993;9:254-257.
5. National High Blood Pressure Education Program Working Group on High Blood Pressure in Children and Adolescents. The fourth report on the diagnosis, evaluation, and treatment of high blood pressure in children and adolescents. *Pediatrics.* 2004;114(2 suppl 4th report):555-576.
6. Miller K. Pharmacological management of hypertension in paediatric patients. *Drugs.* 1994;46:868-887.
7. Webster MWI, Neutze JM, Calder AL. Acute hemodynamic effects of converting enzyme inhibition in children with intracardiac shunts. *Pediatr Cardiol.* 1992;13:129-135.
8. Sluysmans L, Styns-Cailteux M, Tremouroux-Wattiez M, et al. Intravenous enalaprilat and oral enalapril in congestive heart failure secondary to ventricular septal defect in infancy. *Am J Cardiol.* 1992;70:959-961.
9. Rheuban KS, Carpenter MA, Ayers CA, et al. Acute hemodynamic effects of converting enzyme inhibition in infants with congestive heart failure. *J Pediatr.* 1990;117:668-670.
10. Wells TG, Ilyas M. Antihypertensive agents. In: Yaffe SJ, Aranda JV, eds. *Neonatal and Pediatric Pharmacology.* 3rd ed. Philadelphia, PA: Lippincott Williams & Wilkins; 2005:683.
11. *Physicians' Desk Reference.* 60th ed. Montvale, NJ: Thomson PDR; 2006.
12. American Society of Health-System Pharmacists. American Hospital Formulary System. Available at: http://ahfsfirst.firstdatabank.com/AHFSfirst/NSAHFSFirstSearchmain.asp. Accessed June 25, 2006.
13. MacFadyen RJ, Meredith PA, Elliott HL. Enalapril clinical pharmacokinetics and pharmacokinetic-pharmacodynamic relationships. *Clin Pharmacokinet.* 1993;25:274-282.
14. Aronoff A, Brier M, Bennett W. *The Renal Book, 2002.* Available at: http://www.kdp-baptist.louisville.edu/renalbook/. Accessed June 25, 2006.
15. Rouine-Rapp K, Mello DM, Hanley FL, et al. Effect of enalaprilat on postoperative hypertension after surgical repair of coarctation of the aorta. *Pediatr Crit Care Med.* 2003;4:327-332.
16. Young TE, Mangum B. In: *Neofax®: A Manual of Drugs Used in Neonatal Care.* 18th ed. Raleigh, NC: Acorn Publishing; 2005.
17. American Academy of Pediatrics Committee on Drugs. "Inactive" ingredients in pharmaceutical products: update. *Pediatrics.* 1997;99:268-278.
18. Hall CM, Milligan DWA, Berrington J. Probably adverse reaction to a pharmaceutical excipient. *Arch Dis Child Fetal Neonatal Ed.* 2004;89:F184.
19. Hiller JL, Benda GI, Rahatzad M, et al. Benzyl alcohol toxicity: impact on mortality and intraventricular hemorrhage among very low birth weight infants. *Pediatrics.* 1986;77:500-506.

20. Grant JA, Bilodeau PA, Guernsey BG, et al. Unsuspected benzyl alcohol hypersensitivity. *N Engl J Med.* 1982;306:108.
21. Wilson JP, Solimando DA, Edwards MS. Parenteral benzyl alcohol-induced hypersensitivity reaction. *Drug Intell Clin Pharm.*1986;20:689-691.

Enoxaparin Sodium

1. Monagle P, Chan A, Massicotte P, et al. Antithrombotic therapy in children: the seventh ACCP conference on antithrombotic and thrombolytic therapy. *Chest.* 2004;126:645S-647S.
2. Merkel N, Gunther G, Schobess R. Long-term treatment of thrombosis with enoxaparin in pediatric and adolescent patients. *Acta Haematol.* 2006;115:230-236.
3. Michaels LA, Gurian M, Hegyi T, et al. Low molecular weight heparin in the treatment of venous and arterial thromboses in the premature infant. *Pediatrics.* 2004;114:703-707.
4. Dix D, Andrew M, Marzinotto V, et al. The use of low molecular weight heparin in pediatric patients: a prospective cohort study. *J Pediatr.* 2000;136:439-445.
5. Massicotte P, Adams M, Marzinotto V, et al. Low-molecular-weight heparin in pediatric patients with thrombotic disease: a dose finding study. *J Pediatr.* 1996;128:313-318.
6. Burak CR, Bowen MD, Barron TF. The use of enoxaparin in children with acute, nonhemorrhagic ischemic stroke. *Pediatr Neurol.* 2003;29:295-298.
7. Streif W, Goebel G, Chan AK, et al. Use of low molecular mass heparin (enoxaparin) in newborn infants: a prospective cohort study of 62 patients. *Arch Dis Child Fetal Neonatal Ed.* 2003;88:F365-F370.
8. Ho SH, Wu JK, Hamilton DP, et al. An assessment of published pediatric dosage guidelines for enoxaparin: a retrospective review. *J Pediatr Hematol Oncol.* 2004;26:561-566.
9. Massicotte MP, Adams M, Leaker M, et al. A nomogram to establish therapeutic levels of the low molecular weight heparin (LMWH), clivarine in children requiring treatment for venous thromboembolism (VTE) [abstract]. *Thromb Haemost.* 1997;(suppl):282-283.
10. Michelson AD, Bovill E, Monagle P, et al. Antithrombotic therapy in children. *Chest.* 1998;114:748S-769S.
11. Lovenox [package insert]. Bridgewater, NJ: Aventis Pharmaceuticals Inc; November 2005.
12. McEvoy GK, ed. *AHFS Drug Information Essentials 2005–06.* Bethesda, MD: American Society of Health-System Pharmacists; 2005.
13. American Academy of Pediatrics Committee on Drugs. "Inactive" ingredients in pharmaceutical products: update. *Pediatrics.* 1997;99:268-278.
14. Hall CM, Milligan DWA, Berrington J. Probably adverse reaction to a pharmaceutical excipient. *Arch Dis Child Fetal Neonatal Ed.* 2004;89: F184.
15. Hiller JL, Benda GI, Rahatzad M, et al. Benzyl alcohol toxicity: impact on mortality and intraventricular hemorrhage among very low birth weight infants. *Pediatrics.* 1986;77:500-506.
16. Grant JA, Bilodeau PA, Guernsey BG, et al. Unsuspected benzyl alcohol hypersensitivity. *N Engl J Med.* 1982;306:108.
17. Wilson JP, Solimando DA, Edwards MS. Parenteral benzyl alcohol-induced hypersensitivity reaction. *Drug Intell Clin Pharm.* 1986;20:689-691.
18. Dager WE, White RH. Low-molecular weight heparin-induced thrombocytopenia in a child. *Ann Pharmacother.* 2004;38:247-250.
19. Dager WE, Gosselin RC, King JH, et al. Anti-Xa stability of diluted enoxaparin for use in pediatrics. *Ann Pharmacother.* 2004;38:569-573.
20. Dunaway KK, Gal P, Ransom JL. Use of enoxaparin in a preterm infant. *Ann Pharmacother.* 2000;34:1410-1413.

Epinephrine HCl

1. McEvoy GK, ed. *American Hospital Formulary Service Drug Information 2006.* Bethesda, MD: American Society of Health-System Pharmacists; 2006.
2. American Academy of Pediatrics. In: Pickering LK, ed. *2003 Red Book: Report of the Committee on Infectious Diseases.* 26th ed. Elk Grove Village, IL: American Academy of Pediatrics; 2003.
3. American Academy of Pediatrics Committee on Drugs. Drugs for Pediatric Emergencies. *Pediatrics.* 1998; 101:e1-e11.
4. http://www.nhlbi.nih.gov/guidelines/asthma/asthupdt.htm. Accessed July 18, 2006.
5. American Heart Association. 2005 Guidelines for cardiopulmonary resuscitation and emergency cardiovascular care. Part 10.5: Near-Fatal Asthma. *Circulation.* 2005;112(suppl 1):139-142.
6. American Heart Association. 2005 Guidelines for cardiopulmonary resuscitation and emergency cardiovascular care. Part 12: Pediatric advanced life support. *Circulation.* 2005;112(suppl 1):167-187.
7. Berg RA, Otto CW, Kern KB, et al. High-dose epinephrine results in greater early mortality after resuscitation from prolonged cardiac arrest in pigs: a prospective, randomized study. *Crit Care Med.* 1994;22:282-290.
8. Perondi M, Reis A, Paiva E, et al. A comparison of high-dose and standard-dose epinephrine in children with cardiac arrest. *N Engl J Med.* 2004;350:1722-1730.
9. Berg RA, Otto CW, Kern KB, et al. A randomized, blinded trial of high-dose epinephrine versus standard-dose epinephrine in a swine model of pediatric asphyxial cardiac arrest. *Crit Care Med.* 1996;24:1695-1700.
10. Tang W, Weil MH, Sun S, et al. Epinephrine increases the severity of postresuscitation myocardial dysfunction. *Circulation.* 1995;92:3089-3093.
11. Rivers EP, Wortsman J, Rad MY et al. The effect of the total cumulative epinephrine dose administered during human CPR on hemodynamic, oxygen transport, and utilization variables in the postresuscitation period. *Chest.* 1994;106:1499-1507.
12. American Heart Association. 2005 Guidelines for cardiopulmonary resuscitation and emergency cardiovascular care. Part 13: Neonatal Resuscitation Guidelines. *Circulation.* 2005;112(suppl 1):188-195.
13. Goetting MG, Paradis NA. High dose epinephrine in refractory pediatric cardiac arrest. *Crit Care Med.* 1989;17:1258-1262.
14. Goetting MG, Paradis NA. High dose epinephrine improves outcome from pediatric cardiac arrest. *Ann Emerg Med.* 1991;20:22-26.
15. Dieckmann RA, Vardis R. High-dose epinephrine in pediatric out-of-hospital cardiopulmonary arrest. *Pediatrics.* 1995;95:901-913.
16. Barach EM, Nowak RM, Lee TG, et al. Epinephrine for treatment of anaphylactic shock. *JAMA.* 1984;251:2118-2122.
17. Trissel LA, ed. *Handbook on Injectable Drugs.* 13th ed. Bethesda, MD: American Society of Health-System Pharmacists; 2005.
18. Rich DS. New JCAHO medication management standards for 2004. *Am J Health-Syst Pharm.* 2004;61:1349-1358.
19. Epinephrine injection, USP 1:1000, So. El Monte, CA: International Medication Systems Limited; April 2000.
20. Taketomo CK, Hodding JH, Kraus DM. *Pediatric Dosage Handbook.* 12th ed. Hudson, OH: Lexi-Comp Inc; 2005-2006.
21. Horak A, Raine R, Opie LH, et al. Severe myocardial ischemia induced by intravenous adrenaline. *Br Med J.* 1983;286:519.
22. Sullivan TJ. Cardiac disorders in penicillin-induced anaphylaxis. Association with intravenous epinephrine therapy. *JAMA.* 1982;248:2161-2162.
23. Levine DH, Levkoff AH, Pappu LD, et al. Renal failure and other serious sequelae of epinephrine toxicity in neonates. *South Med J.* 1985;78:874-877.
24. Gaze NR. Tissue necrosis caused by commonly used intravenous infusions. *Lancet.* 1978; 2:417-419.
25. MacCara ME. Extravasation: a hazard of intravenous therapy. *Drug Intell Clin Pharm.* 1983;17:713-717.
26. Stier PA, Bogner MP, Webster K, et al. Use of subcutaneous terbutaline to reverse peripheral ischemia. *Am J Emerg Med.* 1999;17:91-94.
27. American Academy of Pediatrics Committee on Drugs. "Inactive" ingredients in pharmaceutical products: update. *Pediatrics.* 1997;99:268-278.
28. Smolinske SC. Review of parenteral sulfite reactions. *J Toxicol Clin Toxicol.* 1992;30:597-606.

29. Lester MR. Sulfite sensitivity: significance in human health. *J Am Col Nutr.* 1995;14:229-232.
30. Allen EM, Van Boerum DH, Olsen AF, et al. Difference between the measured and ordered dose of catecholamine infusion. *Ann Pharmacother.* 1995;29:1095-1100.
31. Kuracheck SC, Rockoff MA. Inadvertent intravenous administration of racemic epinephrine. *JAMA.* 1985;253:1441-1442.

Epoetin Alfa

1. Epogen [package insert]. Thousand Oaks, CA: Amgen Inc; May 12, 2006.
2. Rigden SPA, Montini G, Morris M, et al. Recombinant human erythropoietin therapy in children maintained on hemodialysis. *Pediatr Nephrol.* 1990;4:618-622.
3. Montini G, Zacchello G, Baraldi E, et al. Benefits and risks of anemia correction with recombinant human erythropoietin in children maintained on hemodialysis. *J Pediatr.* 1990;117:556-560.
4. Bianchetti MG, Hammerli I, Roduit C, et al. Epoetin alfa in anemic children or adolescents on regular dialysis. *Eur J Pediatr.* 1991;150:509-512.
5. Campos A, Garin EH. Therapy of renal anemia in children and adolescents with recombinant human erythropoietin (rHuEPO). *Clin Pediatr.* 1992;31:94-99.
6. Tenbrock K, Muller-Berghaus J, Michalk D, et al. Intravenous iron treatment of renal anemia in children on hemodialysis. *Pediatr Nephrol.* 1999;13:580-582.
7. Mak RH. Effect of recombinant human erythropoietin on insulin, amino acid, and lipid metabolism in uremia. *J Pediatr.* 1996;129:97-104.
8. Offner G, Hoyer PF, Latta K, et al. One year's experience with recombinant erythropoietin in children undergoing continuous ambulatory or cycling peritoneal dialysis. *Pediatr Nephrol.* 1990;4:498-500.
9. Caselli D, Maccabruni A, Zuccotti GV, et al. Recombinant erythropoietin for treatment of anaemia in HIV-infected children. *AIDS.* 1996;10:929-31.
10. Zoubek A, Kronberger M. Early epoetin alfa treatment in children with solid tumors. *Med Pediatr Oncol.* 2002;39:459-462.
11. Shannon KM, Mentzer WC, Abels RI, et al. Recombinant human erythropoietin in the anemia of prematurity: results of a placebo-controlled pilot study. *J Pediatr.* 1991;118:949-955.
12. Carnielli V, Montini G, Da Riol R, et al. Effect of high doses of human recombinant erythropoietin on the need for transfusions in preterm infants. *J Pediatr.* 1992;121:98-102.
13. Wandstrat TL, Maxwell SR. Erythropoietin to treat anemia or prematurity. *Ann Pharmacother.* 1997;31:645-646.
14. Carnielli VP, da Riol R, Montini G. Iron supplementation enhances response to high doses of recombinant human erythropoietin in preterm infants. *Arch Dis Child Fetal Neonatal Ed.* 1998;79:F44-F48.
15. Ohls RK, Harcum J, Schibler KR, et al. The effect of erythropoietin on the transfusion requirements of preterm infants weighing 750 grams or less: a randomized, double-blind, placebo-controlled study. *J Pediatr.* 1997;131:661-665.
16. Ohls RK, Veerman MW, Christensen RD. Pharmacokinetics and effectiveness of recombinant erythropoietin administered to preterm infants by continuous infusion in total parenteral nutrition solution. *J Pediatr.* 1996;128:518-523.
17. Maier RF, Obladen M, Muller-Hansen I et al. Early treatment with erythropoietin beta ameliorates anemia and reduces transfusion requirements in infants with birth weights below 1000g. *J Pediatr.* 2002;141:8-15.
18. Reiter PD, Rosenberg AA, Valuck R, et al. Effect of short-term erythropoietin therapy in anemic premature infants. *J Perinatol.* 2005;25:125-129.
19. Donato H, Vain N, Rendo P, et al. Effect of early versus late administration of human recombinant erythropoietin on transfusion requirements in premature infants: results of a randomized, placebo-controlled, multicenter trial. *Pediatrics.* 2000;5:1066-1072.
20. Fridge JL, Vichinsky EP. Correction of the anemia of epidermolysis bullosa with intravenous iron and erythropoietin. *J Pediatr.* 1998;132:871-873.
21. Thomson PDR, ed. *Physicians' Desk Reference.* 60th ed. Montvale, NJ: Thomson Healthcare; 2006.
22. McEvoy GK, ed. *American Hospital Formulary Service Drug Information 2006.* Bethesda, MD: American Society of Health-System Pharmacists; 2006.
23. Shimpo H, Mizumoto T, Kouji O, et al. Erythropoietin in pediatric cardiac surgery. *Chest.* 1997;111:1565-1570.
24. Chikada M, Furuse A, Kotsuka Y, et al. Open-heart surgery in Jehovah's Witness patients. *Cardiovascular Surg.* 1996;4:311-314.
25. Gumy-Pause F, Ozsahin H, Mermillod B, et al. Stepping up versus standard doses of erythropoietin in preterm infants. *Pediatr Hematol Onc.* 2005;22:667-678.
26. Huynh-Delerme C, Penaud JF, Lacombe C. Stability and biological activity of epoietin beta in parenteral nutrition solutions. *Biol Neonate.* 2002;81:158-162.
27. Ohls RK, Christensen RD. Stability of human recombinant epoetin alfa in commonly used neonatal intravenous solutions. *Ann Pharmacother.* 1996;5:466-468.
28. American Academy of Pediatrics Committee on Drugs. "Inactive" ingredients in pharmaceutical products: update. *Pediatrics.* 1997;99:268-278.
29. Hall CM, Milligan DWA, Berrington J. Probable adverse reaction to a pharmaceutical excipient. *Arch Dis Child Fetal Neonatal Ed.* 2004;89: F184.
30. Grant JA, Bilodeau PA, Guernsey BG, et al. Unsuspected benzyl alcohol hypersensitivity. *N Engl J Med.* 1982;306:108.
31. Hiller JL, Benda GI, Rahatzad M, et al. Benzyl alcohol toxicity: inpact on mortality, intraventricular hemorrhage among very low birth weight infants. *Pediatrics.* 1986;77:500-506
32. Wilson JP, Solimando DA, Edwards MS. Parenteral benzyl alcohol-induced hypersensitivity reaction. *Drug Intell Clin Pharm.* 1986;20:689-691.
33. Brandt JR, Avner ED, Hickman RO, et al. Safety and efficacy of erythropoietin in children with chronic renal failure. *Pediatr Nephrol.* 1999;13:143-147.
34. Delanty N, Vaughan C, Frucht S, et al. Erythropoietin-associated hypertensive posterior leukoencephalopathy. *Neurology.* 1997;49:686-689.
35. Latini G, Rosati G. Transient neutropenia may be a risk of treating preterm neonates with high doses of recombinant erythropoietin. *Eur J Pediatr.* 1998;157:443-444.
36. Snanoudj R, Beaudreuil S, Arzouk N. Recovery from pure red cell aplasia caused by anti-erythropoietin antibodies after kidney transplantation. *Am J Transplant.* 2004;4:274-277.

Ertapenem

1. *Physicians' Desk Reference.* 60th ed. Montvale, NJ: Thomson PDR; 2006.
2. Arguedas A, Wang J, Snyder T, et al. Safety and efficacy in a double-blind study of ertapenem vs. ceftriaxone in pediatric patients with complicated urinary tract infections, community acquired pneumonia, or skin and soft tissue infections. Washington, DC: Abstracts of the 45th Interscience Conference on Antimicrobial Agents and Chemotherapy; December 16–19; 2005:254.
3. Mistry G, Blumer J, Topelberg S, et al. Single dose pharmacokinetics of ertapenem in pediatric patients. Washington, DC: Abstracts of the 45th Interscience Conference on Antimicrobial Agents and Chemotherapy; December 16–19;2005:1.
4. Nix DE, Majumdar AK, DiNubile MJ. Pharmacokinetics and pharmacodynamics of ertapenem: an overview for clinicians. *J Antimicrob Chemother.* 2004 Jun;53(suppl 2):ii23-ii28.
5. Keating GM, Perry CM. Ertapenem: a review of its use in the treatment of bacterial infections. *Drugs.* 2005;65:2151-2178.

References

6. Legua P, Lema J, Moll J. Safety and local tolerability of intramuscularly administered ertapenem diluted in lidocaine: a prospective, randomized, double-blind study versus intramuscular ceftriaxone. *Clin Ther.* 2002;24:434-444.
7. Norrby SR. Neurotoxicity of the carbapenem antibacterials. *Drug Safety.* 1996;15:87-90.
8. Norrby SR. Carbapenems in serious infections: a risk-benefit assessment. *Drug Safety.* 2000;22:191-194.
9. Calandra G, Lydick E, Carrigan J, et al. Factors predisposing to seizures in seriously ill infected patients receiving antibiotics: experience with imipenem/cilastatin. *Am J Med.* 1988;84:911-918.

Erythromycin Gluceptate/Lactobionate

1. Erythrocin lactobionate IV [package insert]. Lake Forrest, IL: Hospira Inc; 2004.
2. American Academy of Pediatrics. In: Pickering LK, ed. *2003 Red Book: Report of the Committee on Infectious Diseases.* 26th ed. Elk Grove Village, IL: American Academy of Pediatrics; 2003.
3. Inglesby TV, O'Toole T, Henderson DA, et al. For the Working Group on Civilian Biodefense. Anthrax as a biological weapon 2002: updated recommendations for management. *JAMA.* 2002;287:2236-2252.
4. Centers for Disease Control and Prevention. Update: Investigation of bioterrorism-related anthrax and interim guidelines for exposure management and antimicrobial therapy, October 2001. *MMWR Morb Mortal Wkly Rep.* 2001;50:909-919.
5. Sexually Transmitted Diseases Treatment Guidelines—2006. Available at: http://www.cdc.gov/std/treatment. Accessed September 16, 2006.
6. American Society of Health-System Pharmacists. American Hospital Formulary System. Available at: http://ahfsfirst.firstdatabank.com/AHFSfirst/NSAHFSFirstSearchmain.asp. Accessed September 16, 2006.
7. Patole S, Rao S, Doherty D. Erythromycin as a prokinetic agent in preterm neonates: a systematic review. *Arch Dis Child Fetal Neonatal Ed.* 2005:90:F301-F306.
8. Stenson BJ, Middlemist L, Lyon AJ. Influence of erythromycin on establishment of feeding in preterm infants: observations from a randomised controlled trial. *Arch Dis Child Fetal Neonatal Ed.* 1998;79:F212-F214.
9. Simkiss DE, Adams IP, Myrdal U, et al. Erythromycin in neonatal postoperative intestinal dysmotility. *Arch Dis Child.* 1994;71:F128-F129.
10. Cucchiara S, Minella R, Scoppa A, et al. Antroduodenal motor effects of intravenous erythromycin in children with abnormalities of gastrointestinal motility. *J Pediatr Gastrointest Nutr.* 1997;24:411-418.
11. Di Lorenzo C, Lucanto C, Flores AF, et al. Effect of sequential erythromycin and octreotide on antroduodenal manometry. *J Pediatr Gastrointest Nutr.* 1999;29:293-296.
12. Aronoff A, Brier M, Bennett W. *The Renal Book, 2002.* http://www.kdp-baptist.louisville.edu/renalbook/. Accessed August 6, 2006.
13. Barre J, Mallat A, Rosenbaum J, et al. Pharmacokinetics of erythromycin in patients with severe cirrhosis. Respective influence of decreased serum binding and impaired liver metabolic capacity. *Br J Clin Pharmacol.* 1987;23:753-757.
14. Trissel LA, ed. *Handbook on Injectable Drugs.* 13th ed. [CD-ROM version 1.5]. Bethesda, MD: American Society of Health-System Pharmacists; 2005.
15. Nelson JS, Bradley JS. *Nelson's Pocketbook of Pediatric Antimicrobial Therapy.* 14th ed. Philadelphia, PA: Lippincott Williams & Wilkins; 2000.
16. Eichenwald HF. Adverse reactions to erythromycin. *Pediatr Infect Dis.* 1986;5:147-150.
17. Schweitzer VG. Ototoxic effect of erythromycin therapy. *Arch Otolaryngol.* 1984;110:258-260.
18. McComb JM, Campbell NP, Cleland J. Recurrent ventricular tachycardia associated with QT prolongation after mitral valve replacement and its association with intravenous administration of erythromycin. *Am J Cardiol.* 1984;54:922-923.
19. Farrar HC, Walsh-Sukys MC, Kyllonen K, et al. Cardiac toxicity associated with erythromycin lactobionate: two case reports and a review of the literature. *Pediatric Infect Dis J.* 1993;12:688-691.
20. Sims PJ, Waites KB, Crouse DT. Erythromycin lactobionate toxicity in preterm neonates. *Pediatr Infect Dis J.* 1994;13:166-167.
21. Farrar HC, Walsh-Sukys MC, Kyllonen K, et al. Erythromycin lactobionate toxicity in preterm neonates (reply). *Pediatr Infect Dis J.* 1994;13:166-167.
22. Dan M, Feigll D. Erythromycin associated hypotension. *Pediatr Infect Dis J.* 1993;12:692.
23. American Academy of Pediatrics Committee on Drugs. "Inactive" ingredients in pharmaceutical products: update. *Pediatrics.* 1997;99:268-278.
24. Hall CM, Milligan DWA, Berrington J. Probably adverse reaction to a pharmaceutical excipient. *Arch Dis Child Fetal Neonatal Ed.* 2004;89:F184.
25. Hiller JL, Benda GI, Rahatzad M, et al. Benzyl alcohol toxicity: impact on mortality and intraventricular hemorrhage among very low birth weight infants. *Pediatrics.* 1986;77:500-506.
26. Grant JA, Bilodeau PA, Guernsey BG, et al. Unsuspected benzyl alcohol hypersensitivity. *N Engl J Med.* 1982;306:108.
27. Wilson JP, Solimando DA, Edwards MS. Parenteral benzyl alcohol-induced hypersensitivity reaction. *Drug Intell Clin Pharm.* 1986;20:689-691.
28. Haydon RC, Thelin JW, Davis WE. Erythromycin ototoxicity: analysis and conclusions based on 22 case reports. *Otolaryngol Head Neck Surg.* 1984;92:678-684.
29. Kroboth PD, McNeil MA, Kreeer A, et al. Hearing loss and erythromycin pharmacokinetics in a patient receiving hemodialysis. *Arch Intern Med.* 1983;143:1263-1265.
30. Schweitzer VG. Ototoxic effect of erythromycin therapy. *Arch Otolaryngol.* 1984;110:258-260.
31. Brummett RE, Fox FE. Vancomycin- and erythromycin-induced hearing loss in humans. *Antimicrob Agents Chemother.* 1989;33:791-796.

Esmolol HCl

1. Wiest DB, Garner SS, Uber WE, et al. Esmolol for the management of pediatric hypertension after cardiac operations. *J Thorac Cardiocasc Surg.* 1998;115:890-897.
2. Trippel DI, Wiest DB, Gillette PC. Cardiovascular and antiarrhythmic effects of esmolol in children. *J Pediatr.* 1991;119:142-147.
3. Cuneo BF, Zales VR, Blahunka PC, et al. Pharmaco-dynamics and pharmacokinetics of esmolol, a short-acting beta-blocking agent, in children. *Pediatr Cardiol.* 1994;15:296-301.
4. Luyt D, Dance M, Litmanovitch M, et al. Esmolol in the treatment of severe tachycardia in neonatal tetanus. *Anaesth Intensive Care.* 1994;22:303-304.
5. Wiest DB, Trippel DL, Gillette PC, et al. Pharmacokinetics of esmolol in children. *Clin Pharmacol Ther.* 1991;49:6186-6123.
6. Temple ME, Nahata MC. Treatment of pediatric hypertension. *Pharmacotherapy.* 2000;20:140-150.
7. Wells TG, Ilyas M. Antihypertensive agents. In: Yaffe SJ, Aranda JV, eds. *Neonatal and Pediatric Pharmacology.* 3rd ed. Philadelphia, PA: Lippincott Williams & Wilkins; 2005:683.
8. Smerling A, Gersony WM. Esmolol for severe hypertension following repair of aortic coarctation. *Crit Care Med.* 1990;18:1288-1290.
9. National High Blood Pressure Education Program Working Group on High Blood Pressure in Children and Adolescents. The fourth report on the diagnosis, evaluation, and treatment of high blood pressure in children and adolescents. *Pediatrics..* 2004 Aug;114(2 suppl 4th Report):555-576.
10. Grossman E, Ironi AN, Messerli FH. Comparative tolerability profile of hypertensive crisis treatments. *Drug Safety.* 1998;19:99-122.
11. Aronoff A, Brier M, Bennett W. *The Renal Book, 2002.* Available at: http://www.kdp-baptist.louisville.edu/renalbook/. Accessed July 20, 2006.
12. American Society of Health-System Pharmacists. American Hospital Formulary System. Available at: http://ahfsfirst.firstdatabank.com/AHFSfirst/NSAHFSFirstSearchmain.asp. Accessed July 20, 2006.

13. Wiest DB, Garner SS, Childress LM. Stability of esmolol hydrochloride in 5% dextrose injection. *Am J Health Syst Pharm.* 1995;52:716-718.
14. Trissel LA, ed. *Handbook on Injectable Drugs.* 13th ed. [CD-ROM version 1.5]. Bethesda, MD: American Society of Health-System Pharmacists; 2005.
15. *Physicians' Desk Reference.* 60th ed. Montvale, NJ: Medical Economics Company; 2006.
16. Louis S, Kutt H, McDowell F. The cardiocirculatory changes caused by intravenous Dilantin and its solvent. *Am Heart J.* 1967;74:523-529.
17. American Academy of Pediatrics Committee on Drugs. "Inactive" ingredients in pharmaceutical products: update. *Pediatrics.* 1997;99:268-278.
18. Glasgow AM, Boeckx RL, Miller MK, et al. Hyper-osmolality in small infants due to propylene glycol. *Pediatrics.* 1983;72:353-355.
19. MacDonald MG, Getson PR, Glasgow AM, et al. Propylene glycol: increased incidence of seizures in low birth weight infants. *Pediatrics.* 1987;79:622-625.
20. Leih-Lai M, Sarnaik AP. Therapeutic applications in pediatric intensive care. In: Yaffe SJ, Aranda JV, eds. *Neonatal and Pediatric Pharmacology.* 3rd ed. Philadelphia, PA: Lippincott Williams & Wilkins; 2005:262.

Ethacrynate Sodium

1. Thomson Healthcare, Inc. *USP DI® Drug Information for the Health Care Professional.* Available at: http://www.thomsonhc.com-MICROMEDEX® Healthcare Series [database on the Internet]. Accessed April 10, 2006.
2. Intravenous sodium Edecrin [package insert]. Whitehouse Station, NJ: Merck & Co Inc; February 2005.
3. Loggie JMH, Kleinman LI, Maanen EFV. Renal function and diuretic therapy in infants and children. Part III. *J Pediatr.* 1975;86:825-832.
4. Friedman WF, George BL. New concepts and drugs in the treatment of congestive heart failure. *Pediatr Clin North Am.* 1984;31:1197-1227.
5. Whitman V, Stern RC, Bellet P, et al. Studies on cor pulmonale in cystic fibrosis: I. Effects of diuresis. *Pediatrics.* 1975;55:83-85.
6. Sparrow AW, Friedberg DZ, Nadas AS. The use of ethacrynic acid in infants and children with congestive heart failure. *Pediatrics.* 1968;42:291-302.
7. Chemtob S, Doray JL, Laudignon N, et al. Alternating sequential dosing with furosemide and ethacrynic acid in drug tolerance in the newborn. *Am J Dis Child.* 1989;143:850-854.
8. Scalais E, Papageorgiou A, Aranda JV. Effects of ethacrynic acid in the newborn infant. *J Pediatr.* 1984;104:947-950.
9. Serratto M. Diagnosis and management of heart failure in infants and children. *Comprehensive Ther.* 1992;18:11-19.
10. Trissel LA, ed. *Handbook on Injectable Drugs.* 13th ed. Bethesda, MD: American Society of Health-System Pharmacists; 2005.
11. Robertson CMT, Tyebkhan JM, Peliowski A, et al. Ototoxic drugs and sensorineural hearing loss following severe neonatal respiratory failure. *Acta Paediatrica.* 2006;95:214-223.
12. Kjellstrand CM. Ethacrynic acid in acute tubular necrosis: indications and effect on the natural course. *Nephron.* 1972;9:337-348.
13. Slone D, Jick H, Lewis GP, et al. Intravenously given ethacrynic acid and gastrointestinal bleeding. *JAMA.* 1969;209:1668-1671.
14. VanDerLinde LP, Campbell RK, Jackson E. Guidelines for the intravenous administration of drugs. *Drug Intell Clin Pharm.* 1977;11:30-55.
15. Raymond G, Day P, Rabb M. Sodium content of commonly administered intravenous drugs. *Hosp Pharm.* 1982;17:560-561.

Etomidate

1. American Society of Health-System Pharmacists. American Hospital Formulary System. Available at: http://ahfsfirst.firstdatabank.com/AHFSfirst/NSAHFSFirstSearchmain.asp. Accessed September 3, 2006.
2. Kienstra AJ, Ward MA, Sasan F, et al. Etomidate versus pentobarbital for sedation of children for head and neck CT imaging. *Pediatr Emerg Care.* 2004;20:499-506.
3. Deitch S, Davis DP, Schatteman J, et al. The use of etomidate for prehospital rapid-sequence intubation. *Prehosp Emerg Care.* 2003;7:380-383.
4. Guldner G, Schultz J, Sexton P, et al. Etomidate for rapid-sequence intubation in young children: hemodynamic effects and adverse events. *Acad Emerg Med.* 2003;10:134-139.
5. Levy ML, Aranda M, Zelman V, et al. Propylene glycol toxicity following continuous etomidate infusion for the control of refractory cerebral edema. *Neurosurgery.* 1995;37:363-371.
6. Bozeman WP, Young S. Etomidate as a sole agent for endotracheal intubation in the prehospital air medical setting. *Air Med J.* 2002;21:2-35.
7. Trissel LA, ed. *Handbook on Injectable Drugs.* 13th ed. [CD-ROM version 1.5]. Bethesda, MD: American Society of Health-System Pharmacists; 2005.
8. Louis S, Kutt H, McDowell F. The cardiocirculatory changes caused by intravenous Dilantin and its solvent. *Am Heart J.* 1967;74:523-529.
9. American Academy of Pediatrics Committee on Drugs. "Inactive" ingredients in pharmaceutical products: update. *Pediatrics.* 1997;99:268-278.
10. Glasgow AM, Boeckx RL, Miller MK, et al. Hyperosmolality in small infants due to propylene glycol. *Pediatrics.* 1983;72:353-355.
11. MacDonald MG, Getson PR, Glasgow AM, et al. Propylene glycol: increased incidence of seizures in low birth weight infants. *Pediatrics.* 1987;79:622-625.
12. Dedichek E, Kirschbaum B. A case of propylene glycol toxic reaction associated with etomidate infusion. *Arch Intern Med.* 1991;151:2297-2298.

Etoposide

1. Taketomo CK, ed. *Lexi-Comp's Pediatric Dosage Handbook.* 12th ed. Hudson, OH: Lexi-Comp; 2005:523-525.
2. Dahl GV, Lacayo NJ, Brophy N, et al. Mitoxantrone, etoposide, and cyclosporine therapy in pediatric patients with recurrent or refractory acute myeloid leukemia. *J Clin Oncol.* 2000;18(9):1867-1875.
3. Wells RJ, Adams MT, Alonzo TA, et al. Mitoxantrone and cytarabine induction, high-dose cytarabine, and etoposide intensification for pediatric patients with relapsed or refractory acute myeloid leukemia: Children's Cancer Group Study 2951. *J Clin Oncol.* 2003;21(15):2940-2947.
4. Massimo M, Gandola L, Luksch R, et al. Sequential chemotherapy, high-dose thiotepa, circulating progenitor cell rescue and radiotherapy for childhood high-grade glioma. *Neuro-Oncol.* 2005;7(1):41-48.
5. Coze C, Hartmann O, Michon J, et al. NB87 induction protocol for stage 4 neuroblastoma in children over 1 year of age: a report from the French Society of Pediatric Oncology. *J Clin Oncol.* 1997;15(12):3433-3440.
6. Rodriguez-Galindo C, Daw NC, Kaste SC, et al. Treatment of refractory osteosarcoma with fractionated cyclophosphamide and etoposide. *J Pediatr Hematol Oncol.* 2002;24(4):250-255.
7. Ayas M, Al-Seraihi A, Al-Mahr M, et al. The outcome of children with acute myeloid leukemia (AML) post-allogeneic stem cell transplantation (SCT) is not improved by the addition of etoposide to the conditioning regimen. *Pediatr Blood Cancer.* 2006;47(7):926-930. Epub ahead of print.
8. Sandler ES, Hagg R, Coppes MJ, et al. Hematopoietic stem cell transplantation (HSCT) with a conditioning regimen of busulfan, cyclophosphamide, and etoposide for children with acute myelogenous leukemia (AML): a phase I study of the Pediatric Blood and Marrow Transplant Consortium. *Med Pediatr Oncol.* 2000;35(4):403-409.
9. VePesid [package insert]. Princeton, NJ: Bristol-Myers Squibb; November 2004.
10. Aronoff GR, Berns JS, Brier ME, et al. *Drug Prescribing in Renal Failure: Dosing Guidelines for Adults.* 4th ed. Philadelphia, PA: American College of Physicians; 1999:73.

References

11. American Society of Health-System Pharmacists. American Hospital Formulary System. Available at: http://ahfsfirst.firstdatabank.com/AHFSfirst/NSAHFSFirstSearchmain.asp. Accessed May 10, 2006.
12. Solimando DA, ed. *Lexi-Comp's Drug Information Handbook for Oncology*. 4th ed. Hudson, OH: Lexi-Comp; 2004:313-319.
13. Trissel LA, ed. *Handbook on Injectable Drugs.* 13th ed. [CD-ROM version 1.5]. Bethesda, MD: American Society of Health-System Pharmacists; 2005.
14. Damon LE, Johnston LJ, Ries CA, et al. Treatment of acute leukemia with idarubicin, etoposide, and cytarabine (IDEA). A randomized study of etoposide schedule. *Cancer Chemother Pharmacol.* 2004;53(6):468-474.
15. American Academy of Pediatrics Committee on Drugs. "Inactive" ingredients in pharmaceutical products: update. *Pediatrics.* 1997;99:268-278.
16. Hall CM, Milligan DWA, Berrington J. Probably adverse reaction to a pharmaceutical excipient. *Arch Dis Child Fetal Neonatal Ed.* 2004;89:F184.
17. Hiller JL, Benda GI, Rahatzad M, et al. Benzyl alcohol toxicity: impact on mortality and intraventricular hemorrhage among very low birth weight infants. *Pediatrics.* 1986;77:500-506.
18. Grant JA, Bilodeau PA, Guernsey BG, et al. Unsuspected benzyl alcohol hypersensitivity. *N Engl J Med.* 1982;306:108.
19. Wilson JP, Solimando DA, Edwards MS. Parenteral benzyl alcohol-induced hypersensitivity reaction. *Drug Intell Clin Pharm.* 1986;20:689-691.
20. National Comprehensive Cancer Network (NCCN) Antiemesis Panel Members. NCCN Clinical Practice Guidelines in Oncology. Antiemesis, v.1.2006. Available at: www.nccn.org. Accessed March 29, 2006.
21. Roila F, Feyer P, Maranzamo E, et al. Antiemetics in children receiving chemotherapy. *Support Care Cancer.* 2005;13:129-131.

Famotidine

1. James LP, Marotti T, Stowe CD, et al. Pharmacokinetics and pharmacodynamics of famotidine in infants. *J Clin Pharmacol.* 1998;38:1089-1095.
2. Behrens R, Hofbeck M, Singer H, et al. Frequency of stress lesions of the upper gastrointestinal tract in paediatric patients after cardiac surgery: effects of prophylaxis. *Br Heart J.* 1994;72:186-189.
3. Kraus G, Krishna DR, Chmerlarsch D, et al. Famotidine. Pharmacokinetic properties and suppression of acid secretion in paediatric patients following cardiac surgery. *Clin Pharmacokinet.* 1990;18:77-81.
4. Treem WR, Davis PM, Hyams JS. Suppression of gastric acid secretion by intravenous administration of famotidine in children. *J Pediatr.* 1991;118:812-816.
5. James LP, Kearns GL. Pharmacokinetics and pharmacodynamics of famotidine in paediatric patients. *Clin Pharmacokinet.* 1996;31:103-110. Review.
6. James LP, Marshall JD, Heulitt MJ, et al. Pharmacokinetics and pharmacodynamics of famotidine in children. *J Clin Pharmacol.* 1996;36:48-54.
7. Santeiro ML, Riggs CD, Weibley RE. Famotidine pharmacodynamics and dosing requirements in critically ill children. *Pharmacotherapy.* 1997;17:1103, A175.
8. Jahr JS, Burckart G, Smith SS, et al. Effects of famotidine on gastric pH and residual volume in pediatric injury. *Acta Anaesthesiol Scand.* 1991;35:457-460.
9. Nagita A, Manago M, Aoki S, et al. Pharmacokinetics and pharmacodynamics of famotidine in children with gastroduodenal ulcers. *Ther Drug Monit.* 1994;16:444-449.
10. Maples HD, James LP, Stowe CD, et al. Famotidine Disposition in Children and Adolescents with Chronic Renal Insufficiency. *J Clin Pharmacol* 2003;43:7-14.
11. Aronoff A, Brier M, Bennett W. *The Renal Book, 2002.* Available at: http://www.kdp-baptist.louisville.edu/renalbook/. Accessed August 6, 2006.
12. *Physicians' Desk Reference.* 60th ed. Montvale, NJ: Thomson PDR; 2006.
13. Trissel LA, ed. *Handbook on Injectable Drugs.* 13th ed. [CD-ROM version 1.5]. Bethesda, MD: American Society of Health-System Pharmacists; 2005.
14. American Society of Health-System Pharmacists. American Hospital Formulary System. Available at: http://ahfsfirst.firstdatabank.com/AHFSfirst/NSAHFSFirstSearchmain.asp. Accessed August 6, 2006.
15. Watanabe Y, Tsumura H, Sasaki H, et al. The effects of intermittent and continuous intravenous infusion of famotidine on gastric acidity in patients with peptic ulcers. *Clin Ther.* 1990;12:534-546.
16. DiStefano JE, Mitrano FP, Baptista RJ, et al. Long-term stability of famotidine 20 mg/L in a total parenteral nutrient solution. *Am J Hosp Pharm.* 1989;46:2333-2335.
17. Montoro JB, Pou L, Salvador P, et al. Stability of famotidine 20 and 40 mg/L in total nutrient admixtures. *Am J Hosp Pharm.* 1989;46:2329-2332.
18. American Academy of Pediatrics Committee on Drugs. "Inactive" ingredients in pharmaceutical products: update. *Pediatrics.* 1997;99:268-278.
19. Hall CM, Milligan DWA, Berrington J. Probably adverse reaction to a pharmaceutical excipient. *Arch Dis Child Fetal Neonatal Ed.* 2004;89:F184.
20. Hiller JL, Benda GI, Rahatzad M, et al. Benzyl alcohol toxicity: impact on mortality and intraventricular hemorrhage among very low birth weight infants. *Pediatrics.* 1986;77:500-506.
21. Grant JA, Bilodeau PA, Guernsey BG, et al. Unsuspected benzyl alcohol hypersensitivity. *N Engl J Med.* 1982;306:108.
22. Wilson JP, Solimando DA, Edwards MS. Parenteral benzyl alcohol-induced hypersensitivity reaction. *Drug Intell Clin Pharm.* 1986;20:689-691.
23. Kirch W, Halabi A, Linde M, et al. Negative effects of famotidine on cardiac performance assessed by noninvasive hemodynamic measurements. *Gastroenterology.* 1989;96:1388-1392.
24. Guillet R, Stoll BJ, Cotton CM, et al. Association of H2-blocker therapy and higher incidence of necrotizing enterocolitis in very low birth weight infants. *Pediatrics.* 2006;117:e137-e142.

Fenoldopam

1. Verghese ST, Hammer GB, Lavandosky G, et al. A multicenter, randomized study to determine the pharmacokinetics and pharmacodynamics of fenoldopam mesylate in pediatric patients. *Am J Ther.* 1999;6:283-288.
2. Costello JM, Thiagarajan RR, Dionne RE, et al. Initial experience with fenoldopam after cardiac surgery in neonates with an insufficient response to conventional diuretics. *Pediatr Crit Care Med.* 2006;7:28-33.
3. US Department of Health and Human Services, National Institutes of Health, National Heart, Lung, and Blood Institute. Diagnosis, evaluation, and treatment of high blood pressure in children and adolescents. 4th report. NIH Publication 05-5267. Revised May 2005.
4. Corlopam [prescribing information]. Chicago, IL: Abbott Laboratories; March 2004. Available at: http://www.fda.gov/Medwatch/SAFETY/2004/apr_PI/Corlopam_PI.pdf. Accessed September 13, 2006.
5. Aronoff A, Brier M, Bennett W. *The Renal Book, 2002.* http://www.kdp-baptist.louisville.edu/renalbook/. Accessed August 14, 2006.
6. Karkowsky AM. *Fenoldopam Pediatrics.* Clinical Review for NDA 19-922. http://www.fda.gov/cder/foi/esum/2004/19922_BPCA_Corlopam_Clinical_Review_ltr.pdf#search=%22fenoldopam%20pediatrics%22. Accessed September 13, 2006.

7. Trissel LA, ed. *Handbook on Injectable Drugs.* 13th ed. [CD-ROM version 1.5]. Bethesda, MD: American Society of Health-System Pharmacists; 2005.
8. American Academy of Pediatrics Committee on Drugs. "Inactive" ingredients in pharmaceutical products: update. *Pediatrics.* 1997;99:268-278.
9. Lester MR. Sulfite sensitivity: significance in human health. *J Am Col Nutr.* 1995;14:229-232.
10. Smolinske SC. Review of parenteral sulfite reactions. *J Toxicol Clin Toxicol.* 1992;30:597-606.
11. Lechner BL, Pascual JF, Roscelli JD. Failure of fenoldopam to control severe hypertension secondary to renal graft rejection in a pediatric patient. *Mil Med.* 2005;170:130-132.

Fentanyl Citrate

1. Anand KJ, Sippell WG, Aynsley-Green A. Randomized trial of fentanyl anesthesia in preterm babies undergoing surgery: effects on the stress response. *Lancet.* 1987;243-248.
2. Collins C, Koren G, Crean P, et al. Fentanyl pharmacokinetics and hemodynamic effects in preterm infants during ligation of patient ductus arteriosus. *Anesth Analg.* 1985;64:1078-1080.
3. Friesen R, Henry D. Cardiovascular changes in preterm neonates receiving isofluorane, halothane, fentanyl, and ketamine. *Anesthesiology.* 1986;64:238-242.
4. Hickey PR, Hansen DD, Wessel DL, et al. Pulmonary and systemic hemodynamic responses to fentanyl in infants. *Anesth Analg.* 1985;64:483-486.
5. Robinson S, Gregory G. Fentanyl-air-oxygen anesthesia for ligation of patent ductus arteriosus in preterm infants. *Anesth Analg.* 1981;60:331-334.
6. Yaster M. The dose response of fentanyl in neonatal anesthesia. *Anesthesiology.* 1987;66:433.
7. Koren G, Goresky G, Crean P, et al. Pediatric fentanyl dosing based on pharmacokinetics during cardiac surgery. *Anesth Analg.* 1984;63:577-582.
8. Sandler ES, Weyman C, Conner K, et al. Midazolam versus fentanyl as premedication for painful procedures in children with cancer. *Pediatrics.* 1992;89:631-634.
9. McEvoy GK, ed. *AHFS Drug Information Essentials 2005–06.* Bethesda, MD: American Society of Health-System Pharmacists; 2005.
10. Roth B, Schlunder C, Houben F, et al. Analgesia and sedation in neonatal intensive care using fentanyl by continuous infusion. *Dev Pharmacol Ther.* 1991;17:121-127.
11. Leuschen MP, Willwitt LD, Hoie EB, et al. Plasma fentanyl levels in infants undergoing extracorporeal membrane oxygenation. *J Thorac Cardiovasc Surg.* 1993;105:885-891.
12. Arnold JH, Truog RD, Scavone JM, et al. Changes in the pharmacodynamic response to fentanyl in neonates during continuous infusion. *J Pediatr.* 1991;119:639-643.
13. Koren G, Maurice L. Pediatric uses of opioids. *Pediatr Clin North Am.* 1989;36(5):1141-1157.
14. Robinson S, Gregory G. Fentanyl-air-oxygen anesthesia for ligation of patent ductus arteriosus in preterm infants. *Anesth Analg.* 1981;60:331-334.
15. Lago P, Benini F, Zacchello F. Randomized controlled trial of low dose fentanyl infusion in preterm infants with hyaline membrane disease. *Arch Dis Child Fetal Neonatal Ed.* 1998;79:F194-F197.
16. Buck ML. Pharmacokinetic changes during extracorporeal membrane oxygenation. Implications for drug therapy of neonates. *Clin Pharmacokinet.* 2003;42:403-417.
17. Hanson DD, Hickey PR. Anesthesia for hypoplastic left heart syndrome: use of high-dose fentanyl in 30 neonates. *Anesth Analg.* 1986;65:127-132.
18. Fentanyl citrate injection [USP package insert]. Deerfield, IL: Baxter; November 2003.
19. Billmire DA, Neale HW, Gregory R. Use of IV fentanyl in the outpatient treatment of pediatric facial trauma. *J Trauma.* 1985;25:1079-1080.
20. Koehntop DE, Rodman JH, Brundage DM, et al. Pharmacokinetics of fentanyl in neonates. *Anesth Analg.* 1986;65:227–232.
21. Trissel LA. *Handbook on Injectable Drugs.* 13th ed. Bethesda, MD: American Society of Health-System Pharmacists; 2005.
22. Tobias JD. Subcutaneous administration of fentanyl and midazolam to prevent withdrawal after prolonged sedation in children. *Crit Care Med.* 1999;27:2262-2265.
23. Comstock MK, Schamman FL, Carter JG, et al. Rigidity and hypercarbia on fentanyl–oxygen induction. *Anesthesiology.* 1979;51:328.
24. Jarvis AP, Arancibia CU. A case of difficult neonatal ventilation. *Anesth Analg.* 1987;66:196-199.
25. Wells S, Williamson M, Hooker D. Fentanyl-induced chest wall rigidity in a neonate: a case report. *Heart Lung.* 1994;23:196-198.
26. Lane JC, Tennison MB, Lawless ST, et al. Movement disorder after withdrawal of fentanyl infusion. *J Pediatr.* 1991;119: 649-651.
27. Katz R, Kelly HW, Hsi A. Prospective study on the occurrence of withdrawal in critically ill children who receive fentanyl by continuous infusion. *Crit Care Med.* 1994;22:763-767.
28. Bragonier R, Bartle D, Langton-Hewer S. Acute dystonia in a 14-yr-old following propofol and fentanyl anaesthesia. *Br J Anaesth.* 2000;84:828-829.
29. Aouad MT, Kanzi GE, Siddik-Sayyid SM, et al. Preoperative caudal block prevents emergence agitation in children following sevoflurane anesthesia. *Acta Anaesthesiol Scand.* 2005;49:300-304.
30. Demirbilek S, Togal T, Cicek M, et al. Effects of fentanyl on the incidence of emergence agitation in children receiving desflurane or sevoflurane anaesthesia. *Eur J Anaesthesiol.* 2004;21:538-542.

Ferric Gluconate

1. McEvoy GK, ed. *AHFS Drug Information 2005.* Bethesda, MD: American Society of Health-System Pharmacists; 2005:1429-1433.
2. *Physicians' Desk Reference.* 60th ed. Montvale, NJ: Thomson PDR; 2006:1.
3. Ferrlecit (sodium ferric gluconate complex in sucrose injection) [product information]. Corona CA: Watson Pharma Inc; 2004.
4. Tenbrok K, Muller-Berghaus J, Michalk D, et al. Intravenous iron treatment of renal anemia in children on hemodialysis. *Pediatr Nephrol.* 1999;13:580-582.
5. Yorgin PD, Belson A, Sarwal M, et al. Sodium ferric gluconate therapy in renal transplant and renal failure patients. *Pediatr Nephrol.* 2000;15:171-175.
6. Gillespie RS, Symons JM. Sodium ferric gluconate for post-transplant anemia in pediatric and you adult renal transplant recipients. *Pediatr Transplantation.* 2005;9:43-46.
7. Warady BA, Zobrist RH, Wu J, et al. Sodium ferric gluconate complex therapy in anemic children on hemodialysis. *Pediatr Nephrol.* 2005;20:1320-1327.
8. NKR-DOQI clinical practice guidelines for the treatment of anemia of chronic renal failure. National Kidney Foundation—Dialysis Outcomes Quality Initiative. Available at: http://www.kidney.org/professionals/kdoqi/guidelines_updates/doqiupan_iii.html#8:. Accessed April 21, 2006.
9. Fishbane S, Kowalski EA. The comparative safety of intravenous iron dextran, iron saccharate, and sodium ferric gluconate. *Seminars in Dialysis.* 2000;13(6):381-384.
10. Chertow GM, Mason PD, Vaage-Nilsen O, et al. On the relative safety of parenteral iron formulations. *Nephrol Dial Transplant.* 2004;19:1571-1575.
11. Baile GR, Clark JA, Lane CE, et al. Hypersensitivity reactions and deaths associated with intravenous iron preparations. *Nephrol Dial Transplant.* 2005;20:1443-1449.

References

12. Fishbane S. Safety in iron management. *Am J Kid Disease.* 2003;41(5):S18-S36.
13. Micheal B, Coyne DW, Fishbane S, et al. Sodium ferric gluconate complex in haemodialysis patients: adverse reactions compared to placebo and iron dextran. *Kidney International.* 2002;61:1830-1839.
14. Saadeh C, Srkalovic G. Acute hypersensitivity reaction to ferric gluconate in a premedicated patient. *Ann Pharmacother.* 2005;39:2124-2127.
15. Hiller JL, Benda GI, Rahatzad M, et al. Benzyl alcohol toxicity: impact on mortality and intraventricular hemorrhage among very low birth weight infants. *Pediatrics.* 1986;77:500-506.
16. American Academy of Pediatrics Committee on Drugs. "Inactive" ingredients in pharmaceutical products: update. *Pediatrics.* 1997;99:268-278.
17. Hall CM, Milligan DWA, Berrington J. Probably adverse reaction to a pharmaceutical excipient. *Arch Dis Child Fetal Neonatal Ed.* 2004;89:F1842.
18. Hiller JL, Benda GI, Rahatzad M, et al. Benzyl alcohol toxicity: impact on mortality and intraventricular hemorrhage among very low birth weight infants. *Pediatrics.* 1986;77:500-506.
19. Grant JA, Bilodeau PA, Guernsey BG, et al. Unsuspected benzyl alcohol hypersensitivity. *N Engl J Med.* 1982;306:108.
20. Wilson JP, Solimando DA, Edwards MS. Parenteral benzyl alcohol-induced hypersensitivity reaction. *Drug Intell Clin Pharm.* 1986;20:689-691.

Filgrastim

1. Kojima S, Fukada M, Miyajima Y, et al. Treatment of aplastic anemia in children with recombinant human granulocyte colony-stimulating factor. *Blood.* 1991;77:937-941.
2. Kojima S, Hibi S, Kosaka Y, et al. Immunosuppressive therapy using antithymocyte globulin, cyclosporine, and danazol with or without human granulocyte colony-stimulating factor in children with acquired aplastic anemia. *Blood.* 2000;96:2049-2054.
3. McEvoy GK, ed. *American Hospital Formulary Service Drug Information 2004.* Bethesda, MD: American Society of Health-System Pharmacists; 2004.
4. Neupogen (filgrastim) [product information]. Thousand Oaks, CA: Amgen Inc; December 2004.
5. Little MA, Morland B, Chisholm J, et al. A randomized study of prophylactic G-CSF following MRC UKALL XI intensification regimen in childhood ALL and T-NHL. *Med Pediatr Oncol.* 2002;38:98-103.
6. Alonzo TA, Kobrinsky NL, Aledo A, et al. Impact of granulocyte colony-stimulating factor use during induction for acute myelogenous leukemia in children: a report from the Children's Cancer Group. *J Pediatr Hematol Oncol.* 2002;24:627-635.
7. Furman WL, Crist WM. Biology and clinical applications of hemopoietins in pediatric practice. *Pediatrics.* 1992;90:716-728.
8. Riikonen P, Rahiala J, Salonvarra M, et al. Prophylactic administration of granulocyte colony-stimulating factor (filgrastim) after conventional chemotherapy in children with cancer. *Stem Cells.* 1995;13:289-294.
9. Hawkins DS, Felgenhauer J, Park J, et al. Peripheral blood stem cell support reduces the toxicity of intensive chemotherapy for children and adolescents with metastatic sarcomas. *Cancer.* 2002;95:1354-1365.
10. Welte K, Zeidler C, Reiter A, et al. Differential effects of granulocyte-macrophage colony-stimulating factor and granulocyte colony-stimulating factor in children with severe congenital neutropenia. *Blood.* 1990;75:1056-1063.
11. Bonilla MA, Gillio AP, Ruggeiro M, et al. Effects of recombinant human granulocyte colony-stimulating factor on neutropenia in patients with congenital agranulocytosis. *N Engl J Med.* 1989;320:1574-1580.
12. Gillan ER, Christensen RD, Suen Y, et al. A randomized, placebo-controlled trial of recombinant human granulocyte colony-stimulating factor administration in newborn infants with presumed sepsis: significant induction of peripheral and bone marrow neutrophilia. *Blood.* 1994;84:1427-1433.
13. Makhlouf RA, Doron MW, Bose CL, et al. Administration of granulocyte colony-stimulating factor to neutropenic low birth weight infants of mothers with pre-eclampsia. *J Pediatr.* 1995;126:454-456.
14. Kucukoduk S, Sezer T, Yildiran A, et al. Randomized, double-blinded, placebo-controlled trial of early administration of recombinant human granulocyte colony-stimulating factor to non-neutropenic preterm newborns between 33 and 36 weeks with presumed sepsis. *Scand J Infect Dis.* 2002;34:893-897.
15. Ahmad A, Laborada G, Bussel J, et al. Comparison of recombinant granulocyte colony-stimulating factor, recombinant human granulocyte-macrophage colony-stimulating factor and placebo for treatment of septic preterm infants. *Pediatr Infect Dis J.* 2002;21:1061-1065.
16. Schroten H, Roesler J, Breidenbach T, et al. Granulocyte and granulocyte-macrophage colony-stimulating factors for treatment of neutropenia in glycogen storage disease type Ib. *J Pediatr.* 1991;119:748-754.
17. Calderwood S, Kilpatrick L, Douglas SD, et al. Recombinant human granulocyte colony-stimulating factor therapy for patients with neutropenia and/or neutrophil dysfunction secondary to glycogen storage disease type 1b. *Blood.* 2001;97:376-382.
18. de la Rubia J, Arbona C, de Arriba F, et al. Analysis of factors associated with low peripheral blood progenitor cell collection in normal donors. *Transfusion.* 2002;42:4-9.
19. Madero L, Gonzalez-Vicent M, Molina J, et al. Use of concurrent G-CSF + GM-CSF vs G-CSF alone for mobilization of peripheral blood stem cells in children with malignant disease. *Bone Marrow Transplant.* 2000;26:365-369.
20. Perez-Duenas B, Alcorta I, Estella J, et al. Safety and efficacy of high-dose G-CSF (24 mcg/kg) alone for PBSC mobilization in children. *Bone Marrow Transplant.* 2002;30:987-988.
21. Welte K, Zeidler C, Reiter A, et al. Correction of neutropenia and associated clinical symptoms with recombinant human granulocyte colony-stimulating factor (rhG-CSF) in children with severe congenital neutropenia. *Med Pediatr Oncol.* 1990;18(6):519. (abstract)
22. Medical Economics, ed. *Physicians' Desk Reference.* 54th ed. Oradell, NJ: Medical Economics Company; 2006.
23. Trissel LA. *Handbook on Injectable Drugs.* 13th ed. Bethesda, MD: American Society of Health-System Pharmacists; 2005.

Fluconazole

1. Diflucan [prescribing information]. New York, NY: Pfizer Inc; August 2004.
2. Saxen H, Hoppu K, Pohjavuori M. Pharmacokinetics of fluconazole in very low birth weight infants during the first two weeks of life. *Clin Pharmacol Ther.* 1993;54:269-277.
3. Brammer KW, Coates PE. Pharmacokinetics of fluconazole in pediatric patients. *Eur J Clin Microbiol Infect Dis.* 1994;13:325-329.
4. Viscoli C, Castagnola E, Corsini M, et al. Fluconazole therapy in an underweight infant. *Eur J Clin Microbiol Infect Dis.* 1989;8:925-926.
5. Wiest DB, Flower SL, Garner SS, et al. Fluconazole in neonatal disseminated candidiasis. *Arch Dis Child.* 1991;66:1002.
6. Bergman KA, Meis JF, Horrevorts AM, et al. Acute renal failure in a neonate due to pelviureteric candidal bezoars successfully treated with long-term systemic fluconazole. *Acta Pediatr.* 1992;81:709-711.
7. Huttova M, Hartmanova I, Kralinsky K, et al. Candida fungemia in neonates treated with fluconazole: report of forty cases, including eight with meningitis. *Pediatr Infect Dis J.* 1998;17:1012-1015.
8. Novelli V, Holzel H. Safety and tolerability of fluconazole in children. *Antimicrob Agents Chemother.* 1999;43:1955-1960.
9. Driessen M, Ellis JB, Cooper PA, et al. Fluconazole vs. amphotericin B for the treatment of neonatal fungal septicemia: a prospective randomized trial. *Pediatr Infect Dis J.* 1996;15:1107-1112.
10. Wainer S, Cooper PA, Gouws H, et al. Prospective study of fluconazole therapy in systemic neonatal fungal infection. *Pediatr Infect Dis J.* 1997;16:763-767.
11. Bliss JM, Wellington M, Gigliotti F. Antifungal Pharmacotherapy for Neonatal Candidiasis. *Semin Perinatol.* 2003;27(5):365-374.

12. Kaufman D, Boyle R, Hazen KC, et al. Fluconazole Prophylaxis Against Fungal Colonization and Infection in Preterm Infants. *N Engl J Med.* 2001;345:1660-1666.
13. Kicklighter SD, Springer SC, Cox T, et al. Fluconazole for prophylaxis against candidal rectal colonization in the very low birth weight infant. *Pediatrics.* 2001;107:293-298.
14. Viscoli C, Castagnola E, Fioredda F, et al. Fluconazole in the treatment of candidiasis in immunocompromised children. *Antimicrob Agents Chemother.* 1991;35:365-367.
15. Lee JW, Seibel NL, Amantea M, et al. Safety and pharmacokinetics of fluconazole in children with neoplastic diseases. *J Pediatr.* 1992;120:987-993.
16. Santeiro ML, Riggs D, Weibley RE. Fluconazole therapy in a child with candida tropicalis fungemia. *Ann Pharmacother.* 1992;26:840. Letter.
17. American Academy of Pediatrics. In: Pickering LK, ed. *Red Book: 2006 Report of the Committee on Infectious Diseases.* 27th ed. Elk Grove Village, IL: American Academy of Pediatrics; 2006.
18. Simon G, Simon G, Erdos M, et al. Invasive Cryptococcus laurentii disease in a nine-year-old boy with X-linked Hyper-immunoglobulin M syndrome. *Pediatr Infect Dis J.* 2005;24:935-937.
19. Seay RE, Larson TA, Toscano JP, et al. Pharmacokinetics of fluconazole in immune-compromised children with leukemia or other hematologic diseases. *Pharmacotherapy.* 1995;15:52-58.
20. Humphrey MJ, Jevons S, Tarbit MH. Pharmacokinetic evaluation of UK-49858, a metabolically stable triazole antifungal agent, in animals and humans. *Antimicrob Agents Chemother.* 1985;28:648-653.
21. Dudley MN. Clinical pharmacology of fluconazole. *Pharmacotherapy.* 1990;10(suppl):141-145.
22. Aronoff A, Brier M, Bennett W. *The Renal Book, 2002.* Available at: http://www.kdp-baptist.louisville.edu/renalbook/. Accessed August 10, 2006.
23. Nicolau DP, Crowe H, Nightingale CH, et al. Effect of continuous arteriovenous hemodiafiltration on the pharmacokinetics of fluconazole. *Pharmacotherapy.* 1994;14:502-505.
24. Bafeltowska JJ, Buszman E. Pharmacokinetics of fluconazole in the cerebrospinal fluid of children with hydrocephalus. *Chemother.* 2005;51:370-376.
25. Trissel LA. *Handbook on Injectable Drugs.* 13th ed. Bethesda, MD: American Society of Hospital Pharmacists; 2005.
26. Debruyne D, Rycelynck JP. Clinical pharmacokinetics of fluconazole. *Clin Pharmacokinet.* 1993;24:10-27.

Flumazenil

1. Sugarman JM, Paul RI. Flumazenil: a review. *Pediatr Emerg Care.* 1994;10:37-43.
2. *Physicians' Desk Reference.* 60th ed. Montvale, NJ: Medical Economics Company; 2006.
3. Jones RD, Lawson AD, Andrew LJ, et al. Antagonism of the hypnotic effect of midazolam in children: a randomized, double blind study of placebo and flumazenil administered after midazolam-induced anesthesia. *Br J Anaesth.* 1991;66:660-666.
4. Jones RDM, Chan K, Roulson CJ, et al. Pharmacokinetics of flumazenil and midazolam. *Brit J Anaesthes.* 1993;70:286-292.
5. Negus BH, Street NE. Midazolam-opioid combination and postoperative upper airway obstruction in children. *Anaesthesia Int Care.* 1994;22:232-233.
6. Shannon M, Albers G, Burkhart K, et al. Safety and efficacy of flumazenil in the reversal of benzodiazepine-induced conscious sedation. *J Pediatr.* 1997;131:582-586.
7. Peters JM, Tolia V, Simpson P, et al. Flumazenil in children after esophagogastroduodenoscopy. *Am J Gastroenterol.* 1999;94:1857-1861.
8. American Society of Health-System Pharmacists. American Hospital Formulary System. Available at: http://ahfsfirst.firstdatabank.com/AHFSfirst/NSAHFSFirstSearchmain.asp. Accessed May 10, 2006.
9. American Academy of Pediatrics Committee on Drugs. Emergency drug doses for infants and children. *Pediatrics.* 1998;101:e1-e11.
10. Baktai G, Szekely E, Marialigeti T, et al. Use of midazolam (Dormicum) and flumazenil (Anexate) in paediatric bronchology. *Curr Med Res Opin.* 1992;12:552-559.
11. Collins S, Carter JA. Resedation after bolus administration of midazolam to an infant and its reversal by flumazenil. *Anaesthesia.* 1991;46:471-472.
13. Clark RF, Sage TA, Tunget CL, et al. Delayed onset lorazepam poisoning successfully reversed by flumazenil in a child: case report and review of the literature. *Pediatr Emerg Care.* 1995;11:32-34.
14. Kelly C, Egner J, Rubin J. Successful treatment of triazolam overdose with Ro 15-1788 (Anexate). *S Afr Med J.* 1988;73:442.
15. Roald OK, Dahl V. Flunitrazepam intoxication in a child successfully treated with the benzodiazepine antagonist flumazenil. *Crit Care Med.* 1989;17:1355-1356.
16. Richard P, Autret E, Bardon J, et al. The use of flumazenil in a neonate. *Clin Toxicol.* 1991;29:137-140.
17. Aronoff A, Brier M, Bennett W. *The Renal Book, 2002.* Available at: http://www.kdp-baptist.louisville.edu/renalbook/. Accessed May 26, 2006.
18. Trissel LA, ed. *Handbook on Injectable Drugs.* 13th ed. [CD-ROM version 1.5]. Bethesda, MD: American Society of Health-System Pharmacists; 2005. Accessed May 26, 2006.
19. Hoffman EJ, Warren EW. Flumazenil: a benzodiazepine antagonist. *Clin Pharm.* 1993;12:614-656.
20. L. O'Brien [personal communication]. Roche Laboratories; May 1995.
21. Soni MG, Taylor SL, Greenberg NA, et al. Evaluation of the health aspects of methyl paraben: a review of the published literature. *Food Chem Toxicol.* 2002;40:1335-1373.
22. Nagel JE, Fuscaldo JT, Firemen P. Paraben allergy. *JAMA.* 1977;237:1594-1595.
23. Spivey WH. Flumazenil and seizures. Analysis of 43 cases. *Clin Ther.* 1992;14:292-305.

Fomepizole

1. Antizole [package insert]. Minnetonka, MN: Orphan Medical Inc; December 2000.
2. Mégarbane B, Borron SW, Baud FJ. Current recommendations for treatment of severe toxic alcohol poisonings. *Intensive Care Med.* 2005;31:189-195.
3. Casavant MJ. Fomepizole in the treatment of poisoning. *Pediatrics.* 2001;107:170.
4. Mycyk MB, Leikin JB. Antidote review: fomepizole for methanol poisoning. *Am J Ther.* 2003;10:68-70.
5. Brophy PD, Tenenbein M, Gardner J, et al. Childhood diethylene glycol poisoning treated with alcohol dehydrogenase inhibitor fomepizole and hemodialysis. *Am J Kidney Dis.* 2000;35:958-962.
6. Baum CR, Langman CB, Oker EE, et al. Fomepizole treatment of ethylene glycol poisoning in an infant. *Pediatrics.* 2000;106:1489-1491.
7. De Brabander N, Wojciechowski M, De Decker K, et al. Fomepizole as a therapeutic strategy in paediatric methanol poisoning. A case report and review of the literature. *Eur J Pediatr.* 2005;164:158-161.
8. Benitez JG, Swanson-Biearman B, Krenzelok EP. Nystagmus secondary to fomepizole administration in a pediatric patient. *Clin Toxicol.* 2000;38:795-798.
9. Faessel H, Houze P, Baud FJ, et al. 4-methylpyrazole monitoring during haemodialysis of ethylene glycol intoxicated patients. *Eur J Clin Pharmacol.* 1995;49:211-213.
10. Jobard E, Harry P, Turcant A, et al. 4-Methylpyrazole and hemodialysis in ethylene glycol poisoning. *J Toxicol Clin Toxicol.* 1996;34:373-377.
11. Brent J. Current management of ethylene glycol poisoning. *Drugs.* 2001;61:979-988.

References

Foscarnet, Trisodium Phosphonoformate

1. American Academy of Pediatrics. In: Pickering LK, ed. *Red Book: 2006 Report of the Committee on Infectious Diseases.* 27th ed. Elk Grove Village, IL: American Academy of Pediatrics; 2006.
2. McEvoy GK, ed. *Drug Information Essentials 2005–06*. Bethesda, MD: American Society of Health-System Pharmacists; 2005.
3. Walton RC, Whitcup SM, Mueller BU, et al. Combined intravenous ganciclovir and foscarnet for children with recurrent cytomegalovirus retinitis. *Ophthalmology.* 1995;102:1865-1870.
4. Sastry SM, Epps CH, Walton RC, et al. Combined ganciclovir and foscarnet in pediatric cytomegalovirus retinitis. *J Natl Med Assoc.* 1996;88:661-662.
5. Tejada P, Sarmiento B, Ramos JT, et al. Report of a case of aggressive cytomegalovirus retinitis in an infant with AIDS. *Int Ophthalmol.* 1996–1997;333-337.
6. Khurana RN, Charonis A, Samuel MA, et al. Intravenous foscarnet in the management of acyclovir-resistant herpes simplex virus type 2 in acute retinal necrosis in children. *Med Sci Monit.* 2005;11:CS75-CS78.
7. Bryant P, Sasadeusz J, Carapetis J, et al. Successful treatment of foscarnet-resistant herpes simplex stomatitis with intravenous cidofovir in a child. *Pediatr Infect Dis J.* 2001;20:1083-1086.
8. Crassard N, Souillet AL, Morfin F, et al. Acyclovir-resistant varicella infection with atypical lesions in a non-HIV leukemic infant. *Acta Paediatr.* 2000;89:1497-1499.
9. Levin MJ, Dahl KM, Weinberg A, et al. Development of resistance to acyclovir during chronic infection with the Oka vaccine strain of varicella-zoster virus, in an immunosuppressed child. *J Infect Dis.* 2003;188:954-959.
10. Aronoff GR, Berns JS, Brier ME, et al. *Drug Prescribing in Renal Failure: Dosing Guidelines for Adults.* 4th ed. Philadelphia, PA: American College of Physicians; 1999.
11. Trissel LA, ed. *Handbook on Injectable Drugs.* 13th ed. [CD-ROM version 1.5]. Bethesda, MD: American Society of Health-System Pharmacists; 2005.
12. Hainaut M, Gerard M, Peltier CA, et al. Effectiveness of rescue antiretroviral therapy including intravenously administered zidovudine and foscarnet in a child with HIV-1 enteropathy. *Eur J Pediatr.* 2003;162:528-529.

Fosphenytoin

1. American Society of Health-System Pharmacists. American Hospital Formulary System. Available at: http://ahfsfirst.firstdatabank.com/AHFSfirst/NSAHFSFirstSearchmain.asp. Accessed July 1, 2006.
2. Abernethy DR, Greenblatt DJ. Phenytoin disposition in obesity: determination of loading dose. *Arch Neurol.* 1985;42:468-471.
3. Gustafson MC, Ritter FJ. Fosphenytoin loading for status epilepticus in the neonate. *Epilepsia.* 1999;40:S124.
4. Kriel RL, Cifuentes RF. Fosphenytoin in infants of extremely low birth weight. *Pediatr Neurol.* 2001;24:219-221.
5. Pellock JM. Fosphenytoin use in children. *Neurology.* 1996;46:S14-S16.
6. Pfizer Inc. Data on file. New York, NY; 2000.
7. Meek PD, Davis SN, Collins DM, et al. Guidelines for nonemergency use of parenteral phenytoin products: proceedings of an expert panel consensus process. Panel on Nonemergency Use of Parenteral Phenytoin Products. *Arch Intern Med.* 1999;159:2639-2644.
8. Takeoka M, Krishnamoorthy KS, Soman TB, et al. Fosphenytoin in infants. *J Child Neurol.* 1998;13:537-540.
9. Koul R, Deleu D. Subtherapeutic free phenytoin levels following fosphenytoin therapy in status epilepticus. *Neurology.* 2002;58:147-148.
10. Lewis RJ, Yee L, Inkelis SH, et al. Clinical predictors of post-traumatic seizures in children with head trauma. *Ann Emerg Med.* 1993;22:1114-1118.
11. Tilford JM, Simpson PM, Yeh TS, et al. Variation in therapy and outcome for pediatric head trauma patients. *Crit Care Med.* 2001;29:1056 1061.
12. Adelson PD, Bratton SL, Carney NA, et al. Guidelines for the acute medical management of severe traumatic brain injury in infants, children, and adolescents. Chapter 19. The role of anti-seizure prophylaxis following severe pediatric traumatic brain injury. *Pediatr Crit Care Med.* 2003;4(3 suppl):S72-S75.
13. Stowe CD, Lee KR, Storgion SA, et al. Altered phenytoin pharmacokinetics in children with severe, acute traumatic brain injury. Status epilepticus. *J Clin Pharmacol.* 2000;40:1452-1461.
14. Sjoholm I, Kober A, Odar-Cedelof I, et al. Protein binding in uremia and normal serum: the role of endogenous binding inhibitors. *Biochem Pharmacol.* 1976;25:1205-1213.
15. Liponi DL, Winter ME, Tozer TN. Renal function and therapeutic concentrations of phenytoin. *Neurology.* 1984;34:395-397.
16. Beck DE, Farringer JA, Ravis WR, et al. Accuracy of three methods for predicting concentrations of free phenytoin. *Clin Pharm.* 1987;6:888-894.
17. Pryor FM, Gidal B, Ramsay RE, et al. Fosphenytoin: pharmacokinetics and tolerance of intramuscular loading doses. *Epilepsia.* 2001;42:245-250.
18. Jamerson BD, Dukes GE, Brouwer KL, et al. Venous irritation related to intravenous administration of phenytoin versus fosphenytoin. Pharmacotherapy. 1994;14:47–52.
19. Boucher BA. Fosphenytoin: a novel phenytoin prodrug. *Pharmacotherapy.* 1996;16:777-791.
20. Anderson GD. A mechanistic approach to antiepileptic drug interactions. *Ann Pharmacother.* 1998;32:554-563.
21. Kugler AR, Annesley TM, Nordblom GD, et al. Cross-reactivity of fosphenytoin in two human plasma phenytoin immunoassays. *Clin Chem.* 1998;44:1474-1480.
22. McBryde KD, Wilcox J, Kher KK. Hyperphosphatemia due to fosphenytoin in a pediatric ESRD patient. *Pediatr Nephrol.* 2005;20:1182-1185.

Furosemide

1. McEvoy GK, ed. *AHFS Drug Information Essentials 2005–06*. Bethesda, MD: American Society of Health-System Pharmacists; 2005.
2. Eades SK, Christensen ML. The clinical pharmacology of loop diuretics in the pediatric patient. *Pediatr Nephrol.* 1998;12:603-616.
3. Mirochnick MH, Miceli JJ, Kramer PA, et al. Furosemide pharmacokinetics in very low birth weight infants. *J Pediatr.* 1988;112:653-657.
4. Singh NC, Kissoon N, Mofada SA, et al. Comparison of continuous versus intermittent furosemide administration in postoperative pediatric cardiac patients. *Crit Care Med.* 1992;20:17-21.
5. Battista G, Nichani S, Chang AC, et al. Continuous versus intermittent furosemide infusion in critically ill infants after open heart operations. *Ann Thorac Surg.* 1997;64:1133-1139.
6. Copeland JG, Campbell DW, Plachetka JR, et al. Diuresis with continuous infusion of furosemide after cardiac surgery. *Am J Surg.* 1983;146:796-799.
7. Wells TG. The pharmacology and therapeutics of diuretics in the pediatric patient. *Pediatr Clin North Am.* 1990;37:463-504.
8. Ross BS, Pollak A, Oh W. The pharmacologic effects of furosemide therapy in the low-birth-weight infant. *J Pediatr.* 1978;92:149-152.
9. Engle MA, Lewy JE, Lewy PR, et al. The use of furosemide in the treatment of edema in infants and children. *Pediatrics.* 1978;62:811-818.
10. Yeh TF, Wilks A, Singh J, et al. Furosemide prevents the renal side effects of indomethacin therapy in premature infants with patent ductus arteriosus. *J Pediatr.* 1982;101:433-437.
11. Woo WC, Dupont C, Collinge J, et al. Effects of furosemide in the newborn. *Clin Pharmacol Ther.* 1978;23:266-271.
12. Peterson RG, Simmons MA, Rumack BH. Pharmacology of furosemide in the premature newborn infant. *J Pediatr.* 1980;97:139-143.
13. Schwartz GH, David DS, Riggio RR, et al. Ototoxicity induced by furosemide. *N Engl J Med.* 1970;282:1413-1414.

14. Diuretics. Specific diuretic agents. In: Roberts RJ, ed. *Drug Therapy in Infants: Pharmacologic Principles and Clinical Experience.* Philadelphia, PA: WB Saunders Company; 1984:233-234.
15. Aranda JV, Perez J, Sitar DS, et al. Pharmacokinetic disposition and protein binding of furosemide in newborn infants. *J Pediatr.* 1978;93:507-511.
16. Chemtob S, Papageorgiou A, du Souich P, et al. Cumulative increase in serum furosemide concentration following repeated doses in the newborn. *Am J Perinatol.* 1987;4:203-205.
17. Prandota J. Pharmacodynamic determinants of furosemide diuretic effect in children. *Dev Pharmacol Ther.* 1986;9:88-101.
18. Serratto M. Diagnosis and management of heart failure in infants and children. *Comprehensive Ther.* 1992;18:11-19.
19. Dettorre MD, Stidham GL, Watson DC, et al. Enhanced diuresis with continuous furosemide infusion in post-operative pediatric cardiac surgery patients. *Crit Care Med.* 1993;22:A183.
20. Luciani G, Nichani S, Chang AC, et al. Continuous versus intermittent furosemide infusion in critically ill infants after open heart operations. *Ann Thorac Surg.* 1998;64:1133-1139.
21. Chemtob S, Doray JL, Laudignon N, et al. Alternating sequential dosing with furosemide and ethacrynic acid in drug tolerance in the newborn. *Am J Dis Child.* 1989;143:850-854.
22. Weiss RA, Schoeneman M, Greifer I. Treatment of severe nephrotic edema with albumin and furosemide. *NY State J Med.* 1984;84:384-386.
23. Melvin T, Bennett W. Management of nephrotic syndrome in childhood. *Drugs.* 1991;42:30-51.
24. Baliga R, Lewy JE. Pathogenesis and treatment of edema. *Pediatr Nephrol.* 1987;34:639-647.
25. Haws RM, Baum M. Efficacy of albumin and diuretic therapy in children with nephrotic syndrome. *Pediatrics.* 1993;91:1142-1146.
26. Kelsch RC, Sedman AB. Nephrotic syndrome. *Pediatr Rev.* 1993;14:30-38.
27. Robson WLM, Leung AKC. Nephrotic syndrome in childhood. *Pediatr Rev.* 1993;40:287-323.
28. Scala JL, Jew RK, Poon CY, et al. In vitro analysis of furosemide disposition during neonatal extracorporeal membrane oxygenation (ECMO). *Pediatr Res.* 1996;39(suppl):78A.
29. Trissel LA, ed. *Handbook on Injectable Drugs.* 13th ed. Bethesda, MD: American Society of Health-System Pharmacists; 2005.
30. Loggie JMH, Kleinman LI, Maanen EFV. Renal function and diuretic therapy in infants and children. Part III. *J Pediatr.* 1975;86:825-832.
31. Gallagher KL, Jones JK. Furosemide-induced ototoxicity. *Ann Intern Med.* 1979;91:744-745.
32. Borradori C, Fawer CL, Buelin T, et al. Risk factors of sensorineural hearing loss in preterm infants. *Biol Neonate.* 1997;71:1-10.
33. Rybak LP. Furosemide ototoxicity: clinical and experimental aspects. *Laryngoscope.* 1985;95:1-14.
34. Brummett RE, Bendrick T, Himes D. Comparative ototoxicity of bumetanide and furosemide when used in combination with kanamycin. *J Clin Pharmacol.* 1981;21:628-636.
35. Rybak LP. Pathophysiology of furosemide ototoxicity. *J Otolaryngol.* 1982;11:127-133.
36. Green TP, Thompson TR, Johnson DE, et al. Furosemide promotes patent ductus arteriosus in premature infants with respiratory-distress syndrome. *N Engl J Med.* 1983;308:743-748.
37. Hufnagle KG, Khan SN, Penn D, et al. Renal calcifications: a complication of long term furosemide therapy in preterm infants. *Pediatrics.* 1982;70:360-363.
38. Saarela T, Lanning P, Koivisto M, et al. Nephrocalcinosis in full-term infants receiving furosemide treatment for congestive heart failure: a study of the incidence and 2-year follow up. *Eur J Pediatr.* 1999;158:668-772.
39. Pope JC, Trusler LA, Klein AM, et al. The natural history of nephrocalcinosis in premature infants treated with loop diuretics. *J Urol.* 1996;156:709-712.
40. Alpert SA, Noe HN. Furosemide nephrolithiasis causing ureteral obstruction and urinoma in a preterm neonate. *Urology.* 2004;64:589.e9–589.e11.
41. Turmen T, Thom P, Louridas AT, et al. Protein binding and bilirubin displacing properties of bumetanide and furosemide. *J Clin Pharmacol.* 1982;22:551-556.

Ganciclovir Sodium

1. Singhal S, Mehta J, Powles R, et al. Three weeks of ganciclovir for cytomegaloviraemia after allogenic bone marrow transplant. *Bone Marrow Transplant.* 1995;15:777-781.
2. Bilgrami S, Aslanzadeh J, Feingold JM, et al. Cytomegalovirus viremia, viruria, and disease after autologous peripheral blood stem cell transplantation: no need for surveillance. *Bone Marrow Transplant.* 1999;24:69-73.
3. Atkinson K, Arthur C, Bradstock K, et al. Prophylactic ganciclovir is more effective in HLA-identical family member marrow transplant recipients than in more heavily immune-suppressed HLA-identical unrelated donor marrow transplant recipients. *Bone Marrow Transplant.* 1995;15:401-405.
4. Schmidt GM, Horak DA, Niland JC, et al. A randomized controlled trial of prophylactic ganciclovir for cytomegalovirus pulmonary infection in recipients of allogeneic bone marrow transplants. *N Engl J Med.* 1991;324:1005-1011.
5. American Academy of Pediatrics. In: Pickering LK, ed. *Red Book: 2006 Report of the Committee on Infectious Diseases.* 27th ed. Elk Grove Village, IL: American Academy of Pediatrics; 2006.
6. Green M, Reyes J, Nour B, et al. Randomized trial of ganciclovir followed by high-dose oral acyclovir vs. ganciclovir alone in the prevention of cytomegalovirus disease in pediatric liver transplant recipients: preliminary analysis. *Transplant Proc.* 1994;25:173-174.
7. Prokurat S, Drabik E, Grenda R. Ganciclovir in cytomegalovirus prophylaxis in high-risk pediatric renal transplant recipients. *Transplant Proc.* 1993;24:2577.
8. Canpolat C, Culbert S, Gardner M, et al. Ganciclovir prophylaxis for cytomegalovirus infection in pediatric allogeneic bone marrow transplant recipients. *Bone Marrow Transplant.* 1996;17:589-593.
9. Gerbase MW, Dubois D, Rothmeier C, et al. Cost and outcomes of prolonged cytomegalovirus prophylaxis to cover the enhanced immunosuppression phase following lung transplantation. *Chest.* 1999;116:1265-1272.
10. Gajarski RJ, Rosenblatt HW, Schowengerdt KO, et al. Outcomes among pediatric heart transplant recipients. *Tex Heart Inst J.* 1997;24:97-104.
11. Seu P, Winston DJ, Holt CD, et al. Long-term ganciclovir prophylaxis for successful prevention of primary cytomegalovirus (CMV) disease in CMV-seronegative liver transplant recipients with CMV-seropositive donors. *Transplantation.* 1997;4:1614-1617.
12. *Physicians' Desk Reference.* 60th ed. Montvale, NJ: Thomson PDR; 2006.
13. Gudnason T, Belani KK, Balfour HH Jr. Ganciclovir treatment of cytomegalovirus disease in immunocompromised children. *Pediatr Infect Dis J.* 1989;8:436-440.
14. King SM, Petric M, Superina R, et al. Cytomegalovirus infections in pediatric liver transplantation. *Am J Dis Child.* 1990;144:1307-1310.
15. Megison SM, Andrews WS. Combination therapy with ganciclovir and intravenous IgG for cytomegalovirus infections in pediatric liver transplant recipients.
16. Reusser P, Einsele H, Lee J, et al. Randomized multicenter trial of foscarnet versus ganciclovir for preemptive therapy of cytomegalovirus infection after allogeneic stem cell transplantation. *Blood.* 2002;99:1159-1164.
17. Tanaka-Kitajima N, Sugaya N, Fuatani T, et al. Ganciclovir therapy for congenital cytomegalovirus infection in six infants. *Pediatr Infect Dis J.* 2005;24:782-785.
18. Rojo P, Ramos JT. Ganciclovir treatment of children with congenital cytomegalovirus infection. *Pediatr Infect Dis J.* 2004;23:88-89.
19. Kimberlin DW, Lin CY, Sanchez PJ, et al. Effect of ganciclovir therapy on hearing in symptomatic congenital cytomegalovirus disease involving the central nervous system: a randomized, controlled trial. *J Pediatr.* 2003;143:16-25.
20. Michaels MG, Greenberg DP, Sabo DL, et al. Treatment of children with congenital cytomegalovirus infection with ganciclovir. *Pediatr Infect Dis J.* 2003;22:504-508.

References

21. Demmler GJ. Congenital cytomegalovirus infection treatment. *Pediatr Infect Dis J.* 2003;22:1005-1006.
22. Whitley RJ, Cloud G, Gruber W, et al. Ganciclovir treatment of symptomatic congenital cytomegalovirus infection: results of a phase II study. NATIONAL INSTITUTE OF ALLERGY AND INFECTIOUS DISEASES COLLABORATIVE ANTIVIRAL STUDY GROUP. *J Infect Dis.* 1997;175:1080-1086.
23. Nigro G, Scholz H, Bartmann U. Ganciclovir therapy for symptomatic congenital cytomegalovirus infection in infants: a two-regimen experience. *J Pediatr.* 1994;124:318-322.
24. Trang JM, Kidd L, Gruber W, et al. Linear single-dose pharmacokinetics of ganciclovir in newborns with congenital cytomegalovirus infections. *Clin Pharmacol Ther.* 1993;53:15-21.
25. Whitley RJ, Pass RF, Stagna SB, et al. Pharmacodynamic evaluation of ganciclovir (DHPG) in the treatment of symptomatic congenital cytomegalovirus (CMV) infection. *Pediatr Res.* 1991;29:188A. Abstract.
26. Saitoh A, Viani RM, Schrier RD, et al. Treatment of infants coinfected with HIV-1 and cytomegalovirus with combination antiretrovirals and ganciclovir. *J Allergy Clin Immunol.* 2004;114:983-985.
27. Tokimasa S, Hara J, Osugi Y, et al. Ganciclovir is effective for prophylaxis and treatment of human herpes-virus-6 in allogenic stem cell transplantation. *Bone Marrow Transplant.* 2002;29:595-598.
28. Aronoff GR, Berns JS, Brier ME, et al. *Drug Prescribing in Renal Failure: Dosing Guidelines for Adults.* 4th ed. Philadelphia, PA: American College of Physicians; 1999.
29. Trissel LA. *Handbook on Injectable Drugs.* 10th ed. Bethesda, MD: American Society of Health-Sytem Pharmacists; 1998.
30. Ghosh K, Muirhead D, Christine B, et al. Ultrastructural changes in peripheral blood neutrophils in a patient receiving ganciclovir for CMV pneumonitis following allogenic bone marrow transplantation. *Bone Marrow Transplant.* 1999;24:429-431.
31. Fischler B, Casswall TH, Malmborg P, et al. Ganciclovir treatment in infants with cytomegalovirus infection and cholestasis. *J Pediatric Gastroent Nutr.* 2002;34:154-157.
32. Iwanaga M, Zaitsu M, Ishii E, et al. Protein-losing gastroenteropathy and retinitis associated with cytomegalovirus infection in an immunocompetent infant: a case report. *Eur J Pediatr.* 2004;163:81-84.
33. Rongkavilit C, Bedard M, Ang JY, et al. Severe cytomegalovirus enterocolitis in an immunocompetent infant. *Pediatr Infect Dis J.* 2004;23:579-581.
34. Brady RC, Schleiss MR, Witte DP, et al. Placental transfer of ganciclovir in a woman with acquired immunodeficiency syndrome and cytomegalovirus disease. *Pediatr Infect Dis J.* 2002;21:796-797.

Gentamicin Sulfate

1. Schwartz SN, Pazin GJ, Lyon JA, et al. A controlled investigation of the pharmacokinetics of gentamicin and tobramycin in obese subjects. *J Infect Dis.* 1978;138:499-505.
2. Watterberg KL, Kelly W, Angelus P, et al. The need for a loading dose of gentamicin in neonates. *Ther Drug Monit.* 1989;11:16-20.
3. Semchuk W, Borgmann J, Bowman L. Determination of a gentamicin loading dose in neonates and infants. *Ther Drug Monit.* 1993;15:47-51.
4. Glover ML, Shaffer CL, Rubino CM, et al. A multicenter evaluation of gentamicin therapy in the neonatal intensive care unit. *Pharmacotherapy.* 2001;21:7-10.
5. Prober CG, Stevenson DK, Benitz WE. The use of antibiotics in neonates weighing less than 1200 grams. *Pediatr Infect Dis J.* 1990;9:111-121.
6. American Academy of Pediatrics. In: Pickering LK, ed. *2006 Red Book: Report of the Committee on Infectious Diseases.* 27th ed. Elk Grove Village, IL: American Academy of Pediatrics; 2006.
7. Nelson JS, Bradley JS. *Nelson's Pocketbook of Pediatric Antimicrobial Therapy.* 14th ed. Philadelphia, PA. Lippincott Williams & Wilkins; 2000.
8. Garfunkel JM. Use of gentamicin in newborn infants. *J Infect Dis.* 1971;124:S247-S248.
9. Paisley JW, Smith AL, Smith DH. Gentamicin in newborn infants. *Am J Dis Child.* 1973;126:473-477.
10. McCracken GH Jr, Threlkeld N, Thomas ML. Intravenous administration of kanamycin and gentamicin in newborn infants. *Pediatrics.* 1977;60:463-466.
11. Assael BM, Gianni V, Marini A, et al. Gentamicin dosage in preterm and term neonates. *Arch Dis Child.* 1977;52:883-886.
12. Szefler SJ, Wynn RJ, Clarke DF, et al. Relationship of gentamicin serum concentrations to gestational age in preterm and term neonates. *J Pediatr.* 1980;97:312-315.
13. Zenk KE, Miwa L, Cohen JL, et al. Effect of body weight on gentamicin pharmacokinetics in neonates. *Clin Pharm.* 1984;3:170-173.
14. Mullhall A, De Louvois J, Hurley R. Incidence of potentially toxic concentrations of gentamicin in the neonate. *Arch Dis Child.* 1983;58:897-900.
15. Koren G, Leeder S, Harding E, et al. Optimization of gentamicin therapy in very low birth weight infants. *Pediatr Pharmacol.* 1985;5:79-87.
16. Miranda JC, Schimmel MM, James LS, et al. Gentamicin kinetics in the neonate. *Pediatr Pharmacol.* 1985;5:57-61.
17. Edwards C, Low DC, Bissenden JG. Gentamicin dosage for the newborn. *Lancet.* 1986;1:508-509. Letter.
18. Dahl LB, Melby K, Gutteberg TJ, et al. Serum levels of ampicillin and gentamicin in neonates of varying gestational age. *Eur J Pediatr.* 1986;145:218-221.
19. Zarowitz BJ, Wynn RJ, Buckwald S, et al. High gentamicin trough concentrations in neonates of less than 28 weeks gestational age. *Dev Pharmacol Ther.* 1982;5:68-75.
20. Hindmarsh KW, Nation RL, Williams GL, et al. Pharmacokinetics of gentamicin in very low birth weight preterm infants. *Eur J Clin Pharmacol.* 1983;24:649-653.
21. Young TE, Mangum B, eds. *Neofax.* 18th ed. Raleigh, NC: Acorn Publishing Inc; 2005:36.
22. McAllister TA. Gentamicin in paediatrics. *Postgrad Med J.* 1974;50(suppl 7):45-52.
23. McCracken GH Jr, Eichenwald HF. Antimicrobial therapy: therapeutic recommendations and a review of the newer drugs. Part II. *J Pediatr.* 1974;85:451-456.
24. Taylor M, Keane C. Gentamicin dosage in children. *Arch Dis Child.* 1976;51:369-372.
25. Evans WE, Feldman S, Ossi M, et al. Gentamicin dosage in children: a randomized prospective comparison of body weight and body surface area as dose determinants. *J Pediatr.* 1979;94:139-143.
26. Contopoulos-Ioannidis DG, Giotis ND, Baliatsa DV, et al. Extended-Interval AMINOglycoside ADMINistration for CHILDREN: A META-analysis. *Pediatrics.* 2004;114:e111-e118.
27. Marik PE, Lipman J, Kobilski S, et al. A prospective randomized study comparing once- versus twice-daily amikacin dosing in critically ill adult and paediatric patients. *J Antimicrob Chemother.* 1991;28:753-764.
28. Kafetzis DA, Sianidou L, Vlachos E, et al. Clinical and pharmacokinetic study of a single daily dose of amikacin in paediatric patients with severe gram-negative infections. *J Antimicrob Chemother.* 1991;27:105-112.
29. Trujillo H, Robledo J, Robledo C, et al. Single dose amikacin in paediatric patients with severe gram-negative infections. *J Antimicrob Chemother.* 1991;27:141-147.
30. Viscoli C, Dudley M, Ferrea G, et al. Serum concentration and safety of a single daily dose of amikacin in children undergoing bone marrow transplantation. *J Antimicrob Chemother.* 1991;27:113-120.
31. Sung L, Dupuis LL, Bliss B, et al. Randomized controlled trial of once- versus thrice-daily tobramycin in febrile neutropenic children undergoing stem cell transplantation. *J Natl Cancer Inst.* 2003;95:1869-1877.
32. Dupuis LL, Sung L, Taylor T, et al. Tobramycin pharmacokinetics in children with febrile neutropenia undergoing stem cell transplantation: once-daily versus thrice-daily administration. *Pharmacotherapy.* 2004;24:564-573.
33. Bouffet E, Fuhrmann C, Frappaz D, et al. Once daily antibiotic regimen in paediatric oncology. *Arch Dis Child.* 1994;70:484-487.
34. International Antimicrobial Therapy Cooperative Group of the European Organization for Research and Treatment of Cancer. Efficacy and toxicity of single daily doses of amikacin and ceftriaxone versus multiple daily doses of amikacin and ceftazidime for infection in patients with

cancer and granulocytopenia. *Ann Intern Med.* 1993;119:584-593.
35. Krivoy N, Postovsky S, Elhasid R, et al. Pharmacokinetic analysis of amikacin twice and single daily dosage in immunocompromised pediatric patients. *Infection.* 1998;26:396-398.
36. Chicella M. Once-daily aminoglycoside dosing in pediatrics. What is its role? *J Pediatr Pharm Pract.* 2000:5;98-103.
37. Wakkace AW, Bertino JS. Use of once-daily aminoglycosides in children—rational or inappropriate? *J Pediatr Pharmacol Ther.* 2001;6:380-383.
38. Tobramycin. In: Kucer A, Crowe SM, Grayson ML, Hoy JF, eds. *The Use of Antibiotics: A Clinical Review of Antibacterial, Antifungal and Antiviral Drugs.* 5th ed. Boston, MA: Butterworth Heinemann; 1997:490-503.
39. Baddour LM, Wilson WR, Bayer AS, et al. Infective endocarditis: diagnosis, antimicrobial therapy, and management of complications: a statement for healthcare professionals from the Committee on Rheumatic Fever, Endocarditis, and Kawasaki Disease, Council on Cardiovascular Disease in the Young, and the Councils on Clinical Cardiology, Stroke, and Cardiovascular Surgery and Anesthesia, American Heart Association: endorsed by the Infectious Diseases Society of America. *Circulation.* 2005;111:e394-e434.
40. Aronoff A, Brier M, Bennett W. *The Renal Book, 2002.* http://www.kdp-baptist.louisville.edu/renalbook/. Accessed August 19, 2006.
41. Beringer PM, Vinks AA, Jelliffe RW, et al. Pharmacokinetics of tobramycin in adults with cystic fibrosis: implications for once-daily administration. *Antimicrob Agents Chemother.* 2000;44:809-813.
42. Bates RD, Nahata MC, Jones JW, et al. Pharmacokinetics and safety of tobramycin after once-daily administration in patients with cystic fibrosis. *Chest.* 1997;112:1208-1213.
43. Bragonier R, Brown NM. The pharmacokinetics and toxicity of once-daily tobramycin therapy in children with cystic fibrosis. *J Antimicrob Chemother.* 1998;42:103-106.
44. Master V, Roberts GW, Coulthard KP, et al. Efficacy of once-daily tobramycin monotherapy for acute pulmonary exacerbations of cystic fibrosis: a preliminary study. *Pediatr Pulmonol.* 2001;3:367-376.
45. Loirat P, Rohan J, Baillet A, et al. Increased glomerular filtration rate in patients with major burns and its effect on the pharmacokinetics of tobramycin. *N Engl J Med.* 1978;299:915-919.
46. Armstrong DK, Hidalgo HA, Eldadah M. Vancomycin and tobramycin clearance in an infant during continuous hemo-filtration. *Ann Pharmacother.* 1993;27:224-227.
47. Buck ML. Pharmacokinetic changes during extracorporeal membrane oxygenation. *Clin Pharmacokinet.* 2003;42:403-417.
48. Mendelson J, Portnoy J, Dick V, et al. Safety of the bolus administration of gentamicin. *Antimicrob Agents Chemother.* 1976;9:633-638.
49. Barza M, Brown RB, Shen D, et al. Predictability of blood levels of gentamicin in man. *J Infect Dis.* 1975;132:165-174.
50. Gillett AP, Falk RH, Andrews J, et al. Rapid intravenous injection of tobramycin: suggested dosage schedule and concentrations in serum. *J Infect Dis.* 1976;134:S110-S113.
51. Powell SH, Thompson WL, Luthe MA, et al. Once daily vs. continuous aminoglycoside dosing: efficacy and toxicity in animal and clinical studies of gentamicin, netilmicin and tobramycin. *J Infect Dis.* 1983;147:918-932.
52. Trissel LA, ed. *Handbook on Injectable Drugs.* 13th ed. [CD-ROM version 1.5]. Bethesda, MD: American Society of Health-System Pharmacists; 2005.
53. Bodey GP, Chang HY, Rodriguez V, et al. Feasibility of administering aminoglycoside antibiotics by continuous intravenous infusion. *Antimicrob Agents Chemother.* 1975;8:328-333.
54. Giacoia GP, Schentag JJ. Pharmacokinetics and nephrotoxicity of continuous intravenous infusion of gentamicin in low birth weight infants. *J Pediatr.* 1986;109:715-719.
55. Buchholz U, Richards C, Murthy R, et al. Pyrogenic reactions associated with single daily dosing of intravenous gentamicin. *Infect Control Hosp Epidemiol.* 2000;21:771-774.
56. Fanning MM, Wassel R, Piazza-Hepp T. Pyrogenic reactions to gentamicin therapy. *N Engl J Med.* 2000;343;1658-1659.
57. American Academy of Pediatrics Committee on Drugs. "Inactive" ingredients in pharmaceutical products: update. *Pediatrics.* 1997;99:268-278.
58. Smolinske SC. Review of parenteral sulfite reactions. *J Toxicol Clin Toxicol.* 1992;30:597-606.
59. Lester MR. Sulfite sensitivity: significance in human health. *J Am Col Nutr.* 1995;14:229-232.
60. Soni MG, Taylor SL, Greenberg NA, et al. Evaluation of the health aspects of methyl paraben: a review of the published literature. *Food Chem Toxicol.* 2002;40:1335-1373.
61. Nagel JE, Fuscaldo JT, Firemen P. Paraben allergy. *JAMA.* 1977;237:1594-1595.
62. American Society of Health-System Pharmacists. American Hospital Formulary System. Available at: http://ahfsfirst.firstdatabank.com/AHFSfirst/NSAHFSFirstSearchmain.asp. Accessed August 19, 2006.
63. Massey KL, Hendeles L, Neims A. Identification of children for whom routine monitoring of aminoglycoside serum concentrations is not cost effective. *J Pediatr.* 1986;109:897-901.
64. Logsdon BA, Phelps SJ. Routine monitoring of gentamicin serum concentrations in pediatric patients with normal renal function is unnecessary. *Ann Pharmacother.* 1997;31:1514-1518.
65. Franson TR, Ritch PS, Quebbeman EJ. Aminoglycoside serum concentration sampling via central venous catheters: a potential source of clinical error. *JPEN J Parenter Enteral Nutr.* 1987;11:77-79.
66. McLaughlin JE, Reeves DS. Clinical and laboratory evidence for inactivation of gentamicin by carbenicillin. *Lancet.* 1971;1(7693):261-264.
67. Riff LJ, Jackson GG. Laboratory and clinical conditions for gentamicin inactivation by carbenicillin. *Arch Intern Med.* 1972;130:887-891.
68. Manian FA, Stone WJ, Alford RH. Adverse antibiotic effects associated with renal insufficiency. *Rev Infect Dis.* 1990;12:236-249.
69. Davies M, Morgan JR, Anand C. Interactions of carbenicillin and ticarcillin with gentamicin. *Antimicrob Agents Chemother.* 1975;7:431-434.
70. Weibert R, Keane W, Shapiro F. Carbenicillin inactivation of aminoglycosides in patients with severe renal failure. *Trans Amer Soc Artif Int Organs.* 1976;22:439-443.
71. Beaubien AR, Desjardins S, Ormsby E, et al. Incidence of amikacin ototoxicity: a sigmoid function of total drug exposure independent of plasma levels. *Am J Otolaryngol.* 1989;10:234-243.
72. Beaubien AR, Ormsby E, Bayne A, et al. Evidence that amikacin ototoxicity is related to total perilymph area under the concentration-time curve regardless of concentration. *Antimicrob Agents Chemother.* 1991;35:1070-1074.
73. Snavely SR, Hodges GR. The neurotoxicity of antibacterial agents. *Ann Intern Med.* 1984;101:92-104.

Glycopyrrolate

1. Glycopyrrolate injection, USP [package insert]. Shirley, NY: American Regent Laboratories Inc; July 1998.
2. Annila P, Rorarius M, Reonikainen P, et al. Effect of pre-treatment with intravenous atropine or glycopyrrolate on cardiac arrhythmias during halothane anaesthesia for adenoidectomy in children. *Br J Anaesth.* 1998;80:756-760.
3. Badgwell JM, Heavner JE, Cooper MW, et al. The cardiovascular effects of anticholinergic agents administered during halothane anaesthesia in children. *Acta Anaesthesiol Scand.* 1988;32:383-387.
4. Mirakhur RK, Shepherd WF, Jones CJ. Ventilation and the oculocardiac reflex. Prevention of oculocardiac reflex during surgery for squints: role of controlled ventilation and anticholinergic drugs. *Anaesthesia.* 1986;41:825-828.
5. Pokela ML, Koivisto M. Physiological changes, plasma beta-endorphin and cortisol responses to tracheal intubation in neonates. *Acta Paediatr.* 1994;83:151-156.
6. Hardy JF, Charest J, Girouard G, et al. Nausea and vomiting after strabismus surgery in preschool children. *Can Anaesth Soc J.* 1986;33:57-62.
7. Rautakorpi P, Ali-Melkkila T, Kaila T, et al. Pharmacokinetics of glycopyrrolate in children. *J Clin Anesth.* 1994;6:217-220.
8. Wong Ay, Salem MR, Mani M, et al. Glycopyrrolate as a substitute for atropine in reversal of curarization in pediatric cardiac patients. *Anesth*

Analg. 1974;53:412-417.
9. Goldhill DR, Pyne A, Cones CJ. Antagonism of neuromuscular blockade. The cardiovascular effects in children of the combination of edrophonium and glycopyrronium. *Anaesthesia.* 1988;43:930-934.
10. Glycopyrrolate injection, USP. Shirley, NY: American Regent Laboratories Inc; July 1998.
11. Trissel LA, ed. *Handbook on Injectable Drugs.* 13th ed. Bethesda, MD: American Society of Health-System Pharmacists; 2005.
12. AHFSfirst□ Web version 2.03. Bethesda, MD: American Society of Health-System Pharmacists, First Databank Inc; 2002. Accessed August 9, 2006.
13. Pruitt JW, Goldwasser MS, Sabol SR, et al. Intramuscular ketamine, midazolam, glycopyrrolate for pediatric sedation in the emergency department. *J Oral Maxillofac Surg.* 1995;53:13-17.
14. American Academy of Pediatrics Committee on Drugs. "Inactive" ingredients in pharmaceutical products: update. *Pediatrics.* 1997;99:268-278.
15. Hall CM, Milligan DWA, Berrington J. Probably adverse reaction to a pharmaceutical excipient. *Arch Dis Child Fetal Neonatal Ed.* 2004;89: F184.
16. Hiller JL, Benda GI, Rahatzad M, et al. Benzyl alcohol toxicity: impact on mortality and intraventricular hemorrhage among very low birth weight infants. *Pediatrics.* 1986;77:500-506.
17. Grant JA, Bilodeau PA, Guernsey BG, et al. Unsuspected benzyl alcohol hypersensitivity. *N Engl J Med.* 1982;306:108.
18. Wilson JP, Solimando DA, Edwards MS. Parenteral benzyl alcohol-induced hypersensitivity reaction. *Drug Intell Clin Pharm.* 1986;20:689-691.

Granisetron HCl

1. Thomson PDR, ed. *Physicians' Desk Reference.* 60th ed. Montvale, NJ: Thomson Healthcare; 2006.
2. Miyamima Y, Numata S, Katayama I, et al. Prevention of chemotherapy-induced emesis with granisetron in children with a malignant disease. *Am J Pediatr Hematol Oncol.* 1994;16:236-241.
3. Lemerle J, Amaral D, Southall DP, et al. Efficacy and safety of granisetron in the prevention of chemotherapy-induced emesis in paediatric patients. *Eur J Cancer.* 1991;27:1081-1083.
4. Palmer R. Efficacy and safety of granisetron (Kytril) in two special patient populations: children and adults with impaired hepatic function. *Sem Oncol.* 1994;21:22-25.
5. Jacobson SJ, Shore RW, Greenberg M, et al. The efficacy and safety of granisetron in pediatric cancer patients who had failed standard antiemetic therapy during anticancer chemotherapy. *Am J Pediatr Hematol Oncol.* 1994;16:231-235.
6. Hahlen K, Quintana E, Pinkerton CR, et al. A randomized comparison of intravenously administered granisetron versus chlorpromazine plus dexamethasone in the prevention of ifosfamide-induced emesis in children. *J Pediatr.* 1995;126:309-313.
7. Craft AW, Price L, Eden OB, et al. Granisetron as antiemetic therapy in children with cancer. *Med Pediatr Oncol.* 1995;25:28-32.
8. Komada Y, Matsuyama T, Takao A, et al. A randomized dose-comparison trial of granisetron in preventing emesis in children with leukaemia receiving emetogenic chemotherapy. *Eur J Cancer.* 1999;35:1095-1101.
9. Fujii Y, Tanaka H, Ito M. Ramosetron compared with granisetron for the prevention of vomiting following strabismus surgery in children. *Br J Ophthalmol.* 2001;85:670-672.
10. Fujii Y, Tanaka H. Comparison of granisetron, droperidol, and metoclopramide for prevention of postoperative vomiting in children with a history of motion sickness undergoing tonsillectomy. *J Pediatr Surg.* 2001;36:460-462.
11. Tsuchida Y, Hayashi Y, Asami K, et al. Effects of granisetron in children undergoing high-dose chemotherapy: a multi-institutional, cross-over study. *Int J Oncol.* 1999;14:673-679.
12. Orchard PJ, Rogosheske J, Burns L, et al. A prospective randomized trial of the anti-emetic efficacy of ondansetron and granisetron during bone marrow transplantation. *Biol Blood Marrow Transplant.* 1999;5:386-393.
13. Kalaycio M, Mendez Z, Pohlman B, et al. Continuous-infusion granisetron compared to ondansetron for the prevention of nausea and vomiting after high-dose chemotherapy. *J Cancer Res Clin Oncol.* 1998;124:265-269.
14. Cieslak GD, Watcha MF, Phillips MB, et al. The dose-response relationship and cost-effectiveness of granisetron for the prophylaxis of pediatric postoperative emesis. *Anesthesiology.* 1996;85:1076-1085.
15. Fujii Y, Toyooka H, Tanaka H. Effective dose of granisetron for preventing postoperative emesis in children. *Can J Anaesth.* 1996;43:660-664.
16. Fujii Y, Toyooka H, Tanaka H. A granisetron-droperidol combination prevents postoperative vomiting in children. *Anesth Analg.* 1998;87:761-765.
17. Fujii Y, Tanaka H. Granisetron reduces post-operative vomiting in children: a dose-ranging study. *Eur J Anesthesiology.* 1999;16:62-65.
18. Fujii Y, Saitoh, Y, Tanaka H, et al. Prophylactic therapy with combined granisetron and dexamethasone for the prevention of post-operative vomiting in children. *Eur J Anesthesiology.* 1999;16:376-379.
19. Fujii Y, Tanaka H, Toyooka H. Granisetron and dexamethasone provide more improved prevention of postoperative emesis than granisetron alone in children. *Can J Anaesth.* 1996;43:229-232.
20. Trissel LA. *Handbook on Injectable Drugs.* 13th ed. Bethesda, MD: American Society of Hospital Pharmacists; 2005.
21. Boike SC, Ilson B, Zariffa N, et al. Cardiovascular effects of i.v. granisetron at two administration rates and of ondansetron in healthy adults. *Am J Health-Syst Pharm.* 1997;54:1172-1176.
22. Buyukavci M, Olgun H, Ceviz N. The effects of ondansetron and granisetron on electrocardiography in children receiving chemotherapy for acute leukemia. *Am J Clin Oncol.* 2005;28:201-204.
23. Contu A, Olmeo N, Piro S, et al. A comparison of the antiemetic efficacy and safety of intramuscular and intravenous formulations of granisetron in patients receiving moderately emetogenic chemotherapy. *Anticancer Drugs.* 1995;6:652-656.
24. The Italian Multicenter Study Group. A double-blind randomized study comparing intramuscular (i.m.) granisetron with i.m. granisetron plus dexamethasone in the prevention of delayed emesis induced by cisplatin. *Anticancer Drugs.* 1999;10:465-470.
25. Watanabe H, Hasegawa A, Shinozaki T, et al. Possible side effects of granisetron, an antiemetic agent, inpatients with bone and soft-tissue sarcomas receiving cytotoxic chemotherapy. *Cancer Chemother Pharmacol.* 1995;35:278-282.
26. Carmichael J, Harris AL. High-dose i.v. granisetron for the prevention of chemotherapy-induced emesis: cardiac safety and tolerability. *Anti-Cancer Drugs.* 2003;14:739-744.
27. American Academy of Pediatrics Committee on Drugs. "Inactive" ingredients in pharmaceutical products: update. *Pediatrics.* 1997;99:268-278.
28. Hall CM, Milligan DWA, Berrington J. Probable adverse reaction to a pharmaceutical excipient. *Arch Dis Child Fetal Neonatal Ed.* 2004;89: F184.
29. Hiller JL, Benda GI, Rahatzad M, et al. Benzyl alcohol toxicity: impact on mortality and intraventricular hemorrhage among very low birth weight infants. *Pediatrics.* 1986;77:500-506.
30. Grant JA, Bilodeau PA, Guernsey BG, et al. Unsuspected benzyl alcohol hypersensitivity. *N Engl J Med.* 1982;306:108.
31. Wilson JP, Solimando DA, Edwards MS. Parenteral benzyl alcohol-induced hypersensitivity reaction. *Drug Intell Clin Pharm.* 1986;20:689-691.
32. Wada I, Takeda T, Sato M, et al. Pharmacokinetics of granisetron in adults and children with malignant diseases. *Biol Pharm Bull.* 2001;244:432-435.

References

Haloperidol Lactate

1. Brown RL, Henke A, Greenhalgh DG, et al. The use of haloperidol in the agitated, critically ill pediatric patient with burns. *J Burn Care Rehabil.* 1996;17:34-38.
2. Ratcliff SL, Meyer WJ, Cuervo LJ, et al. The use of haloperidol and associated complications in the agitated, acutely ill pediatric burn patient. *J Burn Care Rehabil.* 2004;25:472-478.
3. Harrison AM, Lugo RA, Lee WE, et al. The use of haloperidol in agitated critically ill children. *Clin Pediatr.* 2002;41:51-54.
4. McEvoy GK, ed. *AHFS Drug Information Essentials 2005–06.* Bethesda, MD: American Society of Health-System Pharmacists; 2005.
5. Renal failure. Aronoff A, Brier M, Bennett W, eds. *The Renal Book, 2002.* Available at: http://www.kdp-baptist.louisville.edu/renalbook/. Accessed June 21, 2006.
6. American Academy of Pediatrics Committee on Drugs. Emergency drug doses for infants and children. *Pediatrics.* 1998;101:e1-e11.
7. Schieveld JN, Leentjens AF. Delirium in severely ill young children in the pediatric intensive care unit (picu). *J Am Acad Child Adolesc Psychiatry.* 2005;44:392-394.
8. Riker RR, Fraser GL, Cox PM. Continuous infusion of haloperidol controls agitation in critically ill patients. *Crit Care Med.* 1994;22:433-439.
9. Trissel LA. *Handbook on Injectable Drugs.* 13th ed. Bethesda, MD: American Society of Health-System Pharmacists; 2005.
10. Sharma ND, Rosman HS, Padhi D, et al. Torsades de pointes associated with intravenous haloperidol in critically ill patients. *Am J Cardiol.* 1998;81:238-240.
11. Isbister GK, Calit C, Kilham HA. Antipsychotic poisoning in young children. A systematic review. *Drug Safety.* 2005;28:1029-1044.
12. Soni MG, Taylor SL, Greenberg NA, et al. Evaluation of the health aspects of methyl paraben: a review of the published literature. *Food Chem Toxicol.* 2002;40:1335-1373.
13. Nagel JE, Fuscaldo JT, Firemen P. Paraben allergy. *JAMA.* 1977;237:1594-1595.
14. Scialli JV, Thornton WE. Toxic reactions from a haloperidol overdose in two children: thermal and cardiac manifestations. *JAMA.* 1977;239:48-49.

Heparin Sodium

1. Grady RM, Eisenberg PR, Bridges ND. Rational approach to use of heparin during cardiac catheterization in children. *J Am Coll Cardiol.* 1995;25:725-729.
2. Monagle P, Chan A, Masicotte P, et al. Antithrombotic therapy in children: the Seventh ACCP Conference on Antithrombotic and Thrombolytic Therapy. *Chest.* 2004;126(3 suppl):645S-687S.
3. Taketomo CK, Hodding JH, Kraus DM. *Pediatric Dosage Handbook.* 12th ed. Hudson, OH: Lexi-Comp Inc; 2005.
4. Bossert E, Peecroft PC. Peripheral intravenous lock irrigation in children: current practice. *Pediatr Nurs.* 1994;20:346-349, 355.
5. Lombardi TP, Gundersen B, Zammett LO, et al. Efficacy of 0.9% sodium chloride injection with or without heparin sodium for maintaining patency of intravenous catheters in children. *Clin Pharm.* 1988;7:832-836.
6. Kleiber C, Hanrahan K, Fagan CL, et al. Heparin vs. saline for peripheral IV locks in children. *Pediatr Nurs.* 1993;19:376, 405-409.
7. Heilskov J, Kleiber C, Johnson K, et al. A randomized trial of heparin and saline for maintaining intravenous locks in neonates. *JSPN.* 1998;3:111-116.
8. Randolph AG, Cook DJ, Gonzales CA, et al. Benefit of heparin in peripheral venous and arterial catheters: systemic review and meta-analysis of randomized controlled trials. *BMJ.* 1998;16:969-975.
9. Rajani K, Goetzman BW, Wennberg RP, et al. Effect of heparinization of fluids infused through an umbilical artery catheter on catheter patency and frequency of complications. *Pediatrics.* 1979;63:552-556.
10. David RJ, Merten DF, Anderson JC, et al. Prevention of umbilical artery catheter clots with heparinized infusates. *Dev Pharmacol Ther.* 1981;2:117-126.
11. Edwards MS, Buffone GJ, Rench MA, et al. Effect of continuous heparin infusion on bactericidal activity for group B streptococci in neonatal sera. *J Pediatr.* 1983;103:787-790.
12. Bosque E, Weaver L. Continuous versus intermittent heparin infusion of umbilical artery catheters in the newborn infant. *J Pediatr.* 1986;108:141-143.
13. Gilhooly JT, Lindenberg JA, Reynolds JW. Survey of umbilical artery catheter practices. *Clin Res.* 1986;34:142A.
14. Chang GY, Lueder FL, DiMichele DM, et al. Heparin and the risk of intraventricular hemorrhage in premature infants. *J Pediatr.* 1997;131:362-366.
15. Schmidt B, Andrew M. Neonatal thrombotic disease: prevention, diagnosis, and treatment. *J Pediatr.* 1988;113:407-409.
16. Alpan G, Eyal F, Springer C, et al. Heparinization of alimentation solutions administered through peripheral veins in premature infants: a controlled study. *Pediatrics.* 1984;74:375-378.
17. Treas LS, Katinis-Bridges B. Efficacy of heparin in peripheral venous infusion in neonates. *J Obstet Gynecol Neonatal Nurs.* 1991;21:214-219.
18. Moclair A, Bates I. The efficacy of heparin in maintaining peripheral infusions in neonates. *Eur J Pediatr.* 1995;154:567-570.
19. Klenner AF, Fusch C, Rakow A, et al. Benefit and risk of heparin for maintaining peripheral venous catheters in neonates: a placebo-controlled trial. *J Pediatr.* 2004;143:741-745.
20. Ronco C, Brendolan A, Bragantini L, et al. Treatment of acute renal failure in newborns by continuous arterio-venous hemofiltration. *Kidney Int.* 1986;29:908-915.
21. Rais-Bahrami K, Short BL. The current status of neonatal extracorporeal membrane oxygenation. *Semin Perinatol.* 2000;24:406-417.
22. Zaidan H, Dhanireddy R, Hamosh M, et al. Effect of continuous heparin administration on Intralipid clearing in very low birth weight infants. *J Pediatr.* 1982;101:599-602.
23. Spear ML, Stahl GE, Hamosh M, et al. Effect of heparin dose and infusion rate on lipid clearance and bilirubin binding in premature infants receiving intravenous fat emulsions. *J Pediatr.* 1988;112:94-98.
24. Andrew M, Marzinotto V, Massicotte P, et al. Heparin therapy in pediatric patients: a prospective cohort study. *Pediatr Res.* 1994;35:78-83.
25. Gal P, Ransom L. Neonatal thrombosis: treatment with heparin and thrombolytics. *DICP Ann Pharmacother.* 1991;25:853-856.
26. Rasoulpour M, McLean RH. Renal venous thrombosis in neonates. *Am J Dis Child.* 1980;134:276-279.
27. McDonald MM, Jacobson LJ, Hay WW Jr, et al. Heparin clearance in the newborn. *Pediatr Res.* 1981;15:1015-1018.
28. McDonald MM, Hathaway WE. Anticoagulant therapy by continuous heparinization in newborn and older infants. *J Pediatr.* 1982;101:451-457.
29. Coombs CJ, Richardson RW, Dowling GJ, et al. Brachial artery thrombosis in infants: an algorithm for limb salvage. *Plast Reconstr Surg.* 2006;117:1481.
30. McEvoy GK, ed. *AHFS Drug Information Essentials 2005–06.* Bethesda, MD: American Society of Health-System Pharmacists; 2005.
31. Green TP, Isham-Schopf B, Irmiter RJ, et al. Inactivation of heparin during extracorporeal circulation in infants. *Clin Pharmacol Ther.* 1990;48:148-154.
32. Trissel LA. *Handbook on Injectable Drugs.* 13th ed. Bethesda, MD: American Society of Health-System Pharmacists; 2005.
33. Heparin [package insert]. Deerfield, IL: Baxter Healthcare Corporation; December 2004.
34. Lesko SM, Mitchell AA, Epstein MR, et al. Heparin use as a risk factor for intraventricular hemorrhage in low birth weight infants. *N Engl J Med.* 1986;314:1156-1160.
35. Cines DB, Kaywin P, Bina M, et al. Heparin-associated thrombocytopenia. *N Engl J Med.* 1980;303:788-795.
36. Murdoch IA, Beattie RM, Silver DM. Heparin-induced thrombocytopenia in children. *Acta Paediatr.* 1993;82:495-497.
37. American Academy of Pediatrics Committee on Drugs. "Inactive" ingredients in pharmaceutical products: update. *Pediatrics.* 1997;99:268-278.

References

38. Smolinske SC. Review of parenteral sulfite reactions. *J Toxicol Clin Toxicol.* 1992;30:597-606.
39. Lester MR. Sulfite sensitivity: significance in human health. *J Am Col Nutr.* 1995;14:229-232.
41. Hall CM, Milligan DWA, Berrington J. Probably adverse reaction to a pharmaceutical excipient. *Arch Dis Child Fetal Neonatal Ed.* 2004;89: F184.
42. Hiller JL, Benda GI, Rahatzad M, et al. Benzyl alcohol toxicity: impact on mortality and intraventricular hemorrhage among very low birth weight infants. *Pediatrics.* 1986;77:500-506.
43. Grant JA, Bilodeau PA, Guernsey BG, et al. Unsuspected benzyl alcohol hypersensitivity. *N Engl J Med.* 1982;306:108.
44. Wilson JP, Solimando DA, Edwards MS. Parenteral benzyl alcohol-induced hypersensitivity reaction. *Drug Intell Clin Pharm.* 1986;20:689-691.
45. Soni MG, Taylor SL, Greenberg NA, et al. Evaluation of the health aspects of methyl paraben: review of the published literature. *Food Chem Toxicol.* 2002;40:1335-1373.
46. Nagel JE, Fuscaldo JT, Firemen P. Paraben allergy. *JAMA.* 1977;237:1594-1595.
47. Shah PS, Ng E, Sinha AK. Heparin for prolonging peripheral intravenous catheter use in neonates. *Cochrane Database Syst Rev.* 2005;4: CD002774. Review.

Hydralazine HCl

1. Beekman RH, Rocchini AP, Rosenthal A. Hemodynamic effects of hydralazine in infants with a large ventricular septal defect. *Circulation.* 1982;65:523-528.
2. Friedman WF, George BL. Treatment of congestive heart failure by altering loading conditions of the heart. *J Pediatr.* 1985;106:697-706.
3. Fried R, Steinherz LJ, Levin AR. Use of hydralazine for intractable cardiac failure in childhood. *J Pediatr.* 1980;97:1009-1011.
4. Plumer LB, Kaplan GW, Mendoza SA. Hypertension in infants—a complication of umbilical arterial catheterization. *J Pediatr.* 1976;89:802-805.
5. Fleischmann LE. Management of hypertensive crises in children. *Pediatr Ann.* 1977;6:410-414.
6. Friedman WF, George BL. New concepts and drugs in the treatment of congestive heart failure. *Pediatr Clin North Am.* 1984;31:1197-1227.
7. Artman M, Parrish MD, Appleton S, et al. Hemodynamic effects of hydralazine in infants with idiopathic dilated cardiomyopathy and congestive heart failure. *Am Heart J.* 1987;113:144-150.
8. Farine M, Arbus GS. Management of hypertensive emergencies in children. *Pediatr Emerg Care.* 1989;5:51-55.
9. Serratto M. Diagnosis and management of heart failure in infants and children. *Comprehensive Ther.* 1992;18:11-19.
10. Miller K. Pharmacological management of hypertension in paediatric patients. *Drugs.* 1994;48:868-887.
11. American Academy of Pediatrics. Committee on Drugs. Emergency drug doses for infants and children. *Pediatrics.* 1988;81:462-465.
12. Adelman RD, Coppo R, Dillon MJ. The emergency management of severe hypertension. *Pediatr Nephrol.* 2000;14:422-427.
13. Loggie JM. Hypertension in children and adolescents. II. Drug therapy. *J Pediatr.* 1969;74:640-654.
14. American Society of Health-System Pharmacists. American Hospital Formulary System. Available at: http://ahfsfirst.firstdatabank.com/AHFSfirst/NSAHFSFirstSearchmain.asp. Accessed August 5, 2006.
15. *Physicians' Desk Reference.* 60th ed. Montvale, NJ: Thomson PDR; 2006.
16. Fivush B, Neu A, Furth S. Acute hypertensive crises in children: emergencies and urgencies. *Curr Opin Pediatr.* 1997;9:233-236.
17. Adelman RD, Coppo R, Dillon MJ. The emergency management of severe hypertension. *Pediatr Nephrol.* 2000;14:422-427.
18. US Department of Health and Human Services. *The Fourth Report on the Diagnosis, Evaluation, and Treatment of High Blood Pressure in Children and Adolescents.* NIH Publication 05-5267; revised May 2005.
19. Aronoff A, Brier M, Bennett W. *The Renal Book, 2002.* Available at: http://www.kdp-baptist.louisville.edu/renalbook/. Accessed August 5, 2006.
20. Adelman RD. Neonatal hypertension. *Pediatr Clin North Am.* 1978;25:99-110.
21. Hanna JD, Chan JC, Gill JR. Hypertension and the kidney. *J Pediatr.* 1991;118:327-340.
22. Trissel LA, ed. *Handbook on Injectable Drugs.* 13th ed. [CD-ROM version 1.5]. Bethesda, MD: American Society of Health-System Pharmacists; 2005.
23. Deal JE, Barratt TM, Dillion MJ. Management of hypertensive emergencies. *Arch Dis Child.* 1992;67:1089-1092.
24. Pagliaro LA, Pagliaro AM, eds. *Problems in Pediatric Drug Therapy.* 2nd ed. Hamilton, IL: Drug Intelligence Publications Inc; 1987.
25. Taketomo CK, Hodding JH, Kraus DM. *Pediatric Dosage Handbook.* 12th ed. Cleveland, OH: Lexi-Comp Inc; 2005.
26. Young TE, Mangum B, eds. *Neofax.* 18th ed. Raleigh, NC: Acorn Publishing Inc; 2005.
27. Louis S, Kutt H, McDowell F. The cardiocirculatory changes caused by intravenous Dilantin and its solvent. *Am Heart J.* 1967;74:523-529.
28. American Academy of Pediatrics Committee on Drugs. "Inactive" ingredients in pharmaceutical products: update. *Pediatrics.* 1997;99:268-278.
29. Glasgow AM, Boeckx RL, Miller MK, et al. Hyper-osmolality in small infants due to propylene glycol. *Pediatrics.* 1983;72:353-355.
30. MacDonald MG, Getson PR, Glasgow AM, et al. Propylene glycol: increased incidence of seizures in low birth weight infants. *Pediatrics.*1987;79:622-625.
31. Soni MG, Taylor SL, Greenberg NA, et al. Evaluation of the health aspects of methyl paraben: a review of the published literature. *Food Chem Toxicol.* 2002;40:1335-1373.
32. Nagel JE, Fiscal JT, Firemen P. Paraben allergy. *JAMA.* 1977;237:1594-1595.
33. Grossman E, Ironi AN, Messerli FH. Comparative tolerability profile of hypertensive crisis treatments. *Drug Safety.* 1998;19:99-122.

Hydrochloric Acid (HCl)

1. Duffy L, Kerzner B, Gebuw V, et al. Treatment of central venous catheter occlusion with HCl. *J Pediatr.* 1989;114:1002-1004.
2. Breaux CW, Duke D, Georgeson KE, et al. Calcium phosphate crystal occlusion of central venous catheters used for total parenteral nutrition in infants and children: prevention and treatment. *J Pediatr Surg.* 1987;22:829-832.
3. Shulman RJ, Reed T, Pitre D, et al. Use of hydrochloric acid to clear obstructed central venous catheters. *J Parenter Enteral Nutr.* 1988;12:509-510.
4. Holcombe BJ, Forloines-Lynn S, Garmhausen LW. Restoring patency of long-term central venous access devices. *J Intraven Nurs.* 1992;15:36-41.
5. Unger A, Rhenman B, Fuller JK, et al. Treatment of severe metabolic alkalosis in a neonate with hydrochloric acid infusion. *Clin Pediatr.* 1985;24:444-448.
6. Nasimi A, Cardona J, Berthier M, et al. Hydrochloric acid infusion for treatment of severe metabolic alkalosis in a neonate. *Clin Pediatr.* 1996;35:271-272.
7. Martin WF, Matzke GR. Treating severe metabolic alkalosis. *Clin Pharm.* 1982;1:42-48.
8. Galla JH. Metabolic alkalosis. *J Am Soc Nephrol.* 2000;11:369-375.
9. Adrogue HJ, Madias NE. Management of life-threatening acid-base disorders. *N Engl J Med.* 1998;338:107-111.
10. Ingram J, Weitzman S, Greenberg ML, et al. Complications of indwelling venous access lines in the pediatric hematology patient: a prospective comparison of external venous catheters and subcutaneous ports. *Am J Pediatr Hematol Oncol.* 1991;13:130-136.
11. Knutson OH. New method for administration of hydrochloric acid in metabolic alkalosis. *Lancet.* 1983;1:953-956.
12. Kopel RF, Durbin CG. Pulmonary artery catheter deterioration during hydrochloric acid infusion for the treatment of metabolic alkalosis. *Crit Care Med.* 1989;17:688-689.

References

Hydrocortisone Sodium Phosphate/Succinate

1. McEvoy GK, ed. *American Hospital Formulary Service Drug Information 2000.* Bethesda, MD: American Society of Health-System Pharmacists; 2000.
2. Hydrocortone phosphate injection [package insert]. Whitehouse Station, NJ: Merck & Co Inc; November 2001.
3. Solu-Cortef [package insert]. Kalamazoo, MI: Pharmacia & Upjohn Company; April 2003.
4. Taketomo CK, Hodding JH, Kraus DM. *Lexi-Comp's Pediatric Dosage Handbook.* [CD-ROM]. Hudson, OH: Lexi-Comp Inc; 2006.
5. Miller JJ. Prolonged use of large intravenous steroid pulses in the rheumatic diseases of children. *Pediatrics.* 1980;65:989-994.
6. Graham VAL, Milton AF, Knowles GK, et al. Routine antibiotics in hospital management of acute asthma. *Lancet.* 1982;1:418-421.
7. National Heart Lung and Blood Institute. NAEPP expert panel report 2. Guidelines for the diagnosis and management of asthma. National Institutes of Health pub. No. 97-4051. Bethesda, MD, 1997.
8. Klevit HD. Corticosteroid therapy in the neonatal period. *Pediatr Clin North Am.* 1970;17:1003-1113.
9. MacDonald MG, Seshia MM, Mullett MD, eds. *Avery's Neonatology Pathophysiology & Management of the Newborn.* Philadelphia, PA: Lippincott Williams & Wilkins; 2005.
10. American Academy of Pediatrics, Section on Endocrinology and Committee on Genetics. Technical report: Congenital adrenal hyperplasia. *Pediatrics.* 2000;106:1511-1518.
11. Tepper RS, Eigen H, Stevens J, et al. Lower respiratory illness in infants and young children with cystic fibrosis: evaluation of treatment with intravenous hydrocortisone. *Pediatr Pulmonol.* 1997:24:48-51.
12. Seri I, Tan R, Evans J. Cardiovascular effects of hydrocortisone in preterm infants with pressor-resistant hypotension. *Pediatrics.* 2001;107:1070-1074.
13. Helbock HJ, Insoft RM, Conte FA. Glucocorticoid-responsive hypotension in extremely low birth weight newborns. *Pediatrics.* 1993;92:715-717.
14. Trissel LA. *Handbook on Injectable Drugs.* 10th ed. Bethesda, MD: American Society of Health-System Pharmacists; 1998.
15. Goldstein DA, Zimmerman B, Spielberg SP. Anaphylactic response to hydrocortisone in childhood: a case report. *Ann Allergy.* 1985;55:599-600.
16. Peller JS, Bardana EJ. Anaphylactoid reaction to corticosteroid: case report and review of the literature. *Ann Allergy.* 1985;54:302-305.
17. American Academy of Pediatrics Committee on Drugs. "Inactive" ingredients in pharmaceutical products: update. *Pediatrics.* 1997;99:268-278.
18. Smolinske SC. Review of parenteral sulfite reactions. *J Toxicol Clin Toxicol.* 1992;30:597-606.
19. Lester MR. Sulfite sensitivity: significance in human health. *J Am Col Nutr.* 1995;14:229-232.
20. Soni MG, Taylor SL, Greenberg NA, et al. Evaluation of the health aspects of methyl paraben: a review of the published literature. *Food Chem Toxicol.* 2002;40:1335-1373.
21. Nagel JE, Fuscaldo JT, Firemen P. Paraben allergy. *JAMA.* 1977;237:1594-1595.
22. Hall CM, Milligan DWA, Berrington J. Probable adverse reaction to a pharmaceutical excipient. *Arch Dis Child Fetal Neonatal Ed.* 2004;89: F184.
23. Hiller JL, Benda GI, Rahatzad M, et al. Benzyl alcohol toxicity: impact on mortality and intraventricular hemorrhage among very low birth weight infants. *Pediatrics.* 1986;77:500-506.
24. Grant JA, Bilodeau PA, Guernsey BG, et al. Unsuspected benzyl alcohol hypersensitivity. *N Engl J Med.* 1982;306:108.
25. Wilson JP, Solimando DA, Edwards MS. Parenteral benzyl alcohol-induced hypersensitivity reaction. *Drug Intell Clin Pharm.* 1986;20:689-691.
26. Fass B. Glucocorticoid therapy for non-endocrine disorders: withdrawal and coverage. *Pediatr Clin North Am.* 1979;26:251-256.
27. Chamberlin P, Meyer WJ. Management of pituitary-adrenal suppression secondary to corticosteroid therapy. *Pediatrics.* 1981;67:245-251.
28. Landstra AM, Boezen HM, Postma DS, et al. Effect of intravenous hydrocortisone on nocturnal airflow limitation in childhood asthma. *Eur Respir J.* 2003;21:627-632.
29. Watterberg KL, Gerdes JS, Cole CH, et al. Prophylaxis of early adrenal insufficiency to prevent bronchopulmonary dysplasia: a multicenter trial. *Pediatrics.* 2004;114:1649-1657.
30. Botos CM, Kurlat I, Young SM, et al. Disseminated candidal infections and intravenous hydrocortisone in preterm infants. *Pediatrics.* 1995;95:883-887.

Ifosfamide

1. Taketomo CK, ed. *Lexi-Comp's Pediatric Dosage Handbook.* 12th ed. Hudson, OH: Lexi-Comp; 2005:668-669.
2. Ninane J, Baurain R, de Kraker J, et al. Alkylating activity in serum, urine, and CSF following high-dose ifosfamide in children. *Cancer Chemother Pharmacol.* 1989;24(suppl 1):S2-S6.
3. Pinkerton CR, Rogers H, James C, et al. A phase II study of ifosfamide in children with recurrent solid tumours. *Cancer Chemother Pharmacol.* 1985;15(3):258-262.
4. Miser JS, Krailo MD, Tarbell NJ, et al. Treatment of metastatic Ewing's sarcoma or primitive neuroectodermal tumor of bone: evaluation of combination ifosfamide and etoposide—a Children's Cancer Group and Pediatric Oncology Group study. *J Clin Oncol.* 2004;22(14):2873-2876.
5. Goorin AM, Harris MB, Bernstein M, et al. Phase II/III trial of etoposide and high-dose ifosfamide in newly diagnosed metastatic osteosarcoma: a pediatric oncology group trial. *J Clin Oncol.* 2002;20(2):426-433.
6. Aronoff GR, Berns JS, Brier ME, et al. *Drug Prescribing in Renal Failure: Dosing Guidelines for Adults.* 4th ed. Philadelphia, PA: American College of Physicians; 1999:74.
7. Falkson G, Hunt M, Borden EC, et al. An extended phase II trial of ifosfamide plus mesna in malignant mesothelioma. *Invest New Drugs.* 1992;10(4):337-343.
8. Ifex [package insert]. Princeton, NJ: Bristol-Myers Squibb, November 2002.
9. Silies H, Blaschke G, Hohenlochter B, et al. Excretion kinetics of ifosfamide side-chain metabolites in children on continuous and short-term infusion. *Int J Clin Pharmacol Ther.* 1998;36(5):246-252.
10. Boddy AV, Yule SM, Wyllie R, et al. Pharmacokinetics and metabolism of ifosfamide administered as a continuous infusion in children. *Cancer Res.* 1993;53(16):3758-3764.
11. Suarez A, McDowell H, Niaudet P, et al. Long-term follow-up of ifosfamide renal toxicity in children treated with malignant mesenchymal tumors: an International Society of Pediatric Oncology report. *J Clin Oncol.* 1991;9(12):2177-2182.
12. National Comprehensive Cancer Network (NCCN) Antiemesis Panel Members. NCCN Clinical Practice Guidelines in Oncology. Antiemesis, v.1.2006. Available at www.nccn.org. Last accessed March 29, 2006.
13. Roila F, Feyer P, Maranzamo E, et al. Antiemetics in children receiving chemotherapy. *Support Care Cancer.* 2005;13:129-131.

Imipenem–Cilastatin Sodium

1. *Physicians' Desk Reference.* 60th ed. Montvale, NJ: Medical Economics Company; 2006.
2. Prober CG, Stevenson DK, Benitz WE. The use of antibiotics in neonates weighing less than 1200 grams. *Pediatr Infect Dis J.* 1990;9:111-121.
3. American Academy of Pediatrics. In: Pickering LK, ed. *2003 Red Book: Report of the Committee on Infectious Diseases.* 26th ed. Elk Grove Village, IL: American Academy of Pediatrics; 2003.

References

4. Nelson JS, Bradley JS. *Nelson's Pocketbook of Pediatric Antimicrobial Therapy.* 14th ed. Philadelphia, PA. Lippincott Williams & Wilkins; 2000.
5. Ahonkhai VI, Cyhan GM, Wilson SE, et al. Imipenem–cilastatin in pediatric patients: an overview of safety and efficacy in studies conducted in the United States. *Pediatr Infect Dis J.* 1989;8:740-744.
6. Nalin DR, Hart CB, Shih WJ, et al. Imipenem/cilastatin for pediatric infections in hospitalized patients. *Scand J Infect Dis.* 1987;52:56-64.
7. Freij BJ, Kusmiesz H, Shelton S, et al. Imipenem and cilastatin in acute osteomyelitis and suppurative arthritis. Therapy in infants and children. *Am J Dis Child.* 1987;141:335-342.
8. Alpert G, Dagan R, Connor E, et al. Imipenem/cilastatin for the treatment of infections in hospitalized children. *Am J Dis Child.* 1985;139:1153-1156.
9. Riikonen P. Imipenem compared with ceftazidime plus vancomycin as initial therapy for fever in neutropenic children with cancer. *Pediatr Infect Dis J.* 1991;10:918-923.
10. Inglesby TV, O'Toole T, Henderson DA, et al., for the Working Group on Civilian Biodefense. Anthrax as a biological weapon 2002: updated recommendations for management. *JAMA.* 2002;287:2236-2252.
11. Centers for Disease Control and Prevention. Update: Investigation of bioterrorism-related anthrax and interim guidelines for exposure management and antimicrobial therapy, October 2001. *MMWR Morb Mortal Wkly Rep.* 2001;50:909-919.
12. Aronoff A, Brier M, Bennett W. *The Renal Book, 2002.* http://www.kdp-baptist.louisville.edu/renalbook/. Accessed August 6, 2006.
13. Jacobs RF, Kearns GL, Trang JM, et al. Single-dose pharmacokinetics of imipenem in children. *J Pediatr.* 1984;105:996-1001.
14. Reed MD, Stern RC, O'Brien CA, et al. Pharmacokinetics of imipenem and cilastatin in patients with cystic fibrosis. *Antimicrob Agents Chemother.* 1985;27:583-588.
15. Trissel LA, ed. *Handbook on Injectable Drugs.* 13th ed. [CD-ROM version 1.5]. Bethesda, MD: American Society of Health-System Pharmacists; 2005.
16. Norrby SR. Neurotoxicity of the carbapenem antibacterials. *Drug Safety.* 1996;15:87-90.
17. Norrby SR. Carbapenems in serious infections: a risk-benefit assessment. *Drug Safety.* 2000;22:191-194.
18. Stuart RL, Turnidge J, Grayson ML. Safety of imipenem is neonates. *Pediatr Infect Dis J.* 1995;14:804-805.
19. Wong VK, Wright HT Jr, Ross LA, et al. Imipenem/cilastatin treatment of bacterial meningitis in children. *Pediatr Infect Dis J.* 1991;10:122-125.
20. Calandra G, Lydick E, Carrigan J, et al. Factors predisposing to seizures in seriously ill infected patients receiving antibiotics: experience with imipenem/cilastatin. *Am J Med.* 1988;84:911-918.
21. Tartaglione TA, Flint NB. Effect of imipenem-cilastatin and ciprofloxacin on tests for glycosuria. *Am J Hosp Pharm.* 1985;42:602-605.

Immune Globulin Intravenous

1. McEvoy GK, ed. *AHFS Drug Information Essentials 2005–06.* Bethesda, MD: American Society of Health-System Pharmacists; 2005.
2. American Academy of Pediatrics. In: Pickering LK, ed. *2003 Red Book: Report of the Committee on Infectious Diseases.* 26th ed. Elk Grove Village, IL: American Academy of Pediatrics; 2003.
3. Spector SA, Gelber RD, McGrath N, et al. A controlled trial of intravenous immune globulin for the prevention of serious bacterial infections in children receiving zidovudine for advanced human immunodeficiency virus infection. *N Engl J Med.* 1994;331:1181-1187.
4. Sullivan KM, Kopecky KJ, Jocom J, et al. Immuno-modulatory and antimicrobial efficacy of intravenous immunoglobulin in bone marrow transplantation. *N Engl J Med.* 1990;323:705-712.
5. Winston DJ, Antin JH, Wolff SN, et al. A multicenter, randomized, double-blind comparison of different doses of intravenous immunoglobulin for prevention of graft-versus-host disease and infection after allogeneic bone marrow transplantation. *Bone Marrow Transplant.* 2001;28:187-196.
6. Rand KH, Gibbs K, Derendorf H, et al. Pharmacokinetics of intravenous immunoglobulin (Gammagard) in bone marrow transplant patients. *J Clin Pharmacol.* 1991;31:1151-1154.
7. Korinthenberg R, Schessl J, Kirschner J, et al. Intravenously administered immunoglobulin in the treatment of childhood Guillain-Barré syndrome: a randomized trial. *Pediatrics.* 2005;116:8-14.
8. Yata J, Nihei K, Ohya T, et al. High-dose immunoglobulin therapy for Guillain-Barré syndrome in Japanese children. *Pediatr Internat.* 2003;45:543-549.
9. Miqdad AM, Abdelbasit OB, Shaheed MM, et al. Intravenous immunoglobulin G (IVIG) therapy for significant hyperbilirubinemia in ABO hemolytic disease of the newborn. *J Matern Fetal Neonatal Med.* 2004;16:163-166.
10. Tanyer G, Siklar Z, Dallar Y, et al. Multiple dose IVIG treatment in neonatal immune hemolytic jaundice. *J Trop Pediatr.* 2001;47:50-53.
11. ASHP Commission on Therapeutics. ASHP therapeutic guidelines for intravenous immune globulin. *Clin Pharm.* 1992;11:117-136.
12. Dwyer JM. Manipulating the immune system with immune globulin. *N Engl J Med.* 1992;326:107-116.
13. Warrier I, Bussel JB, Valdez L, et al. Safety and efficacy of low-dose intravenous immune globulin (IVIG) treatment for infants and children with immune thrombocytopenic purpura. Low-Dose IVIG Study Group. *J Pediatr Hematol Oncol.* 1997;19:197-201.
14. NIH Consensus Development Conference on Intravenous Immunoglobulin. Prevention and treatment of disease. *JAMA.* 1990;264:3189-3193.
15. Newberger JW, Takahashi M, Beiser AS, et al. A single intravenous infusion of gamma globulin as compared with four infusions in the treatment of acute Kawasaki syndrome. *N Engl J Med.* 1991;324:1633-1639.
16. Rowley AH, Shulman ST. Current therapy for acute Kawasaki syndrome. *J Pediatr.* 1991;118:987-991.
17. Kawasaki T. Kawasaki disease. *Acta Paediatr.* 1995;84:713-715.
18. Tse SM, Silverman ED, McCrindle BW, et al. Early treatment with intravenous immunoglobulin in patients with Kawasaki disease. *J Pediatr.* 2002;140:450-455.
19. Newburger JW, Takahashi M, Gerber MA, et al. Diagnosis, treatment, and long-term management of Kawasaki disease: a statement for health professionals from the Committee on Rheumatic Fever, Endocarditis, and Kawasaki Disease, Council on Cardiovascular Disease in the Young, American Heart Association. *Pediatrics.* 2004;114:1708-1733.
20. Sato N, Sugimura T, Akagi T, et al. Selective high dose gamma-globulin treatment in Kawasaki disease: assessment of clinical aspects and cost effectiveness. *Pediatr Internat.* 1999;41:1-7.
21. Burns JC, Capparelli EV, Brown JA, et al. Intravenous gamma-globulin treatment and retreatment in Kawasaki disease. US/Canadian Kawasaki Syndrome Study Group. *Pediatr Infect Dis J.* 1998;17:1144-1148.
22. Hashino K, Ishii M, Iemura M, et al. Re-treatment for immune globulin-resistant Kawasaki disease: A comparative study of additional immune globulin and steroid pulse therapy. *Pediatr Internat.* 2001;43:211-217.
23. Eijkhout HW, van Der Meer JW, Kallenberg CG, et al. The effect of two different dosages of intravenous immunoglobulin on the incidence of recurrent infections in patients with primary hypogammaglobulinemia. *Ann Intern Med.* 2001;135:165-174.
24. Chirico G, Rondini G, Plebani A, et al. Intravenous gamma globulin therapy for prophylaxis of infection in high-risk neonates. *J Pediatr.* 1987;110:437-442.
25. Fischer GW, Weisman LE, Hemming VG. Directed immune globulin for the prevention or treatment of neonatal group B streptococcal infections: a review. *Clin Immunol Immunopathol.* 1992;62:S92-S97.
26. Baker CJ, Melish ME, Hall RT, et al. Intravenous immune globulin for the prevention of nosocomial infection in low-birth-weight neonates. *N Engl J Med.* 1992;327:213-219.
27. Kyllonen KS, Clapp DW, Kliegman RM, et al. Dosage of intravenously administered immune globulin and dosing interval required to maintain target levels of immunoglobulin G in low birth weight infants. *J Pediatr.* 1989;115:1013-1016.
28. Clapp DW, Kliegman RM, Baley JE, et al. Use of intravenously administered immune globulin to prevent nosocomial sepsis in low birth weight infants: report of a pilot study. *J Pediatr.* 1989;115:973-978.

29. Garvey MA, Snider LA, Leitman SF, et al. Treatment of Sydenham's chorea with intravenous immunoglobulin, plasma exchange, or prednisone. *J Child Neurol.* 2005;20:424-429.
30. Perlmutter SJ, Leitman SF, Garvey MA, et al. Therapeutic plasma exchange and intravenous immunoglobulin for obsessive-compulsive disorder and tic disorders in childhood. *Lancet.* 1999;354:1153-1158.
31. Metry DW, Jung P, Levy ML. Use of intravenous immunoglobulin in children with Stevens-Johnson syndrome and toxic epidermal necrolysis: seven cases and review of the literature. *Pediatrics.* 2003;112:1430-1436.
32. Brennan VM, Salome-Bentley NJ, Chapel HM. Prospective audit of adverse reactions occurring in 459 primary antibody-deficient patients receiving intravenous immunoglobulin. *Clin Exp Immunol.* 2003;133:247-251.
33. Carimune [package insert]. Kankakee, IL: ZLB Behring; January 2005.
34. Octagam [package insert]. Centreville, VA: Octapharma USA Inc; December 2005.
35. Sandoglobulin [package insert]. East Hanover, NJ: Novartis Pharmaceuticals Corp; February 2000.
36. Rao SP, Teitlebaum J, Miller ST. Intravenous immune globulin and aseptic meningitis. *Am J Dis Child.* 1992;146:539-540.
37. Jayabose S, Roseman B, Gupta A. Aseptic meningitis syndrome after IV gamma globulin therapy for ITP. *Am J Pediatr Hematol Oncol.* 1990;12:117. Abstract.
38. Kato E, Shindo S, Eto Y, et al. Administration of immune globulin associated with aseptic meningitis. *JAMA.* 1988;259:3269-3270.
39. Casteels-Van Daele M, Wijndaele L, Hunnick K, et al. Intravenous immune globulin and acute aseptic meningitis. *N Engl J Med.* 1990;323:614-615.
40. Boyce TG, Spearman P. Acute aseptic meningitis secondary to intravenous immunoglobulin in a patient with Kawasaki syndrome. *Pediatr Infect Dis J.* 1998;17:1054-1056.
41. Outbreak of hepatitis C associated with intravenous immunoglobulin administration—United States, October 1993–June 1994. *MMWR.* 1994;43:505-508.
42. Berkovitch M, Dolinski G, Tauber T, et al. Neutropenia as a complication of intravenous immunoglobulin (IVIG) therapy in children with immune thrombocytopenic purpura: common and non-alarming. *Int J Immunopharmacol.* 1999;21:411-415.
43. Nakagawa M, Watanabe N, Okuno M, et al. Severe hemolytic anemia following high-dose intravenous immunoglobulin administration in a patient with Kawasaki disease. *Am J Hematol.* 2000;63:160-161.
44. Renal insufficiency and failure associated with immune globulin intravenous therapy—United States, 1985–1998. *MMWR Morb Mortal Wkly Rep.* 1999;48:518-521.

Inamrinone Lactate (previously amrinone)

1. American Society of Health-System Pharmacists. American Hospital Formulary System. Available at: http://ahfsfirst.firstdatabank.com/AHFSfirst/NSAHFSFirstSearchmain.asp. Accessed July 10, 2006.
2. American Heart Association. Guidelines 2005 for cardiopulmonary resuscitation and emergency cardiovascular care. Part 12: Pediatric advanced life support. *Circulation.* 2005;112:167-187.
3. Lawless ST, Burckart GJ. Amrinone pharmacokinetics in neonates and infants (reply to letter). *Crit Care Med.* 1990;18:1495.
4. Lawless ST, Zaritsky A, Miles M. The acute pharmacokinetics and pharmacodynamics of amrinone in pediatric patients. *J Clin Pharmacol.* 1991;31:800-803.
5. Allen-Webb EM, Ross MP, Pappas JB, et al. Age-related amrinone pharmacokinetics in a pediatric population. *Crit Care Med.* 1994;22:1016-1024.
6. Ross MP, Allen-Webb EM, Pappas JB, et al. Amrinone-associated thrombocytopenia: pharmacokinetic analysis. *Clin Pharmacol Ther.* 1993;53:661-667.
7. Rathmell JP, Prielipp RC, Butterworth JF, et al. A multicenter, randomized, blind comparison of amrinone with milrinone after elective cardiac surgery. *Anesth Analg.* 1998;86:683-690.
8. Bailey JM, Miller BE, Kanter KR, et al. A comparison of the hemodynamic effects of amrinone and sodium nitroprusside in infants after cardiac surgery. *Pediatr Anesth.* 1997;84:294-298.
9. Sorensen SK, Ramamoorthy C, Lynn AM, et al. Hemodynamic effects of amrinone in children after Fontan surgery. *Anesth Analg.* 1996;82:241-246.
10. Lawless S, Burckart G, Diven W, et al. Amrinone in neonates and infants after cardiac surgery. *Crit Care Med.* 1989;17:751-754.
11. Laitinen P, Happonen JM, Sairanen H, et al. Amrinone versus dopamine and nitroglycerine in neonates after arterial switch operation for transposition of the great arteries. *J Cardiothoracic Vascular Anesth.* 1999;13:186-190.
12. Aronoff A, Brier M, Bennett W. *The Renal Book, 2002.* Available at: http://www.kdp-baptist.louisville.edu/renalbook/. Accessed August 1, 2006.
13. Berner M, Jaccard C, Oberhansli I, Rouge JC, Friedli B. Hemodynamic effects of amrinone in children after cardiac surgery. *Inten Care Med.* 1990;16:85-88.
14. Lebovitz DJ, Lawless ST, Weise KL. Fatal amrinone overdose in a pediatric patient. *Crit Care Med.* 1995;23:977-980.
15. Trissel LA, ed. *Handbook on Injectable Drugs.* 13th ed. Bethesda, MD: American Society of Health-System Pharmacists; 2005.
16. American Academy of Pediatrics Committee on Drugs. "Inactive" ingredients in pharmaceutical products: update. *Pediatrics.* 1997;99:268-278.
17. Smolinske SC. Review of parenteral sulfite reactions. *J Toxicol Clin Toxicol.* 1992;30:597-606.
18. Lester MR. Sulfite sensitivity: significance in human health. *J Am Col Nutr.* 1995;14:229-232.

Indomethacin Sodium Trihydrate

1. Rennie JM, Cooke RWI. Prolonged low dose indomethacin for persistent ductus arteriosus of prematurity. *Arch Dis Child.* 1991;66:55-58.
2. Rhodes PG, Ferguson MG, Reddy NS, et al. Effects of prolonged versus acute indomethacin therapy in very low birth-weight infants with patent ductus arteriosus. *Eur J Pediatr.* 1988;147:481-484.
3. Hammerman C, Aramburo MJ. Prolonged indomethacin therapy for the prevention of recurrences of patent ductus arteriosus. *J Pediatr.* 1990;117:771-776.
4. Nakamura T, Tamura M, Kadowaki S. Low-dose continuous indomethacin in early days of age reduce the incidence of symptomatic patent ductus arteriosus without adverse effects. *Am J Perinatol.* 2000;17:271-275.
5. Mahony L, Carnero V, Brett C, et al. Prophylactic indomethacin therapy for patent ductus arteriosus in very-low-birth-weight infants. *N Engl J Med.* 1982;306:506-510.
6. Fowlie PR, Davis PG. Prophylactic indomethacin for preterm infants: a systemic review and meta-analysis. *Arch Dis Child Fetal Neonatal Ed.* 2003;88:F464-F466.
7. *Physicians' Desk Reference.* 60th ed. Montvale, NJ: Thomson PDR; 2006.
8. Gersony WM, Peckham GJ, Ellison RC, et al. Effects of indomethacin in premature infants with patent ductus arteriosus: results of a national collaborative study. *J Pediatr.* 1983;102:895-906.
9. Bada HS, Green RS, Pourcyrous M, et al. Indomethacin reduces the risks of severe intraventricular hemorrhage. *J Pediatr.* 1989;115:631-637.
10. Stefano JL, Abbasi S, Pearlman SA, et al. Closure of the ductus arteriosus with indomethacin in ventilated neonates with respiratory distress syndrome. *Am Rev Respir Dis.* 1991;143:236-239.
11. Wiest DB, Pinson JB, Gal PS, et al. Population pharmacokinetics of intravenous indomethacin in neonates with symptomatic patent ductus

arteriosus. *Clin Pharmacol Ther.* 1991;49:550-557.
12. Hanigan WC, Kennedy G, Roemisch F, et al. Administration of indomethacin for the prevention of periventricular-intraventricular hemorrhage in high-risk neonates. *J Pediatr.* 1988;112:941-947.
13. Renfro WH. Criteria for use of indomethacin injection in neonates. *Clin Pharm.* 1993;12:232-234.
14. Zarfin Y, Koren G, Maresky D. Possible indomethacin—aminoglycoside interaction in preterm infants. *J Pediatr.* 1985;106:511-513.
15. Hammerman C, Glaser J, Schimmel MS, et al. Continuous versus multiple rapid infusion of indomethacin: effect on cerebral blood flow velocity. *Pediatrics.* 1995;95:244-248.
16. Christmann V, Liem KD, Semmekrot BA, et al. Changes in cerebral, renal, and mesenteric blood flow velocity during continuous and bolus infusion of indomethacin. *Acta Paediatr.* 2002;91:440-446.
17. Quinn D, Cooper B, Clyman RI. Factors associated with permanent closure of the ductus arteriosus: a role for prolonged indomethacin therapy. *Pediatrics.* 2002;110:e1-e6.
18. Lee J, Rajadurai VS, Tan KW, et al. Randomized trial of prolonged low-dose versus conventional-dose indomethacin for treating patent ductus arteriosus in very low birth weight infants. *Pediatrics.* 2003;112:345-350.
19. Herrera C. Cochrane Neonatal Group. Cochrane review: prolonged versus short course indomethacin for the treatment of patent ductus arteriosus in preterm infants. *Cochrane Database Systematic Reviews.* 2004;CD003480.
20. Sperandio M, Beedgen B, Feneberg R. Effectiveness and side effects of an escalating, stepwise approach to indomethacin treatment for symptomatic patent ductus arteriosus in premature infants below 33 weeks gestation. *Pediatrics.* 2005;116:1361-1366.
21. Ment LR, Oh W, Ehrenkranz RA, et al. Low-dose indomethacin and prevention of intraventricular hemorrhage: a multicenter randomized trial. *Pediatrics.* 1994;93:543-550.
22. Gal P, Ransom JL, Weaver RL, et al. Indomethacin pharmacokinetics in neonates: the value of volume of distribution as a marker of permanent patent ductus arteriosus closure. *Ther Drug Monitor.* 1991;13:42-45.
23. Yeh TF, Achanti B, Patel H, et al. Indomethacin therapy in premature infants with patent ductus arteriosus—determination of therapeutic plasma levels. *Dev Pharmacol Ther.* 1989;12:169-178.
24. Cowan F. Indomethacin, patent ductus arteriosus, and cerebral blood flow. *J Pediatr.* 1986;109:341-344.
25. Mardoum R, Bejar R, Merritt A, et al. Controlled study of the effects of indomethacin on cerebral blood flow velocities in newborn infants. *J Pediatr.* 1991;118:112-115.
26. Coombs RC, Morgan ME, Durbin GM, et al. Gut blood flow velocities in the newborn: effects of patent ductus arteriosus and parenteral indomethacin. *Arch Dis Child.* 1990;65:1067-1071.
27. Colditz P, Murphy D, Rolfe P, et al. Effect of infusion rate of indomethacin on cerebrovascular response in premature neonates. *Arch Dis Child.* 1989;64:8-12.
28. Van Bel F, Van de Bor M, Stijnen T, et al. Cerebral blood flow velocity changes in preterm infants after a single dose of indomethacin: duration of its effect. *Pediatrics.* 1989;84:802-807.
29. Trissel LA, ed. *Handbook on Injectable Drugs*. 13th ed. [CD-ROM version 1.5]. Bethesda, MD: American Society of Health-System Pharmacists; 2005.
30. Barrington K, Brion LP. Cochrane Neonatal Group. Dopamine versus no treatment to prevent renal dysfunction in indomethacin-treated preterm newborn infants. *Cochrane Database Systematic Reviews.* 2002;3:CD003213.
31. Brash AR, Hickey DE, Graham TP, et al. Pharmacokinetics of indomethacin in the neonate. *N Engl J Med.* 1981;305:67-72.
32. Friedman Z, Whitman V, Maisels MJ, et al. Indomethacin disposition and indomethacin induced platelet dysfunction in premature infants. *J Clin Pharmacol.* 1978;18:272-279.
33. Hosono S, Ohono T, Kimoto H, et al. Reduction in blood glucose values following indomethacin therapy for patent ductus arteriosus. *Pediatr Internat*. 1999;41:525-528.
34. Hosono S, Ohono T, Ojima K, et al. Intractable hypoglycemia following indomethacin therapy for patent ductus arteriosus. *Pediatr Internat.* 2000;42:372-374.
35. Hosono S, Ohono T, Kimoto H, et al. Preventive management of hypoglycemia in very low-birth weight infants following indomethacin therapy for patent ductus arteriosus. *Pediatr Internat.* 2001;43:465-468.

Infliximab

1. Lamireau T, Cezard JP, Dabadie A, et al. Efficacy and tolerance of infliximab in children and adolescents with Crohn's disease. *Inflamm Bowel Dis.* 2004;10:745-750.
2. Lionetti P, Bronzini P, Salvestrini C, et al. Response to infliximab is related to disease duration in paediatric Crohn's disease. *Aliment Pharmacol Ther.* 2003;18:425-431.
3. Serrano MS, Schmidt-Sommerfeld E, Kilbaugh TJ, et al. Use of infliximab in pediatric patients with inflammatory bowel disease. *Ann Pharmacother.* 2001;35:823-828.
4. Hyams JS, Markowitz J, Wyllie R. Use of infliximab in the treatment of Crohn's disease in children and adolescents. *J Pediatr.* 2000;137:192-196.
5. Stephens MC, Shepanski MA, Mamula P, et al. Safety and steroid-sparing experience using infliximab for Crohn's disease at a pediatric inflammatory bowel disease center. *Am J Gastroenterol.* 2003;98:104-111.
6. deRidder L, Escher JC, Bouquet J, et al. Infliximab therapy in 30 patients with refractory pediatric Crohn disease with and without fistulas in The Netherlands. *J Pediatr Gastroenterol Nutr.* 2004;39:46-52.
7. Borrelli O, Bascietto C, Viola F, et al. Infliximab heals intestinal inflammatory lesions and restores growth in children with Crohn's disease. *Dig Liver Dis.* 2004;36:342-347.
8. Cezard JP, Nouaili N, Talbotec C, et al. A prospective study of the efficacy and tolerance of a chimeric antibody to tumor necrosis factors (Remicade) in severe pediatric Crohn disease. *J Pediatr Gastroenterol Nutr.* 2003;632-636.
9. BaldossanoR, Braegger CP, Escher JC. Infliximab (Remicade) therapy in the treatment of pediatric Crohn's disease. *Am J Gastroenterol.* 2003;98:833-838.
10. Lahdenne P, Vahasalo P, Honkanen V. Infliximab or etanercept in the treatment of children with refractory juvenile idiopathic arthritis: an open label study. *Ann Rheum Dis.* 2003;62:245-247.
11. Gerloni V, Pontikaki I, Gattinara M, et al. Efficacy of repeated intravenous infusions of an anti-tumor necrosis factor α monoclonal antibody, infliximab, in persistently active, refractory juvenile idiopathic arthritis. *Arthritis Rheum*. 2005;52:548-553.
12. Richards JC, Tay-Kearney ML, Murray K, et al. Infliximab for juvenile idiopathic arthritis-associated uveitis. *Clin Experiment Ophthalmol.* 2005;33:461-468.
13. Rajaraman RT, Kimura Y, Li S, et al. Retrospective case review of pediatric patients with uveitis treated with infliximab. *Ophthalmology.* 2006;113:308-314.
14. Burns JC, Mason WH, Hauger SB, et al. Infliximab treatments for refractory Kawasaki syndrome. *J Pediatr*. 2005;146:662-667.
15. Mamula P, Markowitz JE, Brown KA, et al. Infliximab as a novel therapy for pediatric ulcerative colitis. *J Pediatr Gastroenterol Nutr.* 2002;34:307-311.
16. Mamula P, Markowitz JE, Cohen LJ. Infliximab in pediatric ulcerative colitis: two-year follow up. *J Pediatr Gastroenterol Nutr.* 2004;38:298-301.
17. Eidelwein AP, Cuffari C, Abadom V, et al. Infliximab efficacy in pediatric ulcerative colitis. *Inflamm Bowel Dis.* 2005;11(3):213-218.
18. Russell GH, Katz AJ. Infliximab is effective in acute but not chronic childhood ulcerative colitis. *J Pediatr Gastroenterol Nutr.* 2004;39:166-170.

19. McEvoy GK, ed. *American Hospital Formulary Service Drug Information 2004.* Bethesda, MD: American Society of Health-System Pharmacists; 2004.
20. Crandall WV, Mackner LM. Infusion reactions to infliximab in children and adolescents: frequency, outcome and a predictive model. *Aliment Pharmacol Ther.* 2003;17:75-84.
21. Medical Economics, ed. *Physicians' Desk Reference*. 59th ed. Oradell, NJ: Medical Economics Company; 2006.
22. Friesen CA, Calabro C, Christenson K, et al. Safety of infliximab treatment in pediatric patients with inflammatory bowel disease. *J Pediatr Gastroenterol Nutr.* 2004;39:265-269.
23. Jacobstein DA, Markowitz JE, Kirschner BS, et al. Premedication and infusion reactions with infliximab: results from a pediatric inflammatory bowel disease consortium. *Inflamm Bowel Dis.* 2005;11:442-446.
24. Miele E, Markowitz JE, Mamula P, et al. Human antichimeric antibody in children and young adults with inflammatory bowel disease receiving infliximab. *J Pediatr Gastroenterol Nutr.* 2004;38:502-508.
25. Costamagna P, Furst K, Tully K, et al. Tuberculosis associated with blocking agents against tumor necrosis factor-alpha—California, 2002–2003. *MMWR Morb Mortal Wkly Rep.* 2004;53(30):683-686.

Insulin

1. Kitabchi AE, Umpierrez GE, Murphy MB, et al. Management of hyperglycemic crises in patients with diabetes. *Diabetes Care.* 2001;24:131-153.
2. American Academy of Pediatrics Committee on Drugs. Emergency drug doses for infants and children. *Pediatrics.* 1998;101:e1-e11.
3. Krane EJ. Diabetic ketoacidosis: biochemistry, physiology, treatment, and prevention. *Pediatr Clin North Am.* 1987;34:935-961.
4. Kecskes SA. Diabetic ketoacidosis. *Pediatr Clin North Am.* 1993;40:355-363.
5. Martin MM, Martin AL. Continuous low-dose infusion of insulin in the treatment of diabetic ketoacidosis in children. *J Pediatr.*1976;89:560-564.
6. Fort P, Waters SM, Lifshitz F. Low-dose insulin infusion in the treatment of diabetic ketoacidosis: bolus vs no bolus. *J Pediatr.* 1980;96:36-40.
7. Lightner ES, Kappy MS, Revsin B. Low-dose insulin infusion in patients with diabetic ketoacidosis: biochemical effects in children. *Pediatrics.* 1977;60:681-688.
8. Weber ME, Abbassi V. Continuous insulin therapy in severe diabetic ketoacidosis: variations in dosage requirements. *J Pediatr.* 1977;91:755-756.
9. Edwards GA, Kohaut EC, Wehring B, et al. Effectiveness of low-dose continuous insulin infusion in diabetic ketoacidosis. *J Pediatr.* 1977; 91:701-705.
10. Drop SL, Duval-Arnould BJ, Gober AE, et al. Low-dose intravenous insulin infusion versus subcutaneous insulin injection: a controlled comparative study of diabetic ketoacidosis. *Pediatrics.* 1977;59:733-738
11. Trachtenbarg DE. Diabetic ketoacidosis. *Am Fam Physician.* 2005;71:1705-1714.
12. Collins JW Jr, Hoppe M, Brown K, et al. A controlled trial of insulin infusion and parenteral nutrition in extremely low birth weight infants with glucose intolerance. *J Pediatr.* 1991;118:921-927.
13. Binder ND, Raschko PK, Benda GI, et al. Insulin infusion with parenteral nutrition in extremely low birth weight infants with hyperglycemia. *J Pediatr.* 1989;114:273-280.
14. Goldman SL, Hirata T. Attenuated response to insulin in very low birth weight infants. *Pediatr Res.* 1980;14:50-55.
15. Fuloria M, Friedberg MA, DuRant RH, et al. Effect of flow rate and insulin priming on the recovery of insulin from microbore infusion tubing. *Pediatrics.* 1998;102:1401-1406.
16. Ng SM, May JE, Emmerson AJB. Continuous insulin infusion in hyperglycaemic extremely-low-birth-weight neonates. *Biol Neonate.* 2005;87:269-272.
17. Thabet F, Bourgeois J, Guy B, et al. Continuous insulin infusion in hyperglycaemic very-low-birth-weight infants receiving parenteral nutrition. *Clin Nutr.* 2004;22:545-547.
18. Lui K, Thungappa U, Nair A, et al. Treatment with hypertonic dextrose and insulin in severe hyperkalemia of immature infants. *Acta Paediatr.* 1992;81:213-216.
19. Malone TA. Glucose and insulin versus cation-exchange resin for the treatment of hyperkalemia in very low birth weight infants. *J Pediatr.* 1991;118:121-123.
20. Aronoff A, Brier M, Bennett W. *The Renal Book, 2002.* Available at: http://www.kdp-baptist.louisville.edu/renalbook/. Accessed May 25, 2006.
21. Mena P, Llanos A, Uauy R. Insulin homeostasis in the extremely low birth weight infant. *Semin Perinatol.* 2001;25:436-446.
22. Genuth SM. Constant intravenous insulin infusion in diabetic ketoacidosis. *JAMA.* 1973;223:1348-1351.
23. McEvoy GK, ed. *AHFS Drug Information Essentials 2005–06.* Bethesda, MD: American Society of Health-System Pharmacists; 2005.
24. Simeon PS, Feggner ME, Levin SR. Continuous insulin infusions in neonates: pharmacologic availability of insulin in intravenous solutions. *J Pediatr.* 1994;124:818- 820.
25. Trissel LA. *Handbook on Injectable Drugs*. 13th ed. Bethesda. MD: American Society of Health-System Pharmacists; 2005.
26. Thomson PDR. *Physicians' Desk Reference.* 60th ed. Montvale, NJ: Medical Economics Company; 2006.
27. Furberg H, Jensen AK, Salbu B. Effect of pretreatment with 0.9% sodium chloride or insulin solutions on the delivery of insulin from an infusion system. *Am J Hosp Pharm.* 1986;43:2209-2213.
28. Bull HB. Adsorption of bovine serum albumin on glass. *Biochemica et Biophysica Acta.* 1956;19:464-472.

Interferon Alfa-2a

1. Roferon [package insert]. Nutley, NJ: Hoffman-LaRoche Inc; June 2005.
2. Dow LW, Raimondi SC, Culbert SJ. Response to alpha-interferon in children with Philadelphia chromosome-positive chronic myelocytic leukemia. *Cancer.* 1991;68:1678-1684.
3. Bortolotti F, Jara P, Barbera C. Long term effect of alpha interferon in children with chronic hepatitis B. *Gut.* 2000;46:715-718.
4. Jonas MM, Ott MJ, Nelson SP. Interferon-alpha treatment of chronic hepatitis C virus infection in children. *Pediatr Infect Dis J.* 1998;17:241-246.
5. Ozen H, Kocak N, Yuce A, et al. Retreatment with higher dose interferon alpha in children with chronic hepatitis B infection. *J Pediatr Infect Dis J.* 1999;18:694-697.
6. White CW, Wolf SJ, Korones DN. Treatment of childhood angiomatous diseases with recombinant interferon alpha-2a. *J Pediatr.* 1991;118:59-66.
7. Bauman NM, Burke DK, Smith RJ. Treatment of massive or life-threatening hemangiomas with recombinant alpha2a-interferon. *Otolaryngol Head and Neck Surg.* 1997;117:99-110.
8. MacArthur CJ, Senders CW, Katz J. The use of interferon alpha-2a for life-threatening hemangiomas. *Arch Otolaryngol Head Neck Surg.* 1995;121:690-693.
9. Ezekowitz RA, Mulliken JB, Folkman J. Interferon alpha-2a therapy for life-threatening hemangiomas of infancy. *N Engl J Med.* 1992;326:1456-1463.
10. Tryfonas GI, Tsikopoulos G, Liasidou E. Conservative treatment of hemangiomas in infancy and childhood with interferon-alpha 2a. *Pediatr Surg Int.* 1998;13:590-593.
11. Greinwald JH, Burke DK, Bonthius DJ. An update on the treatment of hemangiomas in children with interferon alpha2-a. *Arch Otolaryngol*

References

Head Neck Surg. 1999;125:21-27.

12. Jakacki RI, Cohen BH, Jamison C, et al. Phase II evaluation of interferon-alpha-2a for progressive or recurrent craniopharyngiomas. *J Neurosurg.* 2000;92:255-260.
13. Aydin F, Senbil N, Kuyucu N, et al. Combined treatment with subcutaneous interferon-α, oral Isoprinosine, and lamivudine for subacute sclerosing panencephalitis. *J Child Neurol.* 2003;18:104-108.
14. Artan R, Akcam M, Yilmaz A, et al. Interferon alpha monotherapy for chronic hepatitis C viral infection in thalassemics and hemodialysis patients. *J Chemother.* 2005;17:651-655.
15. American Academy of Pediatrics Committee on Drugs. "Inactive" ingredients in pharmaceutical products: update. *Pediatrics.* 1997;99:268-278.
16. Hall CM, Milligan DWA, Berrington J. Probably adverse reaction to a pharmaceutical excipient. *Arch Dis Child Fetal Neonatal Ed.* 2004;89: F184.
17. Hiller JL, Benda GI, Rahatzad M, et al. Benzyl alcohol toxicity: impact on mortality and intraventricular hemorrhage among very low birth weight infants. *Pediatrics.* 1986;77:500-506.
18. Grant JA, Bilodeau PA, Guernsey BG, et al. Unsuspected benzyl alcohol hypersensitivity. *N Engl J Med.* 1982;306:108.
19. Wilson JP, Solimando DA, Edwards MS. Parenteral benzyl alcohol-induced hypersensitivity reaction. *Drug Intell Clin Pharm.* 1986;20:689-691.
20. McEvoy GK, ed. *American Hospital Formulary Service Drug Information 2006.* Bethesda, MD: American Society of Health-System Pharmacists; 2006.
21. Barlow CF, Priebe CJ, Mulliken JB. Spastic diplegia as a complication of interferon alpha-2a treatment of hemangiomas of infancy. *J Pediatr.* 1998;132:527-530.
22. Williams SJ, Baird-Lambert JA, Farrell GC. Inhibition of theophylline metabolism by interferon. *Lancet.* 1987;2:939-941.
23. Comanor L, Minor J, Conjeevaram HS, et al. Impact of chronic hepatitis B and interferon-alpha therapy on growth of children. *J Viral Hepat.* 2001;8:139-147.
24. Sokal EM, Conjeevaram HS, Roberts EA, et al. Interferon alpha therapy for chronic hepatitis B in children: a multinational randomized controlled trial. *Gastroenterology.* 1998;114:988-995.
25. Imagawa A, Itoh N, Hanafusa T, et al. Autoimmune endocrine disease induced by recombinant interferon-alpha therapy for chronic active type C hepatitis. *J Clin Endocrin Metab.* 1995;80:922-926.

Interferon Alfa-2b

1. Intron A [package insert]. Kenilworth, NJ: Schering Corporation; March 2004.
2. Vajro P, Tedesco M, Fontanella A, et al. Prolonged and high dose recombinant interferon alpha-2b alone or after prednisone priming accelerates termination of active viral replication in children with chronic hepatitis B injection. *Pediatr Infect Dis J.* 1996;15:223-231.
3. Gurakan F, Kocak N, Ozen H, et al. Comparison of standard and high dosage recombinant interferon alpha 2b for treatment of children with chronic hepatitis B infection. *Pediatr Infect Dis J.* 2000;19:52-56.
4. Ruiz-Moreno M, Rua MJ, Molina J, et al. Prospective, randomized controlled trial of interferon-alpha in children with chronic hepatitis B. *Hepatology.* 1991;13:1035-1039.
5. Sokal EM, Wirth S, Goyens P. Interferon alpha-2b therapy in children with chronic hepatitis B. *Gut.* 1993;17:S87-S90.
6. Sokal EM, Conjeevaram HS, Roberts EA, et al. Interferon alpha therapy for chronic hepatitis B in children: a multinational randomized controlled trial. *Gastroenterology.* 1998;114:988-995.
7. Bruguera M, Amat L, Garcia O, et al. Treatment of chronic hepatitis B in children with recombinant alpha interferon. *J Clin Gastroenterol.* 1993:17:296-299.
8. Dikici B, Bosnak M, Kara, IH, et al. Lamivudine and interferon-alpha combination treatment of childhood patients with chronic hepatitis B infection. *Pediatr Inject Dis J.* 2001;20:988-992.
9. Dikici B, Ozgenc F, Kalayci AG, et al. Current therapeutic approaches in childhood chronic hepatitis B infection: a multicenter study. *J Gastroenterol Hepatol.* 2004;19:127-133.
10. Dikici B, Bosnak M, Bosnak V, et al. Comparison of treatments of chronic hepatitis B in children with lamivudine and α-interferon combination and α-interferon alone. *Pediatr Internat.* 2002;44:517-521.
11. Di Marco V, Lo Iacono O, Almasio P, et al. Long-term efficacy of alpha-interferon in beta-thalassemics with chronic hepatitis C. *Blood.* 1997;90:2207-2212.
12. Ruiz-Moreno M, Rua MJ, Castillo I, et al. Treatment of children with chronic hepatitis C with recombinant interferon-alpha: a pilot study. *Hepatology.* 1992;16:882-885.
13. Bortolotti F, Giacchino R, Vajro P, et al. Recombinant interferon-alpha therapy in children with chronic hepatitis C. *Hepatology.* 1995;22:1623-1627.
14. Gonzalez-Peralta RP, Kelly DA, Haber B, et al. Interferon alfa-2b in combination with ribavirin for the treatment of chronic hepatitis C in children: efficacy, safety, and pharmacokinetics. *Hepatology.* 2005;42:1010-1018.
15. Matsuoka S, Mori K, Nakano Y, et al. Efficacy of interferons in treating children with chronic hepatitis C. *Eur J Pediatr.* 1997;156:704-708.
16. Navid F, Furman WL, Fleming M, et al. The feasibility of adjuvant interferon α-2b in children with high-risk melanoma. *Cancer.* 2005;103:780-787.
17. Dubois J, Hershon L, Carmant L, et al. Toxicity profile of interferon alpha-2b in children: a prospective evaluation. *J Pediatr.* 1999;135:782-785.
18. Chang E, Boyd A, Nelson CC, et al. Successful treatment of infantile hemangiomas with interferon-alpha-2b. *J Ped Hematol Oncol.* 1997;19:237-244.
19. Tamayo L, Oritz DM, Orozco-Covarrubias L, et al. Therapeutic efficacy of interferon alpha-2b in infants with life-threatening giant hemangiomas. *Arch Dermatol.* 1997;133:1567-1571.
20. Garmendia G, Miranda N, Borroso S, et al. Regression of infancy hemangiomas with recombinant IFN-α2b. *J Interferon Cytokine Res.* 2001;21:31-38.
21. Wananukul S, Nuchprayoon I, Seksarn P. Treatment of Kasabach-Merritt syndrome: a stepwise regimen of prednisolone, dipyridamole, and interferon. *Int J Dermatol.* 2003;42:741-748.
22. Lauer SJ, Ochs J, Pollock BH, et al. Recombinant alpha-2B interferon treatment for childhood T-lymphoblastic disease in relapse. *Cancer.* 1994;74:197-202.
23. Ochs J, Abramowitch M, Rudnick S, et al. Phase I-II study of recombinant alpha-2 interferon against advanced leukemia and lymphoma in children. *J Clin Oncol.* 1986;4:883-887.
24. McEvoy GK, ed. *American Hospital Formulary Service Drug Information 2006.* Bethesda, MD: American Society of Health-System Pharmacists; 2006.
25. Iorio R, Pasqualina P, Botta S, et al. Side effects of alpha-interferon therapy and impact on health-related quality of life in children with chronic viral hepatitis. *Pediatr Infect Dis J.* 1997;16:984-990.
26. Williams SJ, Baird-Lambert JA, Farrell GC. Inhibition of theophylline metabolism by interferon. *Lancet.* 1987;2:939-941.
27. Imagawa A, Itoh N, Hanafusa T, et al. Autoimmune endocrine disease induced by recombinant interferon-alpha therapy for chronic active type C hepatitis. *J Clin Endocrin Metab.* 1995;80:922-926.

References

Irinotecan HCl

1. Taketomo CK, ed. *Lexi-Comp's Pediatric Dosage Handbook.* 12th ed. Hudson, OH: Lexi-Comp; 2005:703-705.
2. Cosetti M, Wexler LH, Calleja E, et al. Irinotecan for pediatric solid tumors: the Memorial Sloan Kettering experience. *J Pediatr Hematol Oncol.* 2002;24(2):101-105.
3. Gajjar A, Chintagumpala MM, Bowers DC, et al. Effect of intrapatient dosage escalation of irinotecan on its pharmacokinetics in pediatric patients who have high-grade gliomas and receive enzyme-inducing anticonvulsant therapy. *Cancer.* 2003;97(suppl 9):2374-2380.
4. Blaney S, Berg SL, Pratt C, et al. A phase I study of irinotecan in pediatric patients: a pediatric oncology group study. *Clin Cancer Res.* 2001;7(1):32-37.
5. Bomgaars L, Kerr J, Berg S, et al. A phase I study of irinotecan administered on a weekly schedule in pediatric patients. *Pediatr Blood Cancer.* 2006;46(1):50-55.
6. Camptosar [package insert]. New York, NY: Pfizer; July 2005.
7. Solimando DA, ed. *Lexi-Comp's Drug Information Handbook for Oncology*. 4th ed. Hudson, OH: Lexi-Comp; 2004:475-482.
8. Clinical Trials.gov. Available at: http://www.clinicaltrials.gov/ct/show/NCT00183846. Last accessed: March 21, 2006.
9. van Riel JM, van Groeningen CJ, de Greve J, et al. Continuous infusion of hepatic arterial irinotecan in pretreated patients with colorectal cancer metastatic to the liver. *Ann Oncol.* 2004;15(1):59-63.
10. National Comprehensive Cancer Network (NCCN) Antiemesis Panel Members. NCCN Clinical Practice Guidelines in Oncology. Antiemesis, v.1.2006. Available at www.nccn.org. Last accessed March 29, 2006.
11. Roila F, Feyer P, Maranzamo E, et al. Antiemetics in children receiving chemotherapy. *Support Care Cancer.* 2005;13:129-131.

Iron Dextran

1. NKR DOQI clinical practice guidelines for the treatment of anemia of chronic renal failure. National Kidney Foundation—Dialysis Outcomes Quality Initiative. Available at: http://www.kidney.org/professionals/kdoqi/guidelines_updates/doqiupan_iii.html#8:. Accessed April 27, 2006.
2. *Physicians' Desk Reference.* 60th ed. Montvale, NJ: Thomson PDR; 2006.
3. Reed MD, Bertino JS, Halpin TC. Use of intravenous iron dextran injection in children receiving total parenteral nutrition. *Am J Dis Child.* 1981;135:829-831.
4. Halpin TC, Bertino JS, Rothstein FC, et al. Iron-deficiency anemia in childhood inflammatory bowel disease: treatment with intravenous iron–dextran. *J Parenter Enteral Nutr.* 1982;6:9-11.
5. Fridge JL, Vichinsky EP. Correction of the anemia of epidermolysis bullosa with intravenous iron and erythropoietin. *J Pediatr.* 1998; 132:871-873.
6. Brandt JR, Avner ED, Hickman RO, et al. Safety and efficacy of erythropoietin in children with chronic renal failure. *Pediatr Nephrol.* 1999; 13:143-147.
7. Ohls RK, Harcum J, Schibler KR, et al. The effect of erythropoietin on the transfusion requirements of preterm infants <750 grams: a randomized, double-blind, placebo controlled study. *J Pediatr.* 1997;131:661-665.
8. Young TE, Mangum B, eds. *Neofax.* 18th ed. Raleigh, NC: Acorn Publishing Inc; 2005.
9. Ohls RK, Ehrenkranz RA, Wright LL, et al. Effects of early erythropoietin therapy on the transfusion requirements of preterm infants below 1250 grams birth weight: a multicenter, randomized controlled trial. *Pediatrics.* 2001;108:934-942.
10. Carnielli VP, da Riol R, Montini G. Iron supplementation enhances response to high doses of recombinant human erythropoietin in preterm infants. *Arch Dis Child Fetal Neonatal Ed.* 1998;79:F44–F48.
11. Pollak A, Hayde M, Hayn M, et al. Effect of intravenous iron supplementation on erythropoiesis in erythropoietin-treated premature infants *Pediatrics.* 2001;107;(1):78-85.
12. Meyer MP, Haworth C, Meyer JH, et al. A comparison of oral and intravenous iron supplementation in preterm infants receiving recombinant erythropoietin. *J Pediatr.* 1996;129:258-263.
13. Gelman CR, Rumack BH, Hess AJ, eds. *DRUGDEX(R) System.* Englewood, CO: MICROMEDEX Inc; accessed April 20, 2006.
14. McEvoy GK, ed. *Drug Information Essentials 2005–06.* Bethesda, MD: American Society of Health-System Pharmacists; 2005.
15. Zlotkin SH, Stallings VA, Penchary PB. Total parenteral nutrition in children. *Pediatr Clin North Am.* 1985;32:381-400.
16. Wan KK, Tsallas G. Dilute iron dextran formulation for addition to parenteral nutrient solutions. *Am J Hosp Pharm.* 1980;37:206-210.
17. Norton JA, Peters ML, Wesley R, et al. Iron supplementation of total parenteral nutrition: a prospective study. *J Parenter Enteral Nutr.* 1983;7:457-461.
18. Warady BA, Kausz A, Lerner G, et al. Iron therapy in the pediatric hemodialysis population. *Pediatr Nephrol.* 2004;19:655-661.
19. Greenbaum LA, Pan CG, Caley C, et al. Intravenous iron dextran and erythropoietin use in pediatric hemodialysis patients. *Pediatr Nephrol.* 2000;14:908-911.
20. Trissel LA, ed. *Handbook on Injectable Drugs*. 13th ed. Bethesda, MD: American Society of Health-System Pharmacists; 2005.
21. Cochran EB, Phelps SJ, Helms RA. Parenteral nutrition in pediatric patients. *Clin Pharm.* 1988;7:351-366.
22. Mayhew SL, Quick MW. Compatibility of iron dextran with neonatal parenteral nutrient solutions. *Am J Health-System Pharm.* 1995;54:570-571.
23. Kumpf VJ. Parenteral iron supplementation. *Nutr Clin Pract.* 1996;11(4):139-146.
24. Fishbane S, Kowalski EA. The comparative safety of intravenous iron dextran, iron saccharate, and sodium ferric gluconate. *Seminars in Dialysis*. 2000;13(6):381-384.
25. Chertow GM, Mason PD, Vaage-Nilsen O, et al. On the relative safety of parenteral iron formulations. *Nephrol Dial Transplant.* 2004;19:1571-1575.
26. Baile GR, Clark JA, Lane CE, et al. Hypersensitivity reactions and deaths associated with intravenous iron preparations. *Nephrol Dial Transplant.* 2005;20:1443-1449.
27. Fishbane S. Safety in iron management. *Am J Kid Disease.* 2003;41(5):S18-S36.
28. Tu Y, Knox NL, Biringer JM, et al. Compatibility of iron dextran with total nutrient admixtures. *Am J Hosp Pharm.* 1992;49:2233-2235.
29. Vaughan LM, Small C, Plunkett V. Incompatibility of iron dextran and a total nutrient admixture. *Am J Hosp Pharm.* 1990;47:1745-1746.

Isoproterenol HCl

1. Isuprel. Isoproterenol Hydrochloride Injection, USP. Lake Forest, IL: Hospira Inc; August 2004.
2. Schleien CL, Setzer NA, McLaughlin GE, et al. Postoperative management of the cardiac surgical patient. In: Rogers MC, ed. *Textbook of Pediatric Intensive Care.* 2nd ed. Baltimore, MD: Lippincott Williams & Wilkins; 1992:(1):467-531.
3. Wetzel RC, Tobin JR. Shock. In: Rogers MC, ed. *Textbook of Pediatric Intensive Care.* 2nd ed. Baltimore, MD: Lippincott Williams & Wilkins; 1992:(1):563-613.
4. Nakazawa M, Takahashi Y, Aiba S, et al. Acute hemodynamic effects of dopamine, dobutamine, and isoproterenol in congested infants or young children with large ventricular septal defect. *Jpn Cir J.* 1987;51:1010-1015.
5. Parry WH, Martorano F, Cotton EK. Management of life-threatening asthma with intravenous isoproterenol infusions. *Am J Dis Child.* 1976;130:39-42.
6. Page R, Gay W, Friday G, et al. Isoproterenol associated myocardial dysfunction during status asthmaticus. *Ann Allergy*. 1987;57:402-404.
7. Reyes G, Schwartz PH, Newth CJL, et al. The pharmacokinetics of isoproterenol in critically ill pediatric patients. *J Clin Pharmacol.* 1993;33:29-34.

References

8. Maguire JF, O'Rourke PP, Colan SD, et al. Cardiotoxicity during treatment of severe childhood asthma. *Pediatrics.* 1991;88:1180-1186.
9. Perkin RM, Anas NG. Cardiovascular evaluation and support in the critically ill child. *Pediatr Ann.* 1986;15:30-41.
10. Perkin RM, Levin DL. Shock in the pediatric patient. Part II. Therapy. *J Pediatr.* 1982;101:319-332.
11. McEvoy GK, ed. *AHFS Drug Information Essentials 2005–06.* Bethesda, MD: American Society of Health-System Pharmacists; 2005.
12. Zaritsky A, Chernow B. Use of catecholamines in pediatrics. *J Pediatr.* 1984;105:341-350.
13. National Asthma Education and Prevention Program Expert Panel Report 2: Guidelines for the Diagnosis and Management of Asthma. Available at: www.nhlbi.nih.gov/guidelines/asthma/asthgdln.htm. Accessed April 20, 2006.
14. Dellinger RP, Carlet JM, Masur H, et al. Surviving Sepsis Campaign guidelines for management of severe sepsis and septic shock. *Crit Care Med.* 2004;32:858-873.
15. Tulloh R. Management and therapeutic options in pediatric pulmonary hypertension. *Expert Rev Cardiovasc Ther.* 2006;4:361-374.
16. American Heart Association. 2005 Guidelines for cardiopulmonary resuscitation and emergency cardiovascular care. Part 12: Pediatric advanced life support. *Circulation.* 2005;112(suppl 1):167-187.
17. Trissel LA, ed. *Handbook on Injectable Drugs.* 13th ed. Bethesda, MD: American Society of Health-System Pharmacists; 2005.
18. Rich DS. New JCAHO medication management standards for 2004. *Am J Health-Syst Pharm.* 2004;61:1349-1358.
19. Wood DW, Downes JJ. Intravenous isoproterenol in the treatment of respiratory failure in childhood status asthmaticus. *Ann Allergy.* 1973;31:607-610.
20. Matson JR, Loughlin GM, Strunk RC. Myocardial ischemia complicating the use of isoproterenol in asthmatic children. *J Pediatr.* 1978; 92:776-778.
21. Kurland G, Williams J, Lewiston NJ. Fatal myocardial toxicity during continuous infusion intravenous isoproterenol therapy of asthma. *J Allergy Clin Immunol.* 1979;63:407.
22. Drislane FW, Samuels MA, Kozakewich H, et al. Myocardial contractions band lesions in patient with fatal asthma: possible neurocardiologic mechanism. *Am Rev Respir Dis.* 1987;135:498-501.
23. American Academy of Pediatrics Committee on Drugs. "Inactive" ingredients in pharmaceutical products: update. *Pediatrics.* 1997;99:268-278.
24. Smolinske SC. Review of parenteral sulfite reactions. *J Toxicol Clin Toxicol.* 1992;30:597-606.
25. Lester MR. Sulfite sensitivity: significance in human health. *J Am Col Nutr.* 1995;14:229-232.

Itraconazole

1. American Academy of Pediatrics. In: Pickering LK, ed. *Red Book: 2006 Report of the Committee on Infectious Diseases.* 27th ed. Elk Grove Village, IL: American Academy of Pediatrics; 2006.
2. Pandya NA, Atra AA, Riley U, et al. Role of itraconazole in haematology/oncology. *Arch Dis Child.* 2003;88:258-260.
3. Zhou H, Goldman M, Wu J, et al. A pharmacokinetic study if intravenous itraconazole followed by oral administration of itraconazole capsules in patients with advanced human immunodeficiency. *J Clin Pharmacol.* 1998;38:593-562.
4. Sporanox injection [prescribing information]. Lake Forest, IL: Hospira Inc; June 2006.
5. Trotman RL, Williamson JC, Shoemaker DM, et al. Antibiotic dosing in critically ill adult patients receiving continuous renal replacement therapy. *Clin Infect Dis.* 2005;41(8):1159-1166.
6. Willems L, van der Geest R, de Beule K. Itraconazole oral solution and intravenous formulations: a review of pharmacokinetics and pharmacodynamics. *J Clin Pharm Ther.* 2001;26:159-169.
7. Louis S, Kutt H, McDowell F. The cardiocirculatory changes caused by intravenous Dilantin and its solvent. *Am Heart J.* 1967;74:523-529.
8. American Academy of Pediatrics Committee on Drugs. "Inactive" ingredients in pharmaceutical products: update. *Pediatrics.* 1997;99:268-278.
9. Glasgow AM, Boeckx RL, Miller MK, et al. Hyperosmolality in small infants due to propylene glycol. *Pediatrics.* 1983;72:353-355.
10. MacDonald MG, Getson PR, Glasgow AM, et al. Propylene glycol: increased incidence of seizures in low birth weight infants. *Pediatrics.* 1987;79:622-625.

Kanamycin Sulfate

1. American Academy of Pediatrics. In: Pickering LK, ed. *2003 Red Book: Report of the Committee on Infectious Diseases.* 26th ed. Elk Grove Village, IL: American Academy of Pediatrics; 2003.
2. Schwartz SN, Pazin GJ, Lyon JA, et al. A controlled investigation of the pharmacokinetics of gentamicin and tobramycin in obese subjects. *J Infect Dis.* 1978;138:499-505.
3. Bauer LA, Blouin RA, Griffen WO, et al. Amikacin pharmacokinetics in morbidly obese patients. *Am J Hosp Pharm.* 1980;37:519-522.
4. Prober CG, Stevenson DK, Benitz WE. The use of antibiotics in neonates weighing less than 1200 grams. *Pediatr Infect Dis J.* 1990;9:111-121.
5. Robertson J, Shilkofski N, eds. *The Harriet Lane Handbook*. 17th ed. Philadelphia, PA: Elsevier Mosby; 2005.
6. Howard JB, McCracken GH. Reappraisal of kanamycin usage in neonates. *J Pediatr.* 1975;86:949-956.
7. McCracken GH, Threlkeld N. Kanamycin dosage in newborn infants. *J Pediatr*. 1976;89:313-314.
8. Kanamycin. In: Kucer A, Crowe SM, Grayson ML, et al., eds. *The Use of Antibiotics: A Clinical Review of Antibacterial, Antifungal and Antiviral Drugs.* 5th ed. Boston, MA: Butterworth Heinemann; 1997:439-449.
9. Aronoff A, Brier M, Bennett W. *The Renal Book, 2002.* Available at: http://www.kdp-baptist.louisville.edu/renalbook/. Accessed May 6, 2006.
10. Yow MD, Tengg NE, Bangs J. The ototoxic effects of kanamycin sulfate in infants and children. *J Pediatr.* 1962;60:230-242.
11. Horrevorts AM, de Witte J, Degener JE, et al. Tobramycin in patients with cystic fibrosis. Adjustments in dosing interval for effective treatment. *Chest.* 1987;92:844-848.
12. Kelly HB, Menendez R, Fan L, et al. Pharmacokinetics of tobramycin in cystic fibrosis. *J Pediatr.* 1982;100:318-321.
13. Loirat P, Rohan J, Baillet A, et al. Increased glomerular filtration rate in patients with major burns and its effect on the pharmacokinetics of tobramycin. *N Engl J Med.* 1978;299:915-919.
14. American Society of Health-System Pharmacists. American Hospital Formulary System. Available at: http://ahfsfirst.firstdatabank.com/AHFSfirst/NSAHFSFirstSearchmain.asp. Accessed May 10, 2006.
15. Gillett AP, Falk RH, Andrews J, et al. Rapid intravenous injection of tobramycin: suggested dosage schedule and concentrations in serum. *J Infect Dis.* 1976;134:S110-S113.
16. Dobbs SM, Mawer GE. Intravenous injection of gentamicin and tobramycin without impairment of hearing. *J Infect Dis.* 1976;134 (Suppl): S114-S117.
17. Mendelson J, Portnoy J, Dick V, et al. Safety of the bolus administration of gentamicin. *Antimicrob Agents Chemother.* 1976;9:633-638.
18. Trissel LA, ed. *Handbook on Injectable Drugs.* 13th ed. [CD-ROM version 1.5]. Bethesda, MD: American Society of Health-System Pharmacists; 2005.
19. Bodey GP, Chang HY, Rodriguez V, et al. Feasibility of administering aminoglycoside antibiotics by continuous intravenous infusion. *Antimicrob Agents Chemother.* 1975;8:328-333.
20. Powell SH, Thompson WL, Luthe MA, et al. Once daily vs. continuous aminoglycoside dosing: efficacy and toxicity in animal and clinical studies of gentamicin, netilmicin and tobramycin. *J Infect Dis.* 1983;147:918-932.
21. Giacoia GP, Schentag JJ. Pharmacokinetics and nephrotoxicity of continuous intravenous infusion of gentamicin in low birth weight infants. *J Pediatr.* 1986;109:715-719.

22. Hieber JP, Kusmiesz H, Nelson JD. Kanamycin in children: pharmacology and lack of toxicity of an increased dosage regimen. *J Pediatr.* 1980;96:1089-1091.
23. McCracken GH Jr, Threlkeld N, Thomas ML. Intravenous administration of kanamycin and gentamicin in newborn infants. *Pediatrics.* 1977;60:463-466.
24. American Academy of Pediatrics Committee on Drugs. "Inactive" ingredients in pharmaceutical products: update. *Pediatrics.* 1997;99:268-278.
25. Lester MR. Sulfite sensitivity: significance in human health. *J Am Col Nutr.* 1995;14:229-232.
26. Franson TR, Ritch PS, Quebbeman EJ. Aminoglycoside serum concentration sampling via central venous catheters: a potential source of clinical error. *JPEN J Parenter Enteral Nutr.* 1987;11:77-79.
27. Massey KL, Hendeles L, Neims A. Identification of children for whom routine monitoring of aminoglycoside serum concentrations is not cost effective. *J Pediatr.* 1986;109:897-901.
28. Logsdon BA, Phelps SJ. Routine monitoring of gentamicin serum concentrations in pediatric patients with normal renal function is unnecessary. *Ann Pharmacother.* 1997;31:1514-1518.
29. Beaubien AR, Desjardins S, Ormsby E, et al. Incidence of amikacin ototoxicity: a sigmoid function of total drug exposure independent of plasma levels. *Am J Otolaryngol.* 1989;10:234-243.
30. Beaubien AR, Ormsby E, Bayne A, et al. Evidence that amikacin ototoxicity is related to total perilymph area under the concentration-time curve regardless of concentration. *Antimicrob Agents Chemother.* 1991;35:1070-1074.
31. Snavely SR, Hodges GR. The neurotoxicity of antibacterial agents. *Ann Intern Med.* 1984;101;92-104.
32. Manian FA, Stone WJ, Alford RH. Adverse antibiotic effects associated with renal insufficiency. *Rev Infect Dis.* 1990;12:236-249.

Ketamine HCl

1. Ketamine hydrochloride Injection, USP [product information]. Bedford, OH: Ben Venue Laboratories Inc; 2004.
2. American Academy of Pediatrics Committee on Drugs. Emergency drug doses for infants and children. *Pediatrics.* 1998;101:e1-e11.
3. Slonim AD, Ognibene FP. Amnestic agents in pediatric bronchoscopy. *Chest.* 1999;116:1802-1808.
4. Tobias JD. Sedation and analgesia in paediatric intensive care units. *Paediatr Drugs.* 1999;1:109-126.
5. Hostetler MA, Davis CO. Prospective age-based comparison of behavioral reactions occurring after ketamine sedation in the ED. *Am J Emerg Med.* 2002;20:463-468.
6. Green SM, Nakamura R, Johnson NE. Ketamine for sedation for pediatric procedures: part 2, review and implications. *Ann Emerg Med.* 1990;19:1033-1046.
7. Lin C, Durieux ME. Ketamine and kids: an update. *Paediatr Anaesth.* 2005;15:91-97.
8. Tugrul M, Camci E, Pembeci K, et al. Ketamine infusion versus isoflurane for the maintenance of anesthesia in the prebypass period in children with tetralogy of Fallot. *J Cardiothorac Vasc Anesth.* 2000;14:557-561.
9. Ramchandra DS, Anisya V, Gourie-Devi M. Ketamine monoanaesthesia for diagnostic muscle biopsy in neuromuscular disorders in infancy and childhood: floppy infant syndrome. *Can J Anaesth.* 1990;37:474-476.
10. Pruitt JW, Goldwasser MS, Sabol SR, et al. Intramuscular ketamine, midazolam, glycopyrrolate for pediatric sedation in the emergency department. *J Oral Maxillofac Surg.* 1995;53:13-17.
11. Petrack EM, Marx CM, Wright MS. Intramuscular ketamine is superior to meperidine, promethazine and chlorpromazine for pediatric emergency department sedation. *Arch Pediatr Adolesc Med.* 1996;150:676-681.
12. Epstein FB. Ketamine dissociative sedation in pediatric emergency medical practice. *Am J Emerg Med.* 1993;11:180-182.
13. Hartvig P, Larsson E, Joachimsson PO. Postoperative analgesia and sedation following pediatric cardiac surgery using a constant infusion of ketamine. *J Cardiothorac Vasc Anesth.* 1993;7:148-153.
14. Tobias JD, Martin LD, Wetzel RC. Ketamine by continuous infusion for sedation in the pediatric intensive care unit. *Crit Care Med.* 1990;18:819-821.
15. Singh A, Girotra S, Mehta Y, et al. Total intravenous anesthesia with ketamine for pediatric interventional cardiac procedures. *J Cardiothorac Vasc Anesth.* 2000;14:36-39.
16. Nehama I, Pass R, Bech Her-Karsch A, et al. Continuous ketamine infusion for the treatment of refractory asthma in a mechanically ventilated infant: case report and review of the pediatric literature. *Pediatr Emerg Care.* 1996;12:294-297.
17. Youssef-Ahmed MZ, Silver P, Nimkoff L, et al. Continuous infusion of ketamine in mechanically ventilated children with refractory bronchospasm. *Intensive Care Med.* 1996;22:972-976.
18. Denmark TK, Crane HA, Brown L. Ketamine to avoid mechanical ventilation in severe pediatric asthma. *J Emerg Med.* 2006;30(2):163-166.
19. Ito H, Sobue K, Hirate J, et al. Use of ketamine to facilitate opioid withdrawal in a child. *Anethesiology*. 2006;104:1113.
20. Trissel LA, ed. *Handbook on Injectable Drugs.* 13th ed. Bethesda, MD: American Society of Health-System Pharmacists; 2005.
21. Green SM, Rothrock SG, Lynch EL, et al. Intramuscular ketamine for pediatric sedation in the emergency department: safety profile in 1,022 cases. *Ann Emerg Med.* 1998;31:688-697.
22. Smith JA, Santer LJ. Respiratory arrest following intramuscular ketamine injection in a 4-year-old child. *Ann Emerg Med.* 1993;22:613-615.
23. Klepstad P, Borchgrevink P, Hval B, et al. Long-term treatment with ketamine in a 12-year-old girl with severe neuropathic pain caused by a cervical spinal tumor. *J Pediatr Hematol Oncol.* 2001;23:616-619.
24. Pandey CK, Mathur N, Singh N, et al. Fulminant pulmonary edema after intramuscular ketamine. *Can J Anesth.* 2000;47:894-896.

Ketorolac Tromethamine

1. US Food and Drug Administration Center for Drug Evaluation and Research. Available at: http://www.fda.gov/cder/drug/infopage/COX2/default.htm. Accessed July 17, 2006.
2. Toradol [prescribing information]. Nutley, NJ: Roche Laboratories Inc; September 2002.
3. Buck ML. Clinical experience with ketorolac in children. *Ann Pharmacother.* 1994;28:1009-1013.
4. Gerhardt RT, Gerhardt DM. Intravenous ketorolac in the treatment of fever. *Am J Emerg Med.* 2000;18:500-501.
5. Park JM, Houck CS, Sethna NF, et al. Ketorolac suppresses postoperative bladder spasms after pediatric ureteral reimplantation. *Anesth Analg.* 2000;91:11-15.
6. Dsida RM, Wheeler M, Birmingham PK, et al. Age-stratified pharmacokinetics of ketorolac tromethamine in pediatric surgical patients. *Anesth Analg.* 2002;94:266-270.
7. Munro HM, Walton S, Malviya S, et al. Low-dose ketorolac improves analgesia and reduces morphine requirements following posterior or spinal fusion in adolescents. *Can J Anesth.* 2002;49:461-466.
8. Hackmann T. Smaller dose of 0.5 mg/kg IV ketorolac is sufficient to provide pain relief in children. *Anesth Analg.* 2004;98:275-276.
9. Watcha MF, Jones MB, Lagueruela RG, et al. Comparison of ketorolac and morphine as adjuvants during pediatric surgery. *Anesthesiology.* 1992;76:368-372.
10. Bean JD, Hunt R, Custer MD. Effects of ketorolac on postoperative analgesia and bleeding time in children. *Anesthesiology.* 1993;79:A1190.
11. Vetter TR, Heiner EJ. Intravenous ketorolac as an adjuvant to pediatric patient-controlled analgesia with morphine. *J Clin Anesth.* 1994;6:110-113.
12. Richter RL, Valley RD, Bailey AG, et al. A comparison of intraoperative ketorolac, morphine and saline on postoperative analgesia in the pediatric patient. *Anesthesiology.* 1992;77:A1161.
13. Splinter WM, Reid CW, Roberts DJ, et al. Reducing pain after inguinal hernia repair in children. *Anesthesiology.* 1997;87:542-546.

References

14. Romsing J, Ostergaard D, Walther-Larsen S, et al. Analgesic efficacy and safety of preoperative versus postoperative ketorolac in paediatric tonsillectomy. *Acta Anaesthesiolol Scand.* 1998;42:770-775.
15. Shende D, Das K. Comparative effects of intravenous ketorolac and pethidine on perioperative analgesia and postoperative nausea and vomiting (PONV) for pediatric strabismus surgery. *Acta Anaesthesiolol Scand.* 1999;43:265-269.
16. Maunuksela EL, Kokki H, Bullingham RES. Comparison of intravenous ketorolac with morphine for postoperative pain in children. *Clin Pharmacol Ther.* 1992;52:436-443.
17. Olkkola KT, Maunuksela EL. The pharmacokinetics of postoperative intravenous ketorolac tromethamine in children. *Br J Clin Pharmacol.* 1991;31:182-184.
18. Lieh-Lai, MW, Kaufmann RE, Uy HG, et al. A randomized comparison of ketorolac tromethamine and morphine for postoperative analgesia in critically ill children. *Crit Care Med.* 1999;27:2786-2791.
19. Gunter JB, Varughese AM, Harrington JF, et al. Recovery and complications after tonsillectomy in children: a comparison of ketorolac and morphine. *Anesth Analg.* 1995;81:1136-1141.
20. Rusy LM, Houck CS, Sullivan LJ, et al. A double-blind evaluation of ketorolac tromethamine versus acetaminophen in pediatric tonsillectomy: analgesia and bleeding. *Anesth Analg.* 1995;80:226-229.
21. Papacci P, De Francisci G, Iacobucci T, et al. Use of intravenous ketorolac in the neonate and premature babies. *Paediatr Anaesth.* 2004;14:487-492.
22. Forrest JB, Heitlinger EL, Revell S. Ketorolac for postoperative pain management in children. *Drug Safety.* 1997;16:309-329.
23. Burd RS, Tobias JS. Ketorolac for pain management after abdominal surgical procedures in infants. *South Med J.* 2002;95:331-333.
24. Hamunen K, Maunuksela EL, Sarvela J, et al. Stereoselective pharmacokinetics of ketorolac in children, adolescents and adults. *Acta Anaesthesiol Scand.* 1999;43:1041-1046.
25. Aronoff A, Brier M, Bennett W. *The Renal Book, 2002.* Available at: http://www.kdp-baptist.louisville.edu/renalbook/. Accessed July 17, 2006.
26. Taketomo CK, Hodding JH, Kraus DM, eds. *Pediatric Dosage Handbook.* 12th ed. [CD-ROM version 2006.1] Hudson, OH: Lexi-Comp; 2006.
27. Trissel LA, ed. *Handbook on Injectable Drugs.* 13th ed. [CD-ROM version 1.5]. Bethesda, MD: American Society of Health-System Pharmacists; 2005.
28. Jung D, Mroszczak E, Bynum L. Pharmacokinetics of ketorolac tromethamine in humans after intravenous, intramuscular, and oral administration. *Eur J Clin Pharmacol.* 1988;35:423-425.
29. Brousseau DC, Duffy SJ, Anderson AC, et al. Treatment of pediatric migraine headaches: a randomized, double-blind trial of prochlorperazine versus ketorolac. *Ann Emerg Med.* 2004;43:256-262.
30. Harwick WE Jr, Givens TG, Monroe KW, et al. Effect of ketorolac in pediatric sickle cell vaso-occlusive pain crisis. *Pediatr Emerg Care.* 1999;15:179-182.
31. Suresh S, Wheeler M, Patel A. Case series: IV regional anesthesia with ketorolac and lidocaine: is it effective for the management of complex regional pain syndrome 1 in children and adolescents? *Anesth Analg.* 2003;96:694-695.

L-Cysteine HCl

1. L-cysteine hydrochloride injection [USP package insert] Irvine, CA: Gensia Sicor Pharmaceuticals Inc; July 2004.
2. Helms RA, Storm MC, Christensen ML, et al. Cysteine supplementation results in normalization of plasma taurine concentrations in children receiving home parenteral nutrition. *J Pediatr.* 1999;134:358-361.
3. Shew SB, Keshen TH, Jahoor F, et al. Assessment of cysteine synthesis in very low-birth weight neonates using a [$^{13}C_6$]glucose tracer. *J Pediatr Surg.* 2005;40:52-56.
4. Heird WC, Hay W, Helms RA, et al. Pediatric parenteral amino acid mixture in low birth weight infants. *Pediatrics.* 1988;81:41-50.
5. Laine L, Shulman RJ, Pitre D, et al. Cysteine usage increases the need for acetate in neonates who receive parenteral nutrition. *Am J Clin Nutr.* 1991;54:565-567.
6. Schmidt GL, Baumgartner TG, Fischlschweiger W, et al. Cost containment using cysteine HCl acidification to increase calcium/phosphate solubility in hyperalimentation solutions. *JPEN J Parenter Enteral Nutr.* 1986;10:203-207.

Labetalol HCl

1. Hanna JD, Chan JC, Gill JR. Hypertension and the kidney. *J Pediatr.* 1991;118:327-340.
2. National High Blood Pressure Education Program Working Group on High Blood Pressure in Children and Adolescents. The fourth report on the diagnosis, evaluation, and treatment of high blood pressure in children and adolescents. *Pediatrics.* 2004:114(2 suppl 4th Report):555-576.
3. Bunchman TE, Lynch RE, Wood EG. Intravenously administered labetalol for treatment of hypertension in children. *J Pediatr.* 1992;120:140-144.
4. American Society of Health-System Pharmacists. American Hospital Formulary System. Available at: http://ahfsfirst.firstdatabank.com/AHFSfirst/NSAHFSFirstSearchmain.asp. Accessed July 22, 2006.
5. Deal JE, Barratt TM, Dillion MJ. Management of hypertensive emergencies. *Arch Dis Child.* 1992;67:1089-1092.
6. Ishisaka DY, Toman CS, Housel BF. Labetalol treatment of hypertension in a child. *Clin Pharm.* 1991;10:500-501.
7. Michael J, Groshong T, Tobuas JD. Nicardipine for hypertensive emergencies in children with renal disease. *Pediatr Nephrol.* 1998;12:40-42.
8. Trissel LA, ed. *Handbook on Injectable Drugs.* 13th ed. [CD-ROM version 1.5]. Bethesda, MD: American Society of Health-System Pharmacists; 2005.
9. Soni MG, Taylor SL, Greenberg NA, et al. Evaluation of the health aspects of methyl paraben: a review of the published literature. *Food Chem Toxicol.* 2002;40:1335-1373.
10. Nagel JE, Fuscaldo JT, Firemen P. Paraben allergy. *JAMA.* 1977;237:1594-1595.

Lansoprazole

1. Kovacs TO, Lee CQ, Chiu YL, et al. Intravenous and oral lansoprazole are equivalent in suppressing stimulated acid output in patient volunteers with erosive esophagitis. *Aliment Pharmacol Ther.* 2004;20:883-889.
2. Faure C, Michaud L, Shaghaghi EK, et al. Lansoprazole in children: pharmacokinetics and efficacy in reflux oesophagitis. *Aliment Pharmacol Ther.* 2001;15:1397-1402.
3. Franco MT, Salvia G, Terrin G, et al. Lansoprazole in the treatment of gastro-oesophageal reflux disease in childhood. *Dig Liver Dis.* 2000;32(8):660-666.
4. Gibbons TE, Gold BD. The use of proton pump inhibitors in children: a comprehensive review. *Pediatr Drugs.* 2003;5(1):25-40.
5. Tran A, Rey E, Pons G. Pharmacokinetic-pharmacodynamic study of oral lansoprazole in children. *Clin Pharmacol Ther.* 2002;71:359-367.
6. Robertson J, Shilkofski N, eds. *The Harriet Lane Handbook.* 17th ed. Philadelphia, PA: Elsevier Mosby; 2005.
7. *Physicians' Desk Reference.* 60th ed. Montvale, NJ: Thomson PDR; 2006.
8. Haber M, Hassall E, Hayman MB, et al. Correlation of endoscopic and histologic findings in children with erosive and nonerosive esophagitis pre- and post-treatment. *J Pediatr Gastroenterol Nutr.* 2001;33(3):423.
9. Tolia V, Fitzgerald J, Hassall E, et al. Safety of lansoprazole in the treatment of gastroesophageal reflux disease in children. *J Pediatr*

Gastroenterol Nutr. 2002;35(4):S300-S307.
10. Tolia V, Ferry G, Gunasekaran T, et al. Efficacy of lansoprazole in the treatment of gastroesophageal reflux disease in children. *J Pediatr Gastroenterol Nutr.* 2002;35(4):S308-S318.
11. Croom KF, Scott LJ. Lansoprazole in the treatment of gastro-oesophageal reflux disease in children and adolescents. *Drugs.* 2005;65(15):2129-2135.
12. Scott LJ. Lansoprazole in the management of gastroesophageal reflux disease in children. *Pediatr Drugs.* 2003;5(1)57-61.
13. Gremse D, Winter H, Tolia V, et al. Pharmacokinetics and pharmacodynamics of lansoprazole in children with gastroesophageal reflux disease. *J Pediatr Gastro Nutr.* 2002;35:S319-S326.
14. Fiedorek S, Tolia V, Gold BD, et al. Efficacy and safety of lansoprazole in adolescents with symptomatic erosive and non-erosive gastroesophageal reflux disease. *J Pediatr Gastroenterol Nutr.* 2005;40:319-327.
15. Aronoff A, Brier M, Bennett W. *The Renal Book, 2002.* http://www.kdp-baptist.louisville.edu/renalbook/. Accessed August 9, 2006.
16. Litalien C, Theoret Y, Faure C. Pharmacokinetics of proton pump inhibitors in children. *Clin Pharmacokinet.* 2005;44:441-466.
17. Metz DC, Amer F, Hunt B, et al. Lansoprazole regimens that sustain intragastric pH >6.0: an evaluation of intermittent oral and continuous intravenous infusion dosages. *Aliment Pharmacol Ther.* 2006;23:985-995.
18. Canani RB, Cirillo P, Roggero P, at al. Therapy with gastric acidity inhibitors increases the risk of acute gastroenteritis and community-acquired pneumonia in children. *Pediatrics.* 2006;117:817-820.

Levocarnitine

1. Carnitor [package insert]. Gaithersburg, MD: Sigma-Tau Pharmaceuticals Inc; March, 2004.
2. Goa, KL, Brogden RN. L-carnitine, a preliminary review of its pharmacokinetics, and its therapeutic use in ischemic cardiac disease and primary and secondary carnitine deficiencies in relationship to its role in fatty acid metabolism. *Drugs.* 1987;34:1-24.
3. Zachwieja J, Duran M, Joles JA, et al. Amino acid and carnitine supplementation in haemodialysed children. *Pediatr Nephrol.* 1994;8:739-743.
4. Berard E, Iordache A, Barrillon D, et al. L-carnitine in dialysed patients: the choice of dosage regimen. *Int J Clin Pharmacol Res.* 1995;15:127-133.
5. Berard E, Iordache A. Effect of low doses of L-carnitine on the response to recombinant human erythropoietin in hemodialyzed children: about two cases. *Nephron.* 992;62:368-369.
6. Gloggler A, Bulla M, Furst P. Effect of low dose supplementation of L-carnitine on lipid metabolism in hemodialyzed children. *Kidney Int Suppl.* 1989;27:256-258.
7. National Kidney Foundation. Clinical practice recommendations for anemia in chronic kidney disease in children. *Am J Kidney Dis.* 2006;47: S86-S108.
8. Van Hove JLK, Kahler D, Millington DS, et al. Intravenous L-carnitine and acetyl-L-carnitine in medium chain acyl-coenzyme A dehydrogenase deficiency and isovaleric acidemia. *Pediatr Res.* 1994;35:96-101.
9. Robertson J, Shilkofski N, eds. *The Harriet Lane Handbook.* 17th ed. Philadelphia, PA: Elsevier Mosby; 2005.
10. Schmidt-Sommerfeld E, Penn D, Wolf H. Carnitine deficiency in premature infants receiving total parenteral nutrition: effect of L-carnitine supplementation. *J Pediatr.* 1983;102:931-935.
11. Bonner CM, DeBrie KL, Hug G, et al. Effects of parenteral L-carnitine supplementation on fat metabolism and nutrition in premature neonates. *J Pediatr.* 1995;126:287-292.
12. Helms RA, Mauer EC, Hay WW, et al. Effect of intravenous L-carnitine on growth parameters and fat metabolism during parenteral nutrition in premature neonates. *J Parenter Enteral Nutr.* 1990;14:448-453.
13. Shortland GJ, Walter JH, Stroud C, et al. Randomised controlled trial of L-carnitine as a nutritional supplement in preterm infants. *Arch Dis Child Fetal Neonatal Ed.* 1998;78:185-188.
14. O'Donnell, Finer NN, Rich W, et al. Role of L-carnitine in apnea of prematurity: a randomized, controlled trial. *Pediatrics.* 2002;109:622-626.
15. Whitfield J, Smith T, Sollohub H, et al. Clinical effects of L-carnitine supplementation on apnea and growth in very low birth weight infants. *Pediatrics.* 2003;111:477-482.
16. Pande S, Brio LP, Campbell DE, et al. Lack of effect of L-carnitine supplementation on weight gain in very preterm infants. *J Perinatol.* 2005;25:470-477.
17. Crill CM, Storm MC, Christensen ML, et al. Carnitine supplementation in premature neonates: effect on plasma and red blood cell total carnitine concentrations, nutrition parameters and morbidity. *Clin Nutr.* 2006;25:886-896.
18. DeVivo DC, Bohan TP, Coulter DL, et al. L-Carnitine supplementation in childhood epilepsy: current perspectives. *Epilepsia.* 1998;1216-1225.
19. Raskind JY, El-Chaar GM. The role of carnitine supplementation during valproic acid therapy. *Ann Pharmacother.* 2000;34:630-638.
20. Bohles H, Sewell AC, Wenzel D, et al. The effect of carnitine supplementation in valproate-induced hyperammonaemia. *Acta Paediatr.* 1996;85:446-449.
21. Sulkers EJ, Lafeber HN, Degenhart HJ, et al. Effects of high carnitine supplementation on substrate utilization in low-birth-weight infants receiving total parenteral nutrition. *Am J Clin Nutr.* 1990;52:889-894.
22. Storm MC, Wang B, Helms RA. Stability of carnitine in pediatric TPN and TNA formulations. *J Parenter Enteral Nutr.* 1998;22:S18.
23. Bullock L, Fitzgerald JF, Walter WV. Emulsion stability in total nutrient admixtures containing a pediatric amino acid formulation. *J Parenter Enteral Nutr.* 1992;16:64-68.
24. Crill CM, Wang B, Storm MC, et al. Carnitine: a conditionally essential nutrient in the neonatal population? *J Pediatr Pharmacol Ther.* 2001;6:225-236.
25. Helton E, Darragh R, Francis P, et al. Metabolic aspects of myocardial disease and a role for L-carnitine in the treatment of childhood cardiomyopathy. *Pediatrics.* 2000;105:1260-1270.
26. Carter RW, Singh J, Archambault C, et al. Severe lactic acidosis in association with reverse transcriptase inhibitors with potential response to L-carnitine in a pediatric HIV-positive patient. *AIDS Patient Care STDS.* 2004;18:131-134.

Levothyroxine Sodium

1. Young TE, Mangum B, eds. *Neofax.* 18th ed. Raleigh, NC: Acorn Publishing Inc; 2005.
2. American Society of Health-System Pharmacists. American Hospital Formulary System. Available at: http://ahfsfirst.firstdatabank.com/AHFSfirst/NSAHFSFirstSearchmain.asp. Accessed July 24, 2006.
3. American Academy of Pediatrics. Update of newborn screening and therapy for congenital hypothyroidism. *Pediatrics.* 2006;117:2290-2303.
4. Levothyroxine sodium for injection [package insert]. Bedford, OH: Bedford Laboratories; May 2003.
5. Robertson J, Shilkofski N, eds. *The Harriet Lane Handbook.* 17th ed. Philadelphia, PA: Elsevier Mosby; 2005.
6. Pagliaro LA, Pagliaro AM, eds. *Problems in Pediatric Drug Therapy*. 2nd ed. Hamilton, IL: Drug Intelligence Publications Inc; 1987.
7. Fisher DA. The importance of early management in optimizing IQ in infants with congenital hypothyroidism. *J Pediatr.* 2000;136:273-274.
8. Dubuis JM, Glorieux J, Richer F, et al. Outcome of severe congenital hypothyroidism: closing the developmental gap with early high dose levothyroxine treatment. *J Clin Endocrin Meta.* 1996;81:222-227.
9. Raghavan S, DiMartino J, Saenger P, et al. Pseudotumor cerebri in an infant and l-thyroxine therapy for transient neonatal hypothyroidism. *J Pediatr.* 1997;120:481-483.
10. Zuppa AF, Nadkarni V, Davis L, et al. The effect of a thyroid hormone infusion on vasopressor support in critically ill children with cessation of neurologic function. *Crit Care Med.* 2004;32:2318-2322.

References

Lidocaine

1. American Heart Association. Guidelines 2005 for cardiopulmonary resuscitation and emergency cardiovascular care. Part 12: Pediatric advanced life support. *Circulation.* 2005;112:167-187.
2. American Academy of Pediatrics Committee on Drugs. Emergency drug doses for infants and children. *Pediatrics.*1998;101:e1-e11.
3. American Society of Health-System Pharmacists. American Hospital Formulary System. Available at: http://ahfsfirst.firstdatabank.com/AHFSfirst/NSAHFSFirstSearchmain.asp. Accessed July 10, 2006.
4. Gelman CR, Rumack BH, Hess AJ (eds.). *DRUGDEX(R) System.* Englewood, CO: MICROMEDEX Inc. Accessed April 12, 2006.
5. Ramsey RE. Treatment of status epilepticus. *Epilepsia.* 1993;34:S71-S81.
6. Aggarwal P, Wali JP. Lidocaine in refractory status epilepticus: a forgotten drug in the emergency department. *Am J Emerg Med.* 1993;2:243-244.
7. van Rooij LG, Toet MC, Rademaker KM, et al. Cardiac arrhythmias in neonates receiving lidocaine as anticonvulsive treatment. *Eur J Pediatr.* 2004;163:637-641.
8. Sawaishi Y, Yano T, Enoki M, et al. Lidocaine-dependent early infantile status epilepticus with highly suppressed EEG. *Epilepsia.* 2002;43:201-204.
9. Kobayashi K, Ito M, Miyajima T, et al. Successful management of intractable epilepsy with intravenous lidocaine and lidocaine tapes. *Pediatr Neurol.* 1999;21:476-480.
10. Hellstrom-Westas L, Westgren U, Svenningsen NW, et al. Lidocaine for treatment of severe seizures in newborn infants. *Acta Pediatr Scand.* 1988;77:79-84.
11. Hamano S, Sugiyama N, Yamashita S, et al. Intravenous lidocaine for status epilepticus during childhood. *Dev Med Child Neurol.* 2006;48:220-222.
12. Pascual J, Ciudad J, Berciano J. Role of lidocaine (lignocaine) in managing status epilepticus. *J Neurol Neurosurg Psychiatry.* 1992;55:49-51.
13. Bedford RF, Persing JA, Pobereskin L, et al. Lidocaine or thiopental for rapid control of intracranial hypertension. *Anesth Analg.* 1980;59:435-437.
14. Brucia JJ, Owen DC, Rudy EB. The effects of lidocaine on intracranial hypertension. *J Neurosci Nurs.* 1992;24:205-214.
15. Wallace MS, Lee J, Sorkin L, et al. Intravenous lidocaine: effects on controlling pain after Anti-GD2 antibody therapy in children with neuroblastoma—a report of a series. *Anesth Analg.* 1997;85:794-796.
16. Pentel P, Benowitz N. Pharmacokinetic and pharmacodynamic considerations in drug therapy of cardiac emergencies. *Clin Pharmacokinet.* 1984;9:273-308.
17. Thomson PD, Melmon KL, Richardson JA, et al. Lidocaine pharmacokinetics in advanced heart failure, liver disease, and renal failure in humans. *Ann Intern Med.* 1973;78:499-508.
18. Aronoff A, Brier M, Bennett W. *The Renal Book, 2002.* Available at: http://www.kdp-baptist.louisville.edu/renalbook/. Accessed July 14, 2006.
19. Xylocaine for ventricular arrhythmias [package insert]. Westborough, MA: Astra USA Inc; July 1993.
20. Orlowski JP. Cardiopulmonary resuscitation in children. *Pediatr Clin North Am.* 1980;27:495-512.
21. Trissel LA, ed. *Handbook on Injectable Drugs.* 13th ed. [CD-ROM version 1.5]. Bethesda, MD: American Society of Health-System Pharmacists; 2005.
22. American Academy of Pediatrics Committee on Drugs. "Inactive" ingredients in pharmaceutical products: update. *Pediatrics.* 1997;99:268-278.
23. Lester MR. Sulfite sensitivity: significance in human health. *J Am Col Nutr.* 1995;14:229-232.
24. Soni MG, Taylor SL, Greenberg NA, et al. Evaluation of the health aspects of methyl paraben: a review of the published literature. *Food Chem Toxicol.* 2002;40:1335-1373.
25. Nagel JE, Fuscaldo JT, Firemen P. Paraben allergy. *JAMA.* 1977;237:1594-1595.
26. Berger I, Steinberg A, Schlesinger Y, et al. Neonatal mydriasis: intravenous lidocaine adverse reaction. *J Child Neurol.* 2002;17:400-401.

Linezolid

1. *Physicians' Desk Reference.* 60th ed. Montvale, NJ: Thomson PDR; 2006.
2. American Academy of Pediatrics. In: Pickering LK, ed. *2006 Red Book: Report of the Committee on Infectious Diseases.* 27th ed. Elk Grove Village, IL: American Academy of Pediatrics; 2006.
3. Kearns GL, Jungbluth GL, Abdel-Rahman SM, et al. Impact of ontogeny on linezolid disposition in neonates and infants. *Clin Pharmacol Ther.* 2003;74:413-422.
4. Kaplan SL, Deville JG, Yogev R, et al. Linezolid Pediatric Study Group. Linezolid versus vancomycin for treatment of resistant Gram-positive infections in children. *Pediatr Infect Dis J.* 2003;22:677-686.
5. Kaplan SL, Afghani B, Lopez P, et al. Linezolid for the treatment of methicillin-resistant Staphylococcus aureus infections in children. *Pediatr Infect Dis J.* 2003;22(9 suppl):S178-S185.
6. Jantausch BA, Deville J, Adler S, et al. Linezolid for the treatment of children with bacteremia or nosocomial pneumonia caused by resistant gram-positive bacterial pathogens. *Pediatr Infect Dis J.* 2003;22(9 suppl):S164-S171.
7. Meissner HC, Townsend T, Wenman W, et al. Hematologic effects of linezolid in young children. *Pediatr Infect Dis J.* 2003;22(9 suppl):S186-S192.
8. Graham PL, Ampofo K, Saiman L. Linezolid treatment of vancomycin-resistant Enterococcus faecium ventriculitis. *Pediatr Infect Dis J.* 2002;21:798-800.
9. Ang JY, Lua JL, Turner DR, et al. Vancomycin-resistant Enterococcus faecium endocarditis in a premature infant successfully treated with linezolid. *Pediatr Infect Dis J.* 2003;22:1101-1103.
10. Castagnola E, Moroni C, Gandullia P, et al. Catheter lock and systemic infusion of linezolid for treatment of persistent Broviac catheter-related staphylococcal bacteremia. *Antimicrob Agents Chemother.* 2006;50:1120-1121.
11. Trissel LA, ed. *Handbook on Injectable Drugs.* 13th ed. [CD-ROM version 1.5]. Bethesda, MD: American Society of Health-System Pharmacists; 2005.
12. Thomas CR, Rosenberg M, Blythe V, et al. Serotonin syndrome and linezolid. *J Am Acad Child Adolesc Psychiatry.* 2004;43:790.
13. Bergeron L, Boule M, Perreault S. Serotonin toxicity associated with concomitant use of linezolid. *Ann Pharmacother.* 2005;39:956-961.
14. Morales-Molina JA, Mateu-de Antonio J, Marin-Casino M, et al. Linezolid-associated serotonin syndrome: what we can learn from cases reported so far. *J Antimicrob Chemother.* 2005;56:1176-1178.
15. Kaplan SL, Patterson L, Edwards KM, et al. Linezolid Pediatric Pneumonia Study Group. Pharmacia and Upjohn. Linezolid for the treatment of community-acquired pneumonia in hospitalized children. Linezolid Pediatric Pneumonia Study Group. *Pediatr Infect Dis J.* 2001;20:488-494.
16. Matson KL, Miller SE. Tooth discoloration after treatment with linezolid. *Pharmacotherapy.* 2003;23:682-685.

Lorazepam

1. Khalil SN, Berry JM, Howard G, et al. The antiemetic effect of lorazepam after outpatient strabismus surgery in children. *Anesthesiology.* 1992;77:915-919.
2. Relling RV, Mulhern RK, Fairclough D, et al. Chlorpromazine with and without lorazepam as antiemetic therapy in children receiving uniform chemotherapy. *J Pediatr.* 1993;12:811-816.
3. Relling MV, Mulhern RK, Johnson D, et al. Lorazepam pharmacodynamics in children with cancer. *J Pediatr.* 1989;114:641-646.

References

4. Robertson J, Shilkofski N, eds. *The Harriet Lane Handbook.* 17th ed. Philadelphia, PA: Elsevier Mosby; 2005:867.
5. American Academy of Pediatrics Committee on Drugs. Emergency drug doses for infants and children. *Pediatrics.* 1998;101:e1-e11.
6. Nahata MC. Sedation in pediatric patients undergoing diagnostic procedures. *Drug Intell Clin Pharm.* 1988;22:711-715.
7. Shankar V, Deshpande JK. Procedural sedation in the pediatric patient. *Anesthesiol Clin N Am.* 2005;23:635-654, viii.
8. Flood RG, Krauss B. Procedural sedation and analgesia for children in the emergency department. *Emerg Med Clin North Am.* 2003;21(1):121-139.
9. Krauss B, Green S. Procedural sedation and analgesia in children. *Lancet.* 2006;367:766-780.
10. Taketomo CK, Hodding JH, Kraus DM, eds. *Pediatric Dosage Handbook.* 12th ed. [CD-ROM version 2006.1] Hudson, OH: Lexi-Comp; 2006
11. American Society of Health-System Pharmacists. American Hospital Formulary System. Available at: http://ahfsfirst.firstdatabank.com/AHFSfirst/NSAHFSFirstSearchmain.asp. Accessed May 10, 2006.
12. Tobias JD. Sedation analgesia in paediatric intensive care units. *Pediatr Drugs.* 1999;1:109-126.
13. Young TE, Mangum B, eds. *Neofax®.* 18th ed. Raleigh, NC: Acorn Publishing Inc; 2005:150.
14. Deshmukh A, Wittert W, Schnitzler E, et al. Lorazepam in the treatment of refractory neonatal seizures. *Am J Dis Child.* 1986;140:1042-1044.
15. Maytal J, Novak GP, King KC. Lorazepam in the treatment of refractory neonatal seizures. *J Child Neurol.* 1991;6:319-323.
16. Roddy SM, McBride MC, Torres CF. Treatment of neonatal seizures with lorazepam. *Ann Neurol.* 1987;22:412. Abstract.
17. McDermott CA, Kowalczyk AL, Schnitzler ER, et al. Pharmacokinetics of lorazepam in critically ill neonates with seizures. *J Pediatr.* 1992;120:479-483.
18. Lacey DJ, Singer WD, Horwitz SJ, et al. Clinical and laboratory observations: lorazepam therapy of status epilepticus in children and adolescents. *J Pediatr.* 1986;108:771-774.
19. Crawford TO, Mitchell WG, Snodgrass SR. Lorazepam in childhood status epilepticus and serial seizures: effectiveness and tachyphylaxis. *Neurology.* 1987;37:190-195.
20. Giang DW, McBride MC. Lorazepam versus diazepam for the treatment of status epilepticus. *Pediatr Neurol.* 1988;4:358-361.
21. Appleton R, Sweeney A, Shoonara I, et al. Lorazepam versus diazepam in the acute treatment of epileptic seizures and status epilepticus. *Dev Med Child Neurol.* 1995;37:682-688.
22. Aronoff A, Brier M, Bennett W. *The Renal Book, 2002.* Available at: http://www.kdp-baptist.louisville.edu/renalbook/. Accessed May 6, 2006.
23. Bhatt-Mehta V, Annich G. Sedative clearance during extracorporeal membrane oxygenation. *Perfusion.* 2005;20:309-315.
24. Reincke HM, Gilmore RL, Kuhn RJ. High-dose lorazepam therapy for status epilepticus in a pediatric patient. *Drug Intell Clin Pharm.* 1988;22:889-890.
25. Maloley PA, Gal P, Mize R, et al. Lorazepam dosing in neonates; application of objective sedation scores. *DICP Ann Pharmacother.* 1990;24:326-327. Letter.
26. Ativan® (lorazepam) injection prescribing information. Philadelphia, PA: Wyeth Laboratories; October 2002.
27. McCollam JS, O'Neil MG, Norcross ED, et al. Continuous infusion of lorazepam, midazolam, and propofol for sedation of the critically ill surgery trauma patient: a prospective, randomized comparison. *Crit Care Med.* 1999;27:2454-2458.
28. Pohlman AS, Simpson KP, Hall JB. Continuous intravenous infusions of lorazepam versus midazolam for sedation during mechanical ventilatory support: a prospective, randomized study. *Crit Care Med.* 1994;22:1241-1247.
29. Watling SM, Johnson M, Yanos J. A method to produce sedation in critically ill patients. *Ann Pharmacother.* 1996;30:1227-1231.
30. Swart EL, Schijndel RJ, van Loenen AC, et al. Continuous infusion of lorazepam versus midazolam in patients in the intensive care unit: sedation with lorazepam is easier to manage and is more cost-effective. *Crit Care Med.* 1999;27:1461-1465.
31. Walker JE, Homan RW, Vasko MR, et al. Lorazepam in status epilepticus. *Ann Neurol.* 1979;6:207-213.
32. American Academy of Pediatrics Committee on Drugs. "Inactive" ingredients in pharmaceutical products: update. *Pediatrics.* 1997;99:268-278.
33. Hall CM, Milligan DWA, Berrington J. Probably adverse reaction to a pharmaceutical excipient. *Arch Dis Child Fetal Neonatal Ed.* 2004;89:F184.
34. Hiller JL, Benda GI, Rahatzad M, et al. Benzyl alcohol toxicity: impact on mortality and intraventricular hemorrhage among very low birth weight infants. *Pediatrics.* 1986;77:500-506.
35. Grant JA, Bilodeau PA, Guernsey BG, et al. Unsuspected benzylalcohol hypersensitivity. *N Engl J Med.* 1982;306:108.
36. Wilson JP, Solimando DA, Edwards MS. Parenteral benzyl alcohol-induced hypersensitivity reaction. *Drug Intell Clin Pharm.* 1986;20:689-691.
37. Louis S, Kutt H, McDowell F. The cardiocirculatory changes caused by intravenous Dilantin and its solvent. *Am Heart J.* 1967;74:523-529.
38. Glasgow AM, Boeckx RL, Miller MK, et al. Hyperosmolality in small infants due to propylene glycol. *Pediatrics.* 1983;72:353-355.
39. MacDonald MG, Getson PR, Glasgow AM, et al. Propylene glycol: increased incidence of seizures in low birth weight infants. *Pediatrics.* 1987;79:622-625.
40. Chicella M, Jansen P, Parthiban A, et al. Propylene glycol accumulation associated with continuous infusion of lorazepam in pediatric intensive care patients. *Crit Care Med.* 2002;30:2752-2756.
41. Riker RR, Fraser GL. Adverse events associated with sedatives, analgesics, and other drugs that provide patient comfort in the intensive care unit. *Pharmacotherapy.* 2005:25(5 Pt 2):8S-18S.
42. Neale BW, Mesler EL, Young M, et al. Proylene glycol-induced lactic acidosis in a patient with normal renal function: a proposed mechanism and monitoring recommendations. *Ann Pharmacother.* 2005;39:1732-1736.
43. Yaucher NE, Fish JT, Smith HW, et al. Propylene glycol-associated renal toxicity from lorazapam infusion. *Pharmacotherapy.* 2003;23:1094-1099.
44. Straaten HL, Rademaker CM, de Vries LS. Comparison of the effect of midazolam or vecuronium on blood pressure and cerebral blood flow velocity in premature newborns. *Dev Pharmacol Ther.* 1992;19:191-195.
45. Sugarman JM, Paul RI. Flumazenil: a review. *Pediatr Emerg Care.* 1994;10:37-43.
46. Cronin CM. Neurotoxicity of lorazepam in a premature infant. *Pediatrics.* 1992;89:1129.
47. Reiter PD, Stiles AD. Lorazepam toxicity in a premature infant. *Ann Pharmacother.* 1993; 27:727-729.
48. Chess PR, D'Angio CT. Clonic movement following lorazepam administration in full-term infants. *Arch Pediatr Adolesc Med.* 1998;152:98-99.

Lymphocyte Immune Globulin–Antithymocyte Globulin (equine)

1. Uittenbogaart CH, Robinson BJ, Malekzadeh MH, et al. Use of antithymocyte globulin (dose by rosette protocol) in pediatric renal allograft recipients. *Transplantation.* 1979;28:291-293.
2. Fitzpatrick MM, Duffy PG, Fernando ON, et al. Cadaveric renal transplantation in children under 5 years of age. *Pediatr Nephrol.* 1992;6:166-171.
3. Whitehead B, Helms P, Goodwin M, et al. Heart-lung transplantation for cystic fibrosis. 2: outcome. *Arch Dis Child.* 1991;6:1022-1026.
4. Bernstein D, Baum D, Berry G, et al. Neoplastic disorders after pediatric heart transplantation. *Circulation.* 1993;5(part 2):230-237.
5. Matloub YH, Bostrom B, Golembe B, et al. Antithymocyte globulin, cyclosporine, and prednisone for the treatment of severe aplastic anemia in children. *Am J Pediatr Hematol Oncol.* 1994;16:104-106.
6. Bunchman TE, Ham JM, Sedman AB, et al. Superior allograft survival in pediatric renal transplant recipients. *Transplant Proc.* 1994;26:24-25.
7. Kawahara K, Storb R, Sanders J, et al. Successful allogeneic bone marrow transplantation in a 6.5-year-old male for severe aplastic anemia complicating orthotopic liver transplantation for fulminant non-A non-B hepatitis. *Blood.* 1991;78:1140-1143.
8. Leichter HE, Ettenger RB, Jordan SC, et al. Short-course antithymocyte globulin for treatment of renal transplant rejection in children. *Transplantation.* 1985;41:133-135.

References

9. Conley SB, al-Urzi A, So S, et al. Prevention of rejection and graft loss with an aggressive quadruple immunosuppressive therapy regimen in children and adolescents. *Transplantation.* 1994;57:540-544.
10. Fang JP, XU HG, Huang SL, et al. Immunosuppressive treatment of aplastic anemia in Chinese children with antithymocyte globulin and cyclosporine. *Pediatr Hematol Oncol.* 2006;23:45-50.
11. Rosenfeld S, Follman D, Nunez O, et al. Antithymocyte globulin and cyclosporine for severe aplastic anemia. *JAMA.* 2003;289:1130-1135.
12. Goldenberg NA, Graham DK, Liang X, et al. Successful treatment of severe aplastic anemia in children using standardized immunosuppressive therapy with antithymocyte globulin and cyclosporine A. *Pediatr Blood Cancer.* 2004;43:718-722.
13. Rosenfeld SJ, Kimball J, Vining D, et al. Intensive immunosuppression with antithymocyte globulin and cyclosporine as treatment for severe acquired aplastic anemia. *Blood.* 1995; 85:3058-3065.
14. Zander AR, Zabelina T, Kroger N, et al. Use of five-agent GVHD prevention regimen in recipients of unrelated donor marrow. *Bone Marrow Transplant.* 1999; 23:889-893.
15. Ayas M, Al-Jefri A, Al-Mahr M, et al. Stem cell transplantation for patients with Fanconi anemia with low-dose cyclophosphamide and antithymocyte globulins without the use of radiation therapy. *Bone Marrow Transplant.* 2005;35:463-466.
16. Abdelkefi A, Othman TB, Ladeb S, et al. Bone marrow transplantation for patients with acquired severe aplastic anemia using cyclophosphamide and antithymocyte globulin: the experience from a single center. *Hemtaol J.* 2003;4:208-213.
17. Lynch BA, Vasef MA, Comito M, et al. Effect of *in vivo* lymphocyte-depleting strategies on development of lymphoproliferative disorders in children post allogeneic bone marrow transplantation. *Bone Marrow Transplant.* 2003;32:527-533.
18. Wall DA, Carter SL, Kernan NA, et al. Busulfan/melphalan/antithymocyte globulin followed by unrelated donor cord blood transplantation for treatment of infant leukemia and leukemia in young children: the cord blood transplantation study (COBLT) experience. *Biol Blood Marrow Transplant.* 2005;11:637-646.
19. MacMillan ML, Weisdorf DJ, Davies SM, et al. Early antithymocyte globulin therapy improves survival in patients with steroid-resistant acute graft-versus-host disease. *Biol Blood Marrow Transplant.* 2002;8:40-46.
20. Whitehead B, James I, Helms P, et al. Intensive care management of children following heart and heart-lung transplantation. *Inten Care Med.* 1990;16:426-430.
21. Khositseth S, Matas A, Cook ME, et al. Thymoglobulin versus ATGAM induction therapy in pediatric kidney transplant recipients: a single-center report. *Transplantation.* 2005;8:958-963.
22. Atgam [product information]. Kalamazoo, MI: Pharmacia & Upjohn Company; January 2003.
23. McEvoy GK, ed. *American Hospital Formulary Service Drug Information 2006.* Bethesda, MD: American Society of Health-System Pharmacists; 2006.
24. Rahman GF, Hardy MA, Cohen DJ. Administration of equine anti-thymocyte globulin via peripheral vein in renal transplant recipients. *Transplantation.* 2000;69:1958-1960.
25. Monchon M, Kaiser B, Palmer JA, et al. Evaluation of OKT3 monoclonal antibody and anti-thymocyte globulin in the treatment of steroid-resistant acute allograft rejection in pediatric renal transplants. *Pediatr Nephrol.* 1993;7:259-262.
26. Dearden C, Foukaneli T, Lee P, et al. The incidence and significance of fevers during treatment with antithymocyte globulin for aplastic anemia. *Br J Hematol.* 1998;103:846-848.

Lymphocyte Immune Globulin–Antithymocyte Globulin (rabbit)

1. DiBona E, Rodeghiero F, Bruno B, et al. Rabbit antithymocyte globulin (r-ATG) plus cyclosporine and granulocyte colony stimulating factor is an effective treatment for aplastic anaemia patients unresponsive to a first course of intensive immunosuppressive therapy. *Br J Haematol.* 1999;107:330-334.
2. Fang JP, Xu HG, Huang SL, et al. Immunosuppressive treatment of aplastic anemia in Chinese children with antithymocyte globulin and cyclosporine. *Pediatr Hematol Oncol.* 2006;23:45-50.
3. Di Filippo S, Boissonnat P, Sassolas F, et al. Rabbit antithymocyte globulin as induction immunotherapy in pediatric heart transplantation. *Transplantation.* 2003;75:354-358.
4. Parisi F, Danesi H, Squitieri C, et al. Thymoglobuline use in pediatric heart transplantation. *J Heart Lung Transplant.* 2003;22:591-593.
5. Remberger M, Storer, B, Ringden O, et al. Association between pretransplant Thymoglobulin and reduced non-relapse mortality rate after marrow transplantation from unrelated donors. *Bone Marrow Transplant.* 2002;29:391-397.
6. Seidel MG, Fritsch G, Matthes-Martin S, et al. Antithymocyte globulin pharmacokinetics in pediatric patients after hematopoietic stem cell transplantation. *J Pediatr Hematol Oncol.* 2005;27:532-536.
7. Bond GJ, Mazariegos GV, Sindhi R, et al. Evolutionary experience with immunosuppression in pediatric intestinal transplantation. *J Pediatr Surg.* 2005;40:274-280.
8. Reyes J, Mazariegos GV, Abu-Elmagd K, et al. Intestinal transplantation under tacrolimus monotherapy after perioperative lymphoid depletion with rabbit anti-thymocyte globulin (Thymoglobulin). *Am J Transplant.* 2005;5:1430-1436.
9. Sindhi R, Magill A, Bentlejewski C, et al. Enhanced donor-specific alloreactivity occurs independently of immunosuppression in children with early liver rejection. *Am J Transplant.* 2005;5:96-102.
10. Ault BH, Honaker MR, Gaber AO, et al. Short-term outcomes of Thymoglobulin induction in pediatric renal transplant recipients. *Pediatr Nephrol.* 2002;17:815-818.
11. Brophy PD, Thomas SE, McBryde KD, et al. Comparison of polyclonal induction agents in pediatric renal transplantation. *Pediatr Transplant.* 2001;5:174-178.
12. Khositseth S, Matas A, Cook ME, et al. Thymoglobulin versus ATGAM induction therapy in pediatric kidney transplant recipients: a single-center report. *Transplantation.* 2005;79:958-963.
13. Bell L, Girardin C, Sharma A, et al. Lymphocyte subsets during and after rabbit anti-thymocyte globulin induction in pediatric renal transplantation: sustained T cell depletion. *Transplant Proc.* 1997;29:6S-9S.
14. Kamel MH, Mohan P, Little DM, et al. Rabbit antithymocyte globulin as induction immunotherapy for pediatric deceased donor kidney transplantation. *J Urol.* 2005;174:703-707.
15. Thymoglobulin [package insert]. Cambridge, MA: Genzyme Corporation; March 2005.
16. McEvoy GK, ed. American Hospital Formulary Service Drug Information 2006. Bethesda, MD: *American Society of Health-System Pharmacists*; 2006.

Magnesium Sulfate

1. Magnesium sulfate injection USP [package insert]. Schaumburg, IL: American Pharmaceutical Partners Inc; November 2002.
2. Tsang RC. Neonatal magnesium disturbances. *Am J Dis Child.* 1972; 124:282-283.
3. Maggioni A, Orzalesi M, Mimouni FB. Intravenous correction of neonatal hypomagnesemia: effect on ionized magnesium. *J Pediatr.* 1998;132:652-655.
4. Slayton W, Anstine D. Tetany in a child with AIDS receiving intravenous tobramycin. *S Med J.* 1996;89:1108-1111.
5. McEvoy GK, ed. *AHFS Drug Information Essentials 2005–06.* Bethesda, MD: American Society of Health-System Pharmacists; 2005.
6. 2005 American Heart Association guidelines for cardiopulmonary resuscitation and emergency cardiovascular care: Part 12: Pediatric advanced life support. *Circulation.* 2005;112(24)(suppl 1):IV167-IV187.
7. Dorman BH, Sade RM, Burnette JS, et al. Magnesium supplementation in the prevention of arrhythmias in pediatric patients undergoing surgery for congenital heart defects. *Am Heart J.* 2000; 139:522-528.

8. DiNicola LK, Monem GF, Gayle MO, et al. Treatment of critical status asthmaticus in children. In: Respiratory medicine 1: current issues. *Pediatr Clin North Am.* 1994;41:1293-1324.
9. Ciarallo L, Sauer AH, Shannon MW. Intravenous magnesium therapy for moderate to severe pediatric asthma: results of a randomized placebo-controlled trial. *J Pediatr.* 1996;129:809-814.
10. Dib JG, Engstrom FM, Sisca TS, et al. Intravenous magnesium sulfate treatment in a child with status asthmaticus. *Am J Health-Syst Pharm.* 1999;56:997-1000.
11. Scarfone RJ, Loiselle JM, Joffe MD, et al. A randomized trial of magnesium in the emergency department treatment of children with asthma. *Ann Emerg Med.* 2000;36:572-578.
12. Pabon H, Monem G, Kissoon N. Safety and efficacy of magnesium sulfate infusion in children with status asthmaticus. *Pediatr Emerg Care.* 1994;10:200-204.
13. Monem GF, Kissoon N, DeNicola L. Use of magnesium sulfate in asthma in childhood. *Pediatr Ann.* 1996;25:136, 139-144.
14. Schiermeyer RP, Finkelstein JA. Rapid infusion of magnesium sulfate obviates need for intubation in status asthmaticus. *Am J Emerg Med.* 1994;12:164-166.
15. Abu-Osba YK, Galal O, Manasra K, et al. Treatment of severe persistent pulmonary hypertension of the newborn with magnesium sulfate. *Arch Dis Child.* 1992;67:31-35.
16. Randall RE, Cohne MD, Spray CC, et al. Hypermagnesemia in renal failure. Etiology and toxic manifestations. *Ann Intern Med.* 1964;61:73-88.
17. Levene M, Blennow M, Witelaw A, et al. Acute effects of two different doses of magnesium sulphate in infants with birth asphyxia. *Arch Dis Child.* 1995;73:F174-F177.
18. Trissel LA, ed. *Handbook on Injectable Drugs.* 13th ed. Bethesda, MD: American Society of Health-System Pharmacists; 2005.

Mannitol

1. Osmitrol injection [package insert]. Deerfield, IL: Baxter Healthcare Corporation; March 2005.
2. Thomson Healthcare Inc. *USP DI® Drug Information for the Health Care Professional.* Available at http://www.thomsonhc.com. MICROMEDEX® Healthcare Series [database on the Internet]. Accessed April 10, 2006.
3. Taketomo CK, ed. *Lexi-Comp's Pediatric Dosage Handbook*. 12th ed. Hudson, OH: Lexi-Comp Inc; 2005:793-794.
4. Lewis MA, Awan A. Mannitol and furosemide in the treatment of diuretic resistant oedema in nephrotic syndrome. *Arch Dis Child.* 1999;80:184-185.
5. Adelson PD, Bratton SL, Carney NA, et al. Guidelines for the acute medical management of severe traumatic brain injury in infants, children, and adolescents. Chapter 11. Use of hyperosmolar therapy in the management of severe pediatric traumatic brain injury. *Pediatr Crit Care Med.* 2003;4:S40-S44.
6. American Academy of Pediatrics Committee on Drugs. Emergency drug doses for infants and children. *Pediatrics.* 1998;101:e1-e11.
7. Shaywitz BA, Rothstein P, Venes JL. Monitoring and management of increased intracranial pressure in Reyes syndrome: results in 29 children. *Pediatrics.* 1980;66:198-204.
8. James HE. Methodology for the control of intracranial pressure with hypertonic mannitol. *Acta Neurochir.* 1980;51:161-172.
9. Marshall LF, Smith RW, Rauscher LA, et al. Mannitol dose requirements in brain-injured patients. *J Neurosurg.* 1978;48:169-172.
10. Trissel LA, ed. *Handbook on Injectable Drugs.* 13th ed. Bethesda, MD: American Society of Health-System Pharmacists; 2005.
11. Goldwasser P, Fotino S. Acute renal failure following massive mannitol infusion. Appropriate response of tubuloglomerular feedback? *Arch Intern Med.* 1984;144:2214-2216.
12. Cottrell JE, Robustelli A, Post K, et al. Furosemide-and mannitol-induced changes in intracranial pressure and serum osmolality and electrolytes. *Anesthesiology.* 1977;47:28-30.

Meperidine HCl

1. Tobias JD. Sedation and analgesia in paediatric intensive care units. A guide to drug selection and use. *Paediatr Drugs.* 1999;1:109-126.
2. McEvoy GK, ed. *AHFS Drug Information Essentials 2005–06.* Bethesda, MD: American Society of Health-System Pharmacists; 2005.
3. Demerol [package insert]. Lake Forest, IL: Hospira Inc; March 2005.
4. Pokela ML, Olkkola KT, Koivisto ME, et al. Pharmacokinetics and pharmacodynamics of intravenous meperidine in neonates and infants. *Clin Pharmacol Ther.* 1992;52:342-349.
5. Bhatt-Mehta V, Rosen DA. Management of acute pain in children. *Clin Pharm.* 1991;10:667-685.
6. Fixler DE, Carrell T, Browne R, et al. Oxygen consumption in infants and children during cardiac catheterization under different sedation regimens. *Circulation.* 1974;50:788-794.
7. Cole TB, Sprinkle RH, Smith SJ, et al. Intravenous narcotic therapy for children with severe sickle cell pain crisis. *Am J Dis Child.* 1986;140:1255-1259.
8. Stanger P, Heymann MA, Tarnoff H, et al. Complications of cardiac catheterization of neonates, infants, and children. A three-year study. *Circulation.* 1974;50:595-608.
9. Atwood GF, Evans MA, Harbison RD. Pharmacokinetics of meperidine in infants. *Pediatr Res.* 1976;10:328. Abstract.
10. Auden SM, Sobczyk WL, Solinger RE, et al. Oral ketamine/midazolam is superior to intramuscular meperidine, promethazine, and chlorpromazine for pediatric cardiac catheterization. *Anesth Analg.* 2000;90:299-305.
11. Martinez JL, Sutters KA, Waite S, et al. A comparison of oral diazepam versus midazolam, administered with intravenous meperidine, as premedication to sedation for pediatric endoscopy. *J Pediatr Gastroenterol Nutr.* 2002;35:51-58.
12. Szeto HH, Inturrisi CE, Houde R. Accumulation of normeperidine, an active metabolite of meperidine, in patients with renal failure or cancer. *Ann Intern Med.* 1977;86:738-741.
13. Thomas R. Meperidine HCl and heparin sodium precipitation. *Hosp Pharm.* 1974;9:356. Letter.
14. Levy JH, Rockoff MA. Anaphylaxis to meperidine. *Anesth Analg.* 1982;61:301-303.
15. American Academy of Pediatrics Committee on Drugs. "Inactive" ingredients in pharmaceutical products: update. *Pediatrics.* 1997;99:268-278.
16. Smolinske SC. Review of parenteral sulfite reactions. *J Toxicol Clin Toxicol.* 1992;30:597-606.
17. Lester MR. Sulfite sensitivity: significance in human health. *J Am Col Nutr.* 1995;14:229-232.
18. Trissel LA, ed. *Handbook on Injectable Drugs.* 13th ed. Bethesda, MD: American Society of Health-System Pharmacists; 2005.
19. Kaiko RF, Foley KM, Grabinski PY, et al. Central nervous system excitatory effects of meperidine in cancer patients. *Ann Neurol.* 1983;13:180-185.
20. Goetting MG, Thirman MJ. Neurotoxicity of meperidine. *Ann Emerg Med.* 1985;14:1007-1009.
21. Kyff JV, Rice TL. Meperidine-associated seizures in a child. *Clin Pharm.* 1990;9:337-338.
22. Saneto RP, Fitch JA, Cohen BH. Acute neurotoxicity of meperidine in an infant. *Pediatr Neurol.* 1996;14:339-341.
23. Nahata MC, Clotz MA, Krogg EA. Adverse effects of meperidine, promethazine, and chlorpromazine for sedation in pediatric patients. *Clin Pediatr.* 1985;24:558-560.
24. Nahata MC. Sedation in pediatric patients undergoing diagnostic procedures. *Drug Intell Clin Pharm.* 1988;22:711-715.
25. Snodgrass WR, Dodge WF. Lytic/DPT cocktail: time for rational and safer alternatives. *Pediatr Clin North Am.* 1989;36:1285-1291.
26. American Academy of Pediatrics. Committee on Drugs. Reappraisal of lytic cocktail/demerol, phenergan, and thorazine (DPT) for the sedation of children. *Pediatrics.* 1995;95:598-602.

References

Meropenem

1. van Enk JG, Touw DJ, Lafeber HN. Pharmacokinetics of meropenem in preterm neonates. *Ther Drug Monit.* 2001;23:198-201.
2. American Academy of Pediatrics. In: Pickering LK, ed. *2003 Red Book: Report of the Committee on Infectious Diseases.* 26th ed. Elk Grove Village, IL: American Academy of Pediatrics; 2003.
3. Nair PM. Meropenem in neonates. *Indian Pediatr.* 2005;42:963.
4. Vartzelis G, Theodoridou M, Daikos GL, et al. Brain abscesses complicating Staphylococcus aureus sepsis in a premature infant. *Infection.* 2005;33:36-38.
5. *Physicians' Desk Reference.* 60th ed. Montvale, NJ: Thomson PDR; 2006.
6. Nelson JD, Bradley JS, eds. *Pocketbook of Pediatric Antimicrobial Therapy.* 14th ed. Baltimore, MD: Lippincott Williams & Wilkins; 2000–2001.
7. American Academy of Pediatrics Committee on Infectious Diseases. Therapy for children with invasive pneumococcal infections. *Pediatrics.* 1997;99:289-299.
8. Blumer JL, Reed MS, Kearns GL, et al. Sequential, single-dose pharmacokinetic evaluation of meropenem in hospitalized infants and children. *Antimicrob Agents Chemother.* 1995;39:1721-1725.
9. Bradley JS. Meropenem: a new, extremely broad spectrum beta-lactam antibiotic for serious infections in pediatrics. *Pediatr Infect Dis J.* 1997;16:263-268.
10. Klugman KP, Dagan R. The Meropenem Meningitis Study Group. Randomized comparison of meropenem with cefotaxime for treatment of bacterial meningitis. *Antimicrob Agents Chemother.* 1995;39:1140-1146.
11. Tunkel AR, Hartman BJ, Kaplan SL, et al. Practice guidelines for the management of bacterial meningitis. *Clin Infect Dis.* 2004;39:1267-1284.
12. Trissel LA, ed. *Handbook on Injectable Drugs.* 13th ed. [CD-ROM version 1.5]. Bethesda, MD: American Society of Health-System Pharmacists; 2005.
13. Capitano B, Nicolau DP, Potoski BA, et al. Meropenem administered as a prolonged infusion to treat serious gram-negative central nervous system infections. *Pharmacotherapy.* 2004;24:803-807.
14. Thalhammer F, Traunmuller F, El Menyawi I, et al. Continuous infusion versus intermittent administration of meropenem in critically ill patients. *J Antimicrob Chemother.* 1999;43:523-527.
15. Romanelli G, Cravarezza P. Intramuscular meropenem in the treatment of bacterial infections of the urinary and lower respiratory tracts. *J Antimicrob Chemother.* 1995;36 (supplement A):109-119.
16. Norrby SR. Neurotoxicity of the carbapenem antibacterials. *Drug Safety.* 1996;15:87-90.
17. Norrby SR. Carbapenems in serious infections: a risk-benefit assessment. *Drug Safety.* 2000;22:191-194.
18. Calandra G, Lydick E, Carrigan J, et al. Factors predisposing to seizures in seriously ill infected patients receiving antibiotics: experience with imipenem/cilastatin. *Am J Med.* 1988;84:911-918.
19. American Society of Health-System Pharmacists. American Hospital Formulary System. Available at: http://ahfsfirst.firstdatabank.com/AHFSfirst/NSAHFSFirstSearchmain.asp. Accessed September 15, 2006.

Methotrexate

1. Evans WE, Crom WR, Abromowitch M, et al. Clinical pharmacodynamics of high-dose methotrexate in acute lymphocytic leukemia: identification of a relation between concentration and effect. *N Engl J Med.* 1986;314:471-477.
2. Evans WE, Hutson PR, Stewart CF, et al. Methotrexate cerebrospinal fluid and serum concentrations after intermediate dose methotrexate infusion. *Clin Pharmacol Ther.* 1983;33:301-307.
3. Christensen ML, Rivera, GK, Crom WR, et al. Effect of hydration on methotrexate plasma concentrations in children with acute leukemia. *J Clin Oncol.* 1988;6:797-801.
4. Reiter A, Schrappe M, Ludwig WD, et al. Intensive ALL-type therapy without local radiotherapy provides a 90% event-free survival for children with T-cell lymphoblastic lymphoma: a BFM group report. *Blood.* 2000;95:416-421.
5. Poplack DG, Reaman GH, Bleyer WA, et al. Central nervous system (CNS) preventive therapy with high dose methotrexate (HDMTX) in acute lymphoblastic leukemia (ALL); a preliminary report. *Proc Am Soc Clin Oncol.* 1984;3:204-206.
6. Balis FM, Savitch JL, Bleyer WA, et al. Remission induction meningeal leukemia with high dose intravenous methotrexate. *J Clin Oncol.* 1985;3:485-489.
7. Relling MV, Fairclough D, Ayers D, et al. Patient characteristics associated with high risk methotrexate concentrations and toxicity. *J Clin Oncol.* 1994;12:1667-1672.
8. Evans WE, Crom WR, Stewart CF, et al. Methotrexate systemic clearance influences the probability of relapse in children with standard-risk acute lymphocytic leukemia. *Lancet.* 1984;1:359-362.
9. Horning SJ, Hoppe RT, Hancock SL, et al. Vinblastine, bleomycin, and methotrexate: an effective adjuvant in favorable Hodgkin's disease. *J Clin Oncol.* 1988;6:1822-1831.
10. Djerassi I, Sun Kim J. Methotrexate and citrovorum factor rescue in the management of childhood lymphosarcoma and reticulum cell sarcoma (non-Hodgkin's lymphoma). *Cancer.* 1976;38:1043-1051.
11. Murphy SB, Bowman WP, Abromowitch M, et al. Results of treatment of advanced stage Burkitt's lymphoma and B cell (SIg+) acute lymphoblastic leukemia with high dose fractionated cyclophosphamide and coordinated high dose methotrexate and cytarabine. *J Clin Oncol.* 1986;4:1732-1739.
12. Patte C, Bernard A, Hartmann O, et al. High-dose methotrexate and continuous infusion ara-c in children's non-Hodgkin's lymphoma: phase II studies and their use in further protocols. *Pediatric Hematol Oncol.* 1986;3:11-18.
13. Ramirez I, Sullivan MP, Wang Y, et al. Effective therapy for Burkitt's lymphoma: high dose cyclophosphamide + high dose methotrexate with coordinated intrathecal therapy. *Cancer Chemother Pharmacol.* 1979;3:103-109.
14. Bleyer WA. Clinical pharmacology of intrathecal methotrexate. II: an improved dosage regimen derived from age-related pharmacokinetics. *Cancer Treat Rep.* 1977;61:1419-1425.
15. Trissel LA, ed. *Handbook on Injectable Drugs.* 13th ed. [CD-ROM version 1.5]. Bethesda, MD: American Society of Health-System Pharmacists; 2005.
16. Jaffe N, Robertson R, Ayala A, et al. Comparison of intra-arterial cis-diamminedichloroplatinum II with high dose methotrexate and citrovorum factor rescue in the treatment of primary osteosarcoma. *J Clin Oncol.* 1985;3:1101-1104.
17. Rosen G, Caparros B, Huvos AG, et al. Preoperative chemotherapy for osteogenic sarcoma: selection of postoperative adjuvant chemotherapy based on the response of the primary tumor to preoperative chemotherapy. *Cancer.* 1979;43:1221-1230.
18. Pratt CB, Howarth C, Ransom JL, et al. High dose methotrexate used alone and in combination for measurable primary or metastatic osteosarcoma. *Cancer Treat Rep.* 1980;64:11-20.
19. Jaffe N, Traggis D. Toxicity of high dose methotrexate (NSC-740) and citrovorum factor (NSC-3590) in osteogenic sarcoma. *Cancer Chemother Rep.* 1975;6:31-36.
20. Wallace CA, Sherry DD. Preliminary report of higher dose methotrexate treatment in juvenile rheumatoid arthritis. *J Rheumatol.* 1992;19:1604-1607.
21. Reiff A, Shaham B, Wood BP, et al. High dose methotrexate in the treatment of refractory juvenile rheumatoid arthritis. *Clin and Exper Rheum.* 1995;13:113-118.
22. Gabriel S, Creagan E, O'Fallon WM, et al. Treatment of rheumatoid arthritis with higher dose intravenous methotrexate. *J Rheumatol.* 1990;17:460-465.

23. Aronoff GR, Berns JS, Brier ME, et al. *Drug Prescribing in Renal Failure: Dosing Guidelines for Adults.* 4th ed. Philadelphia, PA: American College of Physicians; 1999.
24. Shapiro WR, Young DF, Mehta BM, et al. Methotrexate: distribution in cerebrospinal fluid after intravenous, ventricular and lumbar injections. *N Engl J Med.* 1975;293:161-166.
25. Gregory RE, Pui CH, Crom WR. Raised plasma methotrexate concentrations following intrathecal administration in children with renal dysfunction. *Leukemia.* 1991;5:999-1003.
26. Hande KR, Balow JE, Drake JC, et al. Methotrexate and hemodialysis. *Ann Intern Med.* 1977;87:495-496.
27. Relling MV, Stapelton FB, Ochs J, et al. Removal of methotrexate, leucovorin, and their metabolites by combined hemodialysis and hemoperfusion. *Cancer.* 1988;62:884-888.
28. Gadgil SD, Damle SR, Advani SH, et al. Effect of activated charcoal on the pharmacokinetics of high-dose methotrexate. *Cancer Treat Rep.* 1982;66:1169-1171.
29. Crom WR, Evans WE. Methotrexate. In: Evans WE, Schentag JJ, Jusko WJ, eds. *Applied Pharmacokinetics: Principles of Therapeutic Drug Monitoring.* 3rd ed. Vancouver, WA: Applied Therapeutics Inc; 1992:1-42.
30. American Society of Health-System Pharmacists. American Hospital Formulary System. Available at: http://ahfsfirst.firstdatabank.com/AHFSfirst/NSAHFSFirstSearchmain.asp. Accessed September 25, 2006.
31. Goldberg NH, Romolo JL, Austin EH, et al. Anaphylactoid type reactions in two patients receiving high-dose intravenous methotrexate. *Cancer.* 1978;41:52-55.
32. Methotrexate injection [prescribing information]. Bedford, OH: Bedford Laboratories; April 2005.
33. American Academy of Pediatrics Committee on Drugs. "Inactive" ingredients in pharmaceutical products: update. *Pediatrics.* 1997;99:268-278.
34. Hall CM, Milligan DWA, Berrington J. Probably adverse reaction to a pharmaceutical excipient. *Arch Dis Child Fetal Neonatal Ed.* 2004;89: F184.
35. Hiller JL, Benda GI, Rahatzad M, et al. Benzyl alcohol toxicity: impact on mortality and intraventricular hemorrhage among very low birth weight infants. *Pediatrics.* 1986;77:500-506.
36. Grant JA, Bilodeau PA, Guernsey BG, et al. Unsuspected benzyl alcohol hypersensitivity. *N Engl J Med.* 1982;306:108.
37. Wilson JP, Solimando DA, Edwards MS. Parenteral benzyl alcohol-induced hypersensitivity reaction. *Drug Intell Clin Pharm.* 1986;20:689-691.
38. Lascari AD, Strano AJ, Johnson WW, et al. Methotrexate-induced sudden fatal pulmonary reaction. *Cancer.* 1977;40:1393-1397.
39. Doyle LA, Berg C, Bottino G, et al. Erythema and desquamation after high-dose methotrexate. *Ann Intern Med.* 1983;98:611-612.
40. Von Hoff DD, Penta JS, Helman LJ, et al. Incidence of drug-related deaths secondary to high-dose methotrexate and citrovorum factor administration. *Cancer Treat Rep.* 1977;61:745-748.
41. Ackland SP, Schilsky RL. High-dose methotrexate: a critical reappraisal. *J Clin Oncol.* 1987;5:2017-2031.
42. Nirenberg A, Mosende C, Mehta BM, et al. High-dose methotrexate with citrovorum factor rescue: predictive values of serum methotrexate concentration and corrective measures to avert toxicity. *Cancer Treat Rep.* 1977;61:779-783.
43. Chan H, Evans WE, Pratt CB. Recovery from toxicity associated with high dose methotrexate prognostic factors. *Cancer Treat Rep.* 1977;61:797-804.
44. Stoller RG, Jacobs SA, Drake JC, et al. Pharmacokinetics of high-dose methotrexate (NSC-740). *Cancer Chemother Rep.* 1975;6:19-24.
45. Romolo JL, Goldberg NH, Hande KR, et al. The effect of hydration on plasma methotrexate levels. *Cancer Treat Rep.* 1977;61:1393-1396.
46. Evans WE, Pratt CB, Taylor RH, et al. Pharmacokinetic monitoring of high-dose methotrexate: early recognition of high risk patients. *Cancer Chemother Pharmacol.* 1979;3:161-166.
47. Stoller RC, Hande KR, Jacobs SA, et al. Use of plasma pharmacokinetics to predict and prevent methotrexate toxicity. *N Engl J Med.* 1977;297:630-634.
48. Van Den Berg HW, Murphy RF, Kennedy DG, et al. Rapid plasma clearance and reduced rate and extent of urinary elimination of parenterally administered methotrexate as a result of severe vomiting and diarrhea. *Cancer Chemother Pharmacol.* 1980;4:47-48.
49. Sand TE, Jacobsen S. Effect of urine pH and flow on renal clearance of methotrexate. *Eur J Clin Pharmacol.* 1981;19:453-456.
50. Evans WE, Pratt CB. Effect of pleural effusions on high-dose methotrexate kinetics. *Clin Pharmacol Ther.* 1978;23:68-72.
51. Chabner BA, Stoller RG, Hande K, et al. Methotrexate disposition in humans: case studies in ovarian cancer and following high dose infusion. *Drug Metab Rev.* 1978;8:107-117.
52. Evans WE, Tsiatis A, Crom WR, et al. Pharmacokinetics of sustained serum methotrexate concentrations secondary to gastrointestinal obstruction. *J Pharm Sci.* 1981;70:1194-1198.
53. Crom WR, Pratt CB, Green AA, et al. The effect of prior cisplatin therapy on the pharmacokinetics of high-dose methotrexate. *J Clin Oncol.* 1984;2:655-661.
54. Garré ML, Relling MV, Kalwinsky D, et al. Pharmacokinetics and toxicity of methotrexate in children with Down's syndrome and acute lymphocytic leukemia. *J Pediatr.* 1987;111:606-612.
55. Leigler DG, Henderson ES, Hahn MA, et al. The effect of organic acids on renal clearance of methotrexate in man. *Clin Pharmacol Ther.* 1970;10:849-857.
56. Reid T, Yuen A, Catilico M, et al. Impact of omeprazole on the plasma clearance of methotrexate. *Cancer Chemother Pharmacol.* 1993;33:82-84.
57. Furst DE. Practical clinical pharmacology and drug interactions of low-dose methotrexate therapy in rheumatoid arthritis. *Br J Rheum.* 1995;34:20-25.
58. DuPuis LL, Koren G, Shore A, et al. Methotrexate-nonsteroidal antiinflammatory drug interaction in children with arthritis. *J Rheumatol.* 1990;17:1469-1473.
59. Wallace CA, Smith AL, Sherry DD. Pilot investigation of naproxen/methotrexate interaction in patients with juvenile rheumatoid arthritis. *J Rheumatol.* 1993;20:1764-1768.
60. Ferrazzini G, Klein J, Sulh H, et al. Interaction between trimethoprim-sulfamethoxazole and methotrexate in children with leukemia. *J Pediatr.* 1990;117:823-826.
61. Aherne GW, Piall E, Marks V, et al. Prolongation and enhancement of serum methotrexate concentrations by probenecid. *Br Med J.* 1978;1:1097.
62. Ronchera CL, Hernandez T, Peris E, et al. Pharmacokinetic interaction between high-dose methotrexate and amoxicillin. *Ther Drug Monit.* 1993;15:375-379.
63. National Comprehensive Cancer Network (NCCN) Antiemesis Panel Members. NCCN Clinical Practice Guidelines in Oncology. Antiemesis, v.1.2006. Available at www.nccn.org. Accessed March, 29, 2006.
64. Roila F, Feyer P, Maranzamo E, et al. Antiemetics in children receiving chemotherapy. *Supportive Care Cancer.* 2005;13:129-131.

Methyldopate HCl

1. Loggie JM. Hypertension in children and adolescents. II. Drug therapy. *J Pediatr.* 1969;74:640-654.
2. American Society of Health-System Pharmacists. American Hospital Formulary System. Available at: http://ahfsfirst.firstdatabank.com/AHFSfirst/NSAHFSFirstSearchmain.asp. Accessed August 5, 2006.
3. Adelman RD. Neonatal hypertension. *Pediatr Clin North Am.* 1978;25:99-110.
4. *Physicians' Desk Reference.* 60th ed. Montvale, NJ: Thomson PDR; 2006.
5. Fivush B, Neu A, Furth S. Acute hypertensive crises in children: emergencies and urgencies. *Curr Opin Pediatr.* 1997;9;233-236.
6. Adelman RD, Coppo R, Dillon MJ. The emergency management of severe hypertension. *Pediatr Nephrol.* 2000;14:422-427.

References

7. Aronoff A, Brier M, Bennett W. *The Renal Book, 2002.* Available at: http://www.kdp-baptist.louisville.edu/renalbook/. Accessed August 5, 2006.
8. Pagliaro LA, Pagliaro AM, eds. *Problems in Pediatric Drug Therapy.* 2nd ed. Hamilton, IL: Drug Intelligence Publications Inc; 1987.
9. Trissel LA, ed. *Handbook on Injectable Drugs.* 13th ed. [CD-ROM version 1.5]. Bethesda, MD: American Society of Health-System Pharmacists; 2005.
10. American Academy of Pediatrics Committee on Drugs. "Inactive" ingredients in pharmaceutical products: update. *Pediatrics.* 1997;99:268-278.
11. Lester MR. Sulfite sensitivity: significance in human health. *J Am Col Nutr.* 1995;14:229-232.
12. Smolinske SC. Review of parenteral sulfite reactions. *J Toxicol Clin Toxicol.* 1992;30:597-606.
13. Soni MG, Taylor SL, Greenberg NA, et al. Evaluation of the health aspects of methyl paraben: a review of the published literature. *Food Chem Toxicol.* 2002;40:1335-1373.
14. Nagel JE, Fuscaldo JT, Firemen P. Paraben allergy. *JAMA.* 1977;237:1594-1595.

Methylprednisolone Sodium Succinate

1. Miller JJ. Prolonged use of large intravenous steroid pulses in the rheumatic diseases of children. *Pediatrics.* 1980;65:989-994.
2. Ferraris JR, Gallo GE, Ramirez J, et al. Pulse methylprednisolone therapy in the treatment of acute crescentic glomerulonephritis. *Nephron.* 1983;34:207-208.
3. Bolton WK, Couser WG. Intravenous pulse methylprednisolone therapy of acute crescentic rapidly progressive glomerulonephritis. *Am J Med.* 1979;66:495-502.
4. Cole BR, Brocklebank JT, Kienstra RA, et al. Pulse methylprednisolone therapy in the treatment of severe glomerulonephritis. *J Pediatr.* 1976;88:307-314.
5. Kimberly RP, Lockshin MD, Sherman RL, et al. High dose intravenous methylprednisolone pulse therapy in systemic lupus erythematosus. *Am J Med.* 1981;70:817-824.
6. Tunc B, Oner AF, Hicsonmez G. The effect of short-course high-dose methylprednisolone on peripheral blood lymphocyte subsets in children with acute leukemia during remission induction treatment. *Leuk Res.* 2003;27:19-21.
7. Orta-Sibu N, Chantler C, Bewick M, et al. Comparison of high-dose intravenous methylprednisolone with low-dose oral prednisolone in acute renal allograft rejection in children. *Br Med J.* 1982;285:258-260.
8. Bocanegra TS, Castaneda MO, Espinoza LR, et al. Sudden death after methylprednisolone pulse therapy. *Ann Intern Med.* 1981;95:122.
9. Moses RE, McCormick A, Nickey W. Fatal arrhythmia after pulse methylprednisolone therapy. *Ann Intern Med.* 1981;95:781-782.
10. National Asthma Education and Prevention Program. Expert Panel Report: Guidelines for the Diagnosis and Management of Asthma. Update on Selected Topics 2002.
11. Ancona KG, Parker RI, Atlas MP, et al. Randomized trial of high-dose methylprednisolone versus intravenous immunoglobulin for the treatment of acute idiopathic thrombocytopenic purpura in children. *J Pediatr Hematol Oncol.* 2002;24:540-544.
12. Plebani A, Clerici Schoeller M, Pietrogrande MC, et al. Steroids in Pneumocystis carinii pneumonia in HIV seropositive infants. *Eur J Pediatr.* 1989;148:579-584.
13. Kline MW, Shearer WT. A national survey on the care of infants and children with human immunodeficiency virus infection. *J Pediatr.* 1991;118:817-821.
14. Sleasman JW, Hemenway C, Klein AS, et al. Corticosteroids improve survival of children with AIDS and Pneumocystis carinii pneumonia. *Am J Dis Child.* 1993;147:30-34.
15. National Institutes of Health—University of California. Expert Panel for corticosteroids as adjunctive therapy for pneumocystis pneumonia. Consensus statement on the use of corticosteroids as adjunctive therapy for pneumocystis pneumonia in the acquired immunodeficiency syndrome. *N Engl J Med.* 1990;323:1500-1504.
16. McEvoy GK, ed. *AHFS Drug Information Essentials 2005–06.* Bethesda, MD: American Society of Health-System Pharmacists; 2005.
17. Bracken MB, Shepard MJ, Collins WF, et al. A randomized, controlled trial of methylprednisolone or naloxone in the treatment of acute spinal-cord injury. *N Engl J Med.* 1990;322:1405-1411.
18. Bracken MB, Shepard MJ, Holford TR, et al. Administration of methylprednisolone for 24 or 48 hours or tirilazad mesylate for 48 hours in the treatment of acute spinal cord injury. Results of the Third National Acute Spinal Cord Injury Randomized Controlled Trial. National Acute Spinal Cord Injury Study. *JAMA.* 1997;28:1597-1604.
19. Jaffe K, Weddon D. Emergency management of blunt trauma in children. *N Engl J Med.* 1991;324:1477.
20. Fackler JC, Yaster M. Multiple trauma in the pediatric patient. In: Rogers MC, ed. *Textbook of Pediatric Intensive Care.* 2nd ed. Baltimore, MD: Lippincott Williams & Wilkins; 1992:1468.
21. Ino T, Okubo M, Akimoto K, et al. Corticosteroid therapy for ventricular tachycardia in children with silent lymphocytic myocarditis. *J Pediatr.* 1995;126:304-308.
22. Desmarquest P, Tamalet A, Fauroux B, et al. Chronic interstitial lung disease in children: response to high-dose intravenous methylprednisone pulses. *Pediatr Pulmonol.* 1998;26:332-338.
23. Delesalle F, Staumont D, Houmany MA, et al. Pulse methylprednisolone therapy for threatening periocular haemangiomas of infancy. *Acta Derm Venereol.* 2006;86:429-432.
24. Arnoff GR, Berns JS, Brier ME, et al. *Drug Prescribing in Renal Failure: Dosing Guidelines for Adults.* 4th ed. Philadelphia, PA: American College of Physicians; 1999.
25. Medical Economics, ed. *Physicians' Desk Reference.* 54th ed. Oradell, NJ: Medical Economics Company; 2000.
26. Trissel LA, ed. *Handbook on Injectable Drugs.* 13th ed. Bethesda, MD: American Society of Health-System Pharmacists; 2005.
27. Baethge BA, Lidsky MD. Intractable hiccups associated with high dose intravenous methylprednisolone therapy. *Ann Intern Med.* 1986;104:58-59.
28. Garrett R, Paulus H. Complications of intravenous methylprednisolone pulse therapy. *Arthritis Rheum.* 1980;23:677.
29. Freedman MD, Schoket AL, Chapel N, et al. Anaphylaxis after methylprednisolone therapy. *JAMA.* 1981;245:607-608.
30. Schonwald S. Methylprednisolone anaphylaxis. *Am J Emerg Med.* 1999;17:583-585.
31. Thompson JF, Chalmers DHK, Wood RFM, et al. Sudden death following high-dose intravenous methylprednisolone. *Transplantation.* 1983;36:594-596.
32. McDougal BA, Whittier FC, Cross DE. Sudden death after bolus steroid therapy for acute rejection. *Transplant Proc.* 1976;8:493-496.
33. American Academy of Pediatrics Committee on Drugs. "Inactive" ingredients in pharmaceutical products: update. *Pediatrics.* 1997;99:268-278.
34. Hall CM, Milligan DWA, Berrington J. Probable adverse reaction to a pharmaceutical excipient. *Arch Dis Child Fetal Neonatal Ed.* 2004;89: F184.
35. Hiller JL, Benda GI, Rahatzad M, et al. Benzyl alcohol toxicity: impact on mortality and intraventricular hemorrhage among very low birth weight infants. *Pediatrics.* 1986;77:500-506.
36. Grant JA, Bilodeau PA, Guernsey BG, et al. Unsuspected benzyl alcohol hypersensitivity. *N Engl J Med.* 1982;306:108.
37. Wilson JP, Solimando DA, Edwards MS. Parenteral benzyl alcohol-induced hypersensitivity reaction. *Drug Intell Clin Pharm.* 1986;20:689-691.
38. Raymond G, Day P, Rabb M. Sodium content of commonly administered intravenous drugs. *Hosp Pharm.* 1982;17:560-561.
39. Chamberlin P, Meyer WJ. Management of pituitary-adrenal suppression secondary to corticosteroid therapy. *Pediatrics.* 1981;67:245-251.
40. Klein-Gitelman MS, Pachman LM. Intravenous corticosteroids: adverse reactions are more variable than expected in children. *J Rheumatol.* 1998;25:1995-2002.
41. Sun Jo D, Yang JW, Han Hwang P, et al. Stevens-Johnson syndrome in a boy with nephrotic syndrome during prednisolone therapy. *Pediatr Nephrol.* 2003;18:959-961.

References

42. Sheth A, Reddymasu S, Jackson R. Worsening of asthma with systemic corticosteroids: a case report and review of literature. *J Gen Intern Med.* 2006;21:C11-C13.
43. Bone RC, Fisher CJ, Clemmer TP, et al. A controlled clinical trial of high dose methylprednisolone in the treatment of severe sepsis and septic shock. *N Engl J Med.* 1987;317:653-658.
44. The Veterans Administration Systemic Sepsis Cooperative Study Group. Effect of high-dose glucocorticoid therapy on mortality in patients with clinical signs of systemic sepsis. *N Engl J Med.* 1987;317:659-665.
45. Ueda N, Yoshikawa T, Chihara M, et al. Atrial fibrillation following methylprednisone pulse therapy. *Pediatr Nephrol.* 1988;2:29-31.
46. Bettinelli A, Paterlini G, Mazzucchi E, et al. Seizures and transient blindness following intravenous pulse methylprednisone in children with primary glomerulonephritis. *Child Nephrol Urol.* 1991;11:41-43.
47. Kasper WJ, Howe PM. Fatal varicella after a single course of corticosteroids. *Pediatr Infect Dis J.* 1990;9:729-732.
48. Siomou E, Challa A, Tzoufi M, et al. Biochemical markers of bone metabolism in infants and children under intravenous corticosteroid therapy. *Calcif Tissue Int.* 2003;73:319-325.
49. Sundel RP, Baker AL, Fulton DR, et al. Corticosteroids in the initial treatment of Kawasaki Disease: report of a randomized trial. *J Pediatr.* 2003;142:611-616.
50. Lang BA, Yeung RSM, Oen KG, et al. Corticosteroid treatment of refractory Kawasaki Disease. *J Rheumatol.* 2006;33:803-809.

Metoclopramide HCl

1. Metoclopramide Injection [package insert]. Irvine, CA: Sicor Pharmaceuticals Inc; May 2005.
2. Marshall G, Kerr S, Vowels M, et al. Antiemetic therapy for chemotherapy-induced vomiting: metoclopramide, benztropine, dexamethasone, and lorazepam regimens compared with chlorpromazine alone. *J Pediatr.* 1989;115:156-160.
3. Gralla RJ, Tyson LB, Kris MG, et al. The management of chemotherapy induced nausea and vomiting. *Med Clin North Am.* 1987;71:289-301.
4. Taketomo CK, Hodding JH, Kraus DM, eds. *Pediatric Dosage Handbook.* 12th ed. [CD-ROM version 2006.1] Hudson, OH: Lexi-Comp; 2006.
5. Kohli-Kumar M, Pearson ADJ, Sharkey I, et al. Urinary retention—an unusual dystonic reaction to continuous metoclopramide infusion. *DICP Ann Pharmacother.* 1991;25:469-470.
6. De Mulder PHM, Seynaeve C, Vermorken JB, et al. Ondansetron compared with high-dose metoclopramide in prophylaxis of acute and delayed cisplatin-induced nausea and vomiting. *Ann Intern Med.* 1990;113:834-840.
7. Brechot JM, Dupeyron JP, Delattre C, et al. Continuous infusion of high-dose metoclopramide: comparison of pharmacokinetically adjusted and standard doses for the control of cisplatin-induced acute emesis. *Eur J Clin Pharmacol.* 1991;40:283-286.
8. Kearns GL, Fiser Dh. Metoclopramide-induced methemoglobinemia. *Pediatrics.* 1988;82:364-366.
9. Benitz WE, Tatro DS. *The Pediatric Drug Handbook.* Chicago, IL: Year Book; 1988:14.
10. Furst SR, Rodarte A. Prophylactic antiemetic treatment with ondansetron in children undergoing tonsillectomy. *Anesthesiol.* 1994;81:799-803.
11. Lin DM, Furst ST, Rodarte A. A double-blinded comparison of metoclopramide and droperidol for prevention of emesis following strabismus surgery. *Anesthesiol.* 1992;76:357-361.
12. Ferrari LR, Donlon JV. Metoclopramide reduces the incidence of vomiting after tonsillectomy in children. *Anesth Analg.* 1992;75:351-354.
13. Shende D, Mandal NG. Efficacy of ondansetron and metoclopramide for preventing postoperative emesis following strabismus surgery in children. *Anaesthesia.* 1997;52:496-500.
14. Kathirvel S, Shende D, Madan R. Comparison of anti-emetic effects of ondansetron, metoclopromidine or a combination of both in children undergoing surgery for strabismus. *Eur J Anaesthesiol.* 1999;16:761-765.
15. Stene FN, Seay RE, Young LA, et al. Prospective, randomized, double-blind, placebo-controlled comparison of metoclopramide and ondansetron for prevention of posttonsillectomy or adenotonsillectomy emesis. *J Clin Anesth.* 1996;8:540-544.
16. Aronoff A, Brier M, Bennett W. *The Renal Book, 2002.* Available at: http://www.kdp-baptist.louisville.edu/renalbook/. Accessed July 20, 2006.
17. Roila F, Basurto C, Bracarda S, et al. Double-blind crossover trial of single vs divided dose of metoclopramide in a combined regimen for treatment of cisplatin-induced emesis. *Eur J Cancer.* 1991;27:119-121.
18. Gralla RJ, Itri LM, Pisko SE, et al. Antiemetic efficacy of high-dose metoclopramide: randomized trials with placebo and prochlorperazine in patients with chemotherapy-induced nausea and vomiting. *N Engl J Med.* 1981;305:905-909.
19. Robertson J, Shilkofski N, eds. *The Harriet Lane Handbook.* 17th ed. Philadelphia, PA: Elsevier Mosby; 2005.
20. Trissel LA, ed. *Handbook on Injectable Drugs.* 13th ed. [CD-ROM version 1.5]. Bethesda, MD: American Society of Health-System Pharmacists; 2005.
21. Allen JC, Gralla RJ, Reilly C, et al. Metoclopramide: dose-related toxicity and preliminary antiemetic studies in children receiving cancer chemotherapy. *J Clin Oncol.* 1985;3:1135-1141.
22. Terrin BN, McWilliams NB, Maurer HM. Side effects of metoclopramide as an antiemetic in childhood cancer chemotherapy. *J Pediatr.* 198;104:138-140.
23. Howrie DL, Felix C, Wollman M, et al. Metoclopramide as an antiemetic agent in pediatric oncology patients. *Drug Intell Clin Pharm.* 1986;20:122-124.
24. Madani S, Tolia V. Gynecomastia with metoclopramide use in pediatric patients. *J Clin Gastroenterol.* 1997;24:79-81.
25. Chellis MJ, Sanders SV, Dean JM, et al. Bedside transpyloric tube placement in the pediatric intensive care unit. *J Parenter Enteral Nutr.* 1996;20:88-90.
26. Ozucelik DN, Karaca MA, Sivri B. Effectiveness of pre-emptive metoclopramide infusion in alleviating pain, discomfort and nausea associated with nasogastric tube insertion: a randomized, double-blind placebo-controlled trial. *Int J Clin Pract.* 2005;59:1422-1427.

Metronidazole/Metronidazole HCl

1. Jager-Roman E, Doyle PE, Baird-Lambert J, et al. Pharmacokinetics and tissue distribution of metronidazole in the new born infant. *J Pediatr.* 1982;100:651-654.
2. Prober CG, Stevenson DK, Benitz WE. The use of antibiotics in neonates weighing less than 1200 grams. *Pediatr Infect Dis J.* 1990;9:111-121.
3. Nelson JS, Bradley JS. *Nelson's Pocketbook of Pediatric Antimicrobial Therapy.* 14th ed. Philadelphia, PA: Lippincott Williams & Wilkins; 2000.
4. American Academy of Pediatrics. In: Pickering LK, ed. *2003 Red Book: Report of the Committee on Infectious Diseases.* 26th ed. Elk Grove Village, IL: American Academy of Pediatrics; 2003.
5. Hall P, Kaye CM, McIntosh N, et al. Intravenous metronidazole in the newborn. *Arch Dis Child.* 1983;58:529-531.
6. Upadhyaya P, Bhatnagar V, Basu N. Pharmacokinetics of intravenous metronidazole in neonates. *J Pediatr Surg.* 1988;23:263-265.
7. Brook I. Treatment of anaerobic infections in children with metronidazole. *Dev Pharmacol Ther.* 1983;6:187-198.
8. Oldenburg B, Speck WT. Metronidazole. *Pediatr Clin North Am.* 1983;30:71-75.
9. Grundfest-Broniatowski S, Quader M, Alexander F, et al. Clostridium difficile colitis in the critically ill. *Dis Colon Rectum.* 1996;39:619-623.
10. Bouza E, Munoz P, Alonso R. Clinical manifestations, treatment and control of infections caused by Clostridium difficile. *Clin Microbiol Infect.* 2005;11 suppl 4:57-64.
11. Emil S, Laberge JM, Mikhail P, et al. Appendicitis in children: a ten-year update of therapeutic recommendations. *J Pediatr Surg.* 2003;38:236-242.
12. American Society of Health-System Pharmacists. American Hospital Formulary System. Available at: http://ahfsfirst.firstdatabank.com/AHFSfirst/NSAHFSFirstSearchmain.asp. Accessed September 20, 2006.
13. Arnoff GR, Berns JS, Brier ME, et al. *Drug Prescribing in Renal Failure: Dosing Guidelines for Adults.* 4th ed. Philadelphia, PA: American College of Physicians; 1999.

References

14. Trissel LA, ed. *Handbook on Injectable Drugs.* 13th ed. [CD-ROM version 1.5]. Bethesda, MD: American Society of Health-System Pharmacists; 2005.

Micafungin

1. American Academy of Pediatrics. In: Pickering LK, ed. *Red Book: 2006 Report of the Committee on Infectious Diseases.* 27th ed. Elk Grove Village, IL: American Academy of Pediatrics; 2006.
2. Seibel NL, Schwartz C, Arrieta A, et al. Safety, tolerability, and pharmacokinetics of micafungin (FK463) in febrile neutropenic pediatric patients. *Antimicrob Agent Chemother.* 2005;49:3317-3324.
3. Tabata K, Katashima M, Kawamura A, et al. Linear pharmacokinetics of micafungin and its active metabolites in Japanese pediatric patients with fungal infections. *Biol Pharm Bull.* 2006;29:1706-1711.
4. Ostrosky-Zeichner L, Kontoyiannis D, Raffalli J, et al. International, open-label, noncomparative, clinical trial of micafungin alone and in combination for treatment of newly diagnosed and refractory candidemia. *Eur J Clin Microbiol Infect Dis.* 2005;24:654-661.
5. Pannaraj PS, Walsh TJ, Baker CJ. Advances in antifungal therapy. *Pediatr Infect Dis J.* 2005;24:921-922.
6. Steinbach WJ, Benjamin DK. New antifungal agents under development in children and neonates. *Curr Opin Infect Dis.* 2005;18:484-489.
7. van Burik JA, Ratanatharathorn V, Stepan DE., et al. Micafungin versus fluconazole for prophylaxis against invasive fungal infections during neutropenia in patients undergoing hematopoietic stem cell transplantation. *Clin Infect Dis.* 2004;39:1407-1416.
8. Kishino S, Ohno K, Shimanura T, et al. Optimal prophylactic dosage and disposition of micafungin in living donor liver recipients. *Clin Transplant.* 2004;18:676-680.
9. *Physicians' Desk Reference.* 60th ed. Montvale, NJ: Thomson PDR; 2006.
10. Carver PL. Micafungin. *Ann Pharmacother.* 2004;38:1707-1721.
11. Herbert MF, Smith HE, Marbury TC, et al. Pharmacokinetics of micafungin in healthy volunteers, volunteers with moderate liver disease, and volunteers with renal dysfunction. *J Clin Pharm.* 2005;45:1145.
12. Heresi GP, Gerstmann DR, Blumer JL, et al. Pharmacokinetic study of micafungin in premature neonates [abstract]. In: Pediatric Academic Societies' Annual Meeting; May 3–6, 2003; Seattle, WA: The Woodlands, Pediatric Academic Societies. Abstract 83.

Midazolam HCl

1. Versed® (midazolam hydrochloride) [prescribing information]. Nutley, NJ: Roche Laboratories; June 2000.
2. American Society of Health-System Pharmacists. American Hospital Formulary System. Available at: http://ahfsfirst.firstdatabank.com/AHFSfirst/NSAHFSFirstSearchmain.asp. Accessed May 20, 2006.
3. Cole WHJ. Midazolam in paediatric anaesthesia. *Anaesth Intensive Care.*1982;10:36-39.
4. Holloway AM, Jordaan DG, Brock-Utne JG. Midazolam for the intravenous induction of anaesthesia in children. *Anaesth Intensive Care.* 1982;10:340-343.
5. Salonen M, Kanto J, Iisalo E, et al. Midazolam as an induction agent in children: a pharmacokinetic and clinical study. *Anesth Analg.* 1987;66:625-628.
6. Shankar V, Deshpande JK. Procedural sedation in the pediatric patient. *Anesthesiol Clin N Am.* 2005;23:635-654.
7. Flood RG, Krauss B. Procedural sedation and analgesia for children in the emergency department. *Emerg Med Clin North Am.* 2003;21:121-139.
8. Krauss B, Green S. Procedural sedation and analgesia in children. *Lancet.* 2006;367:766-780.
9. Sandler ES, Weyman C, Conner K, et al. Midazolam versus fentanyl as premedication for painful procedures in children with cancer. *Pediatrics.* 1992;89:631-634.
10. Tobias JD. Sedation and analgesia in paediatric intensive care units. *Pediatr Drugs.* 1999;109-125.
11. Sievers TD, Yee JD, Foley ME, et al. Midazolam for conscious sedation during pediatric oncology procedures: safety and recovery parameters. *Pediatrics.* 1992; 88:1172-1179.
12. Manzi SF, Shannon WM. Drug therapy in the pediatric emergency department. In: Yaffe SJ, Aranda JV, eds. *Neonatal and Pediatric Pharmacology.* 3rd ed. Philadelphia, PA: Lippincott Williams & Wilkins; 2005:288-289.
13. Slovis TL, Parks C, Reneau D, et al. Pediatric sedation: short-term effects. *Pediatric Radiology.* 1993;23:345-348.
14. Hartwig S, Roth B, Theisohn M. Clinical experience with continuous intravenous sedation using midazolam and fentanyl in the paediatric intensive care unit. *Eur J Pediatr.* 1991;150:784-788.
15. Jacqz-Aigrain E, Daoud P, Burtin P, et al. Pharmacokinetics of midazolam during continuous infusion in critically ill neonates. *Eur J Clin Pharmacol.* 1992;42:329-332.
16. Silvasi DL, Rosen DA, Rosen KR. Continuous intravenous midazolam infusion for sedation in the pediatric intensive care unit. *Anesth Analg.* 1988;67:286-288.
17. Lloyd-Thomas AR, Booker PD. Infusion of midazolam in paediatric patients after cardiac surgery. *Br J Anaesth.*1986;58:1109-1115.
18. Jacqz-Aigrain E, Daoud P, Burtin P, et al. Placebo-controlled trial of midazolam sedation in mechanically ventilated newborn babies. *Lancet.* 1994;344:646-650.
19. Booker PD, Beechey A, Lloyd-Thomas AR. Sedation of children requiring artificial ventilation using an infusion of midazolam. *Br J Anaesth.* 1986;58:1104-1108.
20. Rivera R, Segnini M, Baltodano A, et al. Midazolam in the treatment of status epilepticus in children. *Crit Care Med.* 1993;21:991-994.
21. Kumar A, Bleck TP. Intravenous midazolam for the treatment of refractory status epilepticus. *Crit Care Med.* 1992;20:483-388.
22. Parent JM, Lowenstein DH. Treatment of refractory generalized status epilepticus with continuous infusion of midazolam. *Neurology.* 1994;44:1837-1840.
23. Igartua J, Silver P, Maytal J, et al. Midazolam coma for refractory status epilepticus in children. *Crit Care Med.* 1999;27:1982-1985.
24. Ozdemir D, Gulez P, Uran N, et al. Efficacy of continuous midazolam infusion and mortality in childhood refractory generalized convulsive status epilepticus. *Seizure.* 2005;14:129-132,
25. Holmes GL, Riviello JJ. Midazolam and pentobarbital for refractory status epilepticus. *Pediatr Neurol.* 1999;20:259-264.
26. Marik PE, Varon J. The management of status epilepticus. *Chest.* 2004;126:582-591.
27. Conde Castro JR, Borges AA, Martinez ED, et al. Midazolam in neonatal seizures with no response to phenobarbital. *Neurology.* 2005;64:876-879.
28. Aronoff A, Brier M, Bennett W. *The Renal Book, 2002.* Available at: http://www.kdp-baptist.louisville.edu/renalbook/. Accessed May 20, 2006.
29. Young TE, Mangum B, eds. *Neofax®.* 18th ed. Raleigh, NC: Acorn Publishing Inc; 2005.
30. Chamberlain JM, Altieri MA, Futterman C, et al. A prospective randomized study comparing intramuscular midazolam with intravenous diazepam for the treatment of seizures in children. *Pediatr Emerg Care.* 1997;13:92-94.
31. Vilke GM, Sharieff GQ, Marino A, et al. Midazolam for the treatment of out-of-hospital pediatric seizures. *Prehosp Emerg Care.* 2002;6:215-217.
32. Yaster M, Nichols DG, Deshpande JK, et al. Midazolam–fentanyl intravenous sedation in children: case report of respiratory arrest. *Pediatrics.* 1990;86:463-467.
33. Bergman I, Steeves M, Burckart G, et al. Reversible neurologic abnormalities associated with prolonged intravenous midazolam and fentanyl administration. *J Pediatr.* 1991;119:644-649.
34. Trissel LA, ed. *Handbook on Injectable Drugs.* 13th ed. [CD-ROM version 1.5]. Bethesda, MD: American Society of Health-System

Pharmacists; 2005.
35. American Academy of Pediatrics Committee on Drugs. "Inactive" ingredients in pharmaceutical products: update. *Pediatrics.* 1997;99:268-278.
36. Hall CM, Milligan DWA, Berrington J. Probably adverse reaction to a pharmaceutical excipient. *Arch Dis Child Fetal Neonatal Ed.* 2004;89: F184.
37. Walker JE, Homan RW, Vasko MR, et al. Lorazepam in status epilepticus. *Ann Neurol.* 1979;6:207-213.
38. Grant JA, Bilodeau PA, Guernsey BG, et al. Unsuspected benzylalcohol hypersensitivity. *N Engl J Med.* 1982;306:108.
39. Wilson JP, Solimando DA, Edwards MS. Parenteral benzyl alcohol-induced hypersensitivity reaction. *Drug Intell Clin Pharm.* 1986;20:689-691.
40. Ng E, Klinger G, Shah V, Taddio A. Safety of benzodiazepines in newborns. *Ann Pharmacother.* 2002;36:1150-1155.
41. van den Anker JN, Sauer PJJ. The use of midazolam in the premature neonate. *Eur J Pediatr.* 1992;151:152.
42. Magny JF, Zupan V, Dehan M, et al. Midazolam and myoclonus in neonate. *Eur J Pediatr.* 1992;153:389-390.
43. Bergman I, Steeves M, Burckart G, et al. Reversible neurologic abnormalities associated with prolonged intravenous midazolam and fentanyl administration. *J Pediatr.* 1991;119:644-649.
44. Sury MR, Billingham I, Russell GN, et al. Acute benzodiazepine withdrawal syndrome after midazolam infusions in children. *Crit Care Med.* 1989;17:301-302.
45. Conway EE Jr, Singer LP. Acute benzodiazepine withdrawal after midazolam in children. *Crit Care Med.* 1990;18:461. Letter.
46. Fonsmark L, Rasmussen YH, Carl P. Occurrence of withdrawal in critically ill children. *Crit Care Med.* 1999;27:196-199.
47. Lieh-Lai M, Sarnaik AP. Therapeutic applications in pediatric intensive care. In: Yaffe SJ, Aranda JV, eds. *Neonatal and Pediatric Pharmacology.* 3rd ed. Philadelphia, PA: Lippincott Williams & Wilkins; 2005:261-277.
48. Sugarman JM, Paul RI. Flumazenil: a review. *Pediatr Emerg Care.* 1994;10:37-43.

Milrinone Lactate

1. Chang AC, Atz AM, Wernovsky G, et al. Milrinone: systemic and pulmonary hemodynamic effects in neonates after cardiac surgery. *Crit Care Med.* 1995;23:1907-1914.
2. Barton P, Garcia J, Kouatli A, et al. Hemodynamic effects of IV milrinone lactate in pediatric patients with septic shock. *Chest.* 1996;109:302-312.
3. Lindsay CA, Barton P, Lawless S, et al. Pharmacokinetics and pharmacodynamics of milrinone lactate in pediatric patients with shock. *J Pediatr.* 1998;132:329-334.
4. Zuppa AF, Nicolson SC, Adamson PC, et al. Population pharmacokinetics of milrinone in neonates with hypoplastic left heart syndrome undergoing stage I reconstruction. *Anesth Analg.* 2006;102:1062-1069.
5. De Oliveira NC, Ashburn DA, Khalid F, et al. Prevention of early sudden circulatory collapse after the Norwood operation. *Circulation.* 2004;110(11 suppl 1):II133-138.
6. Paradisis M, Evans N, Kluckow M, et al. Pilot study of milrinone for low systemic blood flow in very preterm infants. *J Pediatr.* 2006;148:306-313.
7. Bailey JM, Miller BE, Lu W, et al. The pharmacokinetics of milrinone in pediatric patients after cardiac surgery. *Anesthesiology.* 1999;90:1012–1018.
8. Ramamoorthy C, Anderson GD, Williams GD, et al. Pharmacokinetics and side effects of milrinone in infants and children after open heart surgery. *Anesth Analg.* 1998;86:283-289.
9. Watson S, Christian K, Churchwell KB. Use of milrinone in the pediatric critical care unit. *Pediatrics.* 1999;104:S681-S682.
10. Rich N, West N, McMaster P, et al. Milrinone in meningococcal sepsis. *Pediatr Crit Care Med.* 2003;4:394-395.
11. Young RA, Ward A. Milrinone: a preliminary review of its pharmacological properties and therapeutic use. *Drugs.* 1988;36:158-192.
12. Aronoff A, Brier M, Bennett W. *The Renal Book, 2002.* Available at: http://www.kdbaptist.louisville.edu/renalbook/. Accessed June 26, 2006.
13. *Physicians' Desk Reference.* 54th ed. Montvale, NJ: Thomson PDR; 2006.
14. Trissel LA, ed. *Handbook on Injectable Drugs.* 13th ed. [CD-ROM version 1.5]. Bethesda, MD: American Society of Health-System Pharmacists; 2005.
15. Akkerman SR, Zhang H, Mullins RE, et al. Stability of milrinone lactate in the presence of 29 critical care drugs and 4 i.v. solutions. *Am J Health-Syst Pharm.* 1999;56:63-68.

Mivacurium

1. Rowlee SC. Monitoring neuromuscular blockade in the intensive care unit: the peripheral nerve stimulator. *Heart Lung.* 1999;28:352-362.
2. *Physicians' Desk Reference.* 60th ed. Montvale; NJ: Thomson PDR; 2006. 3. American Society of Health-System Pharmacists. American Hospital Formulary System. Available at: http://ahfsfirst.firstdatabank.com/AHFSfirst/NSAHFSFirstSearchmain.asp. Accessed August 19, 2006.
4. Martin LD, Bratton SL, O'Rourke PP. Clinical uses and controversies of neuromuscular blocking agents in infants and children. *Crit Care Med.* 1999;27:1358-1368.
5. McCluskey A, Meakin G. Dose-response and minimum time to satisfactory intubation conditions after mivacurium in children. *Anaesthesia.* 1996;51:438-441.
6. Markakis DA, Lau M, Brown R, et al. The pharmacokinetics and steady state pharmacodynamics of mivacurium in children. *Anesthesiology.* 1998;88:978-983.
7. OStergaard D, Gatke MR, Berg H, et al. The pharmacodynamics and pharmacokinetics of mivacurium in children. *Acta Anaesthiol Scand.* 2002;46:512-518.
8. Trissel LA, ed. *Handbook on Injectable Drugs.* 13th ed. [CD-ROM version 1.5]. Bethesda, MD: American Society of Health-System Pharmacists; 2005.
9. American Academy of Pediatrics Committee on Drugs. "Inactive" ingredients in pharmaceutical products: update. *Pediatrics.* 1997;99:268-278.
10. Hall CM, Milligan DWA, Berrington J. Probably adverse reaction to a pharmaceutical excipient. *Arch Dis Child Fetal Neonatal Ed.* 2004;89:F184.
11. Hiller JL, Benda GI, Rahatzad M, et al. Benzyl alcohol toxicity: impact on mortality and intraventricular hemorrhage among very low birth weight infants. *Pediatrics.* 1986;77:500-506.
12. Grant JA, Bilodeau PA, Guernsey BG, et al. Unsuspected benzyl alcohol hypersensitivity. *N Engl J Med.* 1982;306:108.
13. Wilson JP, Solimando DA, Edwards MS. Parenteral benzyl alcohol-induced hypersensitivity reaction. *Drug Intell Clin Pharm.* 1986;20:689-691.
14. Fox MH, Hunt PC. Prolonged neuromuscular block associated with mivacurium. *Br J Anaesth.* 1995;74:237-238.
15. Kendrick K. Prolonged paralysis related to mivacurium: a case study. *J Perianesth Nur.* 2005;20:7-12.

Morphine Sulfate

1. Morphine sulfate injection [USP package insert]. Paramus, NJ: Mayne Pharma (USA) Inc; April 2004.
2. McEvoy GK, ed. *AHFS Drug Information Essentials 2005-06.* Bethesda, MD: American Society of Health-System Pharmacists; 2005.
3. Lynn AM, Slattery JT. Morphine pharmacokinetics in early infancy. *Anesthesiology.* 1987;66:136-139.
4. Koren G, Butt W, Chinyanga H, et al. Postoperative morphine infusion in newborn infants: assessment of disposition characteristics and safety. *J Pediatr.* 1985;107:963-967.

References

5. Farrington EA, McGuiness GA, Johnson GF, et al. Continuous intravenous morphine infusion in postoperative newborn infants. *Am J Perinatol.* 1993;10:84-87.
6. Scott CS, Riggs KW, Ling EW, et al. Morphine pharmacokinetics and pain assessment in premature newborns. *J Pediatr.* 1999;135:423-329.
7. Lynn A, Nespeca MK, Bratton SL, et al. Clearance of morphine in postoperative infants during intravenous infusion: the influence of age and surgery. *Anesth Analg.* 1998;86:958-963.
8. Saarenmaa E, Neuvonen PJ, Rosenberg P, et al. Morphine clearance and effects in newborn infants in relation to gestational age. *Clin Pharmacol Ther.* 2000;68:160-166.
9. Bray RJ. Postoperative analgesia provided by morphine infusion in children. *Anaesthesia.* 1983;38:1075-1078.
10. Dampier CD, Setty BNY, Logan J, et al. Intravenous morphine pharmacokinetics in pediatric patients with sickle cell disease. *J Pediatr.* 1995;126:461-467.
11. Beasley SW, Tibballs J. Efficacy and safety of continuous morphine infusion for postoperative analgesia in the paediatric surgical ward. *Aust NZ J Surg.* 1987;57:233-237.
12. Miser AW, Miser JS, Clark BS. Continuous intravenous infusion of morphine sulfate for control of severe pain in children with terminal malignancy. *J Pediatr.* 1980;96:930-932.
13. Cole TB, Sprinkle RH, Smith SJ, et al. Intravenous narcotic therapy for children with severe sickle cell pain crisis. *Am J Dis Child.* 1986;140:1255-1259.
14. Lynn AM, Opheim KE, Tyler DC. Morphine infusion after pediatric cardiac surgery. *Crit Care Med.* 1984;12:863-866.
15. Bhatt-Mehta V, Rosen DA. Management of acute pain in children. *Clin Pharm.* 1991;10:667-685.
16. Fixler DE, Carrell T, Browne R, et al. Oxygen consumption in infants and children during cardiac catheterization under different sedation regimens. *Circulation.* 1974;50:788-794.
17. Dahlstrom B, Bolme P, Feychting H, et al. Morphine kinetics in children. *Clin Pharmacol Ther.* 1979;26:354-365.
18. Buck ML. Pharmacokinetic changes during extracorporeal membrane oxygenation. Implications for drug therapy of neonates. *Clin Pharmacokinet.* 2003;42:403-417.
19. Bhatt-Meta V, Annich G. Sedative clearance during extracorporeal membrane oxygenation. *Perfusion.* 2005;20:309-315.
20. Trissel LA. *Handbook on Injectable Drugs.* 10th ed. Bethesda, MD: American Society of Health-System Pharmacists; 1998.
21. American Academy of Pediatrics Committee on Drugs. "Inactive" ingredients in pharmaceutical products: update. *Pediatrics.* 1997;99:268-278.
22. Smolinske SC. Review of parenteral sulfite reactions. *J Toxicol Clin Toxicol.* 1992;30:597-606.
23. Lester MR. Sulfite sensitivity: significance in human health. *J Am Col Nutr.* 1995;14:229-232.
24. Tobias JD. Sedation and analgesia in pediatric intensive care units. A guide to drug selection and use. *Paediatr Drugs.* 1999;1:109-126.
25. Gerber N, Apsoloff G. Death from a morphine infusion during a sickle cell crisis. *J Pediatr.* 1993;322-325.
26. Chay PC, Duffy BJ, Walker JS. Pharmacokinetic pharmacodynamic relationships of morphine in neonates. *Clin Pharmacol Ther.* 1992;51:334-342.
27. Mikkelsen S, Feilberg VL, Christensen CB, et al. Morphine pharmacokinetics in premature and mature newborn infants. *Acta Pediatr.* 1994;83:1025-1028.
28. Hartley R, Green M, Quinn MW, et al. Development of morphine glucuronidation in premature neonates. *Biol Neonate.* 1994;66:1-9.
29. Hartley R, Green M, Quinn M, et al. Pharmacokinetics of morphine infusion in premature neonates. *Arch Dis Child.* 1993;69:55-58.
30. Choonara I, Lawrence A, Michalkiewicz A, et al. Morphine metabolism in neonates and infants. *Br J Clin Pharmacol.* 1992;34:434-437.
31. Hartley R, Quinn M, Green M, et al. Morphine glucuronidation in premature neonates. *Br J Clin Pharmacol.* 1993;35:314-317.
32. Olkkola KT, Maunuksela EL, Korpela R, et al. Kinetics and dynamics of postoperative intravenous morphine in children. *Clin Pharmacol Ther.* 1988;44:128-136.
33. Vicente KJ, Kada-Bekhaled K, Hillel G, et al. Programming errors contribute to death from patient-controlled analgesia: case report and estimate of probability. *Can J Anesth.* 2003;50:328-332.

Multivitamins (Adult)

1. M.V.I. Adult [package insert]. Wilmington, NC: AAIPharma; January 2004.
2. Infuvite ADULT [package insert]. Deerfield, IL: Baxter Healthcare Corporation; June 2002.
3. American Society for Parenteral and Enteral Nutrition (A.S.P.E.N.) 2006 Pediatric Multivitamin Shortage Taskforce. A.S.P.E.N. Update on limited availability of parenteral pediatric multivitamins. March 20, 2006. Available at: www.nutritioncare.org. Accessed May 19, 2006.
4. Multivitamin preparations for parenteral use. A statement by the Nutrition Advisory Group. American Medical Association—Department of Foods and Nutrition, 1975. *J Parenter Enteral Nutr.* 1979;3:258-262.
5. Shils ME, Baker H, Frank O. Blood vitamin levels of long-term adult home total parenteral nutrition patients: the efficacy of the AMA–FDA parenteral multivitamin formulation. *J Parenter Enteral Nutr.* 1985;9:179-188.
6. Trissel LA. *Handbook on Injectable Drugs.* 13th ed. Bethesda, MD: American Society of Health-System Pharmacists; 2005.
7. Glockling MR, Lutomski DM, Youngs CH, et al. Small volume infusion of multiple vitamins. *Clin Pharm.* 1984;3:516-518.
8. Louis S, Kutt H, McDowell F. The cardiocirculatory changes caused by intravenous Dilantin and its solvent. *Am Heart J.* 1967;74:523-529.
9. American Academy of Pediatrics Committee on Drugs. "Inactive" ingredients in pharmaceutical products: update. *Pediatrics.* 1997;99:268-278.
10. Glasgow AM, Boeckx RL, Miller MK, et al. Hyperosmolality in small infants due to propylene glycol. *Pediatrics.* 1983;72:353-355.
11. MacDonald MG, Getson PR, Glasgow AM, et al. Propylene glycol: increased incidence of seizures in low birth weight infants. *Pediatrics.* 1987;79:622-625.
12. Alade SL, Brown RE, Paquet A. Polysorbate 80 and E-Ferol toxicity. *Pediatrics.* 1986;77:593-597.
13. Balistreri WF, Farrell MK, Bove KE. Lessons from the E-Ferol tragedy. *Pediatrics.* 1986;78:503-506. Editorial.
14. Scheiner JM, Araujo MM, DeRitter E. Thiamine destruction by sodium bisulfite in infusion solutions. *Am J Hosp Pharm.* 1981;38:1911-1913.
15. MVI Newsflash. Aluminum toxicity and its control in patients receiving total parenteral nutrition. Available at: http://www.imakenews.com/mvius/e_article000120638.cfm. Accessed May 19, 2006.

Multivitamins (Pediatric)

1. M.V.I. Pediatric [package insert]. Paramus, NJ: Mayne Pharma (USA) Inc; January 2006.
2. Infuvite Pediatric [package insert]. Deerfield, IL: Baxter Healthcare Corporation; February 2001.
3. Moore MC, Greene HL, Phillips B, et al. Evaluation of a pediatric multiple vitamin preparation for total parenteral nutrition in infants and children I. Blood levels of water soluble vitamins. *Pediatrics.* 1986;77:530-538.
4. Greene HL, Moore ME, Phillips B, et al. Evaluation of a pediatric multiple vitamin preparation for total parenteral nutrition II. Blood levels of vitamins A, D, and E. *Pediatrics.* 1986;77:539-547.
5. Greene HL, Phillips BL. Vitamin dosages in premature infants. *Pediatrics.* 1987;79:655. Letter.
6. Greene HL, Hambidge KM, Schanler R, et al. Guidelines for the use of vitamins, trace elements, calcium, magnesium, and phosphorus in infants and children receiving total parenteral nutrition. Report of the Subcommittee on Pediatric Parenteral Nutrient Requirements from the Committee on Clinical Practice Issues of the American Society for Clinical Nutrition. *Am J Clin Nutr.* 1988;48:1324-1342.
7. Collier S, Crouch J, Hendricks K, et al. Use of cyclic parenteral nutrition in infants less than 6 months of age. *Nutr Clin Pract.* 1994;9:65-68.
8. Alade SL, Brown RE, Paquet A. Polysorbate 80 and E-Ferol toxicity. *Pediatrics.* 1986;77:593-597.
9. Balistreri WF, Farrell MK, Bove KE. Lessons from the E-Ferol tragedy. *Pediatrics.* 1986;78:503-506. Editorial.

10. Franck LS, Greene HL, Phillips BL. Alpha tocopheral (E) levels in premature infants during and after intravenous multivitamin supplementation. *Clin Res.* 1987;34:115A.
11. Greene HL, Porchelli P, Adcock E, et al. Vitamins for newborn infant formulas: a review of recommendations with emphasis on data from low birth-weigh infants. *Eur J Clin Nutr.* 1992;46(suppl 4):S1-S8.
12. Levy R, Herzberg GR, Andrews WL, et al. Thiamine, riboflavin, folate, and vitamin B12 status of low birth weight infants receiving parenteral and enteral nutrition. *J Parenter Enteral Nutr.* 1992;16:241-247.
13. MVI Newsflash. Aluminum toxicity and its control in patients receiving total parenteral nutrition. Available at: http://www.imakenews.com/mvius/e_article000120638.cfm. Accessed May 19, 2006.

Muromonab-CD3

1. Schroeder TJ, Ryckman FC, Hurtabaise PE, et al. Immunological monitoring during and following OKT3 therapy in children. *Clin Transplantation.* 1991;5:191-196.
2. Schroeder TJ. Monoclonal antibody therapy in pediatric transplantation. *Transplantation Proc.* 1992;24(suppl 1):2-10.
3. Ettenger RB, Marik J, Rosenthal JT, et al. OKT3 for rejection reversal in pediatric renal transplantation. *Clin Transplantation.* 1988;2:180-184.
4. McDiarmid SV, Millis M, Terashita G, et al. Low serum OKT3 levels correlate with failure to prevent rejection in orthotopic liver transplant patients. *Transplantation Proc.* 1990;22:1774-1776.
5. Piatosa B, Grenda R, Prokurat S. Comparison of adjusted-dose vs. standard-dose OKT3 therapy of acute rejection in pediatric kidney transplant recipients. *Transplantation Proc.* 1993;25:2574.
6. McOmber D, Ibrahim J, Lublin DM, et al. Non-ischemic left ventricular dysfunction after pediatric cardiac transplantation: treatment with plasmapheresis and OKT3. *Pediatr Transplant.* 2004;23:552-557.
7. Wilmot I, Kanter KR, Vincent RN, et al. OKT3 treatment in refractory pediatric heart transplant rejection. *J Heart Lung Transplant.* 2005;24:1793-1797.
8. Younes B, McDiarmid S, Martin M, et al. The effect of immunosuppression on post-transplant lymphoproliferative disease in pediatric liver transplant patients. *Transplant.* 2000;71(1):94-99.
9. Leone MR, Barry JM, Alexander SR, et al. Monoclonal antibody OKT3 therapy in pediatric kidney transplant recipients. *J Pediatr.* 1990;116: S86-S91.
10. Ahdoot J, Galindo A, Alejos JC, et al. Use of OKT3 for acute myocarditis in infants and children. *J Heart Lung Transplant.* 2000;19:1118-1121.
11. Medical Economics, ed. *Physicians' Desk Reference.* 54th ed. Oradell, NJ: Medical Economics Company; 2000.
12. Jeyarajah DR, Thistlethwaite JR. General aspects of cytokine-release syndrome: timing and incidence of symptoms. *Transplantation Proc.* 1993;25(suppl 1):16-20.
13. Ryckman FC, Schroeder TJ, Pederson SH, et al. Use of monoclonal antibody immunosuppressive therapy in pediatric renal and liver transplantation. *Clin Transplantation*. 1991;5:186-190.

Nafcillin Sodium

1. American Academy of Pediatrics. In: Pickering LK, ed. *2003 Red Book: Report of the Committee on Infectious Diseases.* 26th ed. Elk Grove Village, IL: American Academy of Pediatrics; 2003.
2. Prober CG, Stevenson DK, Benitz WE. The use of antibiotics in neonates weighing less than 1200 grams. *Pediatr Infect Dis J.* 1990;9:111-121.
3. McCracken GH Jr, Nelson JD, eds. *Antimicrobial Therapy for Newborns: Practical Application.* 2nd ed. New York, NY: Grune and Stratton; 1983.
4. Greene GR, Cohen E. Nafcillin-induced neutropenia in children. *Pediatrics.* 1978;61:94-97.
5. Kancir LM, Tuazon CU, Cardella TA, et al. Adverse reactions to methicillin and nafcillin during treatment of serious Staphylococcus aureus infections. *Arch Intern Med.* 1978;138:909-911.
6. Rhodes KH, Henry NK. Antibiotic therapy for severe infections in infants and children. *Mayo Clin Proc.* 1992;67:59-68.
7. Baddour LM, Wilson WR, Bayer AS, et al. Infective endocarditis: diagnosis, antimicrobial therapy, and management of complications: a statement for healthcare professionals from the Committee on Rheumatic Fever, Endocarditis, and Kawasaki Disease, Council on Cardiovascular Disease in the Young, and the Councils on Clinical Cardiology, Stroke, and Cardiovascular Surgery and Anesthesia, American Heart Association: endorsed by the Infectious Diseases Society of America. *Circulation.* 2005;111:e394-e434.
8. Tunkel AR, Hartman BJ, Kaplan SL, et al. Practice guidelines for the management of bacterial meningitis. *Clin Infect Dis*. 2004;39:1267-1284.
9. Klein JO, Feigin RD, McCracken GH. Report of American Academy of Pediatrics task force on diagnosis and management of meningitis. *Pediatrics.* 1986;78(suppl):959-982.
10. American Academy of Pediatrics. Committee on Infectious Diseases. Treatment of bacterial meningitis. *Pediatrics.* 1988;6:904-907.
11. American Society of Health-System Pharmacists. American Hospital Formulary System. Available at: http://ahfsfirst.firstdatabank.com/AHFSfirst/NSAHFSFirstSearchmain.asp. Accessed July 10, 2006.
12. Feldman WE, Nelson JD, Stanberry LR. Clinical and pharmacokinetic evaluation of nafcillin in infants and children. *J Pediatr.* 1978;93:1029-1033.
13. *Physicians' Desk Reference*. 60th ed. Montvale, NJ: Medical Economics Company; 2006.
14. Eickhoff TC, Kislak JW, Finland M. Clinical evaluation of nafcillin in patients with severe staphylococcal disease. *N Engl J Med*. 1965; 272:699-708.
15. Trissel LA, ed. *Handbook on Injectable Drugs.* 13th ed. [CD-ROM version 1.5]. Bethesda, MD: American Society of Health-System Pharmacists; 2005.
16. Robinson DC, Cookson TL, Frisafe JA. Concentration guidelines for parenteral antibiotics in fluid-restricted patients. *Drug Intell Clin Pharm.* 1987;21:985-989.
17. Zenk KE, Dungy CI, Greene GR. Nafcillin extravasation injury. *Am J Dis Child.* 1981;135:1113-1114.
18. Tilden SJ, Craft JC, Cano R, et al. Cutaneous necrosis associated with intravenous nafcillin therapy. *Am J Dis Child.* 1980;134:1046-1048.
19. MacCara ME. Extravasation: a hazard of intravenous therapy. *Drug Intell Clin Pharm.* 1983;17:713-717.
20. Kitzing W, Nelson JD, Mohs E. Comparative toxicities of methicillin and nafcillin. *Am J Dis Child.* 1981;135:52-55.
21. McLaughlin JE, Reeves DS. Clinical and laboratory evidence for inactivation of gentamicin by carbenicillin. *Lancet.* 1971;1(7693):261-264.
22. Riff LJ, Jackson GG. Laboratory and clinical conditions for gentamicin inactivation by carbenicillin. *Arch Intern Med.* 1972;130:887-981.
23. Manian FA, Stone WJ, Alford RH. Adverse antibiotic effects associated with renal insufficiency. *Rev Infect Dis.* 1990;12:236-249.
24. Davies M, Morgan JR, Anand C. Interactions of carbenicillin and ticarcillin with gentamicin. *Antimicrob Agents Chemother.* 1975;7:431-434.
25. Weibert R, Keane W, Shapiro F. Carbenicillin inactivation of aminoglycosides in patients with severe renal failure. *Trans Amer Soc Artif Int Organs*. 1976;22:439-443.

References

Naloxone HCl

1. *Physicians' Desk Reference.* 60th ed. Montvale, NJ: Thomson PDR; 2006.
2. American Society of Health-System Pharmacists. American Hospital Formulary System. Available at: http://ahfsfirst.firstdatabank.com/AHFSfirst/NSAHFSFirstSearchmain.asp. Accessed July 21, 2006.
3. McGuire W, Fowie PW. Naloxone for narcotic exposed newborn infants. systematic review. *Arch Dis Child Fetal Neonatal Ed.* 2003;88:F308-F311.
4. American Heart Association. Guidelines 2005 for cardiopulmonary resuscitation and emergency cardiovascular care. Part 12: Pediatric advanced life support. *Circulation.* 2005;112:167-187.
5. American Academy of Pediatrics Committee on Drugs. Emergency drug doses for infants and children. *Pediatrics.*1998;101:e1-e11.
6. Standards and guidelines for cardiopulmonary resuscitation (CPR) and emergency cardiac care (ECC). Part VI: Neonatal advanced life support. *JAMA.* 1986;255:2969-2973.
7. American Academy of Pediatrics. Committee on Drugs. Naloxone use in newborns. *Pediatrics.* 1980;65:667-669.
8. Handal KA, Schauben JL, Salamone FR. Naloxone. *Ann Emerg Med.* 1983;12:438-445.
9. American Academy of Pediatrics. Committee on Drugs. Emergency drug doses for infants and children and naloxone use in newborns: clarification. *Pediatrics.* 1989;83:803.
10. American Academy of Pediatrics. Committee on Drugs. Naloxone dosage and route of administration for infants and children: addendum to emergency drug doses for infants and children. *Pediatrics.* 1990;86:484-485.
11. Bowden CA, Krenzelok EP. Clinical applications of commonly used contemporary antidotes. *Drug Safety.* 1997;16:9-47.
12. Lewis JM, Klein-Schwartz W, Benson BE, et al. Continuous naloxone infusion in pediatric narcotic overdose. *Am J Dis Child.* 1984;138:944-946.
13. Moore RA, Rumack BH, Conner CS, et al. Naloxone: underdosage after narcotic poisoning. *Am J Dis Child.* 1980;134:156-158.
14. Tenenbein M. Continuous naloxone infusion for opiate poisoning in infancy. *J Pediatr.* 1984;105:645-648.
15. Furman WL, Menke JA, Barson WJ, et al. Continuous naloxone infusion in two neonates with septic shock. *J Pediatr.* 1984;105:649-651.
16. Goldfrank L, Kulig K. Opioids/opioid antagonists. In: Rumack BH, ed. *Poisindex Information System.* 86th ed. Denver, CO: MICROMEDEX Inc; Accessed April 17, 2006.
17. Fischer CG, Cook DR. The respiratory and narcotic antagonistic effects of naloxone in infants. *Anesth Analg.* 1974;53:849-852.
18. Groeger JS, Carlon GC, Howland WS. Naloxone in septic shock. *Crit Care Med.* 1983;11:650-654.
19. Hackshaw KV, Parker GA, Roberts JW. Naloxone is septic shock. *Crit Care Med.*1990;18:47-51.
20. Shenep JL. Septic shock. *Adv Pediatr Infect Dis.* 1996;12:209-241.
21. Boeuf B, Gauvin G, Guerguerian AM, et al. Therapy of shock with naloxone: a meta-analysis. *Crit Care Med.* 1998;26:1910-1916.
22. Tiengo M. Naloxone in irreversible shock. *Lancet.* 1980;2:690.
23. Cocchi P, Silenzi M, Calabri G, et al. Naloxone in fulminant meningococcemia. *Pediatr Infect Dis.* 1984;3:187.
24. Aronoff A, Brier M, Bennett W. *The Renal Book, 2002.* Available at: http://www.kdp-baptist.louisville.edu/renalbook/. Accessed July 21, 2006.
25. Chernick V, Manfreda J, DeBooy V, et al. Clinical trial of naloxone in birth asphyxia. *J Pediatr.* 1988;113:519-525.
26. Gober AE, Kearns GL, Yokel RA, et al. Repeated naloxone administration for morphine overdose in a 1-month-old infant. *Pediatrics.* 1979;63:606-608.
27. Romac DR. Safety of prolonged high-dose infusion of naloxone hydrochloride for severe methadone overdose. *Clin Pharm.* 1986;5:251-254.
28. Waldron VD: Methadone overdose treated with naloxone infusion. *JAMA.* 1973;225:53.
29. Davidson GM, Goldes FF, Duncalf D, et al. Effects of n–allyloxymorphone-narcotic mixtures in anesthetized patients. *Anesthesiology.* 1963;24:129-130.
30. Trissel LA, ed. *Handbook on Injectable Drugs.* 13th ed. [CD-ROM version 1.5]. Bethesda, MD: American Society of Health-System Pharmacists; 2005.
31. Soni MG, Taylor SL, Greenberg NA, et al. Evaluation of the health aspects of methyl paraben: a review of the published literature. *Food Chem Toxicol.* 2002;40:1335-1373.
32. Nagel JE, Fuscaldo JT, Firemen P. Paraben allergy. *JAMA.* 1977;237:1594-1595.
33. Prough DS, Roy R, Bumgarner J, et al. Acute pulmonary edema in healthy teenagers following conservative doses of intravenous naloxone. *Anesthesiology.* 1984; 60:485-486.

Nesiritide

1. *Physicians' Desk Reference.* 60th ed. Montvale, NJ: Thomson PDR; 2006.
2. Gelman CR, Rumack BH, Hess AJ (eds). *DRUGDEX® System.* Englewood, CO: MICROMEDEX Inc. Accessed April 20, 2006.
3. American Society of Health-System Pharmacists. American Hospital Formulary System. Available at: http://ahfsfirst.firstdatabank.com/AHFSfirst/NSAHFSFirstSearchmain.asp. Accessed September 3, 2006.
4. BNP Consensus Panel 2004: A clinical approach for the diagnostic, prognostic, screening, treatment monitoring, and therapeutic roles of natriuretic peptides in cardiovascular disease. *Cong Heart Fail.* 2004;10(5):1-30.
5. Costello JM, Goodman DM, Green TP. A review of the natriuretic hormone system's diagnostic and therapeutic potential in critically ill children. *Pediatr Crit Care Med.* 2006:7(4):308-318.
6. Mahle WT, Cuadarado AR, Kirshbom PM, et al. Nesiritide in infants and children with congestive heart failure. *Pediatr Crit Care Med.* 2005;6:543-546.
7. Moffett BS, Jefferies JL, Price JF, et al. Administration of a large nesiritide bolus dose in a pediatric patient: case report and review of nesiritide use in pediatrics. *Pharmacotherapy.* 2006;26(2):277-280.
8. Simsic JM, Reddy VS, Kanter et al. Use of nesiritide (human B-type natriuretic peptide) in infants following cardiac surgery. *Pediatr Cardiol.* 2004(25):668-670.
9. Feingold B, Law YW. Nesiritide use in pediatric patients with congestive heart failure. *J Heart Lung Transplant.* 2004;23:1455-1459.
10. Simsic JM, Scheurer M, Tobias JD, et al. Perioperative effects and safety of nesiritide following cardiac surgery in children. *J Intensive Care Med.* 2006;21(1):22-26.
11. Smith T, Rose DA, Russo P, et al. Nesiritide during extracorporeal membrane oxygenation. *Pediatr Anesthesia.* 2005;15:152-157.
12. Ivy DD, Kinsella JP, Wolfe RR, et al. Atrial natriuretic peptide and nitric oxide in children with pulmonary hypertension after surgical repair of congenital heart disease. *Am J Cardiol.* 1996;77:102-105.
13. Marshall J, Berkenbosch JW, Russo P, et al. Preliminary experience with nesiritide in the pediatric population. *J Intensive Care Med.* 2004;19(3):164-170.
14. Sehra R, Underwood K. Nesiritide improves urine output in severely ill pediatric patients awaiting heart transplant [abstract]. *J Card Fail.* 2003;(5):254.
15. Wheeler AD, Tobias JD. Nesiritide in a pediatric oncology patient with renal insufficiency and myocardial dysfunction following septic shock. *Pediatr Hem Oncol.* 2005;22:323-333.
16. Food and Drug Administration. MedWatch Program. *2005 Safety Alert: Natrecor (nesiritide).* Available from http://www.fda.gov/medwatch/SAFETY/2005/natrecor2_DHCP.htm. Accessed July 15, 2006.
17. Moffett BS, Jefferies JL, Rossano J, et al. Nesiritide therapy in a term neonate with renal disease. *Pharmacotherapy.* 2006;26(2)281-284.

References

Nicardipine

1. Milou C, Debuche-Benouachkou V, Semama DS, et al. Intravenous nicardipine as a first-line antihypertensive drug in neonates. *Intensive Care Med.* 2000;26:956-958.
2. Gouyon JB, Geneste B, Semama DS, et al. Intravenous nicardipine in hypertensive preterm infants. *Arch Dis Child Fetal Neonatal Ed.* 1997;76:F126-F127.
3. Treluyer JM, Hubert P, Jouvet P, et al. Intravenous nicardipine in hypertensive children. *Eur J Pediatr.* 1993;152:712-714.
4. Flynn JT, Mottes TA, Brophy PD, et al. Intravenous nicardipine for treatment of severe hypertension in children. *J Pediatr.* 2001;139:38-43.
5. Tobias JD. Nicardipine to control mean arterial pressure after cardiothoracic surgery in infants and children. *Am J Ther.* 2001;8:3-6.
6. McBride BF, White CM, Campbell M, et al. Nicardipine to control neonatal hypertension during extracorporeal membrane oxygen support. *Ann Pharmacother.* 2003;37:667-670.
7. Temple ME, Nahata MC. Treatment of pediatric hypertension. *Pharmacotherapy.* 2000;20:140-150.
8. Michael J, Groshong T, Tobias JD. Nicardipine for hypertensive emergencies in children with renal disease. *Pediatr Nephrol.* 1998;12:40-42.
9. Tobias JD, Hersey S, Mencio GA, et al. Nicardipine for controlled hypotension during spinal surgery. *J Pediatr Ortho.* 1996;16:370-373.
10. Tobias JD, Pietsch JB, Lynch A. Nicardipine to control mean arterial pressure during extracorporeal membrane oxygenation. *Paediatr Anaesth.* 1996;6:51-60.
11. Tenney F, Sakarcan A. Nicardipine is a safe and effective agent in pediatric hypertensive emergencies. *Am J Kidney Dis.* 2000;35:1-3.
12. US Department of Health and Human Services, National Institutes of Health, National Heart, Lung, and Blood Institute. Diagnosis, evaluation, and treatment of high blood pressure in children and adolescents. 4th report. NIH Publication 05-5267. Revised May 2005.
13. Adelman RD, Coppo R, Dillon MJ. The emergency management of severe hypertension. *Pediatr Nephrol.* 2000;14:422-427.
14. Strauser LM, Groshong T, Tobias JD. Initial experience with isradipine for the treatment of hypertension in children. *South Med J.* 2000;93:287-293.
15. Flynn JT, Pasko DA. Calcium channel blockers: pharmacology and place in therapy of pediatric hypertension. *Pediatr Nephrol.* 2000;15:302-316.
16. Ingu A, Morikawa M, Fuse S, et al. Acute occlusion of a simple aortic coarctation presenting as abdominal angina. *Pediatr Cardiol.* 2003;24:488-489.
17. Nakagawa TA, Sartori SC, Morris A, et al. Intravenous nicardipine for treatment of postcoarctectomy hypertension in children. *Pediatr Cardiol.* 2004;25:26-30.
18. McEvoy GK, ed. *AHFS Drug Information Essentials 2005–06.* Bethesda, MD: American Society of Health-System Pharmacists; 2005.
19. *Physicians' Desk Reference.* 60th ed. Montvale, NJ: Thomson PDR; 2006.
20. Fivush B, Neu A, Furth S. Acute hypertensive crises in children: emergencies and urgencies. *Curr Opin Pediatr.* 1997;9:233-236.
21. Aronoff A, Brier M, Bennett W. *The Renal Book, 2002.* http://www.kdp-baptist.louisville.edu/renalbook/. Accessed August 14, 2006.
22. Larson A, Tobias JD. Nicardipine for the treatment of hypertension following cardiac transplantation in a 14-year-old boy. *Clin Pediatr.* 1994;25:309-311.
23. Trissel LA, ed. *Handbook on Injectable Drugs.* 13th ed. [CD-ROM version 1.5]. Bethesda, MD: American Society of Health-System Pharmacists; 2005.
24. Levene MI, Gibson NA, Fenton AC, et al. The use of a calcium-channel blocker, nicardipine, for severely asphyxiated newborn infants. *Dev Med Child Neurol.* 1990;32:567-574.
25. Aya AG, Bruelle P, Lefrant JY, et al. Accidental nicardipine overdosage without serious maternal or neonatal consequence. *Anaesth Intensive Care.* 1996;24:99-101.

Nitroglycerin

1. Nitroglycerin injection, USP. Shirley, NY: American Regent Laboratories Inc; October 2002.
2. McEvoy GK, ed. *Drug Information Essentials 2005–06.* Bethesda, MD: American Society of Health-System Pharmacists; 2005.
3. Friedman WF, George BL. New concepts and drugs in the treatment of congestive heart failure. *Pediatr Clin North Am.* 1984;31:1197 1227.
4. Benson LN, Bohn D, Edmonds JF, et al. Nitroglycerin therapy in children with low cardiac index after heart surgery. *Cardiovasc Med.* 1979;4:207-215.
5. Ilbawi MN, Idriss FS, DeLeon SY, et al. Hemodynamic effects of intravenous nitroglycerin in pediatric patients after heart surgery. *Circulation.* 1985;72:101-107.
6. Schleien CL, Setzer NA, McLaughlin GE, et al. Postoperative management of the cardiac surgical patient. In: Rogers MC, ed. *Textbook of Pediatric Intensive Care.* Baltimore, MD: Williams & Wilkins; 1992:467-531.
7. Adelman RD, Coppo R, Dillon MJ. The emergency management of severe hypertension. *Pediatr Nephrol.* 2000;14:422-427.
8. Trissel LA, ed. *Handbook on Injectable Drugs.* 13th ed. Bethesda, MD: American Society of Health-System Pharmacists; 2005.
9. Louis S, Kutt H, McDowell F. The cardiocirculatory changes caused by intravenous Dilantin and its solvent. *Am Heart J.* 1967;74:523-529.
10. American Academy of Pediatrics Committee on Drugs. "Inactive" ingredients in pharmaceutical products: update. *Pediatrics.* 1997;99:268-278.
11. Glasgow AM, Boeckx RL, Miller MK, et al. Hyperosmolality in small infants due to propylene glycol. *Pediatrics.* 1983;72:353-355.
12. MacDonald MG, Getson PR, Glasgow AM, et al. Propylene glycol: increased incidence of seizures in low birth weight infants. *Pediatrics.* 1987;79:622-625.
13. Elkayam U. Tolerance to organic nitrates: evidence, mechanisms, clinical relevance, and strategies for prevention. *Ann Intern Med.* 1991;114:667-677.
14. Herling IM. Intravenous nitroglycerin: clinical pharmacology and therapeutic considerations. *Am Heart J.* 1984;108:141-149.
15. Gibson GR, Hunter JB, Raabe DS, et al. Methemoglobinemia induced by high-dose intravenous nitroglycerin. *Ann Intern Med.* 1982; 96:615-616.
16. Williams RS, Mickell JJ, Young ES, et al. Methemoglobin levels during prolonged combination nitroglycerin and sodium nitroprusside infusion in infants after cardiac surgery. *J Cardiothorac Vasc Anesth.* 1994;8:658-662.

Norepinephrine Bitartrate

1. McEvoy GK, ed. *Drug Information Essentials 2005–06.* Bethesda, MD: American Society of Health-System Pharmacists; 2005.
2. American Heart Association. 2005 Guidelines for cardiopulmonary resuscitation and emergency cardiovascular care. Part 12: Pediatric advanced life support. *Circulation.* 2005; 112(suppl 1):167-187.
3. Schleien CL, Kuluz JW, Shaffner DH, et al. Cardiopulmonary resuscitation. In: Rogers MC, ed. *Textbook of Pediatric Intensive Care.* Baltimore, MD: Williams & Wilkins; 1992.
4. Norepinephrine Bitartrate injection USP [package insert]. Bedford, OH: Bedford Laboratories; April 2004.
5. Taketomo CK, Hodding JH, Kraus DM. *Pediatric Dosage Handbook.* 12th ed. Hudson, OH: Lexi-Comp Inc; 2005-2006.
6. Trissel LA. *Handbook on Injectable Drugs.* 13th ed. Bethesda, MD: American Society of Health-System Pharmacists; 2005.
7. Zaritsky A, Chernow B. Use of catecholamines in pediatrics. *J Pediatr.* 105:341-350.
8. MacCara ME. Extravasation: a hazard of intravenous therapy. *Drug Intell Clin Pharm.* 1983;17:713-717.
9. Gaze NR. Tissue necrosis caused by commonly used intravenous infusions. *Lancet.* 1978;2:417-419.
10. American Academy of Pediatrics Committee on Drugs. "Inactive" ingredients in pharmaceutical products: update. *Pediatrics.* 1997;99:268-278.

References

11. Smolinske SC. Review of parenteral sulfite reactions. *J Toxicol Clin Toxicol.* 1992;30:597-606.
12. Lester MR. Sulfite sensitivity: significance in human health. *J Am Col Nutr.* 1995;14:229-232.

Octreotide Acetate

1. Roehr CC, Jung A, Proquitte H, et al. Somatostatin or octreotide as treatment options for chylothorax in young children: a systematic review. *Intensive Care Med.* 2006;32:650-657.
2. Rosti L, De Battisti F, Butera G, et al. Octreotide in the management of postoperative chylothorax. *Pediatr Cardiol.* 2005;26:440-443.
3. Mohseni-Bod H, Macrae D, Slavik Z. Somatostatin analog (octreotide) in management of neonatal postoperative chylothorax: is it safe? *Pediatr Crit Care Med.* 2004;5:356-357.
4. Lauterbach R, Sczaniecka B, Koziol J, et al. Somatostatin treatment of spontaneous chylothorax in an extremely low birth weight infant. *Eur J Pediatr.* 2005;164:195-196.
5. Lam JC, Aters S, Tobias JD. Initial experience with octreotide in the pediatric population. *Am J Ther.* 2001;8:409-415.
6. Bhatia C, Pratap U, Slavik Z. Octreotide therapy: a new horizon in treatment of iatrogenic chyloperitoneum. *Arch Dis Child.* 2001; 85:234-235.
7. Andreou A, Papouli M, Papavasasiliou V, et al. Postoperative chylous ascites in a neonate treated successfully with octreotide: bile sludge and cholestasis. *Am J Perinatol.* 2005;8:401-404.
8. Hwang JB, Choi SO, Park WH. Resolution of refractory chylous ascites after Kasai portoenterostomy using octreotide. *J Pediatr Surg.* 2004;39:1806-1807.
9. Goyal A, Smith NP, Jesudason EC, et al. Octreotide for treatment of chylothorax after repair of congenital diaphragmatic hernia. *J Pediatr Surg.* 2003;38:1-2.
10. Cheung YF, Leung MP, Yip MM. Octreotide for treatment of postoperative chylothorax. *J Pediatr.* 2001;139:157-159.
11. Jaros W, Biller J, Greer S, et al. Successful treatment of idiopathic secretory diarrhea of infancy with the somatostatin analogue SMS 201-995. *Gastroenterology.* 1988;94:189-193.
12. Ohlbaum P, Galperine RI, Demarquez JL, et al. Use of a long-acting somatostatin analogue (SMS 201-995) in controlling a significant ileal output in a 5-year-old child. *J Pediatr Gastroenterol Nutr.* 1987;6:466-470.
13. Smith SS, Shulman DI, O'Dorisio TM, et al. Watery diarrhea, hypokalemia, achlorhydria syndrome in an infant: effect of the long-acting somatostatin analogue SMS 201-995 on the disease and linear growth. *J Pediatr Gastroenterol Nutr.* 1987;6:710-716.
14. Lamireau T, Galperine RI, Ohlbaum P, et al. Use of a long acting somatostatin analogue in controlling ileostomy diarrhea in infants. *Acta Paediatr Scand.* 1990;79:871-872.
15. Couper RT, Berzen A, Berall G, et al. Clinical response to the long acting somatostatin analogue SMS 201-995 in a child with congenital microvillus atrophy. *Gut.* 1989;30:1020-1024.
16. Tauber MT, Harris AG, Rochiccioli P. Clinical use of the long acting somatostatin analogue octreotide in pediatrics. *Eur J Pediatr.* 1994;153:304-310.
17. Beckman RA, Siden R, Yanik GA, et al. Continuous octreotide infusion for the treatment of secretory diarrhea caused by acute intestinal graft-versus-host disease in a child. *J Pediatr Hematol Oncol.* 2000;22:344-350.
18. Nanto-Salonen K, Koskinen P, Sonninen P, et al. Suppression of GH secretion in pituitary gigantism by continuous subcutaneous octreotide infusion in a pubertal boy. *Acta Paediatr.* 1999;88:29-33.
19. Hindmarsh PC, Pringle PJ, Di Silvio L, et al. A preliminary report on the role of somatostatin analogue (SMS 201-995) in the management of children with tall stature. *Clinical Endocrinology.* 1990;32:83-91.
20. Wallace AM, Newman K. Successful closure of intestinal fistulae in an infant using the somatostatin analogue SMS 201-995. *J Pediatr Surg.* 1991;26:1097-1100.
21. Inamdar S, Slim MS, Bostwick H, et al. Treatment of duodenocutaneous fistula with somatostatin analog in a child with dermatomyositis. *J Pediatr Gastroenterol Nutr.* 1990;10:402-404.
22. Mahomed A. Subcutaneously administered somatostatin analogue in traumatic pancreatic fistula. *Pediatr Surg Int.* 1997;12:231. Letter.
23. Siafakas C, Fox VL, Nurko S. Use of octreotide for the treatment of severe gastrointestinal bleeding in children. *J Pediatr Gastroenterol Nutr.* 1998;26:356-359.
24. Eroglu Y, Emerick KM, Whitington PF, et al. Octreotide therapy for control of acute gastrointestinal bleeding in children. *J Pediatr Gastroenterol Nutr.* 2004;38:41-47.
25. Heikenen JB, Pohl JF, Werlin SL, et al. Octreotide in pediatric patients. *J Pediatr Gastroenterol Nutr.* 2002;35:600-609.
26. Zellos A, Schwartz KB. Efficacy of octreotide in children with chronic gastrointestinal bleeding. *J Pediatr Gastroenterol Nutr.* 2000;30:442-446.
27. Glaser B, Hirsch HJ, Landau H. Persistent hyperinsulinemic hypoglycemia of infancy: long-term octreotide treatment without pancreatectomy. *J Pediatr.* 1993;123:644-650.
28. Thornton PS, Alter CA, Katz LE, et al. Short and long-term use of octreotide in the treatment of congenital hyperinsulinism. *J Pediatr.* 1993;123:637-643.
29. Barrons RW. Octreotide in hyperinsulinism. *Ann Pharmacotherapy.* 1997;31:239-241.
30. Stanley CA. Hyperinsulinism in infants and children. *Ped Clin N Am.* 1997;44:363-373.
31. Apak RA, Yurdakok M, Oran O, et al. Preoperative use of octreotide in a newborn with persistent hyperinsulinemic hypoglycemia of infancy. *J Pediatr Endocrinol Metab.* 1998;11:143-145.
32. Jackson JA, Hahn HB, Oltorf CE. Long-acting somatostatin analog in refractory neonatal hypoglycemia: follow-up information. *J Pediatr.* 1988;113:1118.
33. Jackson JA, Hahn HB, Oltorf CE, et al. Long-term treatment of refractory neonatal hypoglycemia with long-acting somatostatin analog. *J Pediatr.* 1987;111:548-551.
34. DeClue TJ, Malone JI, Bercu BB. Linear growth during long-term treatment with somatostatin analog (SMS 201-995) for persistent hyperinsulinemic hypoglycemia of infancy. *J Pediatr.* 1990;116:747-749.
35. Bosman-Vermeeren JM, Veereman-Wauters G, Broos P, et al. Somatostatin in the treatment of a pancreatic pseudocyst in a child. *J Pediatr Gastroenterol Nutr.* 1996;23:422-425.
36. Yaffe MR, Gutenberger JE. Chronic pancreatitis and pancreas divisum in an infant: diagnosed by endoscopic retrograde cholangiopancreatography and treated with somatostatin analog. *J Pediatr Gastroenterol Nutr.* 1989;9:108-111.
37. Spiller HA. Management of sulfonylurea ingestions. *Pediatr Emerg Care.* 1999;15:227-230.
38. Tenenbein M. Recent advancements in pediatric toxicology. *Ped Clin N Am.* 1999;46:1179-1188.
39. Mordel A, Sivilotti ML, Old AC, et al. Octreotide for pediatric sulfonylurea poisoning. *J Clin Toxicol.* 1998;36:437.
40. Little GL, Boniface KS. Are one or two dangerous? Sulfonylurea exposure in toddlers. *J Emerg Med.* 2005;28:305-310.
41. Carr R, Zed PJ. Octreotide for sulfonylurea-induced hypoglycemia following overdose. *Ann Pharmacother.* 2002;36:1727-1732.
42. *Physicians' Desk Reference.* 60th ed. Montvale, NJ: Thomson PDR; 2006.
43. Trissel LA, ed. *Handbook on Injectable Drugs.* 13th ed. [CD-ROM version 1.5]. Bethesda, MD: American Society of Health-System Pharmacists; 2005.
44. Seidner DL, Speerhas R. Can octreotide be added to parenteral nutrition solutions? *Point-Counterpoint. Nutr Clin Pract.* 1998;13:84-88.
45. Hunziker UA, Superti-Furga A, Zachmann M, et al. Effects of the long-acting somatostatin analogue SMS 201-995 in an infant with intractable diarrhea. *Helv Paediatr Acta.* 1988;43:103-109.

References

Ondansetron HCl

1. Thomson PDR, ed. *Physicians' Desk Reference*. 60th ed. Montvale, NJ: Thomson Healthcare; 2006.
2. Alvarez O, Freeman A, Bedros AM, et al. Randomized double-blind crossover ondansetron-dexamethasone versus ondansetron-placebo study for the treatment of chemotherapy-induced nausea and vomiting in pediatric patients with malignancies. *J Pediatr Hematol Oncol.* 1995;17:145-150.
3. Vermeulen LC, Matsuzewski KA, Ratko TA, et al. Evaluation of ondansetron prescribing in U.S. academic medical centers. *Arch Intern Med.* 1994;154:1733-1740.
4. Holdsworth MT, Raisch DW, Duncan MH, et al. Assessment of chemotherapy-induced emesis and evaluation of a reduced-dose intravenous ondansetron regimen in pediatric patients. *Ann Pharmacother.* 1995;29:16-21.
5. McQueen KD, Milton JD. Multicenter postmarketing surveillance of ondansetron therapy in pediatric patients. *Ann Pharmacother*. 1994;28:8-92.
6. Sandoval C, Corbi D, Strobino B, et al. Randomized double-blind comparison of single high-dose ondansetron and multiple standard-dose ondansetron in chemotherapy-naïve pediatric oncology patients. *Cancer Invest.* 1999;17:309-313.
7. Nahata MC, Nui LN, Koepke J. Efficacy and safety of ondansetron in pediatric patients undergoing bone marrow transplantation. *Clin Ther.* 1996;18:466-476.
8. Brock P, Brichard B, Reichnitzer C, et al. An increasing loading dose of ondansetron: a North European double-blind randomized study in children, comparing 5 mg/m2 with 10 mg/m2. *Eur J Cancer.* 1996;32A:1744-1748.
9. Parker RI, Prakash D, Mahan Ra et al. Randomized, double-blind, crossover, placebo-controlled trial of intravenous ondansetron for the prevention of intrathecal chemotherapy-induced vomiting in children. *J Pediatr Hematol Oncol.* 2001;23:578-581.
10. Kalaycio M, Mendez Z, Pohlman B, et al. Continuous-infusion granisetron compared to ondansetron for the prevention of nausea and vomiting after high-dose chemotherapy. *J Cancer Res Clin Oncol.* 1998;124:265-269.
11. Furst SR, Rodarte A. Prophylactic antiemetic treatment with ondansetron in children undergoing tonsillectomy. *Anesthesiol*. 1994;81:799-803.
12. Watcha MF, Bras PJ, Cieslak GD, et al. The dose-response relationship of ondansetron in preventing postoperative emesis in pediatric patients undergoing ambulatory surgery. *Anesthesiology.* 1995;82:47-52.
13. Ummenhofer W, Frei FJ, Urwyler A, et al. Effect of ondansetron in the prevention of postoperative nausea and vomiting in children. *Anesthesiology.* 1994;81:804-810.
14. Rose JB, Martin TM, Corddry DH, et al. Ondansetron reduced the incidence and severity of poststrabismus repair vomiting in children. *Anesth Analg.* 1994;79:486-489.
15. Spahr-Schopfer IA, Lerman J, Sikich N, et al. Pharmacokinetics of intravenous ondansetron in healthy children undergoing ear, nose, and throat surgery. *Clin Pharm Ther.* 1995;58:316-321.
16. Patel RI, Davis PJ, Orr RJ, et al. Single-dose ondansetron prevents postoperative vomiting in pediatric outpatients. *Anesth Analg.* 1997;85:538-545.
17. Sadhasivam S, Shende D, Madan R. Prophylactic ondansetron in prevention of postoperative nausea and vomiting following pediatric strabismus surgery. *Anesthesiology.* 2000;92:1035-1042.
18. Sukhani R, Pappas AL, Lurie J, et al. Ondansetron and dolasetron provide equivalent postoperative vomiting control after ambulatory tonsillectomy in dexamethasone-pretreated children. *Anesth Analg.* 2002;95:1230-1235.
19. Khalil SN, Roth AG, Cohen IT, et al. A double-blind comparison of intravenous ondansetron and placebo for preventing postoperative emesis in 1- to 24-month-old pediatric patients after surgery under general anesthesia. *Anesth Analg.* 2005;101:356-361.
20. Reeves JJ, Shannon MW, Fleisher GR. Ondansetron decreases vomiting associated with acute gastroenteritis: a randomized, controlled trial. *Pediatrics.* 2002;109:1-6.
21. Trissel LA. *Handbook on Injectable Drugs.* 13th ed. Bethesda, MD: American Society of Health-System Pharmacists; 2005.
22. Ross AK, Ferrero-Conover D. Anaphylactoid reaction due to the administration of ondansetron in a pediatric neurosurgical patient. *Anesth Analg.* 1998;87:779-780.
23. Boike SC, Ilson B, Zariffa N, Jorkasky DK. Cardiovascular effects of i.v. granisetron at two administration rates and of ondansetron in healthy adults. *Am J Health-Syst Pharm.* 1997;54:1172–1176.
24. Soni MG, Taylor SL, Greenberg NA, et al. Evaluation of the health aspects of methyl paraben: a review of the published literature. *Food Chem Toxicol.* 2002;40:1335-1373.
25. Nagel JE, Fuscaldo JT, Firemen P. Paraben allergy. *JAMA.* 1977;237:1594-1595.
26. Hansten PD, Horn JR. Drug interactions analysis and management. In: Kastrup EK, Olin BR, eds. *Drug Facts and Comparisons*. St. Louis, MO: Facts and Comparisons, A Wolters Kluwer Co; 2000.

Oxacillin Sodium

1. Prober CG, Stevenson DK, Benitz WE. The use of antibiotics in neonates weighing less than 1200 grams. *Pediatr Infect Dis J.* 1990;9:111-121.
2. American Academy of Pediatrics. In: Pickering LK, ed. *2003 Red Book: Report of the Committee on Infectious Diseases.* 26th ed. Elk Grove Village, IL: American Academy of Pediatrics; 2003.
3. Nelson JD, Bradley JS, eds. *Pocketbook of Pediatric Antimicrobial Therapy.* 14th ed. Baltimore, MD: Williams & Wilkins; 2000-2001.
4. McCracken GH Jr, Nelson JD, eds. *Antimicrobial Therapy for Newborns: Practical Application.* 2nd ed. New York, NY: Grune and Stratton; 1983.
5. Rhodes KH, Henry NK. Antibiotic therapy for severe infections in infants and children. Mayo Clin Proc 1992;67:59-68.
6. Leventhal JM, Silken AB. Oxacillin-induced neutropenia in children. *J Pediatr.* 1976; 89:769-771.
7. Howrie DL, Felix C, Wollman M, et al. Metoclopramide as an antiemetic agent in pediatric oncology patients. *Drug Intell Clin Pharm.* 1986;20:122-124.
8. McCracken GH, Eichenwald HF. Antimicrobial therapy: therapeutic recommendations and a review of newer drugs. Part I. Therapy of infectious conditions. *J Pediatr.* 1974;85:297-312.
9. Bulger RJ, Lindholm DD, Murray JS, et al. Effect of uremia on methicillin and oxacillin blood levels. *JAMA.* 1964;187:319-322.
10. American Society of Health-System Pharmacists. American Hospital Formulary System. Available at: http://ahfsfirst.firstdatabank.com/AHFSfirst/NSAHFSFirstSearchmain.asp. Accessed July 9, 2006.
11. Trissel LA, ed. *Handbook on Injectable Drugs.* 13th ed. [CD-ROM version 1.5]. Bethesda, MD: American Society of Health-System Pharmacists; 2005.
12. Klein JO, Sabath LD, Steinhauer BW, et al. Oxacillin treatment of severe staphylococcal infection. *N Engl J Med.* 1963;269:1215-1225
13. Olans RN, Weiner LB. Reversible oxacillin hepatotoxicity. *J Pediatr.* 1976;89:835-838.
14. Oxacillin [package insert]. Bloomfield, CO: Sandoz Inc; January 2004.
15. Dahlgren AF. Adverse drug reactions in home care patients receiving nafcillin or oxacillin. *Am J Health-Syst Pharm.* 1997;54:1176-1179.
16. Stewart GT. Cross allergenicity of penicillin G and related substances. *Lancet.* 1962;1:509-510.
17. Grieco MH. Cross-allergenicity of the penicillins and the cephalosporins. *Arch Intern Med.* 1967;119:141-146.
18. Saxon A. Immediate hypersensitivity reactions to B-lactam antibiotics. *Rev Infect Dis.* 1983;5(suppl 2):S368-S378.
19. Sher TH. Penicillin hypersensitivity—a review. In: Symposium on anti-infective therapy I. Speck WT, Blummer JL, eds. *Pediatr Clin North Am.* 1983;30:161-177.
20. McLaughlin JE, Reeves DS. Clinical and laboratory evidence for inactivation of gentamicin by carbenicillin. *Lancet.*1971;1(7693):261-264.
21. Riff LJ, Jackson GG. Laboratory and clinical conditions for gentamicin inactivation by carbenicillin. *Arch Intern Med.* 1972;130:887-891.

References

22. Manian FA, Stone WJ, Alford RH. Adverse antibiotic effects associated with renal insufficiency. *Rev Infect Dis.* 1990;12:236-249.
23. Davies M, Morgan JR, Anand C. Interactions of carbenicillin and ticarcillin with gentamicin. *Antimicrob Agents Chemother.* 1975;7:431-434.
24. Weibert R, Keane W, Shapiro F. Carbenicillin inactivation of aminoglycosides in patients with severe renal failure. *Trans Amer Soc Artif Int Organs.* 1976;22:439-443.

Palivizumab

1. Groothius JR. Safety of palivizumab in preterm infants 29 to 32 weeks' gestational age without chronic lung disease to prevent serious respiratory syncytial virus infection. *Eur J Clin Microbiol Infect Dis.* 2003;22:414-417.
2. Null D, Pllara B, Dennehy PH, et al. Safety and immunogenicity of palivizumab (Synagis) administered for two seasons. *Pediatr Infect Dis J.* 2005;24:1021-1023.
3. Groothuis JR. Safety and tolerance of palivizumab administration in a large northern hemisphere trial. *Pediatr Infect Dis J.* 2001;20:628-630.
4. The IMpact-RSV Study Group. Palivizumab, a humanized respiratory syncytial virus monoclonal antibody, reduces hospitalization from respiratory syncytial virus infection in high-risk infants. *Pediatrics.* 1998;102:531-537.
5. Palivizumab [package insert]. Gaithersburg, MD: Medimmune Inc; July 23, 2004.
6. Saez-Llorens X, Castano E, Null D, et al. Safety and pharmacokinetics of an intramuscular humanized monoclonal antibody to respiratory syncytial virus in premature infants and infants with bronchopulmonary dysplasia. *Pediatr Infect Dis J.* 1998;17:787-791.
7. Siva Subramanian KN, Weisman LE, Rhodes T, et al. Safety, tolerance, and pharmacokinetics of a humanized monoclonal antibody to respiratory syncytial virus in premature infants and infants with bronchopulmonary dysplasia. *Pediatr Infect Dis J.* 1998;17:110-115.
8. Cox RA, Rao P, Brandon-Cox C. The use of palivizumab monoclonal antibody to control an outbreak of respiratory syncytial virus infection in a special care baby unit. *J Hosp Infect.* 2001;48:186-192.
9. Abadesso C, Almeida HI, Virella D, et al. Use of palivizumab to control an outbreak of syncytial respiratory virus in a neonatal intensive care unit. *J Hosp Infect.* 2004;58:38-41.
10. Wu SY, Bonaparte J, Pyati S. Palivizumab use in very premature infants in the neonatal intensive care unit. *Pediatrics.* 2004;114:554-556.
11. Saez-Llorens X, Moreno MT, Ramilo O, et al. Safety and pharmacokinetics of palivizumab therapy in children hospitalized with respiratory syncytial virus infection. *Pediatr Infect Dis J.* 2004;23:707-712.
12. Malley R, DeVincenzo J, Ramilo O. Reduction or respiratory syncytial virus (RSV) in tracheal aspirates in intubated infants by use of humanized monoclonal antibody to RSV F protein. *J Infect Dis.* 1998;178:1555-1561.
13. Feltes TF, Cabalka AK, Meissner C, et al. Palivizumab prophylaxis reduces hospitalization due to respiratory syncytial virus in young children with hemodynamically significant congenital heart disease. *J Pediatr.* 2003;143:532-540.

Pamidronate

1. Lteif AN, Zimmerman D. Biphosphonates for treatment of childhood hypercalcemia. *Pediatrics.* 1998;102:990-993.
2. Profumo RJ, Reese JC, Foy TM, et al. Severe immobilization-induced hypercalcemia in a child after liver transplantation successfully treated with pamidronate. *Transplantation.* 1994;57:301-303.
3. Schmid I, Stachel D, Schon C, et al. Pamidronate and calcitonin as therapy of acute cancer-related hypercalcemia in children. *Klin Padiatr.* 2001;213:30-34.
4. De Schepper J, de Pont S, Smitz J, et al. Metabolic disturbances after a single dose of 30 mg pamidronate for leukaemia-associated hypercalcemia in a 11-year-old boy. *Eur J Pediatr.* 1999;158:765-766.
5. Khan N, Licata A, Rogers D. Intravenous bisphosphonate for hypercalcemia accompanying subcutaneous fat necrosis: a novel treatment approach. *Clin Pediatr.* 2001;40:217-219.
6. Attard TM, Dhawan A, Kaufman SS, et al. Use of disodium pamidronate in children with hypercalcemia awaiting liver transplantation. *Pediatr Transplant.* 1998;2:157-159.
7. Boudailliez BR, Pautard BJ, Sebert JL, et al. Leukaemia-associated hypercalcemia in a 10-year-old boy: effectiveness of aminohydroxypropylidene biphosphonate. *Pediatr Nephrol.* 1990;4:510-511.
8. Sellers E, Sharma A, Rodd C. The use of pamidronate in three children with renal disease. *Pediatr Nephrol.* 1998;12:778-781.
9. Glorieux FH, Bishop NJ, Plotkin H, et al. Cyclic administration of pamidronate in children with severe osteogenesis imperfecta. *N Engl J Med.* 1998;339:947-952.
10. Fujiwara I, Ogawa E, Igarashi Y, et al. Intravenous pamidronate treatment in osteogenesis imperfecta. *Eur J Pediatr.* 1998;157:261-262.
11. Bembi B, Parma A, Bottega M, et al. Intravenous pamidronate treatment in osteogenesis imperfecta. *J Pediatr.* 1997;131:662-665.
12. Astrom E, Soderhall S. Beneficial effect of biphosphonate during five years of treatment of severe osteogenesis imperfecta. *Acta Paediatr.* 1998;87:64-68.
13. Zacharin M, Kanumakala S. Pamidronate treatment of less severe forms of osteogenesis imperfecta in children. *J Pediatr Endocrinol Metabol.* 2004;17:1511-1517.
14. Falk MJ, Heeger S, Lynch KA, et al. Intravenous bisphosphonate therapy in children with osteogenesis imperfecta. *Pediatrics.* 2003;111:573-578.
15. Lee YS, Low SL, Lim LA, et al. Cyclic pamidronate infusion improves bone mineralization and reduces fracture incidence in osteogenesis imperfecta. *Eur J Pediatr.* 2001;160:641-644.
16. Rauch F, Munns C, Land C, Glorieux FH. Pamidronate in children and adolescents with osteogenesis imperfecta: effect of treatment discontinuation. *J Clin Endocrinol Metabol.* 2006;91:1268-1274.
17. Matarazzo P, Lala R, Masi G, et al. Pamidronate treatment in bone fibrous dysplasia in children and adolescents with McCune-Albright syndrome. *J Pediatr Endocrinol Metabol.* 2002;15:929-937.
18. Zacharin M, O'Sullivan M. Intravenous pamidronate treatment of polyostotic fibrous dysplasia associated with the McCune Albright syndrome. *J Pediatr.* 2000;137:403-409.
19. Shaw NJ, White CP, Fraser WB, et al. Osteopenia in cerebral palsy. *Arch Dis Child.* 1994;71:235-238.
20. Henderson RC, Lark RK, Kecskemetby HH, et al. Bisphosphonates to treat osteopenia in children with quadriplegic cerebral palsy: a randomized, placebo-controlled clinical trial. *J Pediatr.* 2002;141:644-651.
21. Acott PD, Wong JA, Lang BA, Crocker JFS. Pamidronate treatment of pediatric fracture patients on chronic steroid therapy. *Pediatr Nephrol.* 2005;20:368-373.
22. Pamidronate disodium injection [package insert]. Bedford, OH: Bedford Laboratories Inc; May 2005.
23. McEvoy GK, ed. *AHFS Drug Information Essentials 2005–06.* Bethesda, MD: American Society of Health-System Pharmacists; 2005.

Pancuronium Bromide

1. American Society of Health-System Pharmacists. American Hospital Formulary System. Available at: http://ahfsfirst.firstdatabank.com/AHFSfirst/NSAHFSFirstSearchmain.asp. Accessed June 26, 2006.
2. Martin LD, Bratton SL, O'Rourke PP. Clinical uses and controversies of neuromuscular blocking agents in infant and children. *Crit Care Med.* 1999;27:1358-1368.
3. Levene MI, Quinn MW. Use of sedatives and muscle relaxants in newborn babies receiving mechanical ventilation. *Arch Dis Child.* 1992;67:870-873.

4. Shaw NJ, Cooke RW, Gill AB, et al. Randomized trial of routine versus selective paralysis during ventilation for neonatal respiratory syndrome. *Arch Dis Child.* 1993;69:479-482.
5. Stark AR, Bascom R, Frantz ID. Muscle relaxation in mechanically ventilated infants. *J Pediatr.* 1979;94:439-433.
6. Perlman JM, Goodman S, Kreusser KL, et al. Reduction in intraventricular hemorrhage by elimination of fluctuating cerebral blood-flow velocity in preterm infants with respiratory distress syndrome. *N Engl J Med.* 1985;312:1353-1357.
7. Runkle B, Bancalari E. Acute cardiopulmonary effects of pancuronium bromide in mechanically ventilated newborn infants. *J Pediatr.* 1984;104:614.
8. Piotrowski A. Comparison of atracurium and pancuronium in mechanically ventilated neonates. *Intensive Care Med.* 1993;19:401-405.
9. Yamamoto T, Baba H, Shiratsuchi T. Clinical experience with pancuronium bromide in infants and children. *Anesth Analg.* 1973;51:919-924.
10. Maunuksela EL, Fattiker RI. Use of pancuronium in children with congenital heart disease. *Anesth Analg.* 1981;60:798-801.
11. Cunliffe M, Lucero VM, McLeod ME, et al. Neuromuscular blockade for rapid tracheal intubation in children: comparison of succinylcholine and pancuronium. *Can Anaesth Soc J.* 1986;33:760-764.
12. Bennett EJ, Daughety MJ, Bowyer DE, et al. Pancuronium bromide: experiences in 100 pediatric patients. *Anesth Analg.* 1971;50:798-807.
13. Aronoff A, Brier M, Bennett W. *The Renal Book, 2002.* Available at: http://www.kdp-baptist.louisville.edu/renalbook/. Accessed June 26, 2006.
14. Somogyi AA, Shanks CA, Triggs EJ. The effect of renal failure on the disposition and the neuromuscular blocking action of pancuronium bromide. *Eur J Clin Pharmacol.* 1977;12:23-29.
15. Nana A, Cardan E, Leitersdorfer T. Pancuronium bromide: its use in asthmatics and patients with liver disease. *Anaesthesia.* 1972;27:154-158.
16. Costakos DT, Blackwell CE, Krauss AN, et al. Aortic root blood flow increases after pancuronium in neonates with hyaline membrane disease. *Crit Care Med.* 1991;19:187-190.
17. Cabal LA, Siassi B, Artel R, et al. Cardiovascular and catecholamine changes after administration of pancuronium in distressed neonates. *Pediatrics.* 1985;75:284-287.
18. Sinha SK, Levene MI. Pancuronium bromide induced joint contractures in the newborn. *Arch Dis Child.* 1984;59:73-75.
19. Mishima S, Yamamura T. Anaphylactoid reaction to pancuronium. *Anesth Analg.* 1984;63:865-866.
20. Hiller JL, Benda GI, Rahatzad M, et al. Benzyl alcohol toxicity: impact on mortality and intraventricular hemorrhage among very low birth weight infants. *Pediatrics.* 1986;77:500-506.
21. American Academy of Pediatrics Committee on Drugs. "Inactive" ingredients in pharmaceutical products: update. *Pediatrics.* 1997;99:268-278.
22. Hall CM, Milligan DWA, Berrington J. Probably adverse reaction to a pharmaceutical excipient. *Arch Dis Child Fetal Neonatal Ed.* 2004;89:F184.
23. Grant JA, Bilodeau PA, Guernsey BG, et al. Unsuspected benzyl alcohol hypersensitivity. *N Engl J Med.* 1982;306:108.
24. Wilson JP, Solimando DA, Edwards MS. Parenteral benzyl alcohol-induced hypersensitivity reaction. *Drug Intell Clin Pharm.* 1986;20:689-691.
25. Haas JL, Shaefer MS, Miwa LJ, et al. Prolonged paralysis associated with long-term pancuronium use. *Pharmacotherapy.* 1989;9:154-157.
26. Op de Coul AA, Lambregts PC, Koeman J, et al. Neuromuscular complications in patients given pavulon (pancuronium bromide) during artificial ventilation. *Clin Neurol Neurosurg.* 1985;87:17-22.
27. Watling SM, Dasta JF. Prolonged paralysis in intensive care unit patients after the use of neuromuscular blocking agents: a review of the literature. *Crit Care Med.* 1994;22:884-893.
28. Panacek EA, Sherman B. Hydrocortisone and pancuronium bromide: acute myopathy during status asthmaticus. *Crit Care Med.* 1988;16:732.

Pantoprazole

1. *Physicians' Desk Reference.* 60th ed. Montvale, NJ: Thomson PDR; 2006.
2. Litalien C, Theoret Y, Faure C. Pharmacokinetics of proton pump inhibitors in children. *Clin Pharmacokinet.* 2005;44(5):441-466.
3. Ferron G, Schexnayder S, Marshall JD, et al. Pharmacokinetics of IV pantoprazole in pediatric patients. [abstract PII-30]. *Clin Pharmacol Ther.* 2003;73:P37.
4. Kearns GL, Ferron GM, James LP, et al. Pantoprazole disposition in pediatrics [abstract PII-35]. *Clin Pharmacol Ther.* 2003;73:P38.
5. Madrazo de la Garza A, Dibildox M, Vargas A, et al. Efficacy and safety of oral pantoprazole 20 mg given once daily for reflux esophagitis in children. *J Pediatr Gastroenterol Nutr.* 2003;36(2):261-265.
6. Morgan D. Intravenous proton pump inhibitors in the critical care setting. *Crit Care Med.* 2002;30(6):S369-S372.
7. Metz DC, Amer F, Hunt B, et al. Lansoprazole regimens that sustain intragastric pH >6.0: an evaluation of intermittent oral and continuous intravenous infusion dosages. *Aliment Pharmacol Ther.* 2006;23:985-995.
8. Van Rensburg CJ, Hartmann M, Thorpe A, et al. Intragastric pH during continuous infusion with pantoprazole in patients with bleeding peptic ulcer. *Amer J Gastroenterol.* 2003;98(12):2635-2641.
9. Somberg L, Karlstadt R, Blatcher D, et al. Intermittent intravenous pantoprazole maintains control of gastric pH in intensive care unit patients (abstract). *Am J Gastroenterol.* 2002;97:S42.
10. Devlin JW, Walage LS, Olsen KM. Proton pump inhibitor formulary considerations in the acutely ill. Part 1: pharmacology, pharmacodynamics, and available formulations. *Ann Pharmacother.* 2005;39:1667-1677.
11. Sennaroglu E, Karakan S, Kayatas M, et al. Reversible edema in a male patient taking parenteral pantoprazole infusion for pyloric stenosis. *Dig Dis Sci.* 2006;51(1):121-122.
12. Canani RB, Cirillo P, Roggero P, at al. Therapy with gastric acidity inhibitors increases the risk of acute gastroenteritis and community-acquired pneumonia in children. *Pediatrics.* 2006;117:817-820.

Papaverine HCl

1. Griffin MP, Siadaty MS. Papaverine prolongs patency of peripheral arterial catheters in neonates. *J Pediatr.* 2005;146:62-65.
2. Heulitt MJ, Farrington EA, O'Shea TM, et al. Double-blind randomized controlled trial of papaverine-containing solutions to prevent failure of arterial catheters in pediatric patients. *Crit Care Med.* 1993;21:825-829.
3. Young TE, Mangum B. *Neofax®: A Manual of Drugs Used in Neonatal Care.* 18th ed. Raleigh, NC: Acorn Publishing; 2005.
4. Boris JR, Harned RK, Logan LA, et al. The use of papaverine in arterial sheaths to prevent loss of femoral artery pulse in pediatric cardiac catheterization. *Pediatr Cardiol.* 1998;19:390-397.
5. AHFSfirst™ Web version 2.03. American Society of Health-System Pharmacists, First Databank, Inc. 2002. Accessed June 30, 2006.
6. Papaverine hydrochloride injection [USP package insert]. Shirley, NY: American Reagent Laboratories Inc; January 2003.
7. Trissel LA. *Handbook on Injectable Drugs.* 13th ed. Bethesda, MD: American Society of Health-System Pharmacists; 2005.
8. Thomson Healthcare Inc. Micromedex® Healthcare Series. Available at: http//www.micromedex.com. Accessed March 23, 2006.

References

Peginterferon Alfa (alpha-2a, alpha-2b)

1. Kowala-Paskowska A, Sluzewski W, Figlerowicz M, et al. Factors influencing early virological response in children with chronic hepatitis C treated with pegylated interferon and ribavirin. *Hep Res.* 2005;32:224-226.
2. Wirth S, Peper-Boustani H, Lang T, et al. Peginterferon alpha-2b plus ribavirin treatment in children and adolescents with chronic hepatitis C. *Hepatology.* 2005;41:1013-1018.
3. PEG-Intron [package insert]. Kenilworth, NJ: Schering Corporation; February 2005.
4. Castellino S, Lensing S, Riely C, et al. The epidemiology of chronic hepatitis C infection in survivors of childhood cancer: an update of the St Jude Children's Research Hospital hepatitis C seropositive cohort. *Blood.* 2004;103:2460-2466.
5. PEGASYS [package insert]. Nutley, NJ: Hoffman-La Roche Inc; May 2005.
6. American Academy of Pediatrics Committee on Drugs. "Inactive" ingredients in pharmaceutical products: update. *Pediatrics.* 1997;99:268-278.
7. Hall CM, Milligan DWA, Berrington J. Probably adverse reaction to a pharmaceutical excipient. *Arch Dis Child Fetal Neonatal Ed.* 2004;89: F184.
8. Hiller JL, Benda GI, Rahatzad M, et al. Benzyl alcohol toxicity: impact on mortality and intraventricular hemorrhage among very low birth weight infants. *Pediatrics.* 1986;77:500-506.
9. Grant JA, Bilodeau PA, Guernsey BG, et al. Unsuspected benzyl alcohol hypersensitivity. *N Engl J Med.* 1982;306:108.
10. Wilson JP, Solimando DA, Edwards MS. Parenteral benzyl alcohol-induced hypersensitivity reaction. *Drug Intell Clin Pharm.* 1986;20:689-691.

Penicillin G Potassium/Sodium

1. Department of Health and Human Services, Centers for Disease Control and Prevention (CDC). Sexually transmitted diseases treatment guidelines—2002. Available at: http://www.phppo.cdc.gov/cdcRecommends/showarticle.asp?a_artid=1653++++&TopNum=50&CallPg=Adv#CongSyphilis. Accessed May 11, 2006.
2. American Academy of Pediatrics. In: Pickering LK, ed. *2003 Red Book: Report of the Committee on Infectious Diseases.* 26th ed. Elk Grove Village, IL: American Academy of Pediatrics; 2003:701,709.
3. Ikeda MK, Jenson HB. Evaluation and treatment of congenital syphilis. *J Pediatr.* 1990;117:843-852.
4. Azimi PH, Janner D, Berne P, et al. Concentrations of procaine and aqueous penicillin in the cerebrospinal fluid of infants treated for congenital syphilis. *J Pediatr.* 1994;124:649-653.
5. Prober CG, Stevenson DK, Benitz WE. The use of antibiotics in neonates weighing less than 1200 grams. *Pediatr Infect Dis J.* 1990;9:111-121.
6. McCracken GH Jr, Nelson JD, eds. *Antimicrobial Therapy for Newborns: Practical Application.* 2nd ed. New York, NY: Grune and Stratton;1983:16.
7. McCracken GH, Ginsberg C, Chrane DF, et al. Clinical pharmacology of penicillin in newborn infants. *J Pediatr.* 1973;82:692-698.
8. Tunkel AR, Hartman BJ, Kaplan SL, et al. Practice guidelines for the management of bacterial meningitis. *Clin Infect Dis.* 2004;39:1267-1284.
9. Baddour LM, Wilson WR, Bayer AS, et al. Infective endocarditis: diagnosis, antimicrobial therapy, and management of complications: a statement for healthcare professionals from the Committee on Rheumatic Fever, Endocarditis, and Kawasaki Disease, Council on Cardiovascular Disease in the Young, and the Councils on Clinical Cardiology, Stroke, and Cardiovascular Surgery and Anesthesia, American Heart Association: endorsed by the Infectious Diseases Society of America. *Circulation.* 2005;111:e394-e434.
10. Aronoff A, Brier M, Bennett W. *The Renal Book, 2002*. Available at: http://www.kdp-baptist.louisville.edu/renalbook/. Accessed May 16, 2006.
11. Penicillin. In: Kucer A, Crowe SM, Grayson ML, Hoy JF, eds. *The Use of Antibiotics: A Clinical Review of Antibacterial, Antifungal and Antiviral Drugs.* 5th ed. Boston, MA: Butterworth Heinemann; 1997;3-21.
12. Stumpf JL. Cardiac arrest apparently induced by penicillin. *Drug Intell Clin Pharm.* 1987;21:292.
13. Trissel LA, ed. *Handbook on Injectable Drugs.* 13th ed. [CD-ROM version 1.5]. Bethesda, MD: American Society of Health-System Pharmacists; 2005.
14. Bierman CW, Van Arsdel PP Jr. Penicillin allergy in children: the role of immunological tests in its diagnosis. *J Allergy Clin Immunol.* 1969; 43:267-272.
15. Neftel KA, Walti M, Spengler H, et al. Effect of storage of penicillin-G solutions on sensitization to penicillin-G after intravenous administration. *Lancet.* 1982;1:986-988.
16. Pfizer. Pfizerpen® (penicillin G potassium for injection) prescribing information (dated 1987 Apr). In: *Physicians' Desk Reference.* 52nd ed. Montvale, NJ: Medical Economics Company Inc; 1998:2197-2198.
17. Robinson DC, Cookson TL, Frisafe JA. Concentration guidelines for parenteral antibiotics in fluid-restricted patients. *Drug Intell Clin Pharm.* 1987;21:985-989.
18. Inglesby TV, O'Toole T, Henderson DA. et al for the Working Group on Civilian Biodefense. Anthrax as a biological weapon 2002: updated recommendations for management. *JAMA.* 2002;287:2236-2252.
19. Centers for Disease Control and Prevention. Update: Investigation of bioterrorism-related anthrax and interim guidelines for exposure management and antimicrobial therapy, October 2001. *MMWR Morb Mortal Wkly Rep.* 2001;50:909-919.
20. Kurtzman NA, Rogers PW, Harter HR. Neurotoxic reaction to penicillin and carbenicillin. *JAMA.* 1970;214:1320-1321.
21. Smith H, Lerner PI, Weinstein L. Neurotoxicity and massive intravenous therapy with penicillin. A study of possible predisposing factors. *Arch Intern Med.* 1967;120:47-53.
22. American Society of Health-System Pharmacists. American Hospital Formulary System. Available at: http://ahfsfirst.firstdatabank.com/AHFSfirst/NSAHFSFirstSearchmain.asp. Accessed May 16, 2006.

Pentamidine Isethionate

1. American Academy of Pediatrics. In: Pickering LK, ed. *2000 Red Book: Report of the Committee on Infectious Diseases.* 25th ed. Elk Grove Village, IL: American Academy of Pediatrics; 2000.
2. Das VNR, Ranjan A, Sinha AN, et al. A randomized clinical trial of low dosage combination of pentamidine and allopurinol in the treatment of antimony unresponsive cases of visceral leishmaniasis. *J Assoc Physicians India.* 2001;49:605-608.
3. McEvoy GK, ed. *American Hospital Formulary Service Drug Information 2004.* (Version 2.03) Bethesda, MD: American Society of Health-System Pharmacists; 2002.
4. Hughes WT, Price RA, Kim H, et al. Pneumocystis carinii pneumonitis in children with malignancies. *J Pediatr.* 1973;82:404-415.
5. Mofenson LM, Oleske J, Serchuck L, et al. Treating opportunistic infections among HIV-exposed and infected children. *MMWR.* 2004;53(RR-14):1-63.
6. American Academy of Pediatrics, Canadian Paediatric Society Clinical Report. Evaluation and treatment of the human immunodeficiency virus-1-exposed infant. *Pediatrics.* 2004;114:497-505.
7. US Public Health Service (USPHS) and Infectious Diseases Society of America (IDSA) Prevention of Opportunistic Infections Working Group. 2001 USPHS/IDSA guidelines for the prevention of opportunistic infections in persons with human immunodeficiency virus. From the US Department of Health and Human Services HIV/AIDS Information Services (AIDSinfo) website (http://aidsinfo.nih.gov/guidelines). Accessed August 11, 2006.

8. Aronoff A, Brier M, Bennett W. *The Renal Book, 2002.* Available at: http://www.kdp-baptist.louisville.edu/renalbook/. Accessed August 11, 2006.
9. Trissel LA. *Handbook on Injectable Drugs.* 13th ed. Bethesda, MD: American Society of Health-System Pharmacists; 2005.
10. Drake S, Lampasona V, Nicks HL, et al. Pentamidine isethionate in the treatment of Pneumocystis carinii pneumonia. *Clin Pharm.* 1985;4:507-516.
11. Loescher T, Loeschke K, Niebel J. Severe ventricular arrhythmia during pentamidine treatment of AIDS associated Pneumocystis carinii pneumonia. *Infection.* 1987; 15:455.
12. Miller HC. Cardiac arrest after intravenous pentamidine in an infant. *Pediatr Infect Dis J.* 1993;12:694-696.
13. Harel Y, Scott WA, Szeinberg A, et al. Pentamidine-induced torsades de pointes. *Pediatr Infect Dis J.* 1993;12:692-694.
14. Trivedi CD, Pitchumoni CS. Drug-induced pancreatitis. An update. *J Clin Gastroenterol.* 2005;39:709-716.

Pentobarbital Sodium

1. Slovis TL, Parks C, Reneau D, et al. Pediatric sedation: short-term effects. *Pediatr Radiol.* 1993;23:345-348.
2. Pereira JK, Burrows PE, Richards HM, et al. Comparison of sedation regimens for pediatric outpatient CT. *Pediatr Radiol.* 1993;23:341-344.
3. Bloomfield EL, Masaryk TJ, Caplin A, et al. Intravenous sedation for MR imaging of the brain and spine in children: pentobarbital versus propofol. *Radiology.* 1993;186:93-97.
4. Merrick PA, Case BJ, Jagjivan B, et al. Care of pediatric patients sedated with pentobarbital sodium in MRI. *Pediatr Nurs.* 1991;17:34-38.
5. Flood RG, Krauss B. Procedural sedation and analgesia for children in the emergency department. *Emerg Med Clin North Am.* 2003;21:121-139.
6. Malviya S, Voepel-Lewis T, Tait AR, et al. Pentobarbital vs. chloral hydrate for sedation of children undergoing MRI: efficacy and recovery characteristics. *Paediatr Anaesth.* 2004;14:589-595.
7. Mason KP, Zurakowski D, Connor L et al. Infant sedation for MR imaging and CT: oral versus intravenous pentobarbital. *Radiology.* 2004;233:723-728.
8. Sanborn PA, Michna E, Zurakowski D, et al. Adverse cardiovascular and respiratory events during sedation of pediatric patients for imaging examinations. *Radiology.* 2005;237:288-294.
9. Tobias JD, Deshpande JK, Pietsch JB, et al. Pentobarbital sedation for patients in the pediatric intensive care unit. *S Med J.* 1995;88:290-294.
10. Tobias JD. Sedation and analgesia in paediatric intensive care units. *Pediatr Drugs.* 1999;1:109-125.
11. Schaible DH, Cupit GC, Rocci ML. High-dose pentobarbital pharmacokinetics in hypothermic brain-injured children. *J Pediatr.* 1982;100:655-660.
12. Rockoff MA, Marshall LF, Shapiro HM. High-dose barbiturate therapy in humans: a clinical review of 60 patients. *Ann Neurol.* 1979; 6:194-199.
13. Holmes GL, Riviello JJ. Midazolam and pentobarbital for refractory status epilepticus. *Pediatr Neurol.* 1999;20:259-264.
14. Marik PE, Varon J. The management of status epilepticus. *Chest.* 2004;126:582-591.
15. Lowenstein DH, Alldredge BK. Status epilepticus. *New Engl J Med.* 1998;338:970-976.
16. Claassen J, Hirsch LJ, Emerson RG, Mayer SA. Treatment of refractory status epilepticus with pentobarbital, propofol, or midazolam: a systematic review. *Epilepsia.* 2002;43:146-153.
17. Pentobarbital sodium [package insert]. North Chicago, IL: Ovation Pharmaceuticals; July 2003.
18. Kain ZN, Gaal DJ, Kain T, et al. A first-pass cost analysis of propofol versus barbiturates for children undergoing magnetic resonance imaging. *Anesth Analg.* 1994;79:1102-1106.
19. Wermeling DP, Blouin RA, Porter WH, et al. Pentobarbital pharmacokinetics in patients with severe head injury. *Drug Intell Clin Pharm.* 1987;21:459-463.
20. Quandt CM, de los Reyes RA. Pharmacologic management of acute intracranial hypertension. *Drug Intell Clin Pharm.* 1984;18:105-112.
21. Trissel LA, ed. *Handbook on Injectable Drugs.* 13th ed. [CD-ROM version 1.5]. Bethesda, MD: American Society of Health-System Pharmacists; 2005.
22. American Society of Health-System Pharmacists. American Hospital Formulary System. Available at: http://ahfsfirst.firstdatabank.com/AHFSfirst/NSAHFSFirstSearchmain.asp. Accessed May 10, 2006.
23. Louis S, Kutt H, McDowell F. The cardiocirculatory changes caused by intravenous Dilantin and its solvent. *Am Heart J.* 1967;74:523-529.
24. American Academy of Pediatrics Committee on Drugs. "Inactive" ingredients in pharmaceutical products: update. *Pediatrics.* 1997;99:268-278.
25. Glasgow AM, Boeckx RL, Miller MK, et al. Hyper-osmolality in small infants due to propylene glycol. *Pediatrics.* 1983;72:353-355.
26. MacDonald MG, Getson PR, Glasgow AM, et al. Propylene glycol: increased incidence of seizures in low birth weight infants. *Pediatrics.* 1987;79:622-625.
27. Kim SJ, Lee DY, Kim JS. Neurologic outcomes of pediatric epileptic patients with pentobarbital coma. *Pediatr Neurol.* 2001;25:217-220.
28. Young RS, Ropper AH, Hawkes D, et al. Pentobarbital in refractory status epilepticus. *Pediatr Pharmacol.* 1983;3:62-67.
29. Kinoshita H, Nakagawa E, Hanaoka S, et al. Pentobarbital therapy for status epilepticus in children: Timing of tapering. *Pediatr Neurol.* 1995;13:164-168.
30. Butte MJ, Dodson B, Dioun A. Pentobarbital desensitization in a 3-month-old child. *Allergy Asthma Proc.* 2004;25:225-227.

Phenobarbital Sodium

1. Kumar R, Narang A, Kumar P, et al. Phenobarbitone prophylaxis for neonatal jaundice in babies with birth weight 1000–1499 grams. *Indian Pediatr.* 2002;39:945-951.
2. Murki S, Dutta S, Narang A, et al. randomized, triple-blind, placebo-controlled trial of prophylactic oral phenobarbital to reduce the need for phototherapy in G6PD-deficient neonates. *J Perinato.* 2005;25:325-330.
3. Wallin A, Boreus LO. Phenobarbital prophylaxis for hyperbilirubinemia in preterm infants. A controlled study of bilirubin disappearance and infant behavior. *Acta Paediatr Scand.* 1984;73:488-497.
4. Anwar M, Valdivieso J, Hiatt IM, et al. The course of hyperbilirubinemia in the very low birth weight infant treated with phenobarbital. *J Perinatol.* 1987;7:145-148.
5. Osborn DA, Cole MJ, Jeffery HE. Opiate treatment for opiate withdrawal in newborn infants. *Cochrane Database Syst Rev.* 2002;(3):CD002059.
6. Osborn DA, Jeffery HE, Cole MJ. Sedatives for opiate withdrawal in newborn infants. *Cochrane Database Syst Rev.* 2002;(3):CD002053.
7. Finnegan L, Kandall SR. Neonatal abstinence syndrome. In: Yaffe SJ, Aranda JV, eds. *Neonatal and Pediatric Pharmacology.* 3rd ed. Philadelphia, PA: Lippincott Williams & Wilkins; 2005:848-857.
8. Evans DJ, Levene MI. Anticonvulsants for preventing mortality and morbidity in full term newborns with perinatal asphyxia. *Cochrane Database Syst Rev.* 2001;(3):CD001240.
9. Hall RT, Hall FK, Daily DK. High-dose phenobarbital therapy in term newborns infants with severe perinatal asphyxia: a randomized, prospective study with three-year follow-up. *J Pediatr.* 1998;132:345-348.
10. Nahata MC, Masuoka T, Edwards RC. Developmental aspects of phenobarbital dosage requirements in newborn infants with seizures. *J Perinatol.* 1988;8:318-320.
11. Gal P, Toback J, Erkan NV, et al. The influence of asphyxia on phenobarbital dosing requirements in neonates. *Dev Pharmacol Ther.* 1984;7:145-152.

References

12. Painter MJ, Pippenger C, MacDonald H, et al. Phenobarbital and diphenylhydantoin levels in neonates with seizures. *J Pediatr.* 1978;92:315-319.
13. Gal P, Toback J, Boer HR, et al. Efficacy of phenobarbital monotherapy in treatment of neonatal seizures—relationship to blood levels. *Neurology.* 1982;32:1401-1404.
14. Suzuki Y, Cox S, Hayes J, et al. Phenobarbital doses necessary to achieve 'therapeutic' concentration in children. *Dev Pharmacol The.* 1991;17:79-87.
15. Davis AG, Mutchie KD, Thompson JA, et al. Once-daily dosing with phenobarbital in children with seizure disorders. *Pediatrics.* 1981;68:824-827.
16. Walson PD, Mimaki T, Curless R, et al. Once daily doses of phenobarbital in children. *J Pediatr.* 1980;97:303-305.
17. Zupanc ML. Neonatal seizures. *Pediatr Clin North Am.* 2004;51(4):961-978.
18. Pippenger CE, Rosen TS. Phenobarbital plasma levels in neonates. *Clin Perinatol.* 1975;2:111-115.
19. Gilman JT, Gal P, Duchowny MS, et al. Rapid sequential phenobarbital treatment of neonatal seizures. *Pediatrics.* 1989;83:674-678.
20. Donn SM, Grasela TH, Goldstein GW. Safety of a higher loading dose of phenobarbital in the term newborn. *Pediatrics.* 1985;75:1061-1064.
21. Lowenstein DH, Alldredge BK. Status epilepticus. *N Engl J Med.* 1998;338:970-976.
22. American Academy of Pediatrics Committee on Drugs. Emergency drug doses for infants and children. *Pediatrics.* 1998;101:e1-e11.
23. Appleton R, Choonara I, Martland T, et al. The treatment of convulsive status epilepticus in children. The Status Epilepticus Working Party, Members of the Status Epilepticus Working Party. *Arch Dis Child.* 2000;83:415-419.
24. Crawford TO, Mitchell WG, Fishman LS, et al. Very-high-dose phenobarbital for refractory status epilepticus in children. *Neurology.* 1988;38:1035-1040.
25. Lee WK, Liu KT, Young BW. Very-high-dose phenobarbital for childhood refractory status epilepticus. *Pediatr Neurol.* 2006;34:63-65.
26. Aronoff A, Brier M, Bennett W. *The Renal Book, 2002.* Available at: http://www.kdp-baptist.louisville.edu/renalbook/. Accessed May 6, 2006.
27. Porto I, John EG, Heilliczer J. Removal of phenobarbital during continuous cycling peritoneal dialysis in a child. *Pharmacotherapy.* 1997; 17:832-835.
28. Elliott ES, Buck ML. Phenobarbital dosing and pharmacokinetics in a neonate receiving extracorporeal membrane oxygenation. *Ann Pharmacother.* 1999;33:419-422.
29. Dagan O, Kleini J, Gruenwald C, et al. Preliminary studies of the effects of extracorporeal membrane oxygenator on the disposition of common pediatric drugs. *Ther Drug Monitor.* 1993;15:263-266.
30. WD. Status epilepticus. *Pediatr Clin North Am.* 1989;36:383-393.
31. Trissel LA, ed. *Handbook on Injectable Drugs.* 13th ed. [CD-ROM version 1.5]. Bethesda, MD: American Society of Health-System Pharmacists; 2005.
32. Lehy VT, Chugami HT, Aranda JV. Anticonvulsants. In: Yaffe SJ, Aranda JV, eds. *Neonatal and Pediatric Pharmacology*. 3rd ed. Philadelphia, PA: Lippincott Williams & Wilkins; 2005:504-519.
33. Phenobarbital sodium injection USP [package insert]. Cherry Hill, NJ: Elkins-Sinn Inc; August 1987.
34. American Academy of Pediatrics Committee on Drugs. "Inactive" ingredients in pharmaceutical products: update. *Pediatrics.* 1997;99:268-278.
35. Hall CM, Milligan DWA, Berrington J. Probably adverse reaction to a pharmaceutical excipient. *Arch Dis Child Fetal Neonatal Ed.* 2004;89: F184.
36. Hiller JL, Benda GI, Rahatzad M, et al. Benzyl alcohol toxicity: impact on mortality and intraventricular hemorrhage among very low birth weight infants. *Pediatrics.* 1986;77:500-506.
37. Grant JA, Bilodeau PA, Guernsey BG, et al. Unsuspected benzyl alcohol hypersensitivity. *N Engl J Med.* 1982;306:108.
38. Wilson JP, Solimando DA, Edwards MS. Parenteral benzyl alcohol-induced hypersensitivity reaction. *Drug Intell Clin Pharm.* 1986;20:689-691.
39. Louis S, Kutt H, McDowell F. The cardiocirculatory changes caused by intravenous Dilantin and its solvent. *Am Heart J.* 1967;74:523-529.
40. Glasgow AM, Boeckx RL, Miller MK, et al. Hyper-osmolality in small infants due to propylene glycol. *Pediatrics.* 1983;72:353-355.
41. MacDonald MG, Getson PR, Glasgow AM, et al. Propylene glycol: increased incidence of seizures in low birth weight infants. *Pediatrics.* 1987; 79:622-625.
42. Anderson GD. A mechanistic approach to antiepileptic drug interactions. *Ann Pharmacother.* 1998;32:554-563.

Phenytoin Sodium

1. Lewis RJ, Yee L, Inkelis SH, Gilmore D. Clinical predictors of post-traumatic seizures in children with head trauma. *Ann Emer Med.* 1993;22:1114-1118.
2. Tilford JM, Simpson PM, Yeh TS, et al. Variation in therapy and outcome for pediatric head trauma patients. *Crit Care Med.* 2001;29:1056-1061.
3. Adelson PD, Bratton SL, Carney NA, et al. Guidelines for the acute medical management of severe traumatic brain injury in infants, children, and adolescents. Chapter 19. The role of anti-seizure prophylaxis following severe pediatric traumatic brain injury. *Pediatr Crit Care Med.* 2003;4(3 suppl):S72-S75.
4. Stowe CD, Lee KR, Storgion SA, et al. Altered phenytoin pharmacokinetics in children with severe, acute traumatic brain injury. Status epilepticus. *J Clin Pharmacol.* 2000;40:1452-1461.
5. Griebel ML, Kearns GL, Fisher DH, et al. Phenytoin protein binding in pediatric patients with acute traumatic injury. *Crit Care Med.* 1990;18:385-391.
6. Painter MJ, Pippenger C, MacDonald H, et al. Phenobarbital and diphenylhydantoin levels in neonates with seizures. *J Pediatr.* 1978;92:315-319.
7. Loughnan PM, Greenwald A, Purton W, et al. Pharmacokinetic observation of phenytoin disposition in the newborn and young infant. *Arch Dis Child.* 1977;52:302-309.
8. Bourgeois BFD, Dodson WE. Phenytoin elimination in newborns. *Neurology.* 1983;33:173-178.
9. Leff RD, Fisher LJ, Roberts RJ. Phenytoin metabolism in infants following intravenous and oral administration. *Dev Pharmacol Ther.* 1986;9:217-223.
10. Lehr VT, Chugani HT, Aranda JV. Anticonvulsants. In: Yaffe SJ, Aranda JV, eds. *Neonatal and Pediatric Pharmacology.* 3rd ed. Philadelphia, PA: Lippincott Williams & Wilkins; 2005:504-519.
11. Curless RG, Walson PD, Carter DE. Phenytoin kinetics in children. *Neurology.* 1976;26:715-720.
12. Dodson WE. Nonlinear kinetics of phenytoin in children. *Neurology.* 1982;32:42-48.
13. Zalzstein W, Gorodischer R. Cardiovascular Drugs. In: Yaffe SJ, Aranda JV, eds. *Neonatal and Pediatric Pharmacology.* 3rd ed. Philadelphia, PA: Lippincott Williams & Wilkins; 2005:574-594.
14. American Society of Health-System Pharmacists. American Hospital Formulary System. Available at: http://ahfsfirst.firstdatabank.com/AHFSfirst/NSAHFSFirstSearchmain.asp. Accessed July 2, 2006.
15. Phelps SJ, Baldree LA, Boucher BA, et al. Neuropsychiatric toxicity of phenytoin. Importance of monitoring phenytoin levels. *Clin Pediatr.* 1993;32:107-110.
16. Liponi DL, Winter ME, Tozer TN. Renal function and therapeutic concentrations of phenytoin. *Neurology.* 1984;34:395-397.
17. Abernethy DR, Greenblatt DJ. Phenytoin disposition in obesity: determination of loading dose. *Arch Neuro.* 1985;42:468-471.
18. Drugs for epilepsy. *Med Lett Drugs Ther.* 1983;25:81-84.
19. American Academy of Pediatrics Committee on Drugs. Emergency drug doses for infants and children. *Pediatrics.* 1998;101:e1-e11.

20. Shields WD. Status epilepticus. *Pediatr Clin North Am.* 1989;36:383-393.
21. Trissel LA, ed. *Handbook on Injectable Drugs.* 13th ed. [CD-ROM version 1.5]. Bethesda, MD: American Society of Health-System Pharmacists; 2005.
22. Pagliaro LA, Pagliaro AM, eds. *Problems in Pediatric Drug Therapy.* 2nd ed. Hamilton, IL: Drug Intelligence Publications Inc; 1987.
23. Koren G, Brand N, Halkin H, et al. Kinetics of intravenous phenytoin in children. *Pediatr Pharmacol.* 1984;4:31-38.
24. Wheless JW. Pediatric use of intravenous and intramuscular phenytoin: lessons learned. *J Child Neurol.* 1998;13:S11-14, discussion S30-32.
25. Earnest MP, Marx JA, Drury LR. Complications of intravenous phenytoin for acute treatment of seizures. Recommendations for usage. *JAMA.* 1983;249:762-765.
26. American Academy of Pediatrics Committee on Drugs. "Inactive" ingredients in pharmaceutical products: update. *Pediatrics.* 1997;99:268-278.
27. Hall CM, Milligan DWA, Berrington J. Probably adverse reaction to a pharmaceutical excipient. *Arch Dis Child Fetal Neonatal Ed.* 2004;89:F184.
28. Hiller JL, Benda GI, Rahatzad M, et al. Benzyl alcohol toxicity: impact on mortality and intraventricular hemorrhage among very low birth weight infants. *Pediatrics.* 1986;77:500-506.
29. Grant JA, Bilodeau PA, Guernsey BG, et al. Unsuspected benzyl alcohol hypersensitivity. *N Engl J Med.* 1982;306:108.
30. Wilson JP, Solimando DA, Edwards MS. Parenteral benzyl alcohol-induced hypersensitivity reaction. *Drug Intell Clin Pharm.* 1986;20:689-691.
31. Louis S, Kutt H, McDowell F. The cardiocirculatory changes caused by intravenous Dilantin and its solvent. *Am Heart J.* 1967;74:523-529.
32. Glasgow AM, Boeckx RL, Miller MK, et al. Hyper-osmolality in small infants due to propylene glycol. *Pediatrics.* 1983;72:353-355.
33. MacDonald MG, Getson PR, Glasgow AM, et al. Propylene glycol: increased incidence of seizures in low birth weight infants. *Pediatrics.* 1987;79:622-625.
34. Anderson GD. A mechanistic approach to antiepileptic drug interactions. *Ann Pharmacother.* 1998;32:554-563.

Physostigmine Salicylate

1. Physostigmine salicylate injection [package insert]. Decatur, IL: Taylor Pharmaceuticals; August 1998.
2. Rumack BH. Anticholinergic poisoning: treatment with physostigmine. *Pediatrics.* 1973;52:449-451.
3. Shannon M. Toxicology reviews: physostigmine. *Pediatr Emergency Care.* 1998;14:224-226.
4. Bowden CA, Krenzelok EP. Clinical applications of commonly used contemporary antidotes. *Drug Safety.* 1997;16:9-47.
5. Wright SP. Usefulness of physostigmine in imipramine poisoning. *Clin Pediatr.* 1976;15:1123-1128.
6. Ceha LJ, Presperin C, Young E, et al. Anticholinergic toxicity from Nightshade berry poisoning responsive to physostigmine. *J Emerg Med.* 1997;15:65-69.
7. Van Herreweghe I, Mertens K, Maes V, et al. Orphenadrine poisoning in a child: clinical and analytical data. *Intensive Care Med.* 1999;25:1134-1136.
8. Arnold SM, Arnholz D, Garyfallou GT, et al. Two siblings poisoned with diphenhydramine: a case of fictitious disorder by proxy. *Ann Emerg Med.* 1998;32:256-259.
9. Tobis J, Das BN. Cardiac complications in amitriptyline poisoning. Successful treatment with physostigmine. *JAMA.* 1976;235:1474-1476.
10. Smolinske SC. Anticholinergic poisoning. In: Rumack BH, ed. *Poisondex Information System.* Vol. 84. Denver, CO: MICROMEDEX Inc; 1974-2000.
11. Physostigmine. Tricyclic antidepressant poisoning. In: Rumack BH, ed. *Poisondex Information System.* 105th ed. Denver, CO: MICROMEDEX Inc; 1974-2000.
12. Stern TA. Continuous infusion of physostigmine in anticholinergic delirium: case report. *J Clin Psychiatry.* 1983;44:463-464.
13. American Academy of Pediatrics Committee on Drugs. "Inactive" ingredients in pharmaceutical products: update. *Pediatrics.* 1997;99:268-278.
14. Hall CM, Milligan DWA, Berrington J. Probably adverse reaction to a pharmaceutical excipient. *Arch Dis Child Fetal Neonatal Ed.* 2004;89:F184.
15. Hiller JL, Benda GI, Rahatzad M, et al. Benzyl alcohol toxicity: impact on mortality and intraventricular hemorrhage among very low birth weight infants. *Pediatrics.* 1986;77:500-506.
16. Grant JA, Bilodeau PA, Guernsey BG, et al. Unsuspected benzyl alcohol hypersensitivity. *N Engl J Med.* 1982;306:108.
17. Wilson JP, Solimando DA, Edwards MS. Parenteral benzyl alcohol-induced hypersensitivity reaction. *Drug Intell Clin Pharm.* 1986;20:689-691.
18. Lester MR. Sulfite sensitivity: significance in human health. *J Am Col Nutr.* 1995;14:229-232.
19. Smolinske SC. Review of parenteral sulfite reactions. *J Toxicol Clin Toxicol.* 1992;30:597-606.
20. Snyder BD, Blonde L, McWhirter WR. Reversal of amitriptyline intoxication by physostigmine. *JAMA.* 1974;230:1433-1434.
21. Pentel P, Peterson CD. Asystole complicating physostigmine treatment of tricyclic antidepressant overdose. *Ann Emerg Med.* 1980;9:588-590.
22. Schultz U, Idelberger R, Rossaint R, et al. Central anticholinergic syndrome in a child undergoing circumcision. *Acta Anaesthesiol Scand.* 2002;46:224-226.
23. Kulka PJ, Toker H, Heim J, et al. Suspected central anticholinergic syndrome in a 6-week-old infant. *Anesth Analg.* 2004;99:1376-1378.

Piperacillin Sodium

1. Placzek M, Whitelaw A, Want S, et al. Piperacillin in early neonatal infection. *Arch Dis Child.* 1983;58:1006-1009.
2. Kacet N, Roussel-Delvallez M, Gremillet C, et al. Pharmacokinetic study of piperacillin in newborns relating to gestational and postnatal age. *Pediatr Infect Dis. J.* 1992;11:365-369.
3. American Academy of Pediatrics. In: Pickering LK, ed. *Red Book: 2003 Report of the Committee on Infectious Diseases.* 26th ed. Elk Grove Village, IL: American Academy of Pediatrics; 2003.
4. Wilson CB, Koup JR, Opheim KE, et al. Piperacillin pharmacokinetics in pediatric patients. *Antimicrob Agents Chemother.* 1982;22:442-447.
5. Thirumoorthi MC, Asmar BI, Buckley JA, et al. Pharmacokinetics of intravenously administered piperacillin in preadolescent children. *J Pediatr.* 1983;102:941-946.
6. Ciftci AO, Tanyel C, Buyukpamucu N, et al. Comparative trial of four antibiotic combinations for perforated appendicitis in children. *Eur J Surg.* 1997;163:591-596.
7. Prince AS, Neu HC. Use of piperacillin, a semisynthetic penicillin, in the therapy of acute exacerbations of pulmonary disease in patients with cystic fibrosis. *J Pediatr.* 1980;97:148-151.
8. Jackson MA, Kusmiesz H, Shelton S, et al. Comparison of piperacillin vs. ticarcillin plus tobramycin in the treatment of acute pulmonary exacerbation of cystic fibrosis. *Pediatr Infect Dis J.* 1986;5:440-443.
9. Bernig T, Weigel S, Mukodzi S. Antibiotic sequential therapy for febrile neutropenia in pediatric patients with malignancy. *Pediatr Hematol Oncol.* 2000;17:93-98.
10. Mahmood S, Revesz T, Mpofu C. Ferile episodes in children with cancer in the United Arab Emirates. *Pediatr Hematol Oncol.* 1996;13:135-142.
11. Salam IM, Galala KH, Ashaal YI, et al. A randomized prospective study of cefoxitin versus piperacillin in appendectomy. *J Hosp Infect.* 1994;26:133-136.

References

12. Aronoff A, Brier M, Bennett W. *The Renal Book, 2002.* Available at: http://www.kdp-baptist.louisville.edu/renalbook/. Accessed August 6, 2006.
13. DeSchepper PJ, Tjandramaga TB, Mullie A, et al. Comparative pharmacokinetics of piperacillin in normals and in patients with renal failure. *J Antimicrob Chemother.* 1982;9(suppl B):49-57.
14. American Society of Health-System Pharmacists. American Hospital Formulary System. Available at: http://ahfsfirst.firstdatabank.com/AHFSfirst/NSAHFSFirstSearchmain.asp. Accessed August 10, 2006.
15. Trissel LA, ed. *Handbook on Injectable Drugs.* 13th ed. [CD-ROM version 1.5]. Bethesda, MD: American Society of Health-System Pharmacists; 2005.
16. Robinson DC, Cookson TL, Frisafe JA. Concentration guidelines for parenteral antibiotics in fluid-restricted patients. *Drug Intell Clin Pharm.* 1987;21:985-989.
17. Burgess DS, Waldrep T. Pharmacokinetics and pharmacodynamics of piperacillin/tazobactam when administered by continuous infusion and intermittent dosing. *Clin Ther.* 2002;24:1090-1104.
18. Grant EM, Kuti JL, Nicolau DP, et al. Clinical efficacy and pharmacoeconomics of a continuous-infusion piperacillin-tazobactam program in a large community teaching hospital. *Pharmacotherapy.* 2002;22:471-483.
19. Florea NR, Kotapati S, Kuti JL, et al. Cost analysis of continuous versus intermittent infusion of piperacillin-tazobactam: a time-motion study. *Am J Health-Syst Pharm.* 2003;60:2321-2327.
20. Craig WA, Ebert SC. Continuous infusion of beta-lactam antibiotics. *Antimicrob Agents Chemother.* 1992;36:2577-2583.
21. Grieco MH. Cross-allergenicity of the penicillins and the cephalosporins. *Arch Intern Med.* 1967;119:141-146.
22. Sullivan TJ. Pathogenesis and management of allergic reactions to penicillin and other beta-lactam antibiotics. *Pediatr Infect Dis.* 1982;1:344-350.
23. Saxon A. Immediate hypersensitivity reactions to B-lactam antibiotics. *Rev Infect Dis.* 1983;5(suppl 2):S368-S378.
24. Sher TH. Penicillin hypersensitivity—a review. In: Symposium on anti-infective therapy I. Speck WT, Blummer JL, eds. *Pediatr Clin North Am.* 1983;30:161-177.
25. Stewart GT. Cross allergenicity of penicillin G and related substances. *Lancet.* 1962;1:509-510.
26. Wills R, Henry RL, Francis JL. Antibiotic hypersensitivity reactions in cystic fibrosis. *J Paediatr Child Health.* 1998;34:325-329.
27. Rye PJ, Roberts G, Staugas RE, et al. Coagulopathy with piperacillin administration in cystic fibrosis: two case reports. *J Paediatr Child Health.* 1994;30:278-279.
28. Gooding PG, Clark BJ, Sathe SS. Piperacillin: a review of clinical experience. *J Antimicrob Chemother.* 1982;9(suppl B):93-99.
29. Malanga CJ, Kojontis L, Mauzy S. Piperacillin-induced seizures. *Clin Pediatr.* 1997;36:475-478.
30. McLaughlin JE, Reeves DS. Clinical and laboratory evidence for inactivation of gentamicin by carbenicillin. *Lancet.* 1971;1(7693):261-264.
31. Riff LJ, Jackson GG. Laboratory and clinical conditions for gentamicin inactivation by carbenicillin. *Arch Intern Med.* 1972;130:887-891.
32. Manian FA, Stone WJ, Alford RH. Adverse antibiotic effects associated with renal insufficiency. *Rev Infect Dis.* 1990;12:236-249.
33. Davies M, Morgan JR, Anand C. Interactions of carbenicillin and ticarcillin with gentamicin. *Antimicrob Agents Chemother.* 1975;7:431-434.
34. Weibert R, Keane W, Shapiro F. Carbenicillin inactivation of aminoglycosides in patients with severe renal failure. *Trans Amer Soc Artif Int Organs.* 1976;22:439-443.

Piperacillin Sodium–Tazobactam Sodium

1. *Physicians' Desk Reference.* 60th ed. Montvale, NJ: Thomson PDR; 2006.
2. Flidel-Rimon O, Friedman S, Leibovitz E, et al. The use of piperacillin/tazobactam (in association with amikacin) in neonatal sepsis: efficacy and safety data. *Scand J Infect Dis.* 2006;38:36-42.
3. Berger A, Kretzer V, Apfalter P, et al. Safety evaluation of piperacillin/tazobactam in very low birth weight infants. *J Chemother.* 2004;16:166-171.
4. Pillay T, Pillay DG, Adhikari M, et al. Piperacillin/tazobactam in the treatment of Klebsiella pneumoniae infections in neonates. *Am J Perinatol.* 1998;15:47-51.
5. American Academy of Pediatrics. In: Pickering LK, ed. *Red Book: 2006 Report of the Committee on Infectious Diseases.* 27th ed. Elk Grove Village, IL: American Academy of Pediatrics; 2006.
6. Reed MD, Goldfarb J, Yamashita TS, et al. Single-dose pharmacokinetics of piperacillin and tazobactam in infants and children. *Antimicrob Agents Chemother.* 1994;36:2817-2826.
7. Reed MD. The pathophysiology and treatment of cystic fibrosis. *J Pediatr Pharm Pract.* 1997;2:285-305.
8. Manno G, Cruciani M, Romano L, et al. Antimicrobial use and Pseudomonas aeruginosa susceptibility profile in a cystic fibrosis centre. *Int J Antimicrob Agents.* 2005;25:193-197.
9. Arnoff GR, Berns JS, Brier ME, et al. *Drug Prescribing in Renal Failure: Dosing Guidelines for Adults.* 4th ed. Philadelphia, PA: American College of Physicians; 1999.
10. Schoonover LL, Occhipinti DJ, Rodvoid EA, et al. Piperacillin/tazobactam: a new beta-lactam/beta-lactamase inhibitor combination. *Ann Pharmacother.* 1995;29:501-513.
11. Trissel LA, ed. *Handbook on Injectable Drugs.* 13th ed. [CD-ROM version 1.5]. Bethesda, MD: American Society of Health-System Pharmacists; 2005.
12. Burgess DS, Waldrep T. Pharmacokinetics and pharmacodynamics of piperacillin/tazobactam when administered by continuous infusion and intermittent dosing. *Clin Ther.* 2002;24:1090-1104.
13. Grant EM, Kuti JL, Nicolau DP, et al. Clinical efficacy and pharmacoeconomics of a continuous-infusion piperacillin-tazobactam program in a large community teaching hospital. *Pharmacotherapy.* 2002;22:471-483.
14. Florea NR, Kotapati S, Kuti JL, et al. Cost analysis of continuous versus intermittent infusion of piperacillin-tazobactam: a time-motion study. *Am J Health-Syst Pharm.* 2003;60:2321-2327.
15. Wills R, Henry RL, Francis JL. Antibiotic hypersensitivity reactions in cystic fibrosis. *J Paediatr Child Health.* 1998;34:325-329.
16. Rye PJ, Roberts G, Staugas RE, et al. Coagulopathy with piperacillin administration in cystic fibrosis: two case reports. *J Paediatr Child Health.* 1994;30:278-279.
17. Kohler RB, Foerster LA, Wheat LJ, et al. Piperacillin and gentamicin vs carbenicillin and gentamicin for treatment of serious gram-negative infections. *Arch Intern Med.* 1982;142:1335-1337.
18. Gooding PG, Clark BJ, Sathe SS. Piperacillin: a review of clinical experience. *J Antimicrob Chemother.* 1982;9(suppl B):93-99.
19. Malanga CJ, Kojontis L, Mauzy S. Piperacillin-induced seizures. *Clin Pediatr.* 1997;36:475-478.
20. McLaughlin JE, Reeves DS. Clinical and laboratory evidence for inactivation of gentamicin by carbenicillin. *Lancet.* 1971;1(7693):261-264.
21. Riff LJ, Jackson GG. Laboratory and clinical conditions for gentamicin inactivation by carbenicillin. *Arch Intern Med.* 1972;130:887-891.
22. Manian FA, Stone WJ, Alford RH. Adverse antibiotic effects associated with renal insufficiency. *Rev Infect Dis.* 1990;12:236-249.
23. Davies M, Morgan JR, Anand C. Interactions of carbenicillin and ticarcillin with gentamicin. *Antimicrob Agents Chemother.* 1975;7:431-434.
24. Weibert R, Keane W, Shapiro F. Carbenicillin inactivation of aminoglycosides in patients with severe renal failure. *Trans Amer Soc Artif Int Organs.* 1976;22:439-443.

Potassium Chloride

1. Ash SR. The perils of i.v. potassium: are they exaggerated? *Parenterals.* 1987;(Dec/Jan):1, 5-8.
2. Schaber DE, Uden DL, Stone FM, et al. Intravenous KCl supplementation in pediatric cardiac surgical patients. *Pediatr Cardiol.* 1985;6:25-28.

3. Robertson J, Shilkofski, editors. *The Harriet Lane Handbook.* 17th ed. Philadelphia, PA: Elsevier Mosby; 2005.
4. DeFronza RA, Bia M. Intravenous potassium chloride therapy. *JAMA.* 1981;245:2446. (Questions and Answers).
5. Trachtenbarg DE. Diabetic ketoacidosis. *Am Fam Physician.* 2005;71:1705-1714.
6. McEvoy GK, ed. *AHFS Drug Information Essentials 2005–06.* Bethesda, MD: American Society of Health-System Pharmacists; 2005.
7. Trissel LA. *Handbook on Injectable Drugs.* 13th ed. Bethesda, MD: American Society of Health-System Pharmacists; 2005.
8. Potassium chloride [package insert]. Schaumburg, IL: American Pharmaceutical Partners Inc; January 2006.
9. Fisch C, Knoebel SB, Feigen H, et al. Potassium and the monophasic action potential, electrocardiogram, conduction, and arrhythmias. *Prog Cardiovasc Dis.* 1966;8:387-418.
10. Kruse JA, Carlson RW. Rapid correction of hypokalemia using concentrated intravenous potassium chloride infusions. *Arch Intern Med.* 1990;150:613-617.
11. Upton J, Mulliken JB, Murray JE. Major intravenous extravasation injuries. *Am J Surg.* 1979;137:497-506.
12. Soni MG, Taylor SL, Greenberg NA, et al. Evaluation of the health aspects of methyl paraben: a review of the published literature. *Food Chem Toxicol.* 2002;40:1335-1373.
13. Nagel JE, Fuscaldo JT, Firemen P. Paraben allergy. *JAMA.* 1977;237:1594-1595.
14. DeFronzo RA, Taufield PA, Black H, et al. Impaired renal tubular potassium secretion in sickle cell disease. *Ann Intern Med.* 1979;90:310-316.
15. Pucino F, Danielson BD, Carlson JD, et al. Patient tolerance to intravenous potassium chloride with and without lidocaine. *Drug Intell Clin Pharm.* 1988;22:676-679.

Potassium Phosphates

1. Ash SR. The perils of i.v. potassium: are they exaggerated? *Parenterals.* 1987;(Dec/Jan):1, 5-8.
2. Robertson J, Shilkofski, eds. *The Harriet Lane Handbook.* 17th ed. Philadelphia, PA: Elsevier Mosby; 2005.
3. Clark CL, Sacks GS, Dickerson RN, et al. Treatment of hypophosphatemia in patients receiving specialized nutrition support using a graduated dosing scheme: results from a prospective clinical trial. *Crit Care Med.* 1995;23:1504-1511.
4. Trachtenbarg DE. Diabetic ketoacidosis. *Am Fam Physician.* 2005;71:1705-1714.
5. White NH. Diabetic ketoacidosis in children. *Endocrinol Metab Clin North Am.* 2000; 29:657-682.
6. McEvoy GK, ed. *AHFS Drug Information Essentials 2005–06.* Bethesda, MD: American Society of Health-System Pharmacists; 2005.
7. Prestridge LL, Schanler RJ, Shulman RJ, et al. Effect of parenteral calcium and phosphorus therapy on mineral retention and bone mineral content in very low birth weight infants. *J Pediatr.* 1993;122:761-768.
8. Pelegano JF, Rowe JC, Carey DE, et al. Simultaneous infusion of calcium and phosphorus in parenteral nutrition for premature infants: use of physiologic calcium/phosphorus ratio. *J Pediatr.* 1989;114;115-119.
9. Potassium phosphates [package insert]. Schaumburg, IL: American Pharmaceutical Partners Inc; September 2003.
10. Trissel LA. *Handbook on Injectable Drugs.* 13th ed. Bethesda, MD: American Society of Health-System Pharmacists; 2005.
11. Upton J, Mulliken JB, Murray JE. Major intravenous extravasation injuries. *Am J Surg.* 1979;137:497-506.
12. Fisch C, Knoebel SB, Feigen H, et al. Potassium and the monophasic action potential, electrocardiogram, conduction, and arrhythmias. *Prog Cardiovasc Dis.* 1966; 8:387-418.

Pralidoxime Chloride (2-PAM Chloride)

1. American Society of Health-System Pharmacists. American Hospital Formulary System. Available at: http://ahfsfirst.firstdatabank.com/AHFSfirst/NSAHFSFirstSearchmain.asp. Accessed July 20, 2006.
2. Morgan DP, Krenzelok EP, Kulig K, et al. Organophosphates. In: Rumack BH, ed. *Poisondex Information System.* 104th ed. Denver, CO: MICROMEDEX Inc; 1974-2000.
3. Ellenhorn MJ, Barceloux DG. *Medical Toxicology Diagnosis and Treatment of Human Poisoning.* New York, NY: Elsevier; 1988:81-82,1071-1077.
4. Mortensen ML. Management of acute childhood poisonings caused by selected insecticides and herbicides. *Pediatr Clin North Am.* 1986;33:421-445.
5. Zwiener RJ, Ginsburg CM. Organophosphate and carbamate poisoning in infants and children. *Pediatrics.* 1988;81:121-125.
6. Bowden CA, Krenzelok EP. Clinical applications of commonly used contemporary antidotes. *Drug Safety.* 1997;16:9-47.
7. Benitz WE, Tatro DS. *The Pediatric Drug Handbook.* Chicago, IL: Year Book; 1988:14.
8. Farrar HC, Wells TG, Kearns GL. Use of continuous infusion of pralidoxime for treatment of organophosphate poisoning in children. *J Pediatr.* 1990;116:658-661.
9. Schexnayder S, James LP, Kearns GL, et al. The pharmacokinetics of continuous infusion pralidoxime in children with organophosphate poisoning. *Clin Toxicol.* 1998;36:549-555.
10. Namba T, Nolte CT, Jackrel J, et al. Poisoning due to organophosphate insecticides. *Am J Med.* 1971;50:475-492.

Procainamide HCl

1. American Academy of Pediatrics Committee on Drugs. Emergency drug doses for infants and children. *Pediatrics.* 1998;101:e1-e11.
2. American Heart Association. Guidelines 2005 for cardiopulmonary resuscitation and emergency cardiovascular care. Part 12: Pediatric advanced life support. *Circulation.* 2005;112:167-187.
3. American Society of Health-System Pharmacists. American Hospital Formulary System. Available at: http://ahfsfirst.firstdatabank.com/AHFSfirst/NSAHFSFirstSearchmain.asp. Accessed July 10, 2006.
4. Gelman CR, Rumack BH, Hess AJ (eds). *DRUGDEX(R) System.* Englewood, CO: MICROMEDEX Inc; date accessed: April 18, 2006.
5. Mandapati R, Byrum CJ, Kavey RE, et al. Procainamide of rate control of postsurgical junctional tachycardia. *Pediatr Cardiol.* 2000;21:123-128.
6. Luedtke SA, Kuhn RJ, McCaffrey FM. Pharmacologic management of supraventricular tachycardias in children. *Ann Pharmacother.* 1997;21:1347-1359.
7. Trissel LA, ed. *Handbook on Injectable Drugs.* 13th ed. [CD-ROM version 1.5]. Bethesda, MD: American Society of Health-System Pharmacists; 2005.
8. American Academy of Pediatrics Committee on Drugs. "Inactive" ingredients in pharmaceutical products: update. *Pediatrics.* 1997;99:268-278.
9. Lester MR. Sulfite sensitivity: significance in human health. *J Am Col Nutr.* 1995;14:229-232.
10. Smolinske SC. Review of parenteral sulfite reactions. *J Toxicol Clin Toxicol.* 1992;30:597-606.
11. American Academy of Pediatrics Committee on Drugs. "Inactive" ingredients in pharmaceutical products: update. *Pediatrics.* 1997;99:268-278.
12. Hall CM, Milligan DWA, Berrington J. Probably adverse reaction to a pharmaceutical excipient. *Arch Dis Child Fetal Neonatal Ed.* 2004;89: F184.
13. Hiller JL, Benda GI, Rahatzad M, et al. Benzyl alcohol toxicity: impact on mortality and intraventricular hemorrhage among very low birth weight infants. *Pediatrics.* 1986;77:500-506.

References

14. Grant JA, Bilodeau PA, Guernsey BG, et al. Unsuspected benzyl alcohol hypersensitivity. *N Engl J Med.* 1982;306:108.
15. Wilson JP, Solimando DA, Edwards MS. Parenteral benzyl alcohol-induced hypersensitivity reaction. *Drug Intell Clin Pharm.* 1986;20:689-691.
16. Bryson SM, Leson CL, Irwin DB, et al. Therapeutic monitoring and pharmacokinetic evaluation of procainamide in neonates. *DICP Ann Pharmacother.* 1991;25:68-71.
17. Trujillo TC, Nolan PE. Antiarrhythmic agents: drug interactions of clinical significance. *Drug Safety.* 2000;23:509-532.

Promethazine HCl

1. Phenergan Injection [package insert]. Deerfield, IL: Baxter Healthcare Corporation; August, 2005.
2. Ruckman RN, Keane JF, Freed MD, et al. Sedation for cardiac catheterization: a controlled study. *Pediatr Cardiol.* 1980;1:263-268.
3. Fixler DE, Carrell T, Browne R, et al. Oxygen consumption in infants and children during cardiac catheterization under different sedation regimens. *Circulation.* 1974;50:788-794.
4. Khalil S, Philrook L, Rabb M, et al. Ondansetron/promethazine combination or promethazine alone reduces nausea and vomiting after middle ear surgery. *J Clin Anesth.* 1999;11:596-600.
5. Aronoff A, Brier M, Bennett W. *The Renal Book, 2002.* Available at: http://www.kdp-baptist.louisville.edu/renalbook/. Accessed July 21, 2006.
6. Trissel LA, ed. *Handbook on Injectable Drugs.* 13th ed. [CD-ROM version 1.5]. Bethesda, MD: American Society of Health-System Pharmacists; 2005.
7. Mostafavi H, Samimi M. Accidental intra-arterial injection of promethazine HCl during general anesthesia: report of a case. *Anesthesiology.* 1971;35:645-646.
8. *ISMP Safety Newsletter.* August 10, 2006.
9. American Academy of Pediatrics Committee on Drugs. "Inactive" ingredients in pharmaceutical products: update. *Pediatrics.* 1997;99:268-278.
10. Lester MR. Sulfite sensitivity: significance in human health. *J Am Col Nutr.* 1995;14:229-232.
11. Smolinske SC. Review of parenteral sulfite reactions. *J Toxicol Clin Toxicol.* 1992;30:597-606.
12. Starke PR, Weaver J, Chowdhury BA. Boxed warning added to promethazine labeling for pediatric use. *N Engl J Med.* 2005;352:2653.
13. Nahata MC, Clotz MA, Krogg EA. Adverse effects of meperidine, promethazine, and chlorpromazine for sedation in pediatric patients. *Clin Pediatr.* 1985;24:558-560.
14. Nahata MC. Sedation in pediatric patients undergoing diagnostic procedures. *Drug Intell Clin Pharm.* 1988;22:711-715.
15. Cook BA, Bass JW, Nomizu S, et al. Sedation of children for technical procedures: current standards of practice. *Clin Pediatr.* 1992;31:137-142.
16. American Academy of Pediatrics. Committee on Drugs. Reappraisal of lytic cocktail/demerol, phenergan, and thorazine (DPT) for the sedation of children. *Pediatrics.* 1995;95:598-602.
17. Brown ET, Corbett SW, Green SM. Iatrogenic cardiopulmonary arrest during pediatric sedation with meperidine, promethazine, and chlorpromazine. *Pediatr Emerg Care.* 2001;17:351-353.
18. Snodgrass WR, Dodge WF. Lytic/DPT cocktail: time for rational and safer alternatives. *Pediatr Clin North Am.* 1989;36:1285-1291.
19. Ingram DG, Hagemann TM. Promethazine treatment of steroid-induced psychosis in a child. *Ann Pharmacother.* 2003;37:1036-1039.

Propofol

1. Medical Economics, ed. *Physicians' Desk Reference.* 54th ed. Oradell, NJ: Medical Economics Company; 2000.
2. Morton NS, Wee M, Christie G, et al. Propofol for induction of anaesthesia in children. *Anaesthesia.* 1988;43:350-355.
3. Mirakhur RK. Induction characteristics of propofol in children: comparison with thiopentone. *Anaesthesia.* 1988;43:593-598.
4. Patel DK, Keeling PA, Newman GB, et al. Induction dose of propofol in children. *Anaesthesia.* 1988;43:949-952.
5. Martin TM, Nicolson SC, Bargas MS. Propofol anesthesia reduces emesis and airway obstruction in pediatric outpatients. *Anesth Analg.* 1993;76:144-148.
6. Hannallah RS, Britton JT, Schafer PG, et al. Propofol anaesthesia in paediatric ambulatory patients: a comparison with thiopentone and halothane. *Can J Anaesth.* 1994;41:12-18.
7. Borgeat A, Fuchs T, Tassonyi E. Induction characteristics of 2% propofol solution. *Br J Anaesth.* 1997;78:433-435.
8. Pessenbacher K, Gutmann A, Eggenreich U, et al. Two propofol formulations are equivalent in small children aged 1 month to 3 years. *Acta Anaesthesiol Scand.* 2002;46:257-263.
9. Rocca GD, Costa MG, Bruno K, et al. Pediatric renal transplantation: anesthesia and perioperative complications. *Pediatr Surg Int.* 2001;17:175-179.
10. Uezono S, Goto T, Terui K, et al. Emergence agitation after sevoflurane versus propofol in pediatric patients. *Anesth Analg.* 2000;91:563-566.
11. Saricaoglu F, Celebi N, Celik M, et al. The evaluation of propofol dosage for anesthesia induction in children with cerebral palsy with bispectral index (BIS) monitoring. *Paediatr Anaesth.* 2005;15:1048-1052.
12. Cohen IT, Hannallah RS, Goodale DB. The clinical and biochemical effects of propofol infusion with and without EDTA for maintenance anesthesia in healthy children undergoing ambulatory surgery. *Anesth Analg.* 2001;93:106-111.
13. Exil G, Clancy RR, Hyder DJ. Propofol treatment of refractory status epilepticus: a report of five pediatric cases. *Epilepsia.* 1995;36:124.
14. Harrison AM, Lugo RA, Schunk JE. Treatment of convulsive status epilepticus with propofol: a case report. *Pediatr Emer Care.* 1997;13:420-422.
15. Rossetti AO, Logroscino G, Bromfield EB. Refractory status epilepticus: effect of treatment aggressiveness on prognosis. *Arch Neurol.* 2005;62:1698-1702.
16. Harrison AM, Lugo RA, Schunk JE. Treatment of convulsive status epilepticus with propofol: case report. *Pediatr Emerg Care.* 1997;13:420-422.
17. van Gestel JP, Blusse van Oud-Alblas HJ, Malingre M, et al. Propofol and thiopental for refractory status epilepticus in children. *Neurology.* 2005;23:591-592.
18. Dial S, Silver P, Bock K, Sagy M. Pediatric sedation for procedures titrated to a desired degree of immobility results in unpredictable depth of sedation. *Pediatr Emerg Care.* 2001;17:414-420.
19. Vardi A, Salen Y, Padeh S, et al. Is propofol safe for procedural sedation in children? A prospective evaluation of propofol versus ketamine in pediatric critical care. *Crit Care Med.* 2002;30:1231-1236.
20. Gozol D, Rein AJ, Nir A, et al. Propofol does not modify the hemodynamic status of children with intracardiac shunts undergoing cardiac catheterization. *Pediatr Cardiol.* 2001;22:488-90.
21. Hertzog JH, Campbell JK, Dalton HJ, et al. Propofol anesthesia for invasive procedures in ambulatory and hospitalized children: experience in the pediatric intensive care unit. *Pediatrics.* 1999;103(3). Available at: http://www.pediatrics.org/cgi/content/full/103/3/e30.
22. Timpe EM, Eichner SF, Phelps SJ. Propofol-related infusion syndrome in critically ill pediatric patients: coincidence, association, or causation? *J Pediatr Pharmacol Ther.* 2006;11:17-42.
23. Aronoff A, Brier M, Bennett W. *The Renal Book, 2002.* Available at: http://www.kdp-baptist.louisville.edu/renalbook/. Accessed August 13, 2006.
24. American Society of Health-System Pharmacists. American Hospital Formulary System. Available at: http://ahfsfirst.firstdatabank.com/

AHFSfirst/NSAHFSFirstSearchmain.asp. Accessed July 10, 2006.
25. Trissel LA, ed. *Handbook on Injectable Drugs*. 13th ed. [CD-ROM version 1.5]. Bethesda, MD: American Society of Health-System Pharmacists; 2005.
26. Hofer KN, McCarthy MW, Buck ML, et al. Possible anaphylaxis after propofol in a child with food allergy. *Ann Pharmacother*. 2003;37:398-401.
27. American Academy of Pediatrics Committee on Drugs. "Inactive" ingredients in pharmaceutical products: update. *Pediatrics.* 1997;99:268-278.
28. Smolinske SC. Review of parenteral sulfite reactions. *J Toxicol Clin Toxicol.* 1992;30:597-606.
29. Lester MR. Sulfite sensitivity: significance in human health. *J Am Col Nutr.* 1995;14:229-232.
30. Bennett SN, McNeil MM, Bland LA, et al. Postoperative infections traced to contamination of intravenous anesthetic, propofol. *N Engl J Med.* 1995;333:147-154.
31. McHugh GJ, Roper GM. Propofol emulsion and bacterial contamination. *Can J Anaesth.* 1995;42:801-804.
32. Reiter PD, Robles J, Dowell EB. Effect of 24-hour intravenous tubing set change on the sterility of repackaged fat emulsion in neonates. *Ann Pharmacother.* 2004;38:1603-1607.
33. Bragonier R, Bartle D, Langton-Hewer S. Acute dystonia in a 14-yr-old following propofol and fentanyl anaesthesia. *Br J Anaesth*. 2000;84:828-829.
34. Collier C, Kelly K. Propofol and convulsions—the evidence mounts. *Anaesth Intensive Care.* 1991;19:573-575.
35. Harrigan PW, Browne SM, Quail AW. Multiple seizures following re-exposure to propofol. *Anaesth Intensive Care.* 1996;24:261-264.
36. Gelber O, Gal M, Katz Y. Clonic convulsions in a neonate after propofol anaesthesia. *Paediatr Anaesth.* 1997;7:88.
37. Walder B, Tramer MR, Seeck M. Seizure-like phenomena and propofol: a systematic review. *Neurology*. 2002;58:1327-1332.

Propranolol HCl

1. American Society of Health-System Pharmacists. *American Hospital Formulary System.* Available at: http://ahfsfirst.firstdatabank.com/AHFSfirst/NSAHFSFirstSearchmain.asp. Accessed July 23, 2006.
2. American Academy of Pediatrics Committee on Drugs. Emergency drug doses for infants and children. *Pediatrics.* 1998;101:e1-e11.
3. Gelband H, Rosen MR. Pharmacologic basis for the treatment of cardiac arrhythmias. *Pediatrics.* 1975;55:59-67.
4. Roberts RJ, Mueller S, Lauer RM. Propranolol in the treatment of cardiac arrhythmias associated with amitriptyline intoxication. *J Pediatr.* 1973;82:65-67.
5. Guntheroth WG. Disorders of heart rate and rhythm. *Pediatr Clin North Am.* 1978;25:869-890.
6. Serratto M. Diagnosis and management of heart failure in infants and children. *Comprehensive Ther.* 1992;18:11-19.
7. Herndon DN, Barrow RE, Rutan TC, et al. Effect of propranolol on hemodynamic and metabolic response of burned pediatric patients. *Ann Surg.* 1988;208:484-492.
8. Baron PW, Barrow RE, Pierre EJ, et al. Prolonged use of propranolol safely decreases cardiac work in burned children. *J Burn Rehabil.* 1997;18:223-227.
9. National High Blood Pressure Education Program Working Group on High Blood Pressure in Children and Adolescents. The fourth report on the diagnosis, evaluation, and treatment of high blood pressure in children and adolescents. *Pediatrics.* 2004:114(2 suppl 4th Report):555-576.
10. Temple ME, Nahata MC. Treatment of pediatric hypertension. *Pharmacotherapy.* 200;20(2):140-150.
11. Maxwell LG, Colombani PM, Fivush BA. Renal, endocrine and metabolic failure. In: Rogers MC, ed. *Textbook of Pediatric Intensive Care.* 2nd ed. Philadelphia, PA: Williams & Willikins; 1992:1182.
12. American Academy of Pediatrics Committee on Drugs. Drugs for pediatric emergencies. *Pediatrics.* 1998;101:e1-e11.
13. Wensley DF, Karl T, Deanfield JE, et al. Assessment of residual right ventricular outflow tract obstruction following surgery using the response to intravenous propranolol. *Ann Thorac Surg.* 1987;44:633-636.
14. Eades SK. Pharmacotherapy of congenital heart defects. *J Pediatr Pharmacol Ther.* 2004;9:160-178.
15. Aronoff A, Brier M, Bennett W. *The Renal Book, 2002.* Available at: http://www.kdp-baptist.louisville.edu/renalbook/. Accessed July 24, 2006.
16. Propranolol [package insert]. Bedford, OH: Bedford Laboratories; August 2003.
17. Silberbach M, Dunnigan A, Benson W Jr. Effect of intravenous propranolol or verapamil on infant orthodromic reciprocating tachycardia. *Am J Cardiol.* 1989;63:438-442.
18. Trissel LA, ed. *Handbook on Injectable Drugs.* 13th ed. [CD-ROM version 1.5]. Bethesda, MD: American Society of Health-System Pharmacists; 2005.

Protamine Sulfate

1. Protamine sulfate injection, USP [package insert]. Schaumburg, IL: American Pharmaceutical Partners Inc; May 2004.
2. American Society of Health-System Pharmacists. American Hospital Formulary System. Available at: http://ahfsfirst.firstdatabank.com/AHFSfirst/NSAHFSFirstSearchmain.asp. Accessed October 18, 2006
3. Monagle P, Chan A, Massicotte P, et al. Antithrombotic therapy in children: the seventh ACCP conference on antithrombotic and thrombolytic therapy. *Chest.* 2004;126:645S-647S.
4. Trissel LA, ed. *Handbook on Injectable Drugs*. 13th ed. Bethesda, MD: American Society of Health-System Pharmacists; 2005.
5. Stewart WJ, McSweeney SM, Kellett MA, et al. Increased risk of severe protamine reactions in NPH insulin-dependent diabetics undergoing cardiac catheterization. *Circulation*. 1984;70:788-792.
6. Nordstrom L, Fletcher R, Pavek K. Shock of anaphylactoid type induced by protamine: a continuous cardiorespiratory record. *Acta Anaesthesiol Scand*. 1978;22:195-201.
7. Westaby S, Turner MW, Stark J. Complement activation and anaphylactoid response to protamine in a child after cardio-pulmonary bypass. *Br Heart J*. 1985;53:574-576.
8. Wassill VM, Hill GE, Jacoby RM. Antagonism of cardiovascular depressant effect of protamine by calcium. *Anesth Analg*. 1980;59:564. Abstract.
9. Michaels IA, Barash PG. Hemodynamic changes during protamine administration. *Anesth Analg*. 1983;62:831-835.
10. Mayumi H, Toshima Y, Tokunaga K. Pretreatment with H_2 blocker famotidine to ameliorate protamine-induced hypotension in open-heart surgery. *J Cardiovasc Surg*. 1992;33:738-745.
11. Boigner H, Lechner E, Brock H, et al. Life threatening cardiopulmonary failure in an infant following protamine reversal of heparin after cardiopulmonary bypass. *Paediatr Anaesth*. 2001;11:729-732.

Ranitidine

1. Blumer JL, Rothstein FC, Kaplan BS, et al. Pharmacokinetic determination of ranitidine pharmacodynamics in pediatric ulcer disease. *J Pediatr.* 1985;107:301-306.
2. Sarna MS, Saili A, Dutta AK, et al. Stress associated gastric bleeding in newborns: role of ranitidine. *Indian Pediatr.* 1991;28:1305-1308.
3. Rosenthal M, Miller PW. Ranitidine in the newborn. *Arch Dis Child.* 1988;63:88-89.

References

4. *Physicians' Desk Reference.* 60th ed. Montvale, NJ: Thomson PDR; 2006.
5. Kelly EJ, Chatfield SL, Brownlee KG, et al. The effect of intravenous ranitidine on the intragastric pH of preterm infants receiving dexamethasone. *Arch Dis Child.* 1993;69:37-39.
6. Kuusela AL. Long term gastric pH monitoring for determining optimal dose of ranitidine for critically ill preterm and term neonates. *Arch Dis Child Fetal Neonatal Ed.* 1998;78:F151-F153.
7. Wells TG, Heulitt MJ, Taylor BJ, et al. Pharmacokinetics and pharmacodynamics of ranitidine in neonates treated with extracorporeal membrane oxygenation. *J Clin Pharmacol.* 1998;38:402-407.
8. Cid JL, Velasco LA, Codoceo R, et al. Ranitidine prophylaxis in acute gastric mucosal damage in critically ill pediatric patients. *Crit Care Med.* 1988;16:591-593.
9. Wiest DB, O'Neal W, Reigart JR, et al. Pharmacokinetics of ranitidine in critically ill infants. *Dev Pharmacol Ther.* 1989;12:7-12.
10. Cochran EB, Storgion SA, Reiter PR, et al. Effects of continuous vs intermittent ranitidine on gastric pH in critically ill pediatric patients. *Clin Res.* 1991;39:833A. Abstract.
11. Gedeit RG, Weigle CG, Havens PL, et al. Control and variability of gastric pH in critically ill children. *Crit Care Med.* 1993;21:1850-1855.
12. Lugo RA, Harrison M, Cash J, et al. Pharmacokinetics and pharmacodynamics of ranitidine in critically ill children. *Crit Care Med.* 2001;29:759-764.
13. Crill CM, Hak EB. Upper gastrointestinal bleeding in critically ill pediatric patients. *Pharmacotherapy.* 1999;19:162-180.
14. Harrison AM, Lugo RA, Vernon DD. Gastric pH control in critically ill children receiving intravenous ranitidine. *Crit Care Med.* 1998;26:1433-1436.
15. Osteyee JL, Banner W. Effect of two dosing regimens on intravenous ranitidine on gastric pH in critically ill children. *J Crit Care.* 1994;3:267-272.
16. Hyman PE, Garvey TQ III, Abrams CE. Tolerance to intravenous ranitidine. *J Pediatr.* 1987;110:794-796.
17. Dimand RJ, Burckart G, Concepcion W, et al. Continuous infusion ranitidine in post-operative pediatric liver transplant patients: effects on intragastric pH, bleeding and metabolic alkalosis. *Crit Care Med.* 1989;S116. Abstract.
18. Eddleston JM, Booker PD, Green JR. Use of ranitidine in children undergoing cardiopulmonary bypass. *Crit Care Med.* 1989;17:26-29.
19. Aronoff A, Brier M, Bennett W. *The Renal Book, 2002.* Available at: http://www.kdp-baptist.louisville.edu/renalbook/. Accessed August 8, 2006.
20. Smith CL, Bardgett DM, Hunter JM. Haemodynamic effects of the IV administration of cimetidine or ranitidine in the critically ill patient. A double-blind prospective study. *Br J Anaesth.* 1987;59:1397-1402.
21. Trissel LA, ed. *Handbook on Injectable Drugs.* 13th ed. [CD-ROM version 1.5]. Bethesda, MD: American Society of Health-System Pharmacists; 2005.
22. Hatton J, Leur M, Hirsch J, et al. Histamine receptor antagonists and lipid stability in total nutrient admixtures. *JPEN.* 1994;18:308-312.
23. Allwood MC, Martin H. Factors influencing the stability of ranitidine in TPN mixtures. *Clin Nutr.* 1995;14:171-176.
24. Bullock L, Parks RB, Lampasona V, et al. Stability of ranitidine hydrochloride and amino acids in parenteral nutrient solutions. *Am J Hosp Pharm.* 1985;42:2683-2687.
25. Nahum E, Relsh O, Naor N, et al. Ranitidine-induced bradycardia in a neonate—a first report. *Eur J Pediatr.* 1993;152:933-934.
26. Bush A, Busst CM, Shinebourne EA. Cardiovascular effects of tolazoline and ranitidine. *Arch Dis Childhood.* 1987;62:241-246.
27. Guillet R, Stoll BJ, Cotton CM, et al. Association of H2-blocker therapy and higher incidence of necrotizing enterocolitis in very low birth weight infants. *Pediatrics.* 2006;117:e137-e142.

Rasburicase

1. *Physicians' Desk Reference.* 60th ed. Montvale, NJ: Thomson PDR; 2006.
2. Pui CH, Jeha S, Irwin D, et al. Recombinant urate oxidase (rasburicase) in the prevention and treatment of malignancy-associated hyperuricemia in pediatric and adult patients: results of a compassionate-use trial. *Leukemia.* 2001;15:1505-1059.
3. Pui CH, Mahmoud HH, Wiley JM, et al. Recombinant urate oxidase for the prophylaxis or treatment of hyperuricemia in patients with leukemia or lymphoma. *J Clin Oncol.* 2001;19(3):697-704.
4. Goldman SC, Holcengerg JS, Finklestein JZ, et al. A randomized comparison between rasburicase and allopurinol in children with lymphoma or leukemia at high risk for tumor lysis. *Blood.* 2001;97(10):2998-3003.
5. Bosly A, Sonet A, Pinkerton CR, et al. Rasburicase (recombinant urate oxidase) for the management of hyperuricemia in patients with cancer. *Cancer.* 2003;98:1048-1054.
6. Jeha S, Kantarjian, Irwin D, et al. Efficacy and safety of rasburicase, a recombinant urate oxidase (Elitek), in the management of malignancy-associated hyperuricemia in pediatric and adult patients: final results of a multicenter compassionate use trial. *Leukemia.* 2005;19:34-38.
7. Wang LY, Shih LY, Chang H, et al. Recombinant urate oxidase (rasburicase) for the prevention and treatment of tumor lysis syndrome in patients with hematologic malignancies. *Acta Haematol.* 2006;115:35-38.
8. Shin HY, Kang JH, Park ES, et al. Recombinant urate oxidase (Rasburicase) for the treatment of hyperuricemia in pediatric patients with hematologic malignancies: results of a compassionate prospective multicenter study in Korea. *Pediatr Blood Cancer.* 2006;46(4):439-445.
9. Liu CY, Sims-McCallum RP, Schiffer CA. A single dose of rasburicase is sufficient for the treatment of hyperuricemia in patients receiving chemotherapy. *Leukemia Res.* 2005;29:463-465.
10. Hutcherson DA, Gammon DC, Bhatt MS, et al. Reduced-dose rasburicase in the treatment of adults with hyperuricemia associated with malignancy. *Pharmacotherapy.* 2006;26(2):242-247.
11. Van den Berg H, Reintsema AM. Renal tubular damage in rasburicase: risks of alkalinisation. *Ann Oncol.* 2004;15:175-176.

Respiratory Syncytial Virus Immune Globulin Intravenous

1. American Academy of Pediatrics Committee on Infectious Diseases and Committee on Fetus and Newborn. Prevention of respiratory syncytial virus infections: indications for the use of palivizumab and update on the use of RSV-IGIV. *Pediatrics.* 1998;102:1211.
2. Simoes EAF, Sondheimer HM, Top FH Jr, et al. Respiratory syncytial virus immune globulin for prophylaxis against respiratory syncytial virus disease in infants and children with congenital heart disease. *J Pediatr.*1998;133:492-499.
3. RespiGam [package insert]. Gaithersburg, MD: Medimmune Inc; May 2000.
4. The PREVENT Study Group. Reduction of respiratory syncytial virus hospitalization among premature infants and infants with bronchopulmonary dysplasia using respiratory syncytial virus immune globulin prophylaxis. *Pediatrics.* 1997;99:93-99.
5. Groothuis JR, Simoes E, Levin MJ, et al. Prophylactic administration of respiratory syncytial virus immune globulin to high-risk infants and young children. *N Engl J Med.* 1993;329:1524-1530.
6. DeVincenzo JP, Hirsch RL, Fuentes RJ, et al. Respiratory syncytial virus immune globulin treatment of lower respiratory tract infection in pediatric patients undergoing bone marrow transplantation—a compassionate use experience. *Bone Marrow Transplantation.* 2000;25:161-165.
7. Rodriguez WJ, Gruber WC, Welliver RC, et al. Respiratory syncytial virus (RSV) immune globulin intravenous therapy for RSV lower respiratory tract infection in infants and young children at high risk for severe RSV infections. *Pediatrics.* 1997;99:454-461.
8. Rodriguez WJ, Gruber WC, Groothuis JR, et al. Respiratory syncytial virus immune globulin treatment of RSV lower respiratory tract infection in previously healthy children. *Pediatrics.* 1997;100:937-942.
9. American Academy of Pediatrics. In: Pickering LK, ed. *2003 Red Book: Report of the Committee on Infectious Diseases.* 26th ed. Elk Grove Village, IL: American Academy of Pediatrics; 2003.

References

Rifampin

1. Tan TQ, Mason EO, Ou CN, et al. Use of intravenous rifampin in neonates with persistent staphylococcal bacteremia. *Antimicrob Agents Chemother.* 1993;37:2401-2406.
2. Shama A, Patole SK, Whitehall JS. Intravenous rifampicin in neonates with persistent staphylococcal bacteraemia. *Acta Paediatr.* 2002;91:670-673.
3. American Academy of Pediatrics. In: Pickering LK, ed. *Red Book: 2006 Report of the Committee on Infectious Diseases.* 27th ed. Elk Grove Village, IL: American Academy of Pediatrics; 2006.
4. American Academy of Pediatrics Committee on Infectious Diseases. Therapy for children with invasive pneumococcal infections. *Pediatrics.* 1997;99:289-299.
5. Koup HR, Williams WJ, Weber A, et al. Pharmacokinetics of rifampin in children. I. Multiple dose intravenous infusion. *Ther Drug Monit.* 1986;8:11-16.
6. Stover BH, Duff A, Adams G, et al. Emergence and control of methicillin-resistant Staphylococcus aureus in a children's hospital and pediatric long-term care facility. *Am J Infect Control.* 1992;20:248-255.
7. Santos Sanches I, Mato R, de Lencastre H, et al. Patterns of multidrug resistance among methicillin-resistant hospital isolates of coagulase-positive and coagulase-negative staphylococci collected in the international multicenter study. RESIST in 1997 and 1998. *Microb Drug Resist.* 2000;6:199-211.
8. Inglesby TV, O'Toole T, Henderson DA, et al. For the Working Group on Civilian Biodefense. Anthrax as a biological weapon 2002: updated recommendations for management. *JAMA.* 2002;287:2236-2252.
9. Centers for Disease Control and Prevention. Update: Investigation of bioterrorism-related anthrax and interim guidelines for exposure management and antimicrobial therapy, October 2001. *MMWR Morb Mortal Wkly Rep.* 2001;50:909-919.
10. Nahata MC, Fan-Harvard P, Barson WJ, et al. Pharmacokinetics, cerebral fluid concentration, and safety of intravenous rifampin in pediatric patients undergoing shunt placement. *Eur J Clin Pharmacol.* 1990;38:515-517.
11. Rifadin [package insert]. Bedford, OH: Bedford Laboratories; February 2004.
12. Holmberg RE, Pavia AT, Montgomery D, et al. Nosocomial legionella pneumonia in the neonate. *Pediatrics.* 1993;92:450-453.
13. Yzerman EP, Boelens HA, Vogel M, et al. Efficacy and safety of teicoplanin plus rifampicin in the treatment of bacteraemic infections caused by Staphylococcus aureus. *J Antimicrob Chemotherapy.* 1998;42:233-239.
14. Trissel LA, ed. *Handbook on Injectable Drugs.* 13th ed. [CD-ROM version 1.5]. Bethesda, MD: American Society of Health-System Pharmacists; 2005.
15. Chang AB, Grimwood K, Harvey AS, et al. Central nervous system tuberculosis after resolution of miliary tuberculosis. *Pediatr Infect Dis J.* 1998;17:519-523.

Rituximab

1. *Physicians' Desk Reference.* 60th ed. Montvale, NJ: Thomson PDR; 2006.
2. Colombat P, Salles G, Brousee N, et al. Rituximab (anti-CD20 monoclonal antibody) as single first-line therapy for patients with follicular lymphoma with a low tumor burden: clinical and molecular evaluation. *Blood.* 2001;97(1):101-106.
3. Jetsrisuparb A, Wiangnon S, Komvilaisak P, et al. Rituximab combined with CHOP for successful treatment of aggressive recurrent, pediatric B-cell large cell non-Hodgkin's lymphoma. *J Pediatr Hematol Oncol.* 2005;27(4):223-226.
4. Hainsworth JD, Litchy S, Shaffer DW, et al. Maximizing therapeutic benefit of rituximab: maintenance therapy versus re-treatment at progression in patients with indolent non-Hodgkin's lymphoma—a randomized phase II trial of the Minnie Pearl Cancer Research Network. *J Clin Oncol.* 2005;23(6):1088-1095.
5. Kewalramani T, Zelenetz AD, Nimer SD, et al. Rituximab and ICE as second-line therapy before autologous stem cell transplantation for relapsed or primary refractory diffuse large B-cell lymphoma. *Blood.* 2004;103(10):3684-3688.
6. Claviez A, Eckert C, Seeger K, et al. Rituximab plus chemotherapy in children with relapsed or refractory CD20-positive B-cell precursor acute lymphoblastic leukemia. *Haematologica.* 2006;91:272-273.
7. Wiseman GA, Leigh BR, Erwin WD, et al. Radiation dosimetry results from a phase II trial of ibritumomab tiuxetan (Zevalin) radioimmunotherapy for patients with non-Hodgkin's lymphoma and mild thrombocytopenia. *Cancer Biother Radiopharm.* 2003;18(2):165-178.
8. Herman J, Vandenberghe P, van den Heuvel I, et al. Successful treatment with rituximab of lymphoproliferative disorder in a child after cardiac transplantation. *J Heart Lung Transplant.* 2002;21(12):1304-1309.
9. Berney T, Delis S, Kato T, et al. Successful treatment of post-transplant lymphoproliferative disease with prolonged rituximab treatment in intestinal transplant recipients. *Transplantation.* 2002;74(7):1000-1006.
10. Zecca M, Nobili B, Ramenghi U, et al. Rituximab for the treatment of refractory autoimmune hemolytic anemia in children. *Blood.* 2003;101(10):3857-3861.
11. Motto DG, Williams JA, Boxer LA. Rituximab for refractory childhood autoimmune hemolytic anemia. *Isr Med Assoc J.* 2002;4(11):1006-1008.
12. National Comprehensive Cancer Network (NCCN) Antiemesis Panel Members. NCCN Clinical Practice Guidelines in Oncology. Antiemesis, v.1.2006. Available at www.nccn.org. Last accessed March 29, 2006.
13. Roila F, Feyer P, Maranzamo E, et al. Antiemetics in children receiving chemotherapy. *Support Care Cancer.* 2005;13:129-131.

Rocuronium Bromide

1. Rowlee SC. Monitoring neuromuscular blockade in the intensive care unit: the peripheral nerve stimulator. *Heart Lung.* 1999;28:352-362.
2. *Physicians' Desk Reference.* 60th ed. Montvale; NJ: Thomson PDR; 2006.
3. American Society of Health-System Pharmacists. American Hospital Formulary System. Available at: http://ahfsfirst.firstdatabank.com/AHFSfirst/NSAHFSFirstSearchmain.asp. Accessed August 15, 2006.
4. Woloszczuk-Gebicka B, Lapczynski T, Wierzejski W. The influence of halothane, isoflurane and sevoflurane on rocuronium infusions in children. *Acta Anaesthesiol Scand.* 2001;45:73-77.
5. Eikermann M, Kunkemoller I, Peine L, et al. Optimal rocuronium dose for intubation during induction with sevoflurane in children. *Br J Anaesth.* 2002;89:277-281.
6. Martin LD, Bratton SL, O'Rourke PP. Clinical uses and controversies of neuromuscular blocking agents in infants and children. *Crit Care Med.* 1999;27:1358-1368.
7. Wierda JM, Meretoja OA, Taivainen T, et al. Pharmacokinetics and pharmacodynamic modeling of rocuronium in infants and children. *Br J Anaesth.* 1997;78:690-695.
8. Ross AK, Dear GL, Dear RB, et al. Onset and recovery of neuromuscular blockade after two doses of rocuronium in children. *J Clin Anesth.* 1998;10:631-635.
9. Mendez DR, Goto CS, Abramo TJ, et al. Safety and efficacy of rocuronium for controlled intubation with paralytics in the pediatric emergency department. *Pediatr Emerg Care.* 2001;17:233-236.
10. Tobias JD. Continuous infusion of rocuronium in a paediatric intensive care unit. *Can J Anaesth.* 1996;43:353-357.
11. Driessen JJ, Robertson EN, Van Egmond J, Booij LH. Time-course of action of rocuronium 0.3 mg.kg-1 in children with and without endstage renal failure. *Paediatr Anaesth.* 2002;12:507-510.

References

12. Trissel LA, ed. *Handbook on Injectable Drugs.* 13th ed. [CD-ROM version 1.5]. Bethesda, MD: American Society of Health-System Pharmacists; 2005.
13. Kaplan RF, Uejima T, Lobel G, et al. Intramuscular rocuronium in infants and children: a multicenter study to evaluate tracheal intubating conditions, onset, and duration of action. *Anesthesiology.* 1999;91:633-638.
14. Reynolds LM, Lau M, Brown R, et al. Bioavailability of intramuscular rocuronium in infants and children. *Anesthesiology.* 1997;87:1096-1105.

Ropivacaine HCl

1. *Physicians' Desk Reference.* 60th ed. Montvale, NJ: Thomson PDR; 2006.
2. Taketomo CK, Hodding JH, Kraus DM. *Pediatric Dosage Handbook.* 12th ed. Hudson, OH: Lexi-Comp Inc; 2005.
3. Khalil S, Campos C, Farag AM, et al. Caudal block in children: ropivacaine compared with bupivacaine. *Anesthesiology.* 1999;91:1279-1284.
4. Lonnqvist PA, Westrin P, Larsson BA, et al. Ropivacaine pharmacokinetics after caudal block in 1–8-year-old children. *Br J Anaesth.* 2000;85:506-511.
5. Wulf H, Peters C, Behnke H. The pharmacokinetics of caudal ropivacaine 0.2% in children: a study of infants aged less than 1 year and toddlers aged 1–5 years undergoing inguinal hernia repair. *Anaesthesia.* 2000;55:757-760.
6. Hansen TG, Ilett KF, Reid C, et al. Caudal ropivacaine in infants: population pharmacokinetics and plasma concentrations. *Anesthesiology.* 2001;94:579-584.
7. Aguirre-Garay FT, Garcia R, Nava-Ocampo AA. Dose-response of ropivacaine administered caudally to children undergoing surgical procedures under sedation with midazolam. *Clin Exp Pharmacol Physiol.* 2004;31:462-465.
8. Bozkurt P, Arslan I, Bakan M, et al. Free plasma levels of bupivacaine and ropivacaine when used for caudal block in children. *Eur J Anaesth.* 2005;22:634-643.
9. Hansen TG, Ilett KF, Lim SI, et al. Pharmacokinetics and clinical efficacy of long-term epidural ropivacaine infusion in children. *Br J Anaesth.* 2000;85:347-353.
10. Simpson D, Curran MP, Oldfield V, et al. Ropivacaine: a review of its use in regional anaesthesia and acute pain management. *Drugs.* 2005;65:2675-717.
11. Antok E, Bordet F, Duflo F, et al. Patient-controlled epidural analgesia versus continuous epidural infusion with ropivacaine for postoperative analgesia in children. *Anesth Analg.* 2004;97:1608-1611.
12. De Negri P, Ivani G, Tirri T, et al. A comparison of epidural bupivacaine, levobupivacaine, and ropivacaine on postoperative analgesia and motor blockage. *Anesth Analg.* 2004;99:45-48.
13. Trissel LA. *Handbook on Injectable Drugs.* 13th ed. Bethesda, MD: American Society of Health-System Pharmacists; 2005.

Sargramostim

1. American Society of Health-System Pharmacists. American Hospital Formulary System. Available at: http://ahfsfirst.firstdatabank.com/AHFSfirst/NSAHFSFirstSearchmain.asp. Accessed August 16, 2006.
2. Medical Economics, ed. *Physicians' Desk Reference.* 54th ed. Oradell, NJ: Medical Economics Company; 2000.
3. Furman WL, Fairclough DL, Huhn RD, et al. Therapeutic effects and pharmacokinetics of recombinant human granulocyte-macrophage colony-stimulating factor in childhood cancer patients receiving myelosuppressive chemotherapy. *J Clin Oncol.* 1991;9:1022-1028.
4. Furman WL, Crist WM. Biology and clinical applications of hemopoietins in pediatric practice. *Pediatrics.* 1992;90:716-728.
5. Riikonen P, Saarinen UM, Makipernaa A, et al. Recombinant human granulocyte-macrophage colony-stimulating factor in the treatment of febrile neutropenia: a double blind placebo-controlled study in children. *Pediatr Infect Dis J.* 1994;13:197-202.
6. Luksch R, Massimino M, Cefalo G, et al. Effects of recombinant human granulocyte-macrophage colony-stimulating factor in an intensive treatment program for children with Ewing's sarcoma. *Haematologica.* 2001;86:753-760.
7. Saarinen-Pihkala UM, Lanning M, Perkkio M, et al. Granulocyte-macrophage colony-stimulating factor support in therapy of high-risk acute lymphoblastic leukemia in children. *Med Pediatr Oncol.* 2000;34:319-327.
8. Trigg ME, Peters C, Zimmerman MB. Administration of recombinant human granulocyte-macrophage colony-stimulating factor to children undergoing allogenic marrow transplantation: a prospective, randomized, double-masked, placebo-controlled trial. *Pediatr Transplant.* 2000;4:123-132.
9. Welte K, Zeidler C, Reiter A, et al. Differential effects of granulocyte-macrophage colony-stimulating factor and granulocyte colony-stimulating factor in children with severe congenital neutropenia. *Blood.* 1990;75:1056-1063.
10. Venkateswaran L, Wilimas JA, Dancy R, et al. Granulocyte-macrophage colony-stimulating factor in the treatment of neonates with neutropenia and sepsis. *Pediatr Hematol Oncol.* 2000;17:469-473.
11. Ahmad A, Laborada G, Bussel J, et al. Comparison of recombinant granulocyte colony-stimulating factor, recombinant human granulocyte-macrophage colony-stimulating factor and placebo for treatment of septic preterm infants. *Pediatr Infect Dis J.* 2002;21:1061-1065.
12. Guinan EC, Sieff CA, Oette DH, et al. A phase I/II trial of recombinant granulocyte-macrophage colony-stimulating factor in children with aplastic anemia. *Blood.* 1990;76:1077-1082.
13. Jeng MR, Naidu PE, Reiman MD, et al. Granulocyte-macrophage colony stimulating factor and immunosuppression in the treatment of pediatric acquired severe aplastic anemia. *Pediatr Blood Cancer.* 2005;45:170-175.
14. Kushner BH, Kramer K, Cheung NV. Phase II trial of the anti-G_{D2} monoclonal antibody 3F8 and granulocyte-macrophage colony-stimulating factor for neuroblastoma. *J Clin Oncol.* 2001;19(22):4189-4194.
15. American Academy of Pediatrics Committee on Drugs. "Inactive" ingredients in pharmaceutical products: update. *Pediatrics.* 1997;99:268-278.
16. Hall CM, Milligan DWA, Berrington J. Probable adverse reaction to a pharmaceutical excipient. *Arch Dis Child Fetal Neonatal Ed.* 2004;89:F184.
17. Hiller JL, Benda GI, Rahatzad M, et al. Benzyl alcohol toxicity: impact on mortality and intraventricular hemorrhage among very low birth weight infants. *Pediatrics.* 1986;77:500-506.
18. Grant JA, Bilodeau PA, Guernsey BG, et al. Unsuspected benzyl alcohol hypersensitivity. *N Engl J Med.* 1982;306:108.
19. Wilson JP, Solimando DA, Edwards MS. Parenteral benzyl alcohol-induced hypersensitivity reaction. *Drug Intell Clin Pharm.* 1986;20:689-691.
20. Trissel LA. *Handbook on Injectable Drugs.* 13th ed. Bethesda, MD: American Society of Hospital Pharmacists; 2005.
21. Bonig H, Burdach S, Gobel U, et al. Growth factors and hemostasis: differential effects of GM-CSF and G-CSF on coagulation activation—laboratory and clinical evidence. *Ann Hematol.* 2001;80:525-530.

Sodium Bicarbonate

1. American Heart Association in collaboration with the International Liaison Committee on Resuscitation. Guidelines 2000 for cardiopulmonary resuscitation and emergency cardiovascular care. Part 10: Pediatric advanced life support. *Circulation.* 2000;128(suppl 1):1291-1342.
2. American Academy of Pediatrics Committee on Drugs. Emergency drug doses for infants and children. *Pediatrics.* 1998;101:e1-e11.
3. Sagraves R, Kamper C. Controversies in cardiopulmonary resuscitation: pediatric considerations. *DICP Ann Pharmacother.* 1991;25:760-772.
4. Sodium bicarbonate injection, USP. Lake Forest, IL: Hospira Inc; April 2004.
5. McEvoy GK, ed. *AHFS Drug Information Essentials 2005–06.* Bethesda, MD: American Society of Health-System Pharmacists; 2005.

6. Proudfoot AT, Krenzelok EP, Vale JA. Position paper on urine alkalinization. *J Toxicol.* 2004;42:1-26.
7. Kelly KM, Lange B. Oncologic emergencies. *Pediatr Clin NA.* 1997;44:809-830.
8. Simmons MA, Adcock EW, Bard H, et al. Hypernatremia and intracranial hemorrhage in neonates. *N Engl J Med.* 1974;291:6-10.
9. Trissel LA, ed. *Handbook on Injectable Drugs.* 13th ed. Bethesda, MD: American Society of Health-System Pharmacists; 2005.
10. Gaze NR. Tissue necrosis caused by commonly used intravenous infusions. *Lancet.* 1978; 2:417-419.
11. Finberg L. Dangers to infants caused by changes in osmolal concentration. *Pediatrics.* 1967;40:1031-1034.
12. Leuthner SR, Jansen RD, Hageman JR. Cardiopulmonary resuscitation of the newborn. An update. *Pediatr Clin North Am.* 1994;41:893-907.
13. Trachtenbarg DE. Diabetic ketoacidosis. *Am Fam Physician.* 2005;71:1705-1714.
14. Green SM, Rothrock SG, Ho JD, et al. Failure of adjunctive bicarbonate to improve outcome in severe pediatric diabetic ketoacidosis. *Ann Emerg Med.* 1998;31:41-48.
15. Brown CVR, Rhee P, Chan L, et al. Preventing renal failure in patients with rhabdomyolysis: do bicarbonate and mannitol make a difference? *J Trauma.* 2004;56:1191-1196.

Sodium Chloride

1. Deficit therapy. In: Behrman RE, Kliegman RM, Jensen HB, eds. *Nelson Textbook of Pediatrics.* 17th ed. Philadelphia, PA: Saunders; 2004:245-249.
2. Shock. In: Behrman RE, Kliegman RM, Jensen HB, eds. *Nelson Textbook of Pediatrics.* 17th ed. Philadelphia, PA: Saunders; 2004:296-301.
3. Jospe N, Forbes G. Fluids and electrolytes—clinical aspects. *Ped Rev.* 1996;17:395-404.
4. Moritz ML, Ayus JC. Disorders of water metabolism in children: hyponatremia and hypernatremia. *Ped Rev.* 2002;23:371-379.
5. Lin M, Liu SJ, Lim IT. Disorders of water imbalance. *Emerg Med Clin N Am.* 2005;23:749-770.
6. Simma B, Burger R, Falk M, et al. A prospective, randomized, and controlled study of fluid management in children with severe head injury: lactated Ringer's solution versus hypertonic saline. *Crit Care Med.* 1998;26:1265-1270.
7. Khanna S, Davis D, Peterson B, et al. Use of hypertonic saline in the treatment of severe refractory posttraumatic intracranial hypertension in pediatric traumatic brain injury. *Crit Care Med.* 2000;28:1144-1152.
8. Peterson B, Khanna S, Fisher B, et al. Prolonged hypernatremia controls elevated intracranial pressure in head-injured pediatric patients. *Crit Care Med.* 2000;28:1136-1143.
9. Adelson PD, Bratton SL, Carney NA, et al. Guidelines for the acute medical management of severe traumatic brain injury in infants, children, and adolescents. Chapter 11. Use of hyperosmolar therapy in the management of severe pediatric traumatic brain injury. *Pediatr Crit Care Med.* 2003 Jul;4(3 suppl):S40-4.
10. McEvoy GK, ed. *AHFS Drug Information Essentials 2005–06.* Bethesda, MD: American Society of Health-System Pharmacists; 2005.
11. Trissel LA, ed. *Handbook on Injectable Drugs.* 13th ed. Bethesda, MD: American Society of Health-System Pharmacists; 2005.
12. American Academy of Pediatrics Committee on Drugs. "Inactive" ingredients in pharmaceutical products: update. *Pediatrics.* 1997;99:268-278.
13. Hall CM, Milligan DWA, Berrington J. Probable adverse reaction to a pharmaceutical excipient. *Arch Dis Child Fetal Neonatal Ed.* 2004;89:F184.
14. Hiller JL, Benda GI, Rahatzad M, et al. Benzyl alcohol toxicity: impact on mortality and intraventricular hemorrhage among very low birth weight infants. *Pediatrics.* 1986;77:500-506.
15. Grant JA, Bilodeau PA, Guernsey BG, et al. Unsuspected benzyl alcohol hypersensitivity. *N Engl J Med.* 1982;306:108.
16. Wilson JP, Solimando DA, Edwards MS. Parenteral benzyl alcohol-induced hypersensitivity reaction. *Drug Intell Clin Pharm.* 1986;20:689-691.
17. Soni MG, Taylor SL, Greenberg NA, et al. Evaluation of the health aspects of methyl paraben: a review of the published literature. *Food Chem Toxicol.* 2002;40:1335-1373.
18. Nagel JE, Fuscaldo JT, Firemen P. Paraben allergy. *JAMA.* 1977;237:1594-1595.
19. Choski R, Roach ES. Ring-enhancing lesion in central pontine myelinolysis. *Arch Neurol.* 2005;62:1016-1017.
20. Tan H, Onbas O. Central pontine myelinolysis manifesting with massive myoclonus. *Pediatr Neurol.* 2004;31:64-66.
21. Haspolat S, Duman O, Senol U, et al. Extrapontine myelinolysis in infancy: report of a case. *J Child Neurol.* 2004;19:913-15.

Sodium Nitroprusside

1. Nitropress [package insert]. Lake Forest, IL: Hospira Inc; December 2004.
2. McEvoy GK, ed. *Drug Information Essentials 2005–06.* Bethesda, MD: American Society of Health-System Pharmacists; 2005.
3. American Heart Association Guidelines for Cardiopulmonary Resuscitation and Emergency Cardiovascular Care. Part 12: Pediatric Advanced Life Support. *Circulation.* 2005;112(suppl 1):167-187.
4. American Academy of Pediatrics Committee on Drugs. Drugs for Pediatric Emergencies. *Pediatrics.* 1998;101:e1-e11.
5. Perkin RM, Levin DL. Shock in the pediatric patient. Part II. Therapy. *J Pediatr.* 1982;101:319-332.
6. Fleischmann LE. Management of hypertensive crises in children. *Pediatr Ann.* 1977;6:410-414.
7. Benitz WE, Malachowski N, Cohen RS, et al. Use of sodium nitroprusside in neonates: efficacy and safety. *J Pediatr.* 1985;106:102-110.
8. Gordillo-Paniagua G, Velasquez-Jones L, Martini R, et al. Sodium nitroprusside treatment of severe arterial hypertension in children. *J Pediatr.* 1975; 87:799-802.
9. Dillon TR, Janos GG, Meyer RA, et al. Vasodilator therapy for congestive heart failure. *J Pediatr.* 1980;96:623-629.
10. Beverley DW, Hughes CA, Davies DP, et al. Early use of sodium nitroprusside in respiratory distress syndrome. *Arch Dis Child.* 1979;54:403-407.
11. Beekman RH, Rocchini AP, Dick M, et al. Vasodilator therapy in children: acute and chronic effects in children with left ventricular dysfunction or mitral regurgitation. *Pediatrics.* 1984;73:43-51.
12. Appelbaum A, Blackstone EH, Kouchoukos NT, et al. Afterload reduction and cardiac output in infants early after intra-cardiac surgery. *Am J Cardiol.* 1977;39:445-451.
13. Kunathai S, Sholler GF, Celermajer JM, et al. Nitroprusside in children after cardiopulmonary bypass: a study of thiocyanate toxicity. *Pediatr Cardiol.* 1989;10:121-124.
14. Deal JE, Barratt TM, Dillon MJ. Management of hypertensive emergencies. *Arch Dis Child.* 1992;67:1089-1092.
15. Miller K. Pharmacological management of hypertension in paediatric patients. *Drugs.* 1994;48:868-887.
16. National High Blood Pressure Education Program Working Group on High Blood Pressure in Children and Adolescents. The Fourth Report on the Diagnosis, Evaluation, and Treatment of High Blood Pressure in Children and Adolescents. *Pediatrics.* 2004;114:555-576.
17. Young TE, Mangum B, eds. *Neofax.* 18th ed. Raleigh, NC: Acorn Publishing Inc; 2005.
18. Grossman E, Ironi AN, Messerli FH. Comparative tolerability profile of hypertensive crisis treatments. *Drug Safety.* 1998;19:99-122. Review
19. Cottrell JE, Illner P, Kittay MJ, et al. Rebound hypertension after sodium nitroprusside-induced hypotension. *Clin Pharmacol Ther.* 1980;27:32-36.
20. Zubrow AB, Daniel SS, Stark RI, et al. Plasma vasopressin, rennin, and catecholamines during nitroprusside-induced hypotension in the newborn lamb. *J Perinat Med.* 1989:17:271-277.
21. Fivush B, Neu A, Furth S. Acute hypertensive crises in children: emergencies and urgencies. *Curr Opin Pediatr.* 1997;9:233-236.
22. Palmer RF, Lasseter KC. Sodium nitroprusside. *N Engl J Med.* 1975;292:294-297.
23. Trissel LA, ed. *Handbook on Injectable Drugs.* 13th ed. Bethesda, MD: American Society of Health-System Pharmacists; 2005.

References

24. Rich DS. New JCAHO medication management standards for 2004. *Am J Health-Syst Pharm.* 2004;61:1349-1358.
25. Sodorff MM, Galt KA, Galt M, et al. Recommended maximum concentrations of common acute care parenteral admixtures. *Hosp Pharm.* 1999;34:937-942.
26. Raymond G, Day P, Rabb M. Sodium content of commonly administered intravenous drugs. *Hosp Pharm.* 1982;17:560-561.
27. Friedman WF, George BL. New concepts and drugs in the treatment of congestive heart failure. *Pediatr Clin North Am.* 1984;31:1197-1227.
28. Rindone JP, Sloane EP. Cyanide toxicity from sodium nitroprusside: risk and management. *Ann Pharmacother.* 1992;26:515-519.
29. Linakis JG, Lacouture PG, Woolf A. Monitoring cyanide and thiocyanate concentrations during infusion of sodium nitroprusside in children. *Pediatr Cardiol.* 1991;12:214-218.

Succinylcholine Chloride

1. American Society of Health-System Pharmacists. American Hospital Formulary System. Available at: http://ahfsfirst.firstdatabank.com/AHFSfirst/NSAHFSFirstSearchmain.asp. Accessed July 9, 2006.
2. Rowlee SC. Monitoring neuromuscular blockade in the intensive care unit: the peripheral nerve stimulator. *Heart Lung.* 1999;28:352-362.
3. Rose JB, Theroux MC, Katz MS. The potency of succinylcholine in obese adolescents. *Anesth Analg.* 2000;90:576-578.
4. Levy G. Pharmacokinetics of succinylcholine in newborns. *Anesthesiology.* 1970;32:551-552.
5. Cook DR, Fisher CG. Neuromuscular blocking effects of succinylcholine in infants and children. *Anesthesiology.* 1975;42:662-665.
6. Cook DR, Wingard L, Taylor F. Pharmacokinetics of succinylcholine in infants, children and adults. *Clin Pharmacol Ther.* 1976;20:493-498.
7. Jankiewicz AM, Nowakowski P. Ketamine and succinylcholine for emergency intubation of pediatric patients. *DICP Ann Pharmacother.* 1991;2:475-476.
8. Martin LD, Bratton SL, O'Rourke PP. Clinical uses and controversies of neuromuscular blocking agents in infants and children. *Crit Care Med.* 1999;27:1358-1368.
9. Zelicof-Paul A, Smith-Lockridge A, Schnadower D, et al. Controversies in rapid sequence intubation in children. *Curr Opin Pediatr.* 2005;17:355-362.
10. Goudsouzian NG, Liu LM. The neuromuscular response of infants to a continuous infusion of succinylcholine. *Anesthesiology.* 1984;60:97-101.
11. Sullivan M, Thompson WK. Succinylcholine-induced cardiac arrest in children with undiagnosed myopathy. *Can J Anaesth.* 1994;41:497-501.
12. Hiller JL, Benda GI, Rahatzad M, et al. Benzyl alcohol toxicity: impact on mortality and intraventricular hemorrhage among very low birth weight infants. *Pediatrics.* 1986;77:500-506.
13. American Academy of Pediatrics Committee on Drugs. "Inactive" ingredients in pharmaceutical products: update. *Pediatrics.* 1997;99:268-278.
14. Hall CM, Milligan DWA, Berrington J. Probably adverse reaction to a pharmaceutical excipient. *Arch Dis Child Fetal Neonatal Ed.* 2004;89:F184.
15. Grant JA, Bilodeau PA, Guernsey BG, et al. Unsuspected benzyl alcohol hypersensitivity. *N Engl J Med.* 1982;306:108.
16. Wilson JP, Solimando DA, Edwards MS. Parenteral benzyl alcohol-induced hypersensitivity reaction. *Drug Intell Clin Pharm.* 1986;20:689-691.
17. Benzer A, Luz G, Oswald E, et al. Succinylcholine-induced prolonged apnea in a 3-week old newborn: treatment with human plasma cholinesterase. *Anesth Analg.* 1992;74:137-138.
18. Roth F, Wuthrich H. The clinical importance of hyperkalemia following suxamethonium administration. *Br J Anaesth.* 1969;41:311-316.
19. Keneally JP, Bush GH. Changes in serum potassium after suxamethonium in children. *Anaesth Intensive Care.* 1974;2:147-150.
20. Rosenberg H. Intractable cardiac arrest in children given succinylcholine. *Anesthesiology.* 1992;77:105.
21. Larsen U, Juhl B, Hein-Sorenson O, et al. Complications during anesthesia in patients with Duchenne's muscular dystrophy (a retrospective study). *Can J Anaesth.* 1989;36:418-422.

Sufentanil Citrate

1. Schwartz AE, Matteo RS, Ornstein E, et al. Pharmacokinetics of sufentanil in obese patients. *Anesth Analg.* 1991;73:790-793.
2. Guay J, Gaudreault P, Tang A, et al. Pharmacokinetics of sufentanil in normal children. *Can J Anesth.* 1992;39:14-20.
3. Food and Drug Administration. Sufenta (sufentanil citrate) injection [August 28, 2001: Akorn]. MedWatch drug labeling changes. Rockville, MD; October 2001. From FDA website. Available at: (http://www.fda.gov/medwatch/safety/2001/aug01.htm). Accessed August 8, 2006.
4. Sufenta® injection [prescribing information]. Decatur, IL: Taylor Pharmaceuticals; August 1998.
5. Anand KJ, Phil D, Hickey PR. Halothane-morphine compared with high-dose sufentanil for anesthesia and post-operative analgesia in neonatal cardiac surgery. *N Eng J Med.* 1992;326:1-9.
6. Genski JA, Friesen RH, Lane GA, et al. Low-dose sufentanil as a supplement to halothane/N_2O anaesthesia in infants and children. *Can J Anaesth.* 1988;35:379-384.
7. Hickey PR, Hansen DD. Fentanyl- and sufentanil-oxygen-pancuronium anesthesia for cardiac surgery in infants. *Anesth Analgesia.* 1984;63:117-124.
8. American Society of Health-System Pharmacists. American Hospital Formulary System. Available at: http://ahfsfirst.firstdatabank.com/AHFSfirst/NSAHFSFirstSearchmain.asp. Accessed August 10, 2006.
9. Aronoff A, Brier M, Bennett W. *The Renal Book, 2002.* http://www.kdp-baptist.louisville.edu/renalbook/. Accessed August 11, 2006.
10. Moore RA, Yang SS, McNicholas KW, et al. Hemodynamic and anesthetic effects of sufentanil as the sole anesthetic for pediatric cardiovascular surgery. *Anesthesiology.* 1985;62:725-731.
11. Trissel LA, ed. *Handbook on Injectable Drugs.* 13th ed. [CD-ROM version 1.5]. Bethesda, MD: American Society of Health-System Pharmacists; 2005.
12. Albanese J, Durbec O, Viviand X, et al. Sufentanil increases intracranial pressure in patients with head trauma. *Anesthesiology.* 1993;79:493-497.

Tacrolimus

1. McEvoy GK, ed. *Drug Information Essentials 2005–06.* Bethesda, MD: American Society of Health-System Pharmacists; 2005.
2. Prograf [package insert]. Deerfield, IL: Astellas Pharma US Inc; April 2006.
3. McDiarmid SV, Busuttil RW, Ascher NL, et al. FK506 (Tacrolimus) compared with cyclosporine for primary immunosuppression after pediatric liver transplantation. *Transplantation.* 1995;59:530-536.
4. Yasuhara M, Hashida T, Toraguchi M, et al. Pharmacokinetics and pharmacodynamics of FK506 in pediatric patients receiving living-related donor liver transplantations. *Transplant Proc.* 1995;27:1108-1110.
5. McDiarmid SV, Colonna JO, Shaked A, et al. Differences in oral FK506 dose requirements between adult and pediatric liver transplant patients. *Transplantation.* 1993;56:1328-1332.
6. Tzakis AG, Reyes J, Todo S, et al. FK506 versus cyclosporine in pediatric liver transplantation. *Transplant Proc.* 1991;23:3010-3015.
7. Tzakis AG, Reyes J, Todo S, et al. Two-year experience with FK506 in pediatric patients. *Transplant Proc.* 1993;25:619-621.
8. Tzakis AG, Fung JJ, Todo S, et al. Use of FK506 in pediatric patients. *Transplant Proc.* 1991;23:924-927.
9. Busuttil RW, McDiarmid S, Klintmalm GM, et al. A comparison of tacrolimus (FK506) and cyclosporine for immunosuppression in liver transplantation. *N Engl J Med.* 1994;331:1110-1115.
10. Staatz CE, Taylor PJ, Lynch SV, et al. Population pharmacokinetics of tacrolimus in children who receive cut-down or full liver transplants. *Transplantation.* 2001;72:1056-1061.

11. Nash RA, Antin JH, Karanes C, et al. Phase 3 study comparing methotrexate and tacrolimus with methotrexate and cyclosporine for prophylaxis of acute graft-versus-host disease after marrow transplantation from unrelated donors. *Blood.* 2000;96:2062-2068.
12. Osunkwo I, Bessmertny O, Harrison L, et al. A pilot study of tacrolimus and mycophenolate mofetil graft-versus-host disease prophylaxis in childhood and adolescent allogeneic stem cell transplant recipients. *Biol Blood Marrow Transplant.* 2004;10:246-248.
13. Ohashi Y, Minegishi M, Fujie H, et al. Successful treatment of steroid-resistant severe acute GVHD with 24-h continuous infusion of FK506. *Bone Marrow Transplant.* 1997;19:625-627.
14. Robinson BV, Boyle GJ, Miller SA, et al. Optimal dosing of intravenous tacrolimus following pediatric heart transplant. *J Heart Lung Transplant.* 1999;18:786-791.
15. Trissel LA, ed. *Handbook on Injectable Drugs.* 13th ed. Bethesda, MD: American Society of Health-System Pharmacists; 2005.
16. Brown NW, Gonde CE, Adams JE, et al. Low hematocrit and serum albumin concentrations underlie the overestimation of tacrolimus concentrations my microparticle enzyme immunoassay versus liquid chromatography—tandem mass spectrometry. *Clin Chem.* 2005;51:586-592.
17. Taormina D, Abdallah HY, Venkataramanan R, et al. Stability and sorption of FK506 in 5% dextrose injection and 0.9% sodium chloride injection in glass, polyvinyl chloride, and polyolefin containers. *Am J Hosp Pharm.* 1992;49:119-122.
18. Firdaous I, Hassoun A, Otte JB, et al. Pediatric intravenous FK506—how much are we really infusing? *Transplantation.* 1994;57:1821-1823.
19. Nakata Y, Yoshibayashi M, Yonemura T, et al. Tacrolimus and myocardial hypertrophy. *Transplantation.* 2000;69:1960-1962.

Terbutaline Sulfate

1. http://www.nhlbi.nih.gov/guidelines/asthma/asthupdt.htm. Accessed July 18, 2006.
2. Tipton WR, Nelson HS. Frequent parenteral terbutaline in the treatment of status asthmaticus in children. *Ann Allergy.* 1987;252-256.
3. Bremont F, Moisan V, Dutau G. Continuous subcutaneous infusion of Beta 2-agonists in infantile asthma. *Pediatr Pulmonol.* 1992;12:81-83.
4. Fuglsang G, Pedersen S, Borgstrom L. Dose-response relationships of intravenously administered terbutaline in children with asthma. *J Pediatr.* 1989;315-332.
5. Dietrich KA, Conrad SA, Romero MD. Creatine kinase (CK) isoenzymes in pediatric status asthmaticus treated with intravenous terbutaline. *Crit Care Med.* 1991;19:S39. Abstract.
6. DeNicola LK, Monem GF, Gayle MO, et al. Treatment of critical status asthmaticus in children. In: Respiratory medicine 1: current issues. *Pediatr Clin North Am.* 1994;41:1293-1324.
7. Stephanopoulos DE, Monge R, Schell KH, et al. Continuous intravenous terbutaline for pediatric status asthmaticus. *Crit Care Med.* 1998;26:1744-1748.
8. Kambalapalli M, Nichani S, Upadhyayula S. Safety of intravenous terbutaline in acute severe asthma: a retrospective study. *Acta Paediatr.* 2005;94:1214-1217.
9. Payne DNR, Balfour-Lynn IM, Biggart EA. Subcutaneous terbutaline in children with chronic severe asthma. *Pediatric Pulmonol.* 2002;33:356-361.
10. Aronoff A, Brier M, Bennett W. *The Renal Book, 2002.* Available at: http://www.kdp-baptist.louisville.edu/renalbook/. Accessed July 17, 2006.
11. Terbutaline sulfate injection [USP package insert]. Irvine CA: SICOR Pharmaceuticals Inc; February 2004.
12. Hultquist C, Lindberg C, Nyberg L, et al. Pharmacokinetics of intravenous terbutaline in asthmatic children. *Dev Pharmacol Ther.* 1989;13:11-20.
13. McEvoy GK, ed. *American Hospital Formulary Service Drug Information 2006.* Bethesda, MD: American Society of Health-System Pharmacists; 2006.
14. Trissel LA. *Handbook on Injectable Drugs.* 13th ed. Bethesda, MD: American Society of Health-System Pharmacists; 2005.
15. Danziger Y, Garty M, Volwitz B, et al. Reduction of serum theophylline levels by terbutaline in children with asthma. *Clin Pharmacol Ther.* 1985;37:469-471.

Thiopental Sodium

1. Thiopental [package insert]. North Chicago, IL: Abbott Laboratories; February 1991.
2. American Academy of Pediatrics Committee on Drugs. Emergency drug doses for infants and children. *Pediatrics.* 1998;101:e1-11.
3. Morton NS, Wee M, Christie G, et al. Propofol for induction of anaesthesia in children. *Anaesthesia.* 1988;43:350-355.
4. Mirakhur RK. Induction characteristics of propofol in children: comparison with thiopentone. *Anaesthesia.* 1988;43:593-598.
5. Badgwell JM, Cunliffe M, Lerman J. Thiopental attenuates dysrhythmias in children: comparison of induction regimens. *Tex Med.* 1990;86:36-38.
6. Viitanen H, Annila P, Rorarius M, et al. Recovery after halothane anaesthesia induced with thiopental, propofol-alfentanil or halothane for day-case adenoidectomy in small children. *Br J Anaesth.* 1998;81:960-962.
7. Wodey E, Chonow L, Beneux X, et al. Haemodynamic effects of propofol vs thiopental in infants: an echocardiographic study. *Br J Anaesth.* 1999;82:516-520.
8. Jonmarker C, Westrin P, Larsson S, et al. Thiopental requirements for induction of anesthesia in children. *Anesthesiology.* 1987;67:104-107.
9. Westrin P, Jonmarker C, Werner O. Thiopental requirements for induction of anesthesia in neonates and in infants one to six months of age. *Anesthesiology.* 1989;71:344-346.
10. Bhutada A, Sahni R, Rastogi S, et al. Randomised controlled trial of thiopental for intubation in neonates. *Arch Dis Child Fetal Neonatal Ed.* 2000;82:F34-37.
11. Brett CM, Fisher DM. Thiopental dose-response relations in unpremedicated infants, children, and adults. *Anesth Analg.* 1987;66:1024-1027.
12. Demarquez JL, Galperine R, Billeaud C, et al. High-dose thiopental pharmacokinetics in brain injured children and neonates. *Dev Pharmacol Ther.* 1987;10:292-300.
13. Goldberg RN, Moscoso P, Bauer CR, et al. Use of barbiturate therapy in severe perinatal asphyxia: a randomized controlled trial. *J Pediatr.* 1986;109:851-856.
14. Eyre JA, Wilkerson AR. Thiopentone induced comas after severe birth asphyxia. *Arch Dis Child.* 1986;61:1084-1089.
15. Quandt CM, de los Reyes RA. Pharmacologic management of acute intracranial hypertension. *Drug Intell Clin Pharm.* 1984;18:105-112.
16. Sidi A, Cotev S, Hadani M, et al. Long-term barbiturate infusion to reduce intracranial pressure. *Crit Care Med.* 1983;11:478-481.
17. Quandt CM, de los Reyes RA, Diaz FG. Barbiturate-induced coma for the treatment of cerebral ischemia: review of outcome. *Clin Pharm.* 1982;1:549-551.
18. Russo H, Bressolle F, Duboin MP. Pharmacokinetics of high-dose thiopental in pediatric patients with increased intracranial pressure. *Ther Drug Monit.* 1997;19:63-70.
19. Krauss B, Green S. Procedural sedation and analgesia in children. *Lancet.* 2006;367:766-780.
20. Orlowski JP, Erenberg G, Lueders H, et al. Hypothermia and barbiturate coma for refractory status epilepticus. *Crit Care Med.* 1984;12:367-371.
21. Bonati M, Marraro G, Celardo A, et al. Thiopental efficacy in phenobarbital-resistant neonatal seizures. *Dev Pharmacol Ther.* 1990;15:16-20.
22. Amit R, Goitein KJ, Mathot I, et al. Prolonged electrocerebral silent barbiturate coma in intractable seizure disorders. *Epilepsia.* 1988;29:63-66.
23. Young GB, Blume WT, Bolton CF, et al. Anesthetic barbiturates in refractory status epilepticus. *Can J Neurol Sci.* 1980;7:291-292.
24. Aronoff A, Brier M, Bennett W. *The Renal Book, 2002.* Available at: http://www.kdp-baptist.louisville.edu/renalbook/. Accessed June 6, 2006.

References

25. Russo H, Bressolle F. Pharmacodynamics and pharmacokinetics of thiopental. *Clin Pharmacokinet.* 1998;35:95-134.
26. American Society of Health-System Pharmacists. American Hospital Formulary System. Available at: http://ahfsfirst.firstdatabank.com/AHFSfirst/NSAHFSFirstSearchmain.asp. Accessed June 6, 2006.
27. Trissel LA, ed. *Handbook on Injectable Drugs.* 13th ed. [CD-ROM version 1.5]. Bethesda, MD: American Society of Health-System Pharmacists; 2005.
28. Schalen W, Messeter K, Nordstrom H. Complications and side effects during thiopentone therapy in patients with severe head injuries. *Acta Anaesthesiol Scand.* 1992;36:369-377.
29. Sorbo S. The pharmacokinetics of thiopental in pediatric surgical patients. *Anesthesiology.* 1984;61:666-670.

Ticarcillin

1. Prober CG, Stevenson DK, Benitz WE. The use of antibiotics in neonates weighing less than 1200 grams. *Pediatr Infect Dis J.* 1990;9:111–121.
2. American Academy of Pediatrics. In: Pickering LK, ed. *2003 Red Book: Report of the Committee on Infectious Diseases.* 26th ed. Elk Grove Village, IL: American Academy of Pediatrics; 2003.
3. Nelson JD, Bradley JS, eds. *Pocketbook of Pediatric Antimicrobial Therapy.* 14th ed. Baltimore, MD: Williams & Wilkins; 2000–2001.
4. McCracken GH Jr, Nelson JD, eds. *Antimicrobial Therapy for Newborns: Practical Application.* 2nd ed. New York, NY: Grune and Stratton; 1983.
5. Nelson JD. Neonatal ticarcillin dosage. *Pediatrics.* 1979;64:549-550. Letter.
6. Nelson JD, Kusmiesz H, Shelton S, et al. Clinical pharmacology and efficacy of ticarcillin in infants and children. *Pediatrics.* 1978;61:858-863.
7. Rhodes KH, Henry NK. Antibiotic therapy for severe infections in infants and children. *Mayo Clin Proc.* 1992;67:59-68.
8. Ticar prescribing information. Research Triangle Park, NC: GlaxoSmithKline; September 2002.
9. Parry MF, Neu HC, Merlino M, et al. Treatment of pulmonary infections in patients with cystic fibrosis: a comparative study of ticarcillin and gentamicin. *J Pediatr.* 1977;90:144-148.
10. McLaughlin FJ, Matthews WJ, Strieder DJ, et al. Clinical and bacteriological responses to three antibiotic regimens for acute exacerbations of cystic fibrosis: ticarcillin–tobramycin, azlocillin–tobramycin, and azlocillin–placebo. *J Infect Dis.* 1983;147:559-567.
11. Parry MF, Neu HC. Tobramycin and ticarcillin therapy for exacerbations of pulmonary disease in patients with cystic fibrosis. *J Infect Dis.* 1976;134(suppl):S194-S197.
12. Jackson MA, Kusmiesz H, Shelton S, et al. Comparison of piperacillin vs. ticarcillin plus tobramycin in the treatment of acute pulmonary exacerbation of cystic fibrosis. *Pediatr Infect Dis J.* 1986;5:440-443.
13. Shenep JL, Hughes WT, Roberson PK, et al. Vancomycin, ticarcillin, and amikacin compared with ticarcillin–clavulanate and amikacin in the empirical treatment of febrile, neutropenic children with cancer. *N Engl J Med.* 1988;319:1053-1058.
14. Shenep JL, Flynn PM, Baker DK, et al. Oral cefixime is similar to continued intravenous antibiotics in the empirical treatment of febrile neutropenic children with cancer. *Clin Infect Dis.* 2001;32:36-43.
15. Aronoff A, Brier M, Bennett W. *The Renal Book, 2002.* Available at: http://www.kdp-baptist.louisville.edu/renalbook/. Accessed August 5, 2006.
16. Arnoff GR, Berns JS, Brier ME, et al. *Drug Prescribing in Renal Failure: Dosing Guidelines for Adults.* 4th ed. Philadelphia, PA: American College of Physicians; 1999.
17. Parry MF, Neu HC. Pharmacokinetics of ticarcillin in patients with abnormal renal function. *J Infect Dis.* 1976;133:46-49.
18. Kallay MC, Tabechian H, Riley GR, et al. Neurotoxicity due to ticarcillin in patient with renal failure. *Lancet.* 1979;1:608-609. Letter.
19. Trissel LA, ed. *Handbook on Injectable Drugs.* 13th ed. [CD-ROM version 1.5]. Bethesda, MD: American Society of Health-System Pharmacists; 2005.
20. Robinson DC, Cookson TL, Frisafe JA. Concentration guidelines for parenteral antibiotics in fluid-restricted patients. *Drug Intell Clin Pharm.* 1987;21:985–989.
21. American Society of Health-System Pharmacists. American Hospital Formulary System. Available at: http://ahfsfirst.firstdatabank.com/AHFSfirst/NSAHFSFirstSearchmain.asp. Accessed August 5, 2006.
22. Stewart GT. Cross allergenicity of penicillin G and related substances. *Lancet.* 1962;1:509-510.
23. Grieco MH. Cross-allergenicity of the penicillins and the cephalosporins. *Arch Intern Med.* 1967;119:141-146.
24. Sullivan TJ. Pathogenesis and management of allergic reactions to penicillin and other beta-lactam antibiotics. *Pediatr Infect Dis.* 1982;1:344-350.
25. Saxon A. Immediate hypersensitivity reactions to B-lactam antibiotics. *Rev Infect Dis.* 1983;5(suppl 2):S368-S378.
26. Sher TH. Penicillin hypersensitivity—a review. In: Symposium on anti-infective therapy I. Speck WT, Blummer JL, eds. *Pediatr Clin North Am.* 1983;30:161-177.
27. Nanji AA, Lindsay J. Ticarcillin associated hypokalemia. *Clin Biochem.* 1982;15:118-119.
28. McLaughlin JE, Reeves DS. Clinical and laboratory evidence for inactivation of gentamicin by carbenicillin. *Lancet.* 1971;1(7693):261-264.
29. Riff LJ, Jackson GG. Laboratory and clinical conditions for gentamicin inactivation by carbenicillin. *Arch Intern Med.* 1972;130:887-891.
30. Manian FA, Stone WJ, Alford RH. Adverse antibiotic effects associated with renal insufficiency. *Rev Infect Dis.* 1990;12:236-249.
31. Davies M, Morgan JR, Anand C. Interactions of carbenicillin and ticarcillin with gentamicin. *Antimicrob Agents Chemother.* 1975;7:431-434.
32. Weibert R, Keane W, Shapiro F. Carbenicillin inactivation of aminoglycosides in patients with severe renal failure. *Trans Amer Soc Artif Int Organs.* 1976;22:439-443.

Ticarcillin Disodium–Clavulanate Potassium

1. *Physicians' Desk Reference.* 60th ed. Montvale, NJ: Medical Economics Company; 2006.
2. American Academy of Pediatrics. In: Pickering LK, ed. *2003 Red Book: Report of the Committee on Infectious Diseases.* 26th ed. Elk Grove Village, IL: American Academy of Pediatrics; 2003.
3. Foulds G, McBride TJ, Knirsch AK, et al. Penetration of sulbactam and ampicillin into cerebrospinal fluid of infants and young children with meningitis. *Antimicrob Agents Chemother.* 1987;31:1703-1705.
4. Kanra G, Secmeer G, Akalin E, et al. Sulbactam/ampicillin in the treatment of pediatric infections. *Diagn Microbiol Infect Dis.* 1989;12:185S-187S.
5. Kulhanjian J, Dunphy MG, Hamstra S, et al. Randomized comparative study of ampicillin/sulbactam vs. ceftriaxone for treatment of soft tissue and skeletal infections in children. *Pediatr Infect Dis J.* 1989;8:605-610.
6. Meier H, Springsklee M, Wildfeuer A. Penetration of ampicillin and sulbactam into human costal cartilage. *Infection.* 1994;22:152-155.
7. Aronoff SC, Scoles PV, Makley JT, et al. Efficacy and safety of sequential treatment with parenteral sulbactam/ampicillin and oral sultamicillin for skeletal infections in children. *Rev Infect Dis.* 1986;8:S639-S643.
8. Reed MD. A reassessment of ticarcillin/clavulanic acid dose recommendations for infants, children and adults. *Pediatr Infect Dis J.* 1998;17:1195-1199.
9. Begue P, Quiniou F, Quinet B. Efficacy and pharmacokinetics of Timentin in paediatric infections. *J Antimicrob Chemother.* 1986;17:81-91.
10. Reed MD, Yamashita TS, Blummer JL. Pharmacokinetic-based ticarcillin/clavulanic acid dose recommendations for infants and children. *J Clin Pharmacol.* 1995;35:658-665.
11. Reed MD. Rational prescribing of extended-spectrum penicillin β-lactamase inhibitor combinations: focus on ticarcillin/clavulanic acid. *Ann Pharmacother.* 1998;32:S17-S21.
12. Croydon EAP, Hermoso C. An evaluation of the safety and tolerance of Timentin. *J Antimicrob Chemother.* 1986;17:233-240.

13. Kristjansson K, Cox F, Taylor L. Ticarcillin/clavulanic acid combination; treatment of bacterial infections in hospitalized children. *Clin Pediatr.* 1989;28:521-524.
14. Dougherty SH, Sirinek KR, Schauer PR, et al. Ticarcillin/clavulanate compared with clindamycin/gentamicin (with or without ampicillin) for the treatment of intra-abdominal infections in pediatric and adult patients. *Am Surg.* 1995;61:297-303.
15. Jacobs RF, Elser JM. Timentin therapy for staphylococcus aureus infections in children: results of a multi-center trial. *Pediatr Infect Dis J.* 1989;8:441-444.
16. Meier H, Adam D, Heilmann HD. Penetration of ticarcillin/clavulanate into cartilage. *J Antimicrob Chemother.* 1989;24:101-105.
17. Pokorny WJ, Kaplan SL, Mason EO. A preliminary report of ticarcillin and clavulanate versus triple antibiotic therapy in children with ruptured appendicitis. *Surgery.* 1972;172:S54-S56.
18. Sirinek KR, Levine BA. A randomized trial of ticarcillin and clavulanate versus gentamicin and clindamycin in patients with complicated appendicitis. *Surgery.* 1972;172:30-35.
19. Blumer JL. Ticarcillin/clavulanate for the treatment of serious infections in hospitalized pediatric patients. *Pediatric Infect Dis J.* 1998;17:1211-1215.
20. Reed MD, Yamashita TS, Blummer JL. Pharmacokinetic-based ticarcillin/clavulanic acid dose recommendations for infants and children. *J Clin Pharmacol.* 1995; 35:658-665.
21. Shenep JL, Hughes WT, Roberson PK, et al. Vancomycin, ticarcillin, and amikacin compared with ticarcillin–clavulanate and amikacin in the empirical treatment of febrile, neutropenic children with cancer. *N Engl J Med.* 1988;319:1053-1058.
22. Allo MD, Bennion RS, Kathir K, et al. Ticarcillin/clavulanate versus imipenem/cilistatin for the treatment of infections associated with gangrenous and perforated appendicitis. *Amer Surg.* 1999;65:99-104.
23. Schaison G, Reinert P, Leverger G. Timentin (ticarcillin and clavulanic acid) in combination with aminoglycosides in the treatment of febrile episodes in neutropenic children. *J Antimicrob Chemother.* 1986;17C:177-181.
24. Bolton-Maggs PHB, Van Saene HKF, McDowell HP, et al. Clinical evaluation of ticarcillin with clavulanic acid, and gentamicin in the treatment of febrile episodes in neutropenic children. *J Antimicrob Chemother.* 1991;27:669-676.
25. Blumer JL. Ticarcillin/clavulanate for the treatment of serious infections in hospitalized pediatric patients. *Pediatric Infect Dis J.* 1998;17:1211-1215.
26. Arnoff GR, Berns JS, Brier ME, et al. *Drug Prescribing in Renal Failure: Dosing Guidelines for Adults.* 4th ed. Philadelphia, PA: American College of Physicians; 1999.
27. Parry MF, Neu HC. Pharmacokinetics of ticarcillin in patients with abnormal renal function. *J Infect Dis.* 1976;133:46-49.
28. Kallay MC, Tabechian H, Riley GR, et al. Neurotoxicity due to ticarcillin in patient with renal failure. *Lancet.* 1979;1:608-609. Letter.
29. Nelson JS, Bradley JS. *Nelson's Pocketbook of Pediatric Antimicrobial Therapy.* 14th ed. Philadelphia, PA: Lippincott Williams & Wilkins; 2000.
30. Trissel LA, ed. *Handbook on Injectable Drugs.* 13th ed. [CD-ROM version 1.5]. Bethesda, MD: American Society of Health-System Pharmacists; 2005.
31. American Society of Health-System Pharmacists. American Hospital Formulary System. Available at: http://ahfsfirst.firstdatabank.com/AHFSfirst/NSAHFSFirstSearchmain.asp. Accessed September 24, 2006.
32. Munckhof WJ, Carney J, Neilson G, et al. Continuous infusion of ticarcillin-clavulanate for home treatment of serious infections: clinical efficacy, safety, pharmacokinetics and pharmacodynamics. *Int J Antimicrob Agents.* 2005;25:514-522.
33. McLaughlin JE, Reeves DS. Clinical and laboratory evidence for inactivation of gentamicin by carbenicillin. *Lancet.* 1971;1(7693):261-264.
34. Riff LJ, Jackson GG. Laboratory and clinical conditions for gentamicin inactivation by carbenicillin. *Arch Intern Med.* 1972;130:887-891.
35. Manian FA, Stone WJ, Alford RH. Adverse antibiotic effects associated with renal insufficiency. *Rev Infect Dis.* 1990;12:236-249.
36. Davies M, Morgan JR, Anand C. Interactions of carbenicillin and ticarcillin with gentamicin. *Antimicrob Agents Chemother.* 1975;7:431-434.
37. Weibert R, Keane W, Shapiro F. Carbenicillin inactivation of aminoglycosides in patients with severe renal failure. *Trans Amer Soc Artif Int Organs.* 1976;22:439-443.

Tissue Plasminogen Activator (TPA)-Alteplase

1. The Seventh ACCP Conference on Antithrombotic and Thrombolytic Therapy. Antithrombotic therapy in children. *Chest.* 2004;126 (suppl)645S-687S. Available at: www.chestjournal.org/cgi/content/full/126/3_suppl/645S.
2. Dillon PW, Fox PS, Berg CJ, et al. Recombinant tissue plasminogen activator for neonatal and pediatric vascular thrombolytic therapy. *J Pediatr Surg.* 1993;28:1264-1269.
3. Nowak-Gottl U, Schwabe D, Schneider W, et al. Thrombolysis with recombinant tissue-type plasminogen activator in renal venous thrombosis in infancy. *Lancet.* 1992;430:1105. Letter.
4. Farnoux C, Camard O, Pinquier D, et al. Recombinant tissue-type plasminogen activator therapy of thrombosis in 16 neonates. *J Pediatr.* 1998;133:137-140.
5. Levy M, Benson LN, Burrows PE, et al. Tissue plasminogen activator for the treatment of thromboembolism in infants and children. *J Pediatr.* 1991;118:467-472.
6. Van Overmeire B, Van Reempts PJ, Van Acker KJ. Intracardiac thrombosis formation with rapidly progressive heart failure in the neonate: treatment with tissue-type plasminogen activator. *Arch Dis Child.* 1992;67:443-445.
7. Glover ML, Camacho MT, Wolfsdorf J. The use of alteplase in a newborn receiving extracorporeal membrane oxygenation. *Ann Pharmacotherapy.* 1999;33:416-419.
8. Guerin V, Boisseau MR. Efficiency of alteplase in the treatment of venous arterial thrombosis in neonates. *Am J Hematol.* 1993;42:236-237.
9. Gupta AA, Leaker M, Andrew M, et al. Safety and outcomes of thrombolysis with tissue plasminogen activator for treatment of intravascular thrombosis in children. *J Pediatr.* 2001;139:682-688.
10. Kennedy LA, Drummond WH, Knight ME, et al. Successful treatment of neonatal aortic thrombosis with tissue plasminogen activator. *J Pediatr.* 1990;116:798-801.
11. Deeg KH, Wolfel D, Rupprecht T. Diagnosis of neonatal aortic thrombosis by colour coded Doppler sonography. *Pediatr Radiol.* 1992;22:62-63.
12. Smets K, Vanhaesebrouck P, Voet D, et al. Use of tissue type plasminogen activator in neonates: case reports and review of the literature. *Am J Perinatol.* 1996;13:217-222.
13. Zenz W, Muntean W, Beitzke A, et al. Tissue plasminogen activator (alteplase) treatment for femoral artery thrombosis after cardiac catheterization in infants and children. *Br Heart J.* 1993;70:382-385.
14. Pyles LA, Pierpont ME, Steiner ME, et al. Fibrinolysis by tissue plasminogen activator in a child with pulmonary embolism. *J Pediatr.* 1990;116:801-804.
15. Gruber A, Nasel C, Lang W, et al. Intra-arterial thrombolysis for the treatment of perioperative childhood cardioembolic stroke. *Neurology.* 2000;54:1684-1686.
16. Atkinson JB, Bagnall HA, Gomperts E. Investigational use of tissue plasminogen activator for occluded central venous catheters. *J Parenter Enter Nutr.* 1990;4:310-311.
17. Davis SN, Vermeulen L, Banton J, et al. Activity and dosage of alteplase dilution for clearing occlusions of venous-access devices. *Am J Health Syst Pharm.* 2000;57:1039-1045.
18. Deitcher SR, Fesen MR, Kiproff PM, et al. Safety and efficacy of alteplase for restoring function in occluded central venous catheters: results of the cardiovascular thrombolytic to open occluded lines trial. *J Clin Oncol.* 2001;20:317-324.
19. Jacobs BR, Haygood M, Hingl J. Recombinant tissue plasminogen activator in the treatment of central venous catheter occlusion in children. *J Pediatr.* 2001;139:593-596.
20. Choi M, Massicotte MP, Marzinotto V, et al. The use of alteplase to restore patency of central venous lines in pediatric patients: a cohort study. *J Pediatr.* 2001;139:152-156.

References

21. Timoney JP, Malkin MG, Groeger JS, et al. Safe and cost effective use of alteplase for the clearance of occluded central venous access devices. *J Clin Oncol*. 2002;22:1918-1922.
22. Shen V, Li X, Murdock M, et al. Recombinant tissue plasminogen activator (alteplase) for restoration of function to occluded central venous catheters in pediatric patients. *J Pediatr Hematol Oncol*. 2003;25:38-45.
23. Mehta JS, Adams GG. Recombinant tissue plasminogen activator following paediatric cataract surgery. *Br J Ophthalmol*. 2000;84:983-986.
24. Klais CM, Hattenbach LO, Steinkamp GW, et al. Intraocular recombinant tissue-plasminogen activator fibrinolysis of fibrin formation after cataract surgery in children. *J Cataract Refract Surg*. 1999;25:357-362.
25. Zalta AH, Sweeney CP, Zalta AK, et al. Intracameral tissue plasminogen activator use in a large series of eyes with valved glaucoma drainage implants. *Arch Ophthalmol*. 2002;120:1487-1493.
26. Krendel S, Pollack P, Hanly J. Tissue plasminogen activator in pediatric myocardial infarction. *Ann Emerg Med*. 2000;35:502-505.
27. Bishop NB, Pon S, Ushay HM, et al. Alteplase in the treatment of complicated parapneumonic effusion: a case report. *Pediatrics*. 2003;111: E188-E190. Available at: http://www.pediatrics.org/cgi/content/full/111/2/e188.
28. Levitas A, Zucker N, Zalzstein E, et al. Successful treatment of infective endocarditis with recombinant tissue plasminogen activator. *J Pediatr*. 2003;143:649-652.
29. McEvoy GK, ed. *Drug Information Essentials 2005–06*. Bethesda, MD: American Society of Health-System Pharmacists; 2005.
30. Frazin BS. Maximal dilution of Activas. *Am J Hosp Pharm*. 1990;47:1016.
31. Trissel LA. *Handbook on Injectable Drugs*. 13th ed. Bethesda, MD: American Society of Health-System Pharmacists; 2005.
32. Calis KA, Cullinane AM, Horne MK III. Bioactivity of cryopreserved alteplase solutions. *Am J Health-Syst Pharm*. 1999;56:2056-2057.
33. Fasano R, Kent P, Valentino L. Superior vena cava thrombus treated with low-dose, peripherally administered recombinant tissue plasminogen activator in a child. *J Pediatr Hematol Oncol*. 2005;27:692-695.
34. Tan H, Kizilkaya M, Alper F, et al. Thrombolytic therapy with tissue plasminogen activator for superior vena cava thrombosis in an infant with sepsis. *Acta Paediatrica*. 2005;94:239-253.
35. Diamond IR, Wales PW, Connolly B, et al. Tissue plasminogen activator for the treatment of intraabdominal abscesses in a neonate. *J Pediatr Surg*. 2003;38:1234-1236.
36. Wang M, Hays T, Balasa V, et al. Low-dose tissue plasminogen activator thrombolysis in children. *J Pediatr Hematol Oncol*. 2003;25:379-386.
37. Zenz W, Muntean W, Gallist L, et al. Recombinant tissue plasminogen activator treatment in two infants with fulminant meningococcemia. *Pediatrics*. 1995;96:144-147.
38. Zenz W, Zoehrer B, Levin M, et al. Use of recombinant tissue plasminogen activator in children with meningococcal purpura fulminans: a retrospective study. *Crit Care Med*. 2004;32:1777-1780.

Tobramycin Sulfate

1. Blouin RA, Mann HJ, Griffen WO, et al. Tobramycin pharmacokinetics in morbidly obese patients. *Clin Pharmacol Ther.* 1979;26:508-512.
2. Watterberg KL, Kelly W, Angelus P, et al. The need for a loading dose of gentamicin in neonates. *Ther Drug Monit.* 1989;11:16-20.
3. Gal P, Ransom JL, Weaver RL. Gentamicin in neonates: the need for loading doses. *Amer J Perinatol.* 1990;7:254-257.
4. American Academy of Pediatrics. In: Pickering LK, ed. *2003 Red Book: Report of the Committee on Infectious Diseases.* 26th ed. Elk Grove Village, IL: American Academy of Pediatrics; 2003.
5. Prober CG, Stevenson DK, Benitz WE. The use of antibiotics in neonates weighing less than 1200 grams. *Pediatr Infect Dis J.* 1990;9:111-121.
6. McCracken GH Jr, Nelson JD, eds. *Antimicrobial Therapy for Newborns: Practical Application.* 2nd ed. New York, NY: Grune and Stratton; 1983.
7. Nahata MC, Powell DA, Durrell DE, et al. Effect of gestational age and birth weight on tobramycin kinetics in newborn infants. *J Antimicrob Chemother.* 1984;14:59-65.
8. Nahata MC, Powell DA, Gregoire RP, et al. Tobramycin kinetics in newborn infants. *J Pediatr.* 1983;103:136-138.
9. Young TE, Mangum B, eds. *Neofax®*. 18th ed. Raleigh, NC: Acorn Publishing Inc; 2005;66.
10. Kafetzis DA, Sinaniotis CA, Kitsiou-Tzeli S, et al. Tobramycin dosage in infants and children. *Lancet.* 1978; 2:1264. Letter.
11. Tobramycin. In: Kucer A, Crowe SM, Grayson ML, et al., eds. *The Use of Antibiotics: A Clinical Review of Antibacterial, Antifungal and Antiviral Drugs.* 5th ed. Boston, MA: Butterworth Heinemann; 1997;490-503.
12. Contopoulos-Ioannidis DG, Giotis ND, Baliatsa DV, et al. Extended-Interval aminoglycoside administration for children: A meta-analysis. *Pediatrics.* 2004;114:e111-e118.
13. Langhendries JP, Battisti O, Bertrand JM, et al. Once-a-day administration of amikacin in neonates: Assessment of nephrotoxicity and ototoxicity. *Dev Pharmacol Ther.* 1993;20:220-230.
14. Marik PE, Lipman J, Kobilski S, et al. A prospective randomized study comparing once- versus twice-daily amikacin dosing in critically ill adult and paediatric patients. *J Antimicrob Chemother.* 1991;28:753-764.
15. Kafetzis DA, Sianidou L, Vlachos E, et al. Clinical and pharmacokinetic study of a single daily dose of amikacin in paediatric patients with severe gram-negative infections. *J Antimicrob Chemother*. 1991;27:105-112.
16. Trujillo H, Robledo J, Robledo C, et al. Single dose amikacin in paediatric patients with severe gram-negative infections. *J Antimicrob Chemother.* 1991;27:141-147.
17. Viscoli C, Dudley M, Ferrea G, et al. Serum concentration and safety of a single daily dose of amikacin in children undergoing bone marrow transplantation. *J Antimicrob Chemother.* 1991;27:113-120.
18. Sung L, Dupuis LL, Bliss B, et al. Randomized controlled trial of once- versus thrice-daily tobramycin in febrile neutropenic children undergoing stem cell transplantation. *J Natl Cancer Inst.* 2003;95:1869-1877.
19. Dupuis LL, Sung L, Taylor T, et al. Tobramycin pharmacokinetics in children with febrile neutropenia undergoing stem cell transplantation: once-daily versus thrice-daily administration. *Pharmacotherapy*. 2004;24:564-573.
20. Bouffet E, Fuhrmann C, Frappaz D, et al. Once daily antibiotic regimen in paediatric oncology. *Arch Dis Child.* 1994;70:484-487.
21. International Antimicrobial Therapy Cooperative Group of the European Organization for Research and Treatment of Cancer. Efficacy and toxicity of single daily doses of amikacin and ceftriaxone versus multiple daily doses of amikacin and ceftazidime for infection in patients with cancer and granulocytopenia. *Ann Intern Med.* 1993;119:584-593.
22. Krivoy N, Postovsky S, Elhasid R, et al. Pharmacokinetic analysis of amikacin twice and single daily dosage in immunocompromised pediatric patients. *Infection.* 1998;26:396-398.
23. Chicella M. Once-daily aminoglycoside dosing in pediatrics. What is its role? *J Pediatr Pharm Pract.* 2000:5;98-103.
24. Wallace CS, Hall M, Kuhn RJ. Pharmacologic management of cystic fibrosis. *Clin Pharm.* 1993;12:657-674.
25. Smyth A, Tan KH, Hyman-Taylor P, et al. Once versus three-times daily regimens of tobramycin treatment for pulmonary exacerbations of cystic fibrosis—the TOPIC study: a randomized controlled trial. *Lancet.* 2005;365:573-578.
26. Beringer PM, Vinks AA, Jelliffe RW, et al. Pharmacokinetics of tobramycin in adults with cystic fibrosis: implications for once-daily administration. *Antimicrob Agents Chemother.* 2000;44:809-813.
27. Bates RD, Nahata MC, Jones JW, et al. Pharmacokinetics and safety of tobramycin after once-daily administration in patients with cystic fibrosis. *Chest.* 1997;112:1208-1213.
28. Bragonier R, Brown NM. The pharmacokinetics and toxicity of once-daily tobramycin therapy in children with cystic fibrosis. *J Antimicrob Chemother.* 1998;42:103-106.
29. Master V, Roberts GW, Coulthard KP, et al. Efficacy of once-daily tobramycin monotherapy for acute pulmonary exacerbations of cystic fibrosis: a preliminary study. *Pediatr Pulmonol.* 2001;3:367-376.
30. Aronoff A, Brier M, Bennett W. *The Renal Book, 2002*. Available at: http://www.kdp-baptist.louisville.edu/renalbook/. Accessed May 29,

2006.
31. Horrevorts AM, de Witte J, Degener JE, et al. Tobramycin in patients with cystic fibrosis. Adjustments in dosing interval for effective treatment. *Chest.* 1987;92:844-848.
32. Kelly HB, Menendez R, Fan L, et al. Pharmacokinetics of tobramycin in cystic fibrosis. *J Pediatr.* 1982;100:318-321.
33. Loirat P, Rohan J, Baillet A, et al. Increased glomerular filtration rate in patients with major burns and its effect on the pharmacokinetics of tobramycin. *N Engl J Med.* 1978;299:915-919.
34. Armstrong DK, Hidalgo HA, Eldadah M. Vancomycin and tobramycin clearance in an infant during continuous hemo-filtration. *Ann Pharmacother.* 1993;27:224-227.
35. Buck ML. Pharmacokinetic changes during extracorporeal membrane oxygenation. *Clin Pharmacokinet.* 2003;42:403-417.
36. Gillett AP, Falk RH, Andrews J, et al. Rapid intravenous injection of tobramycin: suggested dosage schedule and concentrations in serum. *J Infect Dis.* 1976;134:S110-S113.
37. Dobbs SM, Mawer GE. Intravenous injection of gentamicin and tobramycin without impairment of hearing. *J Infect Dis.* 1976;134 (suppl): S114-S117.
38. Mendelson J, Portnoy J, Dick V, et al. Safety of the bolus administration of gentamicin. *Antimicrob Agents Chemother.* 1976;9:633-638.
39. Trissel LA, ed. *Handbook on Injectable Drugs.* 13th ed. [CD-ROM version 1.5]. Bethesda, MD: American Society of Health-System Pharmacists; 2005.
40. Bodey GP, Chang HY, Rodriguez V, et al. Feasibility of administering aminoglycoside antibiotics by continuous intravenous infusion. *Antimicrob Agents Chemother.* 1975;8:328-333.
41. Powell SH, Thompson WL, Luthe MA, et al. Once daily vs. continuous aminoglycoside dosing: efficacy and toxicity in animal and clinical studies of gentamicin, netilmicin and tobramycin. *J Infect Dis.* 1983;147:918-932.
42. Giacoia GP, Schentag JJ. Pharmacokinetics and nephrotoxicity of continuous intravenous infusion of gentamicin in low birth weight infants. *J Pediatr.* 1986;109:715-719.
43. American Society of Health-System Pharmacists. American Hospital Formulary System. Available at: http://ahfsfirst.firstdatabank.com/AHFSfirst/NSAHFSFirstSearchmain.asp. Accessed May 29, 2006.
44. American Academy of Pediatrics Committee on Drugs. "Inactive" ingredients in pharmaceutical products: update. *Pediatrics.* 1997;99:268-278.
45. Lester MR. Sulfite sensitivity: significance in human health. *J Am Col Nutr.* 1995;14:229-232.
46. Franson TR, Ritch PS, Quebbeman EJ. Aminoglycoside serum concentration sampling via central venous catheters: a potential source of clinical error. *JPEN J Parenter Enteral Nutr.* 1987;11:77-79.
47. Bentur Y, Hummel D, Roifman CM, et al. Interpretation of excessive levels of inhaled tobramycin. *Ther Drug Monit.* 1989;11:109-110.
48. Redmann S, Wainwright C, Stacey S, et al. Misleading high tobramycin plasma concentrations can be caused by skin contamination of fingerprick blood following inhalation of nebulized tobramycin (TOBI): a short report. *Ther Drug Monit.* 2005;27:205-257.
49. Massey KL, Hendeles L, Neims A. Identification of children for whom routine monitoring of aminoglycoside serum concentrations is not cost effective. *J Pediatr.* 1986;109:897-901.
50. Logsdon BA, Phelps SJ. Routine monitoring of gentamicin serum concentrations in pediatric patients with normal renal function is unnecessary. *Ann Pharmacother.* 1997;31:1514-1518.
51. Beaubien AR, Desjardins S, Ormsby E, et al. Incidence of amikacin ototoxicity: a sigmoid function of total drug exposure independent of plasma levels. *Am J Otolaryngol.* 1989;10:234-243.
52. Beaubien AR, Ormsby E, Bayne A, et al. Evidence that amikacin ototoxicity is related to total perilymph area under the concentration-time curve regardless of concentration. *Antimicrob Agents Chemother.* 1991;35:1070-1074.
53. Snavely SR, Hodges GR. The neurotoxicity of antibacterial agents. *Ann Intern Med.* 1984;101;92-104.
54. Manian FA, Stone WJ, Alford RH. Adverse antibiotic effects associated with renal insufficiency. *Rev Infect Dis.* 1990;12:236-249.

Topotecan HCl

1. Walterhouse DO, Lyden ER, Breitfeld PP, et al. Efficacy of topotecan and cyclophosphamide given in a phase II window trial in children with newly diagnosed metastatic rhabdomyosarcoma: a Children's Oncology Group study. *J Clin Oncol.* 2004;22(8):1360-1362.
2. Nitschke R, Parkhurst J, Sullivan J, et al. Topotecan in pediatric patients with recurrent and progressive solid tumors: a Pediatric Oncology Group phase II study. *J Pediatr Hematol Oncol.* 1998;20(4):315-318.
3. Tubergen DG, Stewart CF, Pratt CB, et al. Phase I trial and pharmacokinetic (PK) and pharmacodynamics (PD) study of topotecan using a five-day course in children with refractory solid tumors: a pediatric oncology group study. *J Pediatr Hematol Oncol.* 1996;18(4):352-361.
4. Wells RJ, Reid JM, Ames MM, et al. Phase I trial of cisplatin and topotecan in children with recurrent solid tumors: Children's Oncology Group Study 0942. *J Pediatr Hematol Oncol.* 2002;24(2):89-93.
5. Pratt CB, Stewart CF, Santana VM, et al. Phase I study of topotecan for pediatric patients with malignant solid tumors. *J Clin Oncol.* 1994;12(3):539-543.
6. Santana VM, Zamboni WC, Kirstein MN, et al. A pilot study of protracted topotecan using a pharmacokinetically guided dosing approach in children with solid tumors. *Clin Cancer Res.* 2003;9(2):633-640.
7. Furman WL, Stewart CF, Kirstein M, et al. Protracted intermittent schedule of topotecan in children with refractory acute leukemia: a Pediatric Oncology Group Study. *J Clin Oncol.* 2002;20(6):1617-1624.
8. *Physicians' Desk Reference.* 60th ed. Montvale, NJ: Thomson PDR; 2006.
9. Aronoff GR, Berns JS, Brier ME, eds., et al. *Drug Prescribing in Renal Failure.* 4th ed. Philadelphia, PA: American College of Physicians; 1999:77.
10. Trissel LA, ed. *Handbook on Injectable Drugs.* 13th ed. [CD-ROM version 1.5]. Bethesda, MD: American Society of Health-System Pharmacists; 2005.
11. Taketomo CK, Hodding JH, Kraus DM, eds. *Pediatric Dosage Handbook.* 12th ed. [CD-ROM version 2006.1]. Hudson, OH: Lexi-Comp; 2006.
12. National Comprehensive Cancer Network (NCCN) Antiemesis Panel Members. NCCN Clinical Practice Guidelines in Oncology. Antiemesis, v.1.2006. Available at: www.nccn.org. Accessed March 29, 2006.
13. Roila F, Feyer P, Maranzamo E, et al. Antiemetics in children receiving chemotherapy. *Support Care Cancer.* 2005;13:129-131.

Tromethamine

1. THAM solution [package insert]. North Chicago, IL: Abbott Laboratories; November 2000.
2. McEvoy GK. American Society of Health-System Pharmacists. American Hospital Formulary System. Available at: http://ahfsfirst.firstdatabank.com/AHFSfirst/NSAHFSFirstSearchmain.asp. Accessed October 5, 2006.
3. Gupta JM, Dahlenburg GW, Davis JW. Changes in blood gas tensions following administration of amine buffer THAM to infants with respiratory distress syndrome. *Arch Dis Child.* 1967;42:416-427.
4. Baum JD, Robertson NRC. Immediate effects of alkaline infusion in infants with respiratory distress syndrome. *J Pediatr.* 1975;87:255.
5. Nahas GG, Sutin KM, Fermon C, et al. Guidelines for the treatment of acidaemia with THAM. *Drugs.* 1998;55(2):191-224.
6. Strauss J. Tris (hydroxymethyl) amino-methane (THAM): a pediatric evaluation. *Pediatrics.* 1968;41:667-689.
7. Holmdahl MH, Wiklund L, Wetterberg T, et al. The place of THAM in the management of academia in clinical practice. *Acta Anaesthesiol Scand.* 2000;44:524-527.
8. Roberton NRC. Apnea after THAM administration in the newborn. *Arch Dis Child.* 1970;45:206-214.
9. Hooge MN, Verhoeven BH, Rutten WJ, et al. Irreversible ischemia of the hand after peripheral administration of tromethamol (THAM).

Intensive Care Med. 2003;29:503.
10. Tarail R, Bennett TE. Hypoglycemic activity of TRIS buffer in man and dog. *Proc Soc Exp Biol Med.* 1959;102:208-209.
11. Goldenberg VE, Wiegenstein L, Hopkins GB. Hepatic injury associated with tromethamine. *JAMA.* 1968;205:81-84.

Tubocurarine Chloride

1. American Society of Health-System Pharmacists. American Hospital Formulary System. Available at: http://ahfsfirst.firstdatabank.com/AHFSfirst/NSAHFSFirstSearchmain.asp. Accessed May 10, 2006.
2. Martin LD, Bratton SL, O'Rourke PP. Clinical uses and controversies of neuromuscular blocking agents in infants and children. *Crit Care Med.* 1999;27:1358-1368.
3. Bush GH, Stead A. The use of d-tubocurarine in neonatal anaesthesia. *Br J Anaesth.* 1962;34:721-728.
4. Walts LF, Dillon JB. The response of newborns to succinylcholine and d-tubocurarine. *Anesthesiology.* 1969;31:35-38.
5. Goudsouzian NG, Donlon JV, Savarese JJ, et al. Re-evaluation of dosage and duration of action of d-tubocurarine in the pediatric age group. *Anesthesiology.* 1975;43:416-425.
6. Nightingale DA, Bush GH. A clinical comparison between tubocurarine and pancuronium in children. *Br J Anaesth.* 1973;45:63-69.
7. Fisher DM, O'Keeffe C, Stanski DR, et al. Pharmacokinetics and pharmacodynamics of d-tubocurarine in infants, children, and adults. *Anesthesiology.* 1982;57:203-208.
8. Aronoff A, Brier M, Bennett W. *The Renal Book, 2002.* Available at: http://www.kdp-baptist.louisville.edu/renalbook/. Accessed May 6, 2006.
9. Trissel LA, ed. *Handbook on Injectable Drugs.* 13th ed. [CD-ROM version 1.5]. Bethesda, MD: American Society of Health-System Pharmacists; 2005.
10. Basta SJ, Savarese JJ, Ali HH, et al. Histamine-releasing potencies of atracurium, dimethyltubocurarine and tubocurarine. *Br J Anaesth.* 1983;55:105S-106S.
11. Bush GH, Stead A. The use of d-tubocurarine in neonatal anaesthesia. *Br J Anaesth.* 1962;34:721-728.
12. American Academy of Pediatrics Committee on Drugs. "Inactive" ingredients in pharmaceutical products: update. *Pediatrics.* 1997;99:268-278.
13. Lester MR. Sulfite sensitivity: significance in human health. *J Am Col Nutr.* 1995;14:229-232.
14. Smolinske SC. Review of parenteral sulfite reactions. *J Toxicol Clin Toxicol.* 1992;30:597-606.
15. Hiller JL, Benda GI, Rahatzad M, et al. Benzyl alcohol toxicity: impact on mortality and intraventricular hemorrhage among very low birth weight infants. *Pediatrics.* 1986;77:500-506.
16. Hall CM, Milligan DWA, Berrington J. Probably adverse reaction to a pharmaceutical excipient. *Arch Dis Child Fetal Neonatal Ed.* 2004;89:F184.
17. Grant JA, Bilodeau PA, Guernsey BG, et al. Unsuspected benzyl alcohol hypersensitivity. *N Engl J Med.* 1982;306:108.
18. Wilson JP, Solimando DA, Edwards MS. Parenteral benzyl alcohol-induced hypersensitivity reaction. *Drug Intell Clin Pharm.* 1986;20:689-691.
19. Ostergaard D, Engbaek J, Viby-Mogensen J. Adverse reactions and interactions of the neuromuscular blocking drugs. *Med Toxicol Adverse Drug Ex.* 1989;4:351-368.
20. Durbin CG. Neuromuscular blocking agents and sedative drugs: clinical uses and toxic effects in the critical care unit. *Crit Care Clin.* 1991;7:489-506.

Valproate Sodium

1. American Academy of Pediatrics Committee on Drugs: Valproic acid: benefits and risks. *Pediatrics.* 1982;70:316-319.
2. Dreifuss FE, Santilli N, Langer DH, et al. Valproic acid hepatic fatalities: a retrospective review. *Neurology.* 1987;37:379-385.
3. Dreifuss FE, Langer DH, Moline KA, et al. Valproic acid hepatic fatalities. II. US experience since 1984. *Neurology.* 1989;39:201-207.
4. Bryant AE 3rd, Dreifuss FE. Valproic acid hepatic fatalities. III. U.S. experience since 1986. *Neurology.* 1996;46:465-469.
5. Mathew NT, Kailasam J, Meadors L, et al. Intravenous valproate sodium (depacon) aborts migraine rapidly: a preliminary report. *Headache.* 2000;40:720-723.
6. Schwartz TH, Karpitskiy VV, Sohn RS. Intravenous valproate sodium in the treatment of daily headache. *Headache.* 2002;42:519-522.
7. Stillman MJ, Zajac D, Rybicki LA. Treatment of primary headache disorders with intravenous valproate: initial outpatient experience. *Headache.* 2004;44:65-69.
8. Reiter PD, Nickisch J, Merritt G. Efficacy and tolerability of intravenous valproic acid in acute adolescent migraine. *Headache.* 2005;45:899-903.
9. *Physicians' Desk Reference.* 60th ed. Montvale, NJ: Medical Economics Company; 2006.
10. Redenbaugh JE, Sato S, et al. Sodium valproate: pharmacokinetics and effectiveness in treating intractable seizures. *Neurology.* 1980;30:1-6.
11. Sherard ES, Steiman GS, Couri D. Treatment of childhood epilepsy with valproic acid: results of the first 100 patients in a 6-month trial. *Neurology.* 1980:30:31-35.
12. Braathen G. Theorall K, Persson A, et al. Valproate in the treatment of absence epilepsy in children: a study of dose-response relationships. *Epilepsia.* 1988;29:548-552.
13. Herngren L, Lundberg B, Nergardh A. Pharmacokinetics of total and free valproate during monotherapy in infants. *J Neurol.* 1991;238:315-319.
14. Cloyd JC, Kriel RL, Fishcer JH. Valproic acid pharmacokinetics in children. II. Discontinuation of concomitant antiepileptic drug therapy. *Neurology.* 1985;35:1623-1627.
15. Cloyd JC, Fischer JH, Kriel RL, et al. Valproic acid pharmacokinetics in children. IV. Effects of age and antiepileptic drugs on protein binding and intrinsic clearance. *Clin Pharmacol Ther.* 1993;53:22-29.
16. Marlow N, Cooke RW. Intravenous sodium valproate in the neonatal intensive care unit. *J R Soc Med.* 1989;152:208-210.
17. Alfonso I, Alvarez LA, Gilman J, et al. Intravenous valproate dosing in neonates. *J Child Neurol.* 2000;15:827-829.
18. Hovinga CA, Chicella MF, Rose DF, et al. Use of intravenous valproate in three pediatric patients with convulsive or nonconvulsive status epilepticus. *Ann Pharmacother.* 1999;33:579-584.
19. Hodges BM, Mazur JE. Intravenous valproate in status epilepticus. *Ann Pharmacother.* 2001;35:1465-1470.
20. White JR, Santos CS. Intravenous valproate associated with significant hypotension in the treatment of status epilepticus. *J Child Neurol.* 1999;14:822-823.
21. Uberall MA, Trollmann R, Wunsiedler U, Wenzel D. Intravenous valproate in pediatric epilepsy patients with refractory status epilepticus. *Neurology.* 2000;54:2188-2189.
22. Venkataraman V, Wheless JW. Safety of rapid intravenous infusion of valproate loading doses in epilepsy patients. *Epilepsy Res.* 1999;147-153.
23. Chez MG, Hammer MS, Loeffel M, et al. Clinical experience of three pediatric and one adult case of spike-and-wave status epilepticus treated with injectable valproic acid. *J Child Neurol.* 1999;14:239-242.
24. Aronoff A, Brier M, Bennett W. *The Renal Book, 2002.* Available at: http://www.kdp-baptist.louisville.edu/renalbook/. Accessed May 6, 2006.
25. Brewster D, Muir NC. Valproate plasma protein binding in the uremic condition. *Clin Pharmacol Ther.* 1980;27:76-82.
26. Orr JM, Farrell FS, Abbott FS, et al. The effects of peritoneal dialysis on the single dose and steady state pharmacokinetics of valproic acid in a uremic child. *Eur J of Clin Pharmacol.* 1983;24:387-390.
27. Peters CN, Pohlmann-Eden B. Intravenous valproate as an innovative therapy in seizure emergency situations including status epilepticus—

experience in 102 adult patients. *Seizure.* 2005;14:164-169.
28. Kriel RL, Fischer JH, Cloyd JC, et al. Valproic acid pharmacokinetics in children: III. Very high dosage requirements. *Pediatr Neurol.* 1986;2:202-208.
29. Kumar P, Vallis CJ, Hall CM. Intravenous valproate associated with circulatory collapse. *Ann Pharmacother.* 2003;37:1797-1799.
30. Jha S, Jose M, Patel R. Intravenous sodium valproate in status epilepticus. *Neurol India.* 2003;51:421-422.
31. Birnbaum AK, Kriel RL, Norberg SK, et al. Rapid infusion of sodium valproate in acutely ill children. *Pediatr Neurol.* 2003;28:300-303.
32. Rosenberg HK, Ortega W. Hemorrhagic pancreatitis in a young child following valproic acid therapy. Clinical and ultrasonic assessment. *Clin Pediatr.* 1987;26:98-101.
33. Cooper MA, Groll A. A case of chronic pancreatic insufficiency due to valproic acid in a child. *Can J Gastroenterol.* 2001;15:127-130.
34. Batalden PB, Van Dyne BJ, Cloyd J. Pancreatitis associated with valproic acid therapy. *Pediatrics.*1979;64:520-522.
35. Bohan TP, Helton E, McDonald I, et al. Effect of L-carnitine treatment for valproate-induced hepatotoxicity. *Neurology.* 2001;56:1405-1409.
36. Raskind JY, El-Chaar GM. The role of carnitine supplementation during valproic acid therapy. *Ann Pharmacother.* 2000;34:630-638.
37. DeVivo DC, Bohan TP, Coulter DL, et al. L-Carnitine supplementation in childhood epilepsy: current perspectives. *Epilepsia.* 1998;39:1216-1225.
38. Temkin NR, Dikmen SS, Anderson GD, et al. Valproate therapy for prevention of posttraumatic seizures: a randomized trial. *J Neurosurg.* 1999;91:593-600.
39. Anderson GD. A mechanistic approach to antiepileptic drug interactions. *Ann Pharmacother.* 1998;32:554-563.

Vancomycin HCl

1. Bauer LA, Black DJ, Lill JS. Vancomycin dosing in morbidly obese patients. *Eur J Clin Pharmacol.* 1998;54:621-625.
2. Asbury WH, Darsey EH, Rose B, et al. Vancomycin pharmacokinetics in neonates and infants: a retrospective evaluation. *Ann Pharmacother.* 1993;27:490-494.
3. McDougal A, Ling EW, Levine M. Vancomycin pharmacokinetics and dosing in premature neonates. *Ther Drug Monitor.* 1995;17:319-326.
4. Grimsley C, Thomson AH. Pharmacokinetics and dose requirements of vancomycin in neonates. *Arch Dis Child.* 1999;81:F221-F227.
5. de Hoog M, Schoemaker RC, Mouton JW, et al. Vancomycin population pharmacokinetics in neonates. *Clin Pharmacol Ther.* 2000;67:360-367.
6. American Academy of Pediatrics. In: Pickering LK, ed. *Red Book: 2006 Report of the Committee on Infectious Diseases.* 27th ed. Elk Grove Village, IL: American Academy of Pediatrics; 2006.
7. Prober CG, Stevenson DK, Benitz WE. The use of antibiotics in neonates weighing less than 1200 grams. *Pediatr Infect Dis J.* 1990;9:111-121.
8. Reed MD, Kliegman RM, Weiner JS, et al. The clinical pharmacology of vancomycin in seriously ill preterm infants. *Pediatr Res.* 1987;22:360-363.
9. James A, Koren G, Milliken J, et al. Vancomycin pharmacokinetics and dose recommendations for preterm infants. *Antimicrob Agents Chemother.* 1987;31:52-54.
10. Gabriel MH, Kildoo CW, Gennrich JL, et al. Prospective evaluation of a vancomycin dosage guideline for neonates. *Clin Pharm.* 1991;10:129-132.
11. Schadd UB, McCracken GH, Nelson JD. Clinical pharmacology and efficacy of vancomycin in pediatric patients. *J Pediatr.* 1980;96:119-126.
12. Nelson JD, Bradley JS, eds. *Pocketbook of Pediatric Antimicrobial Therapy*. 14th ed. Baltimore, MD: Lippincott Williams & Wilkins; 2000–2001.
13. Tunkel AR, Hartman BJ, Kaplan SL, et al. Practice guidelines for the management of bacterial meningitis. *Clin Infect Dis.* 2004;39:1267-1284.
14. Baddour LM, Wilson WR, Bayer AS, et al. Infective endocarditis: diagnosis, antimicrobial therapy, and management of complications: a statement for healthcare professionals from the Committee on Rheumatic Fever, Endocarditis, and Kawasaki Disease, Council on Cardiovascular Disease in the Young, and the Councils on Clinical Cardiology, Stroke, and Cardiovascular Surgery and Anesthesia, American Heart Association: endorsed by the Infectious Diseases Society of America. *Circulation.* 2005;111:e394-e434.
15. Calza, L Manfredi R, Chiodo F. Antibiotic Therapy for Infective Endocarditis in Childhood. *J Pediatr Pharmacol Ther.* 2006;11:64-91.
16. Inglesby TV, O'Toole T, Henderson DA, et al. Working Group on Civilian Biodefense. Anthrax as a biological weapon 2002: updated recommendations for management. *JAMA.* 2002;287:2236-2252.
17. Centers for Disease Control and Prevention. Update: Investigation of bioterrorism-related anthrax and interim guidelines for exposure management and antimicrobial therapy, October 2001. *MMWR Morb Mortal Wkly Rep.* 2001;50:909-919.
18. Spafford PS, Sinkin RA, Cox X, et al. Prevention of central venous catheter-related coagulase-negative staphylococcal sepsis in neonates. *J Pediatr.* 1994;125:259-263.
19. Anon. Report from the hospital infection control practices advisory committee; comment period and public meeting. Preventing the spread of vancomycin resistance. Federal Register. May 17, 1994;59:2578-2563.
20. Baier RJ, Bocchini JA, Brown EG. Selective use of vancomycin to prevent coagulase-negative staphylococcal nosocomial bacteremia in high risk very low birth weight infants. *Pediatr Infect Dis J.* 1998;17:179-183.
21. Ocete E, Ruiz-Extremera A, Goicoechea A, et al. Low-dosage prophylactic vancomycin in central-venous catheters for neonates. *Early Human Dev.* 1998;53:S181-S186.
22. Henrickson KJ, Axtell RA, Hoover SM, et al. Prevention of central venous catheter-related infections and thrombotic events in immunocompromised children by the use of vancomycin/ciprofloxacin/heparin flush solution: a randomized, multicenter, double-blind trial. *J Clin Oncol.* 2000;18:1269-1278.
23. Swayne R, Rampling A, Newsom B. Intraventricular vancomycin for treatment of shunt-associated ventriculitis. *J Antimicrob Chemother.* 1987;19:249-253.
24. Pfausler B, Haring H, Wissel K. Cerebrospinal fluid pharmacokinetics of intraventricular vancomycin in patients with staphylococcal ventriculitis associated with CSF drainage. *Clin Infect Dis.* 1997;25:733-735.
25. Al-Jeraisy MA, Einhau S, Christensen ML, et al. Intraventricular vancomycin in pediatric patients with cerebrospinal fluid shunt infection. *J Pediatr Pharmacol Ther.* 2004;36-42.
26. Thompson JB, Einhaus S, Buckingham S, et al. Vancomycin for treating cerebrospinal fluid shunt infections in pediatric patients. *J Pediatr Pharmacol Ther.* 2005;10:14-25.
27. Arnoff GR, Berns JS, Brier ME, et al. *Drug Prescribing in Renal Failure: Dosing Guidelines for Adults.* 4th ed. Philadelphia, PA: American College of Physicians; 1999.
28. Matzke GR, McGory RW, Halstenson CE, et al. Pharmacokinetics of vancomycin in patients with various degrees of renal function. *Antimicrob Agents Chemother.* 1984;25:433-437.
29. Amaker RD, Dipiro JT, Bhatia J. Pharmacokinetics of vancomycin in critically ill infants undergoing extracorporeal membrane oxygenation. *Antimicrob Agents Chemother.* 1996;40:1139-1142.
30. Chang D. Influence of malignancy on the pharmacokinetics of vancomycin in infants and children. *Pediatr Infect Dis J.* 1995;14:667-673.
31. Chang D, Liem L, Malogolowkin M. A prospective study of vancomycin pharmacokinetics and dosage requirements in pediatric cancer patients. *Pediatr Infect Dis J.* 1994;13:969-974.
32. American Society of Health-System Pharmacists. American Hospital Formulary System. Available at: http://ahfsfirst.firstdatabank.com/AHFSfirst/NSAHFSFirstSearchmain.asp. Accessed September 21, 2006.
33. Trissel LA, ed. *Handbook on Injectable Drugs.* 13th ed. [CD-ROM version 1.5]. Bethesda, MD: American Society of Health-System Pharmacists; 2005.
34. Koren G, James A. Vancomycin dosing in preterm infants: prospective verification of new recommendations. *J Pediatr.* 1987;110:797-798.
35. Alpert G, Campos JM, Harris MC, et al. Vancomycin dosage in pediatrics reconsidered. *Am J Dis Child.* 1984;138:20-22.
36. Pawlotsky F, Thomas A, Kergueris MF, et al. Constant rate infusion of vancomycin in premature neonates: a new dosage schedule. *Br J Clin Pharmacol.* 1998;46:163-167.

References

37. Weathers L, Riggs D, Santeiro M, et al. Aerosolized vancomycin for treatment of airway colonization by methicillin-resistant Staphylococcus aureus. *Pediatr Infect Dis J.* 1990;9:220-221.
38. Maiz L, Canton R, Mir N, et al. Aerosolized vancomycin for the treatment of methicillin-resistant Staphylococcus aureus infection in cystic fibrosis. *Pediatr Pulmonol.* 1998;26:287-289.
39. Newfield P, Roizen MF. Hazard of rapid administration of vancomycin. *Ann Intern Med.* 1979;91:581.
40. Glicklich D, Figura I. Vancomycin and cardiac arrest. *Ann Intern Med.* 1984;101:880-881.
41. Healy DP, Sahai JV, Fuller SH, et al. Vancomycin-induced histamine release and "red man syndrome": comparison of 1- and 2-hour infusions. *Antimicrob Agents Chemother.* 1990;34:550-554.
42. Renz CL, Thurn JD, Finn HA, et al. Antihistamine prophylaxis permits rapid vancomycin infusion. *Crit Care Med.* 1999;27:1732-1737.
43. Chicella M, Adkins J, Mancao MY, et al. Impact of pediatric specific guidelines for vancomycin serum concentration monitoring on patient care. *J Pediatr Pharm Pract.* 1999;4:146-151.
44. Lee KR, Phelps SJ. Implementation of vancomycin monitoring criteria in a pediatric hospital. *J Pediatr Pharmacol Ther.* 2004;9:179-186.
45. Somerville AL, Wright DH, Rotschafer JC. Implications of vancomycin degradation products on therapeutic drug monitoring in patients with end-stage renal disease. *Pharmacotherapy.* 1999;9:702-707.
46. Kingery JR, Sowinski KM, Kraus MA, et al. Vancomycin assay performance in patients with end-stage renal disease receiving hemodialysis. *Pharmacotherapy.* 2000;20:653-656.

Vasopressin

1. McDonald JA, Martha PM, Kerrigan J, et al. Treatment of the young child with postoperative central diabetes insipidus. *Am J Dis Child.* 1989; 143:201-204.
2. Weigle CG, Tobin JR. Metabolic and endocrine disease in pediatric intensive care. In: Rogers MC, ed. *Textbook of Pediatric Intensive Care.* 2nd ed. Baltimore, MD: Williams & Wilkins; 1992:(2)1252.
3. Rosenzweig EB, Stare TJ, Chen JM, et al. Intravenous arginine-vasopressin in children with vasodilatory shock after cardiac surgery. *Circulation.* 1999;100:II182-II186.
4. Vasudevan A, Lodha R, Kabra SK. Vasopressin infusion in children with catecholamine-resistant septic shock. *Acta Paediatr.* 2005;94:380-383.
5. Holmes CL, Walley KR. Vasopressin in the ICU. *Curr Opin Crit Care.* 2004;10:442-448.
6. Dellinger RP, Carlet JM, Masur H, et al. Surviving sepsis campaign guidelines for management of severe sepsis and septic shock. *Crit Care Med.* 2004;32:858-873.
7. McEvoy GK, ed. *Drug Information Essentials 2005–06.* Bethesda, MD: American Society of Health-System Pharmacists; 2005.
8. Durbin DR, Liacouras CA. Chapter 93: Gastrointestinal emergencies. In: Fleisher GR, Ludwig S, eds. *Textbook of Pediatric Emergency Medicine.* 4th ed. Philadelphia, PA: Lippincott Williams & Wilkins; 2000:1017-1041.
9. Tuggle DW, Bennett KG, Scott J, et al. Intravenous vasopressin and gastrointestinal hemorrhage in children. *J Pediatr Surg.* 1988;23:627-629.
10. Hyams JS, Leichtner AM, Schwartz AN. Recent advance in diagnosis and treatment of gastrointestinal hemorrhage in infants and children. *J Pediatr.* 1985;106:1-9.
11. Mann K, Berg RA, Nadkarni V. Beneficial effects of vasopressin in prolonged pediatric cardiac arrest: a case series. *Resuscitation.* 2002;52:149-156.
12. American Heart Association guidelines for cardiopulmonary resuscitation and emergency cardiovascular care. Part 12: pediatric advanced life support. *Circulation.* 2005;112 (suppl 1):167-187.
13. Trissel LA. *Handbook on Injectable Drugs.* 13th ed. Bethesda, MD: American Society of Health-System Pharmacists; 2005.

Vecuronium Bromide

1. Rowlee SC. Monitoring neuromuscular blockade in the intensive care unit: the peripheral nerve stimulator. *Heart Lung.* 1999;28:352-362.
2. Martin LD, Bratton SL, O'Rourke PP. Clinical uses and controversies of neuromuscular blocking agents in infants and children. *Crit Care Med.* 1999;27:1358-1368.
3. Eldadah MK, Newth CJ. Vecuronium by continuous infusion for neuromuscular blockade in infants and children. *Crit Care Med.* 1989;17:989-992.
4. Woelfel SK, Dong ML, Brandom BW, et al. Vecuronium infusion requirements in children during halothane-narcotic-nitrous oxide, isoflurane-narcotic-nitrous oxide, and narcotic-nitrous oxide anesthesia. *Anesth Analg.* 1991;73:33-38.
5. Fitzpatrick KT, Black GW, Crean PM, et al. Continuous vecuronium infusion for prolonged muscle relaxation in children. *Can J Anaesth.* 1991;38:169-174.
6. Sloan MH, Lerman J, Bissonnette B. Pharmacodynamics of high dose vecuronium in children during balanced anesthesia. *Anesthesiology.* 1991;74:656-659.
7. Meretoja OA, Taivainen T, Jalkanen L, et al. Synergism between atracurium and vecuronium in infants and children during nitrous oxide-oxygen-alfentanil anesthesia. *Br J Anaesth.* 1994;73:605-607.
8. Vercuronium bromide [package insert]. Bedford, OH: Bedford Laboratories; March 2004.
9. Trissel LA, ed. *Handbook on Injectable Drugs.* 13th ed. [CD-ROM version 1.5]. Bethesda, MD: American Society of Health-System Pharmacists; 2005.
10. American Society of Health-System Pharmacists. American Hospital Formulary System. Available at: http://ahfsfirst.firstdatabank.com/AHFSfirst/NSAHFSFirstSearchmain.asp. Accessed August 2, 2006.
11. Goudsouzian NG, Young ET, Moss J, et al. Histamine release during the administration of atracurium or vecuronium in children. *Br J Anaesth.* 1986;58:1229-1233.
12. Durrani Z, O'Hara J. Histaminoid reaction from vecuronium priming: a case report. *Anesthesiology.* 1987;67:130-132.
13. Hiller JL, Benda GI, Rahatzad M, et al. Benzyl alcohol toxicity: impact on mortality and intraventricular hemorrhage among very low birth weight infants. *Pediatrics.* 1986;77:500-506.
14. American Academy of Pediatrics Committee on Drugs. "Inactive" ingredients in pharmaceutical products: update. *Pediatrics.* 1997;99:268-278.
15. Hall CM, Milligan DWA, Berrington J. Probably adverse reaction to a pharmaceutical excipient. *Arch Dis Child Fetal Neonatal Ed.* 2004;89: F184.
16. Grant JA, Bilodeau PA, Guernsey BG, et al. Unsuspected benzyl alcohol hypersensitivity. *N Engl J Med.* 1982;306:108.
17. Wilson JP, Solimando DA, Edwards MS. Parenteral benzyl alcohol-induced hypersensitivity reaction. *Drug Intell Clin Pharm.* 1986;20:689-691.
18. Margolis BD, Khachikian D, Friedman Y, et al. Prolonged reversible quadriparesis in mechanically ventilated patients who received long-term infusions of vecuronium. *Chest.* 1991;100:877-878.
19. Lagasse RS, Katz RI, Peterson M, et al. Prolonged neuromuscular blockade following vecuronium infusion. *J Clin Anesth.* 1990;2:269-271.
20. Segredo V, Caldwell JE, Matthay MA, et al. Persistent paralysis in critically ill patients after long-term administration of vecuronium. *N Engl J Med.* 1992;327:524-528.
21. Salviati L, Laverda AM, Zancan L, et al. Acute quadriplegic myopathy in a 17-month-old boy. *J Child Neurol.* 2000;15:63-66.
22. Yeaton P, Teba L. Sinus node exit block following administration of vecuronium. *Anesthesiology.* 1988;68:177-178.

23. Panacek EA, Sherman B. Hydrocortisone and pancuronium bromide: acute myopathy during status asthmaticus. *Crit Care Med.* 1988;16:732.
24. Watling SM, Dasta JF. Prolonged paralysis in intensive care unit patients after the use of neuromuscular blocking agents: a review of the literature. *Crit Care Med.* 1994;22:884-893.
25. Dupuic JY, Martin R, Tetrault JP. Atracurium and vecuronium interaction with gentamicin and tobramycin. *Can J Anaesth.* 1989;36:407-411.
26. Kronenfeld MA, Thomas SJ, Turndorf H. Recurrence of neuromuscular blockade after reversal of vecuronium in a patient receiving polymyxin/amikacin sternal irrigation. *Anesthesiology.* 1986;65:93-94.
27. Jeffrey JE, Tamburro RF, Schmidt GM, et al. Dilated nonreactive pupils secondary to neuromuscular blockade. *Anesthesiology.* 2000;92:1476-1487.

Verapmil HCl

1. 2005 American Heart Association Guidelines for Cardiopulmonary Resuscitation and Emergency Cardiovascular Care Part 12: Pediatric Advanced Life Support. *Circulation.* 2005;112(24 suppl):IV-167 to IV-187.
2. American Society of Health-System Pharmacists. American Hospital Formulary System. Available at: http://ahfsfirst.firstdatabank.com/AHFSfirst/NSAHFSFirstSearchmain.asp. Accessed August 7, 2006.
3. Radford D. Side effects of verapamil in infants. *Arch Dis Child.* 1983;58:465-466.
4. Epstein ML, Kiel EA, Victoria BE. Cardiac decompensation following verapamil therapy in infants with supraventricular tachycardia. *Pediatrics.* 1985;75:737-740.
5. Garson A Jr. Medicolegal problems in the management of cardiac arrhythmias in children. *Pediatrics.* 1987;79:84-88.
6. Kirk CR, Gibbs JL, Thomas R, et al. Cardiovascular collapse after verapamil in supraventricular tachycardia. *Arch Dis Child.* 1987;62:1265-1266.
7. Strasburger JF. Cardiac arrhythmias in childhood. Diagnostic considerations and treatment. *Drugs.* 1991;42:974-983.
8. Dick M II, Campbell RM. Advances in the management of cardiac arrhythmias in children. *Pediatr Clin North Am.* 1984;31:1175-1195.
9. Soler-Soler J, Sagrista-Sauleda J, Cabrera A, et al. Effect of verapamil in infants with paroxysmal supraventricular tachycardia. *Circulation.* 1979;59:876-879.
10. Sapire DW, O'Riordan AC, Black IF. Safety and efficacy of short and long-term verapamil therapy in children with tachycardia. *Am J Cardiol.* 1981;48:1091-1097.
11. Dhala A, Lewis DA, Garland J, et al. Verapamil sensitive incessant ventricular tachycardia in the newborn. *PACE.* 1996;19:1652-1654.
12. Porter CJ, Garson A, Gillette PC. Verapamil: an effective calcium blocking agent for pediatric patients. *Pediatrics.* 1983;71:748-755.
13. Shahar E, Barzilay Z, Frand M. Verapamil in the treatment of paroxysmal supraventricular tachycardia in infants and children. *J Pediatr.* 1981;98:323-326.
14. Porter CJ, Gillette PC, Garson A, et al. Effects of verapamil on supraventricular tachycardia in children. *Am J Cardiol.* 1981;48:487-491.
15. Aronoff A, Brier M, Bennett W. *The Renal Book, 2002.* Available at: http://www.kdp-baptist.louisville.edu/renalbook/. Accessed August 7, 2006.
16. Woodcock BG, Rietbrock I, Vohringer HF, et al. Verapamil disposition in liver disease and intensive care patients: kinetics, clearance, and apparent blood flow relationships. *Clin Pharmacol Ther.* 1981;29:27-34.
17. Hamann SR, Blouin RA, McAllister RG. Clinical pharmacokinetics of verapamil. *Clin Pharmacokinet.* 1984;9:26-41.
18. Liao WB, Bullard MJ, Kuo CT, et al. Anticholinergic overdose induced torsade de pointes successfully treated with verapamil. *Jpn Heart J.* 1996;37:925-931.
19. Trissel LA, ed. *Handbook on Injectable Drugs.* 13th ed. Bethesda, MD: American Society of Health-System Pharmacists; 2005.
20. Haug MT, DeRespino J, Zimmerman J, et al. Extended verapamil infusion for recurrent atrial tachyarrhythmias complicating acute myocardial infarction. *Clin Pharm.* 1984;3:540-544.
21. Chew CY, Hecht HS, Collett JT, et al. Influence of severity of ventricular dysfunction on hemodynamic responses to intravenously administered verapamil in ischemic heart disease. *Am J Cardiol.* 1981;47:917-922.
22. Reiter MJ, Shand DG, Aanonsen LM, et al. Pharmacokinetics of verapamil: experience with a sustained intravenous infusion regimen. *Am J Cardiol.* 1982;50:716-721.
23. Rowland TW. Augmented ventricular rate following verapamil treatment for atrial fibrillation with Wolff-Parkinson-White syndrome. *Pediatrics.* 1983;72:245-246.
24. Maiteh M, Daoud AS. Myoclonic seizure following intravenous verapamil injection: case report and review of the literature. *Ann Trop Paediatr.* 2001;21:271-272.
25. Ilan Y, Hillman M, Oren R. Intravenous verapamil for tachyarrhythmia in Duchenne's muscular dystrophy. *Pediatr Cardiol.* 1990;11:177-178.
26. Zalman F, Perloff JK, Durant NN, et al. Acute respiratory failure following intravenous verapamil in Duchenne's muscular dystrophy. *Am Heart J.* 1983;105:510-511.

Vinblastine Sulfate

1. Gadner H, Grois N, Arico M, et al. A randomized trial of treatment for multisystem Langerhans' cell histiocytosis. *J Pediatr.* 2001;138:728-734.
2. Nachman JB, Sposto R, Herzog P, et al. Randomized comparison of low-dose involved-field radiotherapy and no radiotherapy for children with Hodgkin's disease who achieve a complete response to chemotherapy. *J Clin Oncol.* 2002;20:3765-3771.
3. Schneider DT, Hilgenfeld E, Schwabe D, et al. Acute myelogenous leukemia after treatment for malignant germ cell tumors in children. *J Clin Oncol.* 1999;17:3226-3233.
4. Baranzelli MC, Kramar A, Bouffet E, et al. Prognostic factors in children with localized malignant nonseminomatous germ cell tumors. *J Clin Oncol.* 1999;17:1212-1218.
5. American Society of Health-System Pharmacists. American Hospital Formulary System. Available at: http://ahfsfirst.firstdatabank.com/AHFSfirst/NSAHFSFirstSearchmain.asp. Accessed September 26, 2006.
6. Aronoff GR, Berns JS, Brier ME, et al. *Drug Prescribing in Renal Failure: Dosing Guidelines for Adults.* 4th ed. Philadelphia, PA: American College of Physicians; 1999.
7. Perry MC. Hepatotoxicity of chemotherapeutic agents. *Semin Oncol.* 1982;9:65-74.
8. Vinblastine sulfate for injection [package insert]. Bedford, OH: Bedford Laboratories; December 2001.
9. Trissel LA, ed. *Handbook on Injectable Drugs.* 13th ed. [CD-ROM version 1.5]. Bethesda, MD: American Society of Health-System Pharmacists; 2005.
10. Dorr RT, Alberts DS. Vinca alkaloid skin toxicity: antidote and drug disposition studies in the mouse. *J Natl Cancer Inst.* 1985;74:113-120.
11. American Academy of Pediatrics Committee on Drugs. "Inactive" ingredients in pharmaceutical products: update. *Pediatrics.* 1997;99:268-278.
12. Hall CM, Milligan DWA, Berrington J. Probably adverse reaction to a pharmaceutical excipient. *Arch Dis Child Fetal Neonatal Ed.* 2004;89:F184.
13. Hiller JL, Benda GI, Rahatzad M, et al. Benzyl alcohol toxicity: impact on mortality and intraventricular hemorrhage among very low birth weight infants. *Pediatrics.* 1986;77:500-506.
14. Grant JA, Bilodeau PA, Guernsey BG, et al. Unsuspected benzyl alcohol hypersensitivity. *N Engl J Med.* 1982;306:108.
15. Wilson JP, Solimando DA, Edwards MS. Parenteral benzyl alcohol-induced hypersensitivity reaction. *Drug Intell Clin Pharm.* 1986;20:689-691.

References

16. Chan JD. Pharmacokinetic drug interactions of vinca alkaloids: summary of case reports. *Pharmacotherapy*. 1998;18:1304-1307.
17. Weiss HD, Walker MD, Wiernik PH. Neurotoxicity of commonly used antineoplastic agents (second of two parts). *N Engl J Med*. 1974;291:127-133.
18. Kris MG, Pablo D, Gralla RJ, et al. Dyspnea following vinblastine or vindesine administration in patients receiving mitomycin plus vinca alkaloid combination therapy. *Cancer Treat Rep*. 1983;68:1029-1031.
19. Ballen KK, Weiss ST. Fatal acute respiratory failure following vinblastine and mitomycin administration for breast cancer. *Am J Med Sci*. 1988;295:558-560.
20. Hoelzer KL, Harrison BR, Luedke SW, et al. Vinblastine-associated pulmonary toxicity in patients receiving combination therapy with mitomycin and cisplatin. *Drug Intell Clin Pharm*. 1986;20:287-289.
21. Rao SX, Ramaswamy G, Leven M, et al. Fatal acute respiratory failure after vinblastine-mitomycin therapy in lung carcinoma. *Arch Inter Med*. 1985;145:1905-1907.
22. Ozols RF, Hogan WM, Ostchega Y, et al. MVP (mitomycin, vinblastine, and progesterone): a second-line regimen in ovarian cancer with a high incidence of pulmonary toxicity. *Cancer Treat Rep*. 1983;67:721-722.
23. Konits PH, Aisner J, Sutherland JC, et al. Possible pulmonary toxicity secondary to vinblastine. *Cancer*. 1982;50:2771-2774.
24. Israel RH, Olson JP. Pulmonary edema associated with intravenous vinblastine. *JAMA*. 1978;240:1585.
25. National Comprehensive Cancer Network (NCCN) Antiemesis Panel Members. NCCN Clinical Practice Guidelines in Oncology. Antiemesis, v.1.2006. Available at www.nccn.org. Accessed March 29, 2006.
26. Roila F, Feyer P, Maranzamo E, et al. Antiemetics in children receiving chemotherapy. *Support Care Cancer*. 2005;13:129-131.

Vincristine Sulfate

1. Arico M, Valsecchi MG, Conter V, et al. Improved outcome in high-risk childhood acute lymphoblastic leukemia defined by prednisone-poor response treated with double Berlin-Frankfurt-Muenster protocol II. *Blood*. 2002;100:420-426.
2. Nachman JB, Sposto R, Herzog P, et al. Randomized comparison of low-dose involved-field radiotherapy and no radiotherapy for children with Hodgkin's disease who achieve a complete response to chemotherapy. *J Clin Oncol*. 2002;20:3765-3771.
3. American Society of Health-System Pharmacists. American Hospital Formulary System. Available at: http://ahfsfirst.firstdatabank.com/AHFSfirst/NSAHFSFirstSearchmain.asp. Accessed September 26, 2006.
4. Crom WR, Graff SS, Synold T, et al. Pharmacokinetics of vincristine in children and adolescents with acute lymphocytic leukemia. *J Pediatr*. 1994;125:642-649.
5. Dorr VJ, Morris D, Lorber M. Chemotherapy programs. In: Perry MC, ed. *The Chemotherapy Sourcebook*. 2nd ed. Baltimore, MD: Lippincott Williams & Wilkins; 1996:845-887.
6. Whitelaw DM, Cowan DH, Cassidy FR, et al. Clinical experience with vincristine. *Cancer Chemother Rep*. 1963;30:13-20.
7. Perry MC. Hepatotoxicity of chemotherapeutic agents. *Semin Oncol*. 1982;9:65-74.
8. Aronoff GR, Berns JS, Brier ME, et al. *Drug Prescribing in Renal Failure: Dosing Guidelines for Adults*. 4th ed. Philadelphia, PA: American College of Physicians; 1999.
9. Legha SS. Vincristine neurotoxicity: pathophysiology and management. *Med Toxicol*. 1986;1:421-427.
10. Jeannine SM, Lindley C. Appropriateness of maximum-dose guidelines for vincristine. *Am J Health-Syst Pharm*. 1997;54:1755-1758.
11. Trissel LA, ed. *Handbook on Injectable Drugs*. 13th ed. [CD-ROM version 1.5]. Bethesda, MD: American Society of Health-System Pharmacists; 2005.
12. Cohen MR. Hazard warning: deaths due to accidental intrathecal injection of vincristine. *Hosp Pharm*. 1989;24:694.
13. Meggs WJ, Hoffman RS. Fatality resulting from intraventricular vincristine administration. *Clin Toxicol*. 1998;36(3):243-246.
14. MacCara ME. Extravasation: a hazard of intravenous therapy. *Drug Intell Clin Pharm*. 1983;17:713-717.
15. Chan JD. Pharmacokinetic drug interactions of vinca alkaloids: summary of case reports. *Pharmacotherapy*. 1998;18:1304-1307.
16. Hansen MM, Ranek L, Walbom S, et al. Fatal hepatitis following irradiation and vincristine. *Acta Med Scand*. 1982;212:171-174.
17. Hogan-Dann CM, Fellmeth WG, McGuire SA, et al. Polyneuropathy following vincristine therapy in two patients with Charcot-Marie-Tooth syndrome. *JAMA*. 1984;252:2862-2863.
18. Igarashi M, Thompson EJ, Rivera GK. Vincristine neuropathy in type I and type II Charcot-Marie-Tooth disease (hereditary motor sensory neuropathy). *Med Ped Oncol*. 1995;25:113-116.
19. McGuire SA, Gospe SM Jr, Dahl G. Acute vincristine neurotoxicity in the presence of hereditary motor and sensory neuropathy type I. *Med Ped Oncol*. 1989;17:520-523.
20. National Comprehensive Cancer Network (NCCN) Antiemesis Panel Members. NCCN Clinical Practice Guidelines in Oncology. Antiemesis, v.1.2006. Available at www.nccn.org. Last accessed March 29, 2006.
21. Roila F, Feyer P, Maranzamo E, et al. Antiemetics in children receiving chemotherapy. *Support Care Cancer*. 2005;13:129-131.

Vitamin A

1. AHFSfirst™ Web version 2.03. American Society of Health-System Pharmacists, First Databank Inc. 2002. Accessed June 30, 2006.
2. Shenai JP, Kennedy KA, Chytil F, et al. Clinical trial of vitamin A supplementation in infants susceptible to bronchopulmonary dysplasia. *J Pediatr*. 1987;111:269-277.
3. Tyson JE, Wright LL, Oh W, et al. Vitamin A supplementation for extremely-low-birth-weight infants. *N Engl J Med*. 1999;340:1962-1968.
4. Young TE, Mangum B. *Neofax®: A Manual of Drugs Used in Neonatal Care*. 18th ed. Raleigh, NC: Acorn Publishing; 2005.
5. Shenai JP. Vitamin A supplementation in very low birth weight neonates: rationale and evidence. *Pediatrics*. 1999;104(6):1369-1374.
6. Gleghorn EE, Eisenberg LD, Hack S, et al. Observations of vitamin A toxicity in three patients with renal failure receiving parenteral alimentation. *Am J Clin Nutr*. 1986;44(1):107-112.
7. Aquasol [parenteral prescribing information]. Wilmington, DE: Astra Zeneca; April 2001.
8. Alade SL, Brown RE, Paquet A Jr. Polysosrbate 80 and the E-Ferol tragedy. *Pediatrics*. 1986;77:593-597.

Vitamin K_1–Phytonadione

1. McEvoy GK, ed. *AHFS Drug Information Essentials 2005–06*. Bethesda, MD: American Society of Health-System Pharmacists; 2005.
2. Thomson PDR. *Physicians' Desk Reference*. 60th ed. Montvale, NJ: Medical Economics Company; 2006.
3. Lane PA, Hathaway WE. Vitamin K in infancy. *J Pediatr*. 1985;106:351-359.
4. American Academy of Pediatrics. Committee on Nutrition. Vitamin K compounds and water soluble analogues: use in therapy and prophylaxis in pediatrics. *Pediatrics*. 1961;28:501-507.
5. Hathaway WE. The bleeding newborn. *Clin Perinatol*. 1975;2:83-97.
6. Uses and hazards of vitamin K drugs. *Med Lett Drugs Ther*. 1963;5:97-98.
7. American Academy of Pediatrics. Committee on Fetus and Newborn Policy Statement. Controversies concerning vitamin K and the newborn. *Pediatrics*. 2003;112;191-192.
8. Montgomery RR, Hathaway WE. Acute bleeding emergencies. *Pediatr Clin North Am*. 1980;27:327-344.
9. Glader BE, Buchanan GR. The bleeding neonate. *Pediatrics*. 1976;58:548-555.
10. Nammacher MA, Willemin M, Hartmann JR, et al. Vitamin K deficiency in infants beyond the neonatal period. *J Pediatr*. 1970;76:549-554.

11. Walters TR, Koch HF. Hemorrhagic diathesis and cystic fibrosis in infancy. *Am J Dis Child.* 1972;124:641-642.
12. Bolton-Maggs P, Brook L. The use of vitamin K for reversal of over-warfarinization in children. *Br J Haematol.* 2002;118:924-925. Letter.
13. Udall JA. Don't use the wrong vitamin K. *Calif Med.* 1970;112:65-67.
14. Mattea EJ, Quinn K. Adverse reactions after intravenous phytonadione administration. *Hosp Pharm.* 1981;16:224-235.
15. Trissel LA. *Handbook on Injectable Drugs.* 13th ed. Bethesda, MD: American Society of Health-System Pharmacists; 2005.
16. Kumar D, Greer FR, Super DM, et al. Vitamin K status of premature infants: implications for current recommendations. *Pediatrics.* 2001;108:1117-1122.
17. Barash P, Kitahata LM, Mandel S. Acute cardiovascular collapse after intravenous phytonadione. *Anesth Analg.* 1976;55:304-306.
18. American Academy of Pediatrics Committee on Drugs. "Inactive" ingredients in pharmaceutical products: update. *Pediatrics.* 1997;99:268-278.
19. Hall CM, Milligan DWA, Berrington J. Probable adverse reaction to a pharmaceutical excipient. *Arch Dis Child Fetal Neonatal Ed.* 2004;89: F184. Review.
20. Hiller JL, Benda GI, Rahatzad M, et al. Benzyl alcohol toxicity: impact on mortality and intraventricular hemorrhage among very low birth weight infants. *Pediatrics.* 1986;77:500-506.
21. Grant JA, Bilodeau PA, Guernsey BG, et al. Unsuspected benzyl alcohol hypersensitivity. *N Engl J Med.* 1982;306:108.
22. Wilson JP, Solimando DA, Edwards MS. Parenteral benzyl alcohol-induced hypersensitivity reaction. *Drug Intell Clin Pharm.* 1986;20:689-691.
23. Loughnan PM, McDougall PN, Balvin H, et al. Late onset haemorrhagic disease in premature infants who received intravenous vitamin K1. *J Paediatr Child Health.* 1996;32:268-269.

Voriconazole

1. American Academy of Pediatrics. In: Pickering LK, ed. *Red Book: 2006 Report of the Committee on Infectious Diseases.* 27th ed. Elk Grove Village, IL: American Academy of Pediatrics; 2006.
2. Frankenbusch K, Eifinger F, Kribs A, et al. Severe primary cutaneous aspergillosis refractory to amphotericin B and the successful treatment with systemic voriconazole in two premature infants with extremely low birth weight. *J Perinatol.* 2006;26:511-514.
3. Muldrew KM, Maples HD, Stowe CD, et al. Intravenous voriconazole therapy in a preterm infant. *Pharmacotherapy.* 2005;25:893-898.
4. Maples HD, Stowe CD, Saccente SL, et al. Voriconazole serum concentrations in an infant treated for *Trichosporon beigelii* infection. *Pediatr Infect Dis J.* 2003;22:1022-1024.
5. Guzman-Cottrill JA, Zheng X, Chadwick EG. Fusarium solani endocarditis successfully treated with liposomal amphotericin B and voriconazole. *Pediatr Infect Dis J.* 2004;23:1059-1061.
6. Pannaraj PS, Walsh TJ, Baker CJ. Advances in antifungal therapy. *Pediatr Infect Dis J.* 2005;24(10):921-922.
7. Steinbach WJ, Benjamin DK. New antifungal agents under development in children and neonates. *Curr Opin Infect Dis.* 2005;18:484-489.
8. Schwartz S, Ruhnke M, Ribaud P, et al. Improved outcome in central nervous system aspergillosis, using voriconazole treatment. *Blood.* 2005;106:2641-2645.
9. Chakraborty A, Workman MR, Bullock PR. Scedosporium apiospermum brain abscess treated with surgery and voriconazole. *J Neurosurg.* 2005;103:83-87.
10. Walsh TJ, Karlsson MO, et al. Pharmacokinetics and safety of intravenous voriconazole in children after single- or multiple-dose administration. *Antimicrob Agents Chemother.* 2004;48(6):2166-2172.
11. Walsh TJ, Lutsar I, Driscoll T, et al. Voriconazole in the treatment of aspergillosis, scedosporiosis and other invasive fungal infections in children. *Pediatr Infect Dis J.* 2002;21:240-248.
12. *Physicians' Desk Reference.* 60th ed. Montvale, NJ: Thomson PDR; 2006.
13. Peng LW, Lien YH. Pharmacokinetics of single, oral-dose voriconazole in peritoneal dialysis patients. *Am J Kidney Dis.* 2005;45(1):162-166.

Zidovudine

1. AIDSinfo. Recommendations for use of antiretroviral drugs in pregnant HIV-1-infected women for maternal health and interventions to reduce perinatal HIV-1 transmission in the United States—July 6, 2006. Available at: http://aidsinfo.nih.gov/ContentFiles/PerinatalGL.pdf. Accessed September 1, 2006.
2. American Academy of Pediatrics. In: Pickering LK, ed. *Red Book: 2006 Report of the Committee on Infectious Diseases.* 27th ed. Elk Grove Village, IL: American Academy of Pediatrics; 2006.
3. AIDSinfo. Guidelines for the use of antiretroviral agents in pediatric HIV infection—November 03, 2005. Available at: http://aidsinfo.nih.gov/ContentFiles/PediatricGuidelines.pdf. Accessed March 31, 2006.
4. Mirochnick M, Capparelli E, Connor J. Pharmacokinetics of zidovudine in infants: a population analysis across studies. *Clin Pharmacol Ther.* 1999;66:16-24.
5. McKinney RE, Pizzo PA, Scott GB, et al. Safety and tolerance of intermittent intravenous and oral zidovudine therapy in human immunodeficiency virus-infected pediatric patients. *J Pediatr.* 1990;116:640-647.
6. Blanche S, Caniglia M, Fischer A, et al. Zidovudine therapy in children with acquired immunodeficiency syndrome. *Am J Med.* 1988;85:203-207.
7. Connor EM, Pizzo PA, Balis F, et al. Working Group on Antiretroviral Therapy: National Pediatric HIV Resource Center. Antiretroviral therapy and medical management of the human immunodeficiency virus-infected child. *Pediatr Infect Dis J.* 1993;12:513-522.
8. Mueller BU, Jacobsen F, Butler KM, et al. Combination treatment with azidothymidine and granulocyte colony-stimulating factor in children with human immunodeficiency virus infection. *J Pediatr.* 1992;121:797-802.
9. Balis FM, Pizzo PA, Eddy J, et al. Pharmacokinetics of zidovudine administered intravenously and orally in children with human immunodeficiency virus infection. *J Pediatr.* 1989;114:880-884.
10. Pizzo PA, Eddy J, Falloon J, et al. Effect of continuous intravenous infusion of zidovudine (AZT) in children with symptomatic HIV infection. *N Engl J Med.* 1988;319:889-896.
11. Balis FM, Pizzo PA, Murphy RF, et al. The pharmacokinetics of zidovudine administered by continuous infusion in children. *Ann Intern Med.* 1989;110:279-285.
12. Aronoff A, Brier M, Bennett W. The Renal Book, 2002. http://www.kdp-baptist.louisville.edu/renalbook/. Accessed May 6, 2006.
13. *Physicians' Desk Reference.* 60th ed. Montvale, NJ: Thomson PDR; 2006.
14. Trissel LA, ed. *Handbook on Injectable Drugs.* 13th ed. [CD-ROM version 1.5]. Bethesda, MD: American Society of Health-System Pharmacists; 2005.
15. Myers SA, Torrente S, Hinthorn D, et al. Life-threatening maternal and fetal macrocytic anemia from antiretroviral therapy. *Obstet Gynecol.* 2005;106:1189-1191.
16. Scalfaro P, Chesaux JJ, Buchwalder PA, et al. Severe transient neonatal lactic acidosis during prophylactic zidovudine treatment. *Intensive Care Med.* 1998;24:247-250.

Index of Brand and Generic Drug Names

A

Index of Brand and Generic Drug Names

B

C

Index of Brand and Generic Drug Names

D

E

Index of Brand and Generic Drug Names

F

G

H

Index of Brand and Generic Drug Names

I

J

K

L

Index of Brand and Generic Drug Names

Index of Brand and Generic Drug Names

O

P

Index of Brand and Generic Drug Names

Q

R

Index of Brand and Generic Drug Names

S

T

U

Index of Brand and Generic Drug Names

V

X

Z